Pilates

THIRD EDITION

Rael Isacowitz

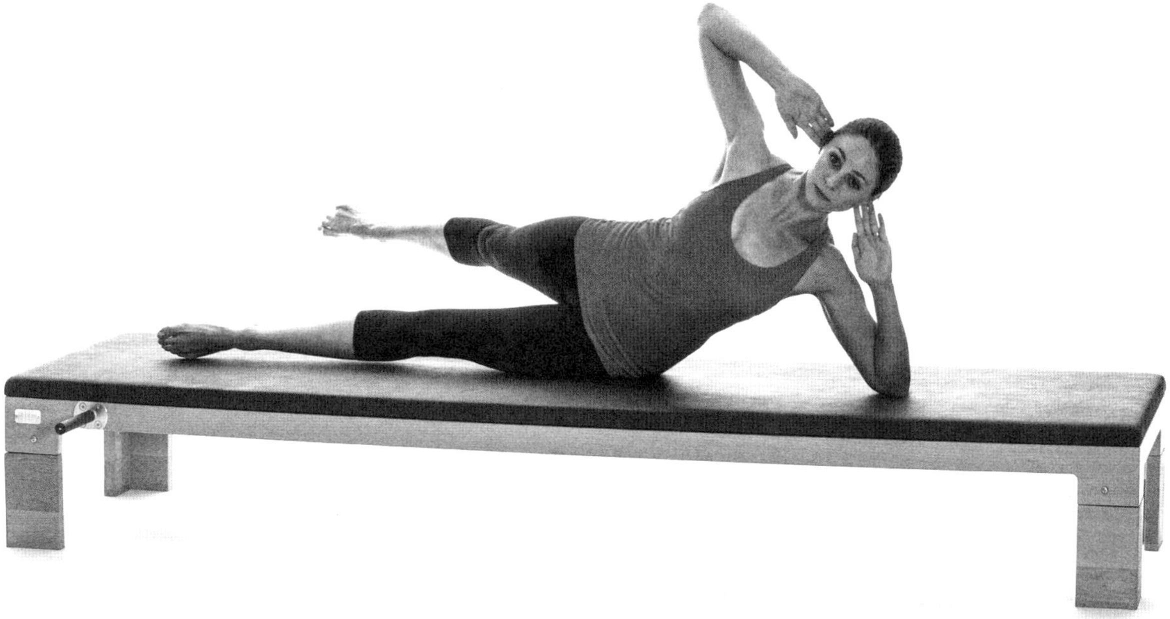

HUMAN KINETICS

Library of Congress Cataloging-in-Publication Data

Names: Isacowitz, Rael, 1955- author.
Title: Pilates / Rael Isacowitz.
Description: Third edition. | Champaign, IL : Human Kinetics, [2023] | Includes bibliographical references and index.
Identifiers: LCCN 2021051350 (print) | LCCN 2021051351 (ebook) | ISBN 9781492598862 (paperback) | ISBN 9781492598879 (epub) | ISBN 9781492598893 (pdf)
Subjects: LCSH: Pilates method.
Classification: LCC RA781.4 .I73 2023 (print) | LCC RA781.4 (ebook) | DDC 613.7/192--dc23/eng/20211029
LC record available at https://lccn.loc.gov/2021051350
LC ebook record available at https://lccn.loc.gov/2021051351

ISBN: 978-1-4925-9886-2 (print)

Senior Acquisitions Editor: Michelle Earle; **Managing Editor:** Hannah Werner; **Copyeditor:** Heather Gauen Hutches; **Indexer:** Andrea J. Hepner; **Permissions Manager:** Martha Gullo; **Graphic Designer:** Julie L. Denzer; **Cover Designer:** Keri Evans; **Cover Design Specialist:** Susan Rothermel Allen; **Photographs (cover and interior):** Kirk Fitzek; **Photo Production Manager:** Jason Allen; **Senior Art Manager:** Kelly Hendren; **Illustrations:** © Human Kinetics; **Printer:** Premier Print Group

Human Kinetics books are available at special discounts for bulk purchase. Special editions or book excerpts can also be created to specification. For details, contact the Special Sales Manager at Human Kinetics.

Printed in the United States of America 10 9 8 7 6 5 4

Human Kinetics
1607 N. Market Street
Champaign, IL 61820
USA

United States and International
Website: **US.HumanKinetics.com**
Email: info@hkusa.com
Phone: 1-800-747-4457

Canada
Website: **Canada.HumanKinetics.com**
Email: info@hkcanada.com

Human Kinetics' authorized representative for product safety in the EU is Mare Nostrum Group B.V., Mauritskade 21D, 1091 GC Amsterdam, The Netherlands.
Email: gpsr@mare-nostrum.co.uk

E8094

I dedicate this work to two people who have helped shape my life in so many ways. Whose unwavering support and unconditional love allow me to discover and rediscover the joys of life every day. My wife, Adelle, who makes the adage "Behind every good man there is a great woman" truer than ever, and my son, Elan, who will always be my ultimate teacher—I see myself in him and through him.

Equally I dedicate this book, and my daily practice, to my BASI family: a global community of tens of thousands of exceptional people who share the common values of passion, compassion, and excellence—you inspire me to be the best that I can be.

> The joy of Pilates is found in the exploration and transformation of body, mind, and spirit.
>
> —Rael Isacowitz

Contents

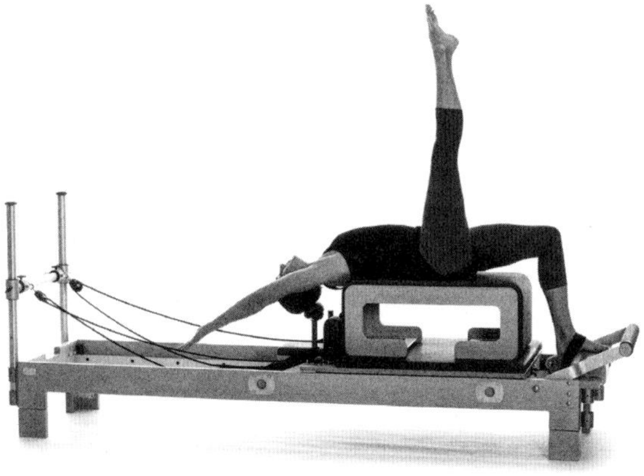

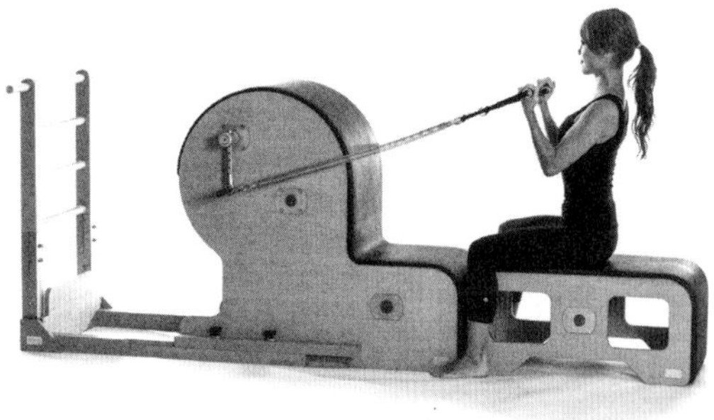

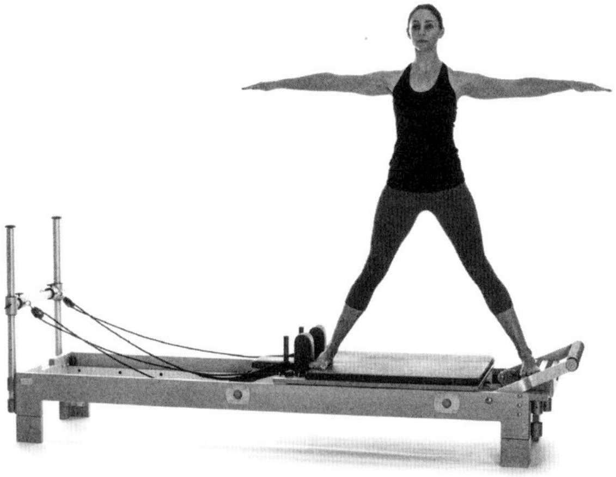

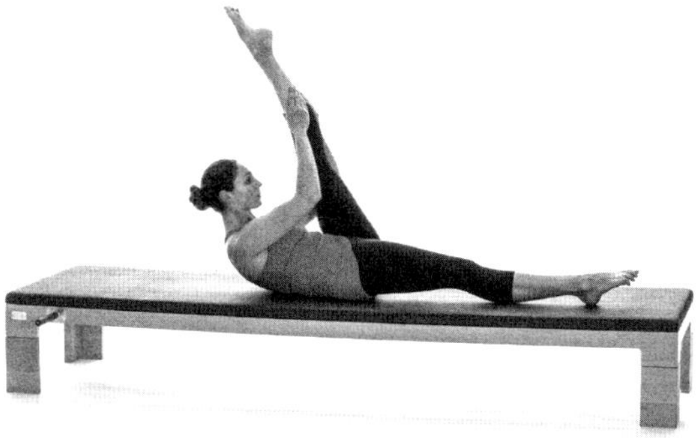

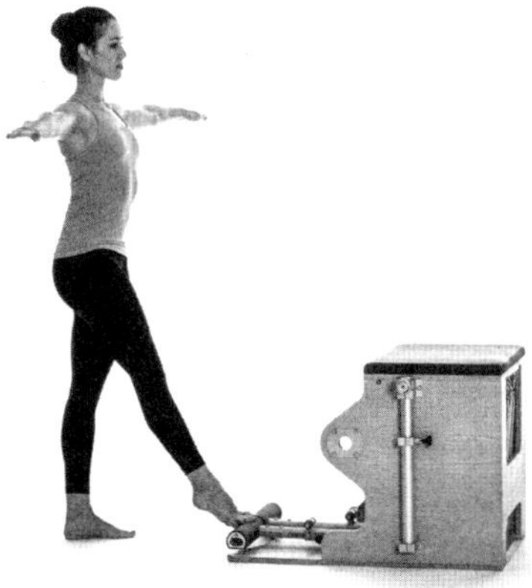

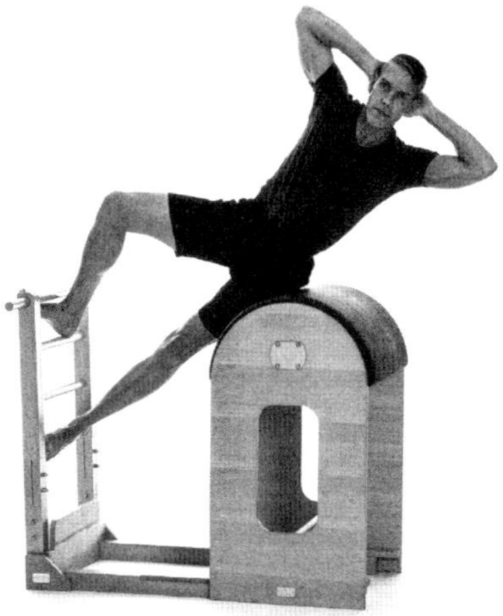

Foreword

Kathleen Stanford Grant (August 1, 1921–May 27, 2010) wrote the following words for the first edition of this book. She is desperately missed by her family, her friends, and by the entire Pilates community. She left an indelible mark on this industry. Personally, I miss our long conversations and casual banter. We provided a safe space for each other to speak our minds, no matter the topic. Kathy continues to guide my Pilates practice and my teaching every single day.

When I first met Rael in Santa Fe, New Mexico, in 1991, the Pilates community was indeed very small. Upon the recommendation of Jean-Claude West, who had studied with me and was running his own studio in New York, I was invited to teach a workshop on the wunda chair, a Pilates apparatus that I had worked on a lot with Joseph Pilates. Until then, I had not been consulted for professional advice by the Pilates community. The gathering in Santa Fe was a breakthrough; first and foremost, in recognizing the first generation of Pilates teachers and also in the sharing of information and drawing on our collective experience and expertise.

I was guided to Mr. Pilates by Pearl Lang, the renowned dancer and choreographer, after undergoing double knee surgery. He used the wunda chair extensively for my knee therapy, believing it to be most beneficial for that purpose. I learned a vast amount about the wunda chair during my rehabilitation and went on to develop my own repertoire. I continued to use the wunda chair in my teaching at Henri Bendel from 1973 to 1988, and I still use it in my teaching today, including the Pilates program I run for the Tisch School of the Arts at NYU.

When I entered the studio in Santa Fe, I was immediately surrounded by a group of seasoned professionals who had come from far and wide, hungry for information and enthusiastic about spending time with me. I noticed a man in the group and when I asked for a volunteer to demonstrate some of the work, he eagerly jumped up. He got on the wunda chair and started demonstrating. I immediately recognized that he was an accomplished mover and that he knew Pilates well. As I started prodding and poking, making intricate adjustments to his alignment and movement, I could see a look of astonishment cross his face. The young male ego! This made me chuckle inside. He was clearly strong, but he relied too much on his strength and athletic ability rather than on his core.

We proceeded to work for several hours together as I taught, demonstrated, adjusted, and corrected. I respected his openness to learning and his humility in the presence of another teacher. That workshop was a pivotal point in the evolution of Pilates. From that point on the wunda chair, which had become all but obsolete, boomed in popularity.

Rael, for the young man was of course him, has often expressed to me that our meeting changed his career. It set him on a path of inner exploration and self-assessment. His work changed and his teaching changed; he discovered how to work from within. Rael and I went on to become, above all else, good friends. I am now regarded as one of the elders of the Pilates community, and Rael as a world-renowned teacher and a leader in his own right. He has developed a fine teacher training program, Body Arts and Science International (BASI Pilates), to which he invited me to serve as honorary advisor.

Back in 1991 Rael requested that I conduct a workshop at his center in Southern California. I made a promise to him that I would do it, but I could not say when. Thereafter, on every occasion we met, he would remind me of my promise. It took 14 years for me to fulfill it. In 2005 I came to Southern California from New York to give a workshop at On Center Conditioning (now BASI Pilates Academy, USA). Although Rael also taught, the students got to witness their mentor being guided by his mentor. This in itself was a valuable lesson, possibly more valuable than the work itself.

Rael performs the work with unique mastery, and he certainly moves from within. At the same time he demonstrates an ever-present youthful desire to continue learning and growing. We need to keep the lineage of Pilates alive, preserving the past and respecting the future, upholding the values and principles of this system—and few have done as much toward that end as Rael. He is the male that Mr. Pilates wished for to continue his work.

Kathy Stanford Grant

First-generation Pilates teacher, Pilates elder

Preface

When the first edition of this book was published, it was the culmination of 16 years of good intentions and three years of actual writing. I wanted to put my work as a student and teacher of Pilates into words. Yet each time I attempted to do so, I found the enormity of the task at hand overwhelming. I knew that in order to offer something profound and valuable to Pilates enthusiasts, I needed more knowledge and experience. So back to the studio I went, to master the repertoire of movements, to explore the work further, and to teach another few thousand sessions. This process of ever-expanding education spanned five continents and more practice hours than I could ever count.

Around 1990, when I first felt the urge to write a book, I had already been doing Pilates for more than 10 years. I had earned a bachelor's degree from the Wingate Institute of Physical Education and Sports in Israel, danced professionally, and completed my master's degree in dance studies at the University of Surrey in England. I had been an avid competitive swimmer since my youth and had practiced yoga since my early teens. Yet, endeavoring to master Pilates felt like learning to walk again. This humbling experience, which taught me how to move with an ease and flow I had never before experienced, inspired me—and at times frustrated me. I had embarked on a lifelong journey of learning and practice that would deepen my understanding of movement and offer me a path to physical and mental well-being.

Now, with the publication of the third edition of *Pilates*, my initial agonizing over the writing of the book seems like time well spent. My own body of work, knowledge, and experience has continued to expand; the number of people who practice Pilates worldwide has grown exponentially; and Pilates has further established itself in the mainstream of fitness, athletic training, and therapy. As a result, the demand for well-trained teachers has also continued to increase, and teachers have become better educated and better equipped to deal with the expanding scope of this method. The educational organization I founded in 1989, Body

Arts and Science International (BASI), now has a global reach of around 45 countries, with a community of tens of thousands of students and graduates, and it continues to grow by the day. BASI Pilates started out being all about movement, and in the process, it has become a movement—a movement for positive change in the world. The BASI family is a diverse collective of people from different cultures, backgrounds, nationalities, religions, and genders who all share common values—values that far exceed the individual and the physical movements themselves, extending to the community, society, and the planet itself. For this I am eternally proud and grateful.

Joseph Pilates dreamed of universal recognition and growth and believed it could happen; yet I doubt that even in his most ambitious dreams, he envisaged the popularity of the Pilates method that we are witnessing today. He wanted to see his method (which he called *Contrology*) embraced by the medical profession and taught in every school because he believed it could benefit society as a whole.

Today, Joseph Pilates' dreams are coming true. His method is indeed being used in schools, and it is increasingly found in clinics and hospitals. Research is substantiating many of his principles and concepts and the medical profession is recognizing its value. I have long believed that if every person on Earth did a Pilates session every day, we would live in a far better world—it simply makes you feel so good!

Joseph Pilates died a disillusioned man, by many accounts. In his short book *Your Health*, he expresses his disdain for the medical profession and people's closed-mindedness. Tragically, he and his wife Clara did not live to witness the development of their method into the phenomenon it has become. Yet the spirit of their teaching lives on, and I feel a deep, personal responsibility to uphold the integrity and high standard of their work. I hope this book makes a valuable contribution to keeping the flame alive and burning bright for generations to come.

Acknowledgments

This third edition of *Pilates* is the culmination of a career that has spanned well over 40 years and has taken me all over the globe as a teacher and presenter. Several pages of acknowledgments would not suffice in thanking all of the students, teachers, colleagues, peers, friends, and dear family members who have helped me along the way. They have taught, inspired, and guided me, and all have been kind to me. Inevitably they impacted my career and influenced the outcome of this book. Each person deserves my deepest gratitude.

As hopeful as I was when the first edition of *Pilates* was published, I could never have dreamed of the success the book has enjoyed. Over 100,000 copies have been sold worldwide and it has been translated into seven languages. Yet it is the positive impact that it has had on so many readers' lives around the globe that brings me the greatest joy, and is my ultimate reward.

I would like, however, to single out several people who have been instrumental in the production and publication of the third edition of *Pilates*.

Michelle Earle, senior acquisitions editor at Human Kinetics, first approached me with the idea of writing a third edition several years ago. I was not immediately convinced that I could take on such a large endeavor at a time when BASI Pilates continued to grow internationally and the demands on my time and resources were immeasurable, along with the myriad other projects I had my hands in. Yet Michelle, in her warm and supportive way, made me feel that it was not only possible but also the right decision. Michelle has kept me on track and has always been willing to adjust the delivery schedule when life has had other plans, such as a global pandemic. I could not ask or wish for a better partner in this venture.

Kirk Fitzek, photographer, designer, and friend for over 25 years, again gave generously of his time, expertise, and enormous talent as he did for the prior editions. He shot over 6,000 photos for this third edition, which includes all-new pictures on BASI Systems equipment. Kirk has an endless supply of patience and manages to be calming and encouraging, even when a shoot drags on and energy is running desperately low. Kirk understands as much about alignment, muscle recruitment, and the BASI teaching methodology as any seasoned BASI teacher.

It is with deep gratitude that I thank the talented models whose commitment and skill are so evident in this book: Ellsworth Howard, Cara Frazier, Ena Kirima, Rina Kirima, Sondra Karman, Christopher Chiles, Latoya McKelvin, and Kristen Stevenson. Each one of them gave generously and tirelessly to the process of taking thousands of pictures. They are active members of the BASI Pilates community who have devoted years to honing their skills. Each represents the BASI family honorably and is a testament to the power of Pilates.

Stella Hull-Lampkin, BASI operations manager and my loyal assistant, has been by my side every step of the way—assisting in the process of photo shoots and edits, being a sounding board for my endless stream of deliberations, and simply making sure I am drinking enough water. The third edition of *Pilates* could not have come to fruition without Stella.

The team at BASI Pilates Academy, USA, the Pilates center in Southern California that I established in 1991, is diverse in talent and skill yet unified in its support and hard work. Also, the international faculty of BASI Pilates, the educational organization that I founded in 1989 and continue to direct, is the backbone of everything I do. I am proud to work with these dedicated faculty members who travel the globe upholding the excellence that BASI is known for. I can't possibly thank them enough for all they do and for all they have given me.

I am honored to have traveled this path of exploration and practice and to have encountered so many soulful and generous people along the way. My hope is that in some small way, this book serves to thank them all.

Introduction

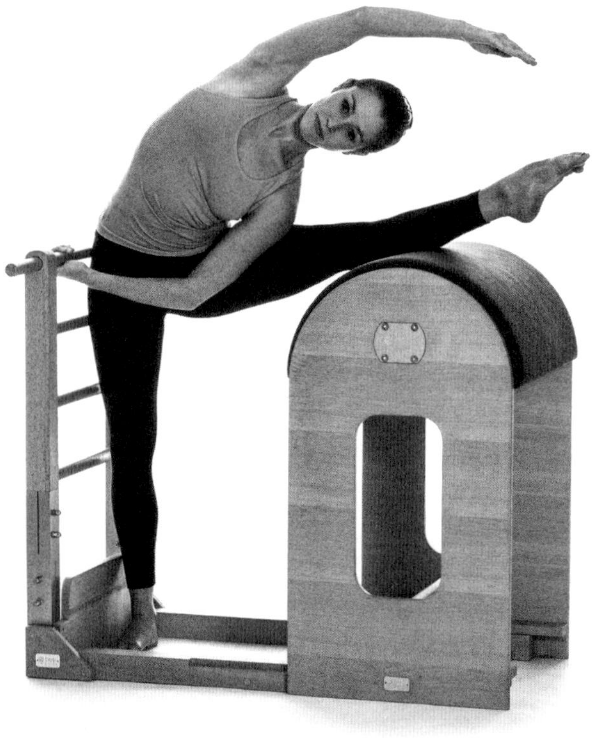

This book is for people who are seeking a comprehensive understanding of the Pilates method—including the underlying philosophy, far-reaching benefits, and much of the vast repertoire. I have endeavored to cover as much ground as possible, with the aim of providing a definitive textbook for those who teach and practice the method with commitment and dedication. At the same time, *Pilates* is not exclusively for the professional; my hope is that it will serve as an informative introduction for anyone interested in delving into the depths of this discipline.

In this third edition, I further expand the offering of modifications, variations, and progressions for many of the exercises. The goal is to make the material more widely accessible to a broader audience, ranging from beginners just starting their Pilates journey, to teachers using Pilates in a therapeutic environment, to veteran instructors working with athletes. In general, modifications make the exercises easier and more accessible, variations offer variety, and progressions introduce more challenge and a higher degree of difficulty.

All references to Pilates and the Pilates method in this book refer to the system of physical and mental conditioning developed by Joseph Hubertus Pilates. Although some of the movements differ from the exact choreography or sequence in which they were originally performed, the intent and text are inspired by, and closely align with, the original works of Mr. Pilates. The legacy of this man, whom the great choreographer George Balanchine called the "genius of the body" (according to first-generation teacher Romana Kryzanowska), remains an invaluable resource for generations of teachers and enthusiasts.

Joseph and his wife Clara set up the first Pilates studio in New York City soon after arriving from Germany in the mid-1920s. The rest is history—and an important and fundamental part of the method itself. Understanding the method's history allows us to understand the exercises and see them in the context of their time, taking into account the lifestyle and general activities of people in the 1920s. At that time, computers did not exist to cause the epidemic of round-shoulder syndrome, fast food was not available to hasten the advance of obesity, the relative scarcity of cars kept people more physically active, and lower back pain did not plague over 80 percent of the population of the Western world, as it does today. It was a very different world with very different needs!

Pilates covers the art and science of human movement as it relates to the Pilates method. I believe that every movement in this method can and should be substantiated both scientifically (through anatomy, physiology, biomechanics, and kinesiology) and artistically (through aesthetics, psychology, inner sensations, and the flow of energy and life force). The significant overlap between the art and science of human movement has been recognized and explored through the ages. The mind and the body share a nourishing, symbiotic relationship that brings about profound and at times inexplicable results. This mind–body relationship lies at the heart of the Pilates method.

An in-depth exploration of each aspect of Pilates would far exceed the parameters of this book; instead, I provide information about the Pilates method as a whole, emphasizing the repertoire and how to approach each exercise, including presentation, description, and analysis. The subjects of anatomy, physiology, and biomechanics are not covered in detail, though a working knowledge of these areas of study is important for Pilates professionals and serious enthusiasts, and therefore further study in these areas is highly recommended. See the selected resources list at the end of the book for suggestions.

Pilates takes you through a range of exercise levels, from fundamental through intermediate and finally touching on the advanced level. The book's 200-plus exercises are conveniently organized by apparatus, with each apparatus addressed in a separate chapter. The exercises in each chapter are grouped into blocks, based on regions of the body and the function of certain muscle groups. Within each block there are individual exercises, as well as series and groups of exercises (described further in chapter 3). The description of each exercise includes its level of difficulty, a recommended resistance range (if applicable), and number of repetitions. I also provide a muscle focus, objectives of the exercise, commentary, some ideas for imagery that may prove valuable in both executing and teaching the movements, and a checklist of points that help ensure a positive outcome. This book includes very little master-level work, which must be taught in an educational setting. For instance, my Legacy Program, taught through BASI Pilates, involves four phases: Mentor, Master I, Master II, and Honors, and delves into the most complex and advanced realms of the Pilates method.

Over the years, several approaches to the practice of the Pilates method have emerged. The classical approach advocates doing the work, manufacturing the apparatus, and sequencing the exercises exactly as Joseph Pilates did. Some other approaches deal primarily with rehabilitation; they have created protocols for specific treatments that use the Pilates apparatus but have changed the repertoire significantly. Often practitioners do not address the original repertoire or the holistic aspect of the work, and at times the relationship to the source is very loose indeed. Still other approaches deal with select populations, such as dancers and athletes, or the aging population and pregnant women, adapting the repertoire to their needs and, again, at times forgoing the original Pilates exercises and philosophy.

A BRIEF HISTORY OF PILATES

Joseph Pilates was born near Düsseldorf, Germany, in 1883. He was a sickly child, plagued with rickets, asthma, and rheumatic fever. His drive to overcome these ailments led him to explore bodybuilding, gymnastics, diving, and other physical pursuits. He studied Eastern and Western philosophies and forms of exercise and was greatly influenced by ancient Greek and Roman regimens. This rich background provided him with the foundation to create a system that he developed throughout his life.

In 1912, Mr. Pilates traveled to England as a circus performer in a living Greek statue act. When World War I broke out, he was interned in a camp on the Isle of Man along with other German nationals. While there, he taught and practiced his physical fitness program and began devising apparatus to aid in the rehabilitation of the disabled and sick. A look at the apparatus of today reveals that certain pieces—most notably the cadillac—must have been fashioned around the frame of a hospital bed. Mr. Pilates is credited with assisting many victims of the influenza epidemic and helping others recover from wartime diseases.

After the war, Mr. Pilates returned to Germany and was invited by the German government to train the new army. Recognizing the implications of such an endeavor, he decided to leave for America. (By certain accounts he was invited to the United States to help train Max Schmeling, the German world-title-holding boxer.) The period before Mr. Pilates' immigration to the United States is not well documented, but he appears to have met some of the great European movement innovators of that time, such as Rudolf von Laban, Kurt Jooss, and Mary Wigman. Although Mr. Pilates was not a dancer, these early encounters may have set the stage for his profound involvement with the dance community later in his career.

On the way to the United States, Joseph met Clara, who soon became his wife and played an integral role in developing and teaching his method. She has been described as a compassionate, knowledgeable, and kind teacher, in some ways a superior teacher to Joseph Pilates himself. In 1926 they set up their first studio in New York City, which attracted a diverse population, including socialites, circus performers, gymnasts, and other athletes.

But those who truly recognized the value of Mr. Pilates' system and his inherent, deep understanding of the workings of the human body were the members of the dance community, including luminaries such as George Balanchine, Ted Shawn, Martha Graham, and Hanya Holm. They embraced the method, often integrating it into their dance technique and training, as they witnessed its positive effects on dancers' bodies in both their performance and injury recovery.

Mr. Pilates was a disciplined man, as his teaching, his physical condition, and his performance clearly illustrate. His work appears to show the influence of other disciplines such as yoga, gymnastics, boxing, martial arts, and Eastern and Western philosophies. Exactly which disciplines he immersed himself in, and how much, is largely unknown, but it is fair to surmise that some other influences crept into his method. He taught and demonstrated his work in many environments, from the studio to his small New York apartment to the outdoors, where he seemed the most comfortable and inspired. He had the drive of a believer and the creativity of a genius. This was a man who believed deeply in his system as a way of life. His guiding philosophy was that achieving good health means that the whole being—body, mind, and spirit—must be addressed. He was convinced that his system could affect every facet of one's being, and therefore society as a whole.

Mr. Pilates dreamed of seeing his work taught in every college and school. He believed that children should be given knowledge of the body, and that the information should be simple and accessible. He revered the simplicity of movement and the elegance of nature's design of the body, both human and animal. Many early articles about Mr. Pilates describe his passion for animals and animal-like movement, which is indicated by the names he gave to several of the exercises.

Over the course of his career Mr. Pilates developed more than 600 exercises for his various apparatus. Pilates equipment is designed to condition the entire body, using positions and movements that simulate functional activities and thereby correct body alignment and balance. Using springs, pulleys, and gravity, the equipment challenges the musculature in diverse ways, with particular focus on the intrinsic muscles. These deep-lying layers of muscle are encouraged to work to achieve optimum movement mechanics and maintain correct positioning and alignment.

Joseph Pilates was ahead of his time in his approach to well-being, his invention of exercise equipment, and his creation of exercises and their integration into everyday life. He created the wunda chair, which doubled as a piece of furniture and could arguably be considered the first home gym. The image of Joseph Pilates extolling the virtues of his equipment in his New York apartment, with Clara looking on, suggests that his presentations exceeded the bounds of mere demonstration. Rare footage corroborates this impression; Mr. Pilates produced a film that explains and promotes the many facets of his system, including personal health tips and even showering techniques. Something between an instructional guide and an infomercial, the film suggests that Mr. Pilates was forward-thinking in his marketing methods as well as his approach to health, fitness, and well-being. Years after his death, his work spearheaded a revolution in the world of fitness and led to an evolution of the wellness industry.

The Pilates method is not merely a physical fitness regimen of mindlessly repeated exercises; it is a holistic approach to well-being and a lifelong process of refinement. In the opening paragraph of his book *Return to Life Through Contrology*, Mr. Pilates wrote, "Physical fitness is the first requisite of happiness. Our interpretation of physical fitness is the attainment and maintenance of a uniformly developed body with a sound mind fully capable of naturally, easily, and satisfactorily performing our many and varied daily tasks with spontaneous zest and pleasure."

Throughout this book, and in my teaching and practice, I strive to remain true to the essence of Joseph Pilates' work while allowing an evolutionary process to take place. This approach incorporates the art and science of human movement as it relates specifically to the Pilates method, viewing it through the prism of contemporary knowledge and modern society. I call this approach *body arts and science*, and it led to the establishment of Body Arts and Science International (BASI), an organization that provides Pilates education to enthusiasts and professionals globally. "Evolution" is at times misconstrued as rejection of the classical work of Joseph Pilates, but nothing could be further from the truth.

Joseph Pilates planted the seeds of a new approach to body conditioning, yet we can surmise that he did not define or even understand many of the concepts as we do today. Computers and sophisticated research methods enable us to scientifically substantiate notions that, for Mr. Pilates and other innovators of that time, were largely based on intuition. This research has given impetus to the adoption and expansion of Pilates into many arenas such as therapeutic work, athletic training, pre- and postnatal conditioning, and exercise for older adults. This evolution of Pilates, which I consider BASI to be, keeps the method as alive and relevant today as it was when Mr. Pilates was alive. Evolution is necessary, and as long as it is soundly grounded in the original works of Joseph Pilates and preserves both his work and intent, it should be referred to as Pilates.

Therapists have long yearned for a system that could take patients from the early stages of rehabilitation to the long-term goal of a well-conditioned, efficiently functioning body. Athletes have searched for ways to gain an extra edge to achieve peak performance in competition. Dancers have looked for a system to improve strength, flexibility, and technique while maintaining the body type and appearance required of dancers. Actors, circus performers, musicians, singers—the list goes on—are constantly seeking to enhance their performance and extend their careers. Pilates is extremely well suited for all these groups.

However, top performers in these disciplines are also now keenly aware of the need to use the mind as well as the body. Herein lies the essence of the Pilates method. Once athletes have reached the upper limits of their physical capabilities, additional training and practice often results in diminishing returns. It is tapping into the potential of the mind and its intricate connection to the body that will likely provide the elusive edge every athlete seeks. Many have found the answer in Pilates; its credibility is now widely accepted.

Pilates cannot transform the body in a few sessions or offer a perfect physique in a matter of weeks (as is sometimes claimed). It takes time, commitment, and consistent work to experience change. But if you are willing to go the distance, the results can be quite profound. Pilates not only offers a bridge between mind and body, between everyday life and optimal performance, between rehabilitation and healthy movement, it offers a system that—when used to its full potential—can enhance every aspect of life. It offers a solution for those with restricted mobility as well as elite athletes. It is as beneficial for an 11-year-old as it is for an 80-year-old and as motivating for men as for women. It is adaptable and diverse. Pilates, in other words, is for anyone (but not necessarily for everyone). As long as there is a drive toward positive change, a world of discovery and untapped potential awaits.

1

Enhancing the Mind and Body

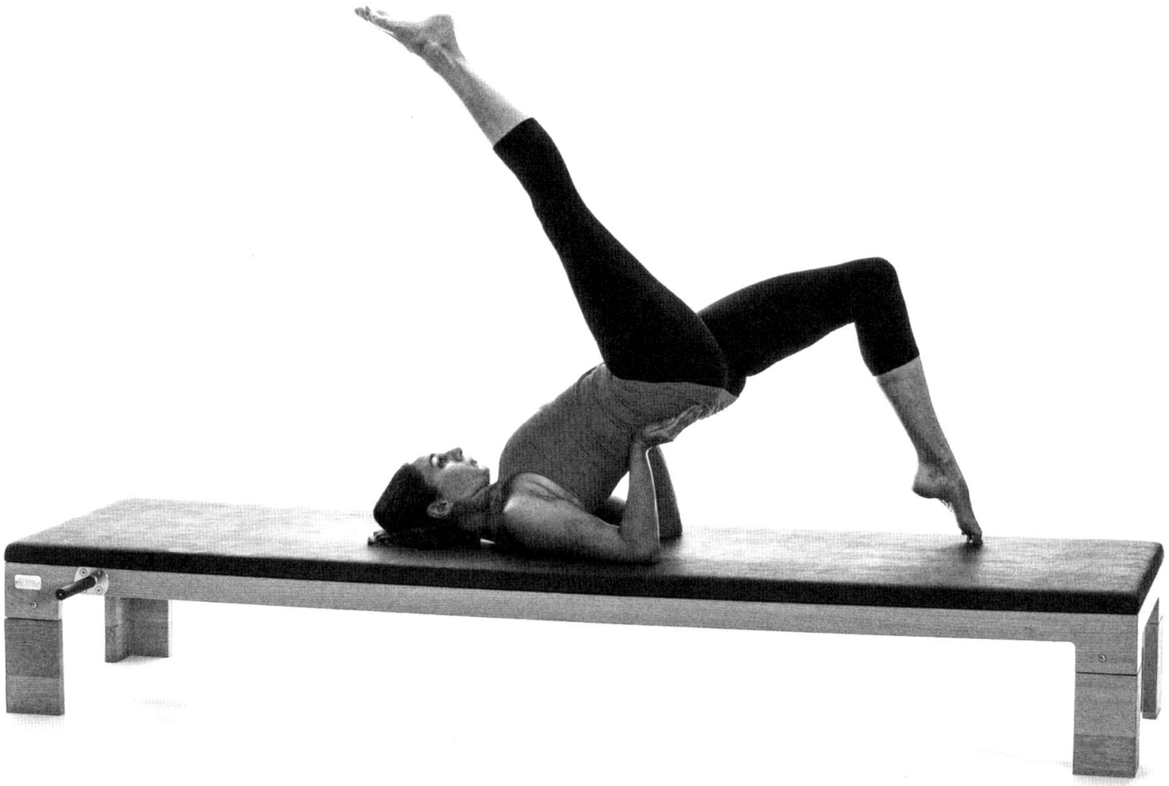

Is the exponential growth of Pilates—a method known by few people before the year 2000—merely hype? Why this sudden growth spurt, which would be characterized as nothing short of an epidemic by Malcolm Gladwell, the author of the widely read book *The Tipping Point*? The reasons for the enormous popularity of Pilates lie in its far-reaching, diverse benefits, which include improved fitness and athletic performance, better function, and a heightened sense of well-being.

The dance community has long benefited from Pilates. Dancers are supreme athletes, as measured by the feats they perform and the level of physical fitness they exhibit. Yet the demand on their bodies is enormous, and they suffer a very high incidence of injury—some studies suggest even higher than that of football players. As a result, dancers need an exceptional conditioning regimen to supplement their dance training and assist with injury prevention and rehabilitation. A dancer myself, I have often maintained that Joseph Pilates is the unsung hero of the dance world, given that many a dance career has been enhanced or saved by his method. Now everyone can benefit from the method that dancers have used as a form of cross-training for so many years and enjoy many of the same results.

Athletes were among the first to recognize the far-reaching rewards of extensive cross-training. Now they are awakening to Pilates and embracing it as a legitimate form of cross-training to enhance performance and prevent injury. The fact that so many athletes elect to practice Pilates out of the many forms of conditioning available to them is a testament to its value. It is embraced by the highest-ranked golfers and the best swimmers in the world; the most elite dancers, figure skaters, and tennis players; the fastest, highest-jumping ball players; and a host of actors, singers, and musicians. At the same time, it is also the best possible choice for people who have never exercised before and is an excellent foray into the world of fitness.

In 2000 I gave a presentation on enhancing athletic performance using the Pilates method. In preparation I informally surveyed some Olympic-level swimmers, asking them what they looked for in a cross-training regimen and how they thought Pilates could help their performance. The answers varied, but most respondents identified two common goals: to improve core strength and to explore the benefits of mind–body control and power. These two concepts encapsulate the essence of Pilates—in fact, very few, if any, training regimens are as effective as Pilates in achieving these goals.

Is Pilates for anyone? Yes. Will everyone select Pilates as their fitness regimen of choice? No. Not everyone will relate to the Pilates approach, and for certain training goals it may not be the most effective choice. For instance, bodybuilders interested in increasing muscle mass are better served by weight training. Sprinters who wish to gain speed and agility may prefer plyometrics or another form of resistance training. (However, even bodybuilders and sprinters can benefit greatly from certain aspects of Pilates, such as the development of core strength, heightened awareness, and flexibility and control.)

Still, the adaptability and wide appeal of Pilates is astounding. It can serve a broad spectrum of the population, because its benefits are not limited to the young, super fit, or super athletic. It has long been my view that the two populations that will ultimately benefit the most from Pilates are youths and older adults—essentially the bookends of life's spectrum. I have witnessed drastic changes in posture, alignment, weight, and body-mass distribution resulting from Pilates that have surprised even me, a devotee of Pilates for the past 40-plus years. I have seen positive changes in self-image, athletic performance, and the ability to perform daily activities. My clients have shared heartwarming stories of improvement in their personal and sexual relations. I have witnessed—and personally experienced—postinjury and postsurgery rehabilitation and neuromuscular reeducation programs incorporating Pilates that were successful beyond all expectations. It sounds too good to be true. Yet these transformations occur time and again throughout the world, and the international community is taking notice. Although more scientific research is needed, the research that has been conducted is beginning to substantiate many of these anecdotal findings, bringing welcome credibility to the practice of Pilates.

Of course, Pilates is not a potion that cures all and brings about miraculous changes immediately. Change takes time, commitment, and discipline. If you are dedicated to regular Pilates sessions (e.g., three times a week for at least six weeks), some positive changes are inevitable. Although certain changes can and often do occur immediately—for instance, a change in body awareness, muscle activation, or alignment—it takes time for most changes and adaptations to become imprinted in the neuromuscular system, for muscles to transform, and for the transformation to be integrated into a person's life.

One of the most gratifying experiences I have had in my Pilates career was working with a woman named Stella, who came to me at age 76 with severe scoliosis and an array of muscular and structural imbalances. The medical literature would say that changes could not be made to this woman's alignment, posture, or even movement at this point in her life. In fact, it would probably say that without either surgery or bracing during her preteen years, no significant changes in her physical alignment could have been achieved at any point in her life. But Stella worked with a commitment and dedication that I have seldom seen. She inspired everyone around her, including me. After my first session with Stella, I realized how unique she was, and she realized that she had found a system that could enhance her life greatly. Within the first few sessions her body awareness improved. After 30 sessions she moved differently, her posture improved, her confidence was elevated—in fact, her whole life changed. She realized early on that these results were only the beginning and that remaining committed for the long haul—not for days, weeks, or months, but for years—was imperative. And remain committed she did!

Was it simply the method, the exercises, and the apparatus that brought about changes? I believe not. It was Stella. She had a positive outlook, determination, and a powerful drive. Pilates provided a vehicle and the tools for change. Did she suddenly have a straight spine? Absolutely not! Such a change to the skeletal structure could not take place at her age. Yet her alignment, muscular control, and efficiency in movement did change. Her level of pain decreased dramatically, and she began to enjoy her daily activities, especially her beloved gardening, relatively pain free. I would not be exaggerating to say that Pilates gave her a new lease on life!

I believe the body is the divine temple of all that lies within. It carries the nucleus of who we are and embodies our true potential. Although I have spent much of my life tuning my body as if it were a fine musical instrument, I knew viscerally from an early age (and later consciously) that physical activity—be it Pilates, swimming, yoga, dance, surfing, windsurfing, kiteboarding, running, paragliding, biking, snowboarding, or skiing—ultimately serves my inner being. The physical benefits are undoubtedly important, but the effects on the inner being carry implications that are infinite and far-reaching. They influence how you function, how you feel, how you relate to yourself and those around you, and how successful you are in every respect. It simply makes you feel good. And if you feel good, you function well, you are fulfilled, and life seems more complete. The old adage that proclaims that within a healthy body lies a healthy mind could be taken one step further: A healthy mind guides a healthy body.

Benefits of Pilates

- Develops many aspects of physical fitness (strength, flexibility, coordination, speed, agility, and endurance)
- Heightens body awareness
- Enhances body control
- Teaches correct muscle activation
- Corrects posture and alignment
- Facilitates optimal function of the internal organs
- Improves balance and proprioception
- Enhances focus on breathing and its related physical and psychological benefits
- Offers a vehicle for concentration and focus
- Promotes relaxation and the release of tension
- Helps keep musculature and bone structure in an optimal state
- Provides a safe, low-impact form of exercise for populations such as pregnant women, those with restrictions, and older adults
- Serves as effective cross-training for athletic pursuits and daily activities
- Distributes body mass aesthetically (people report looking and feeling slimmer)
- Provides a path to inner harmony through a finely tuned body and mind

MIND AND BODY AS ONE

Discussion of the mind–body connection is as old as the ages; it rises up every now and again like a tidal wave. The 1970s and 1980s saw trends that focused on the physical being—hard-driving approaches with infamous mottos such as "no pain, no gain" or "work until you drop." More recently the fitness industry has returned to a mind–body focus—calmer, more introspective, and more refined and integrated systems of exercise and movement. We've seen a surge in the popularity of yoga and Pilates, an emphasis on nurturing the body rather than punishing it, and a renewed focus on the power of the mind–body connection. Proof of this connection continues to accrue, especially in the form of research based on brain-scan imaging that reveals changes in the brain that occur as a result of changes in the body and vice versa.

Joseph Pilates created his system of exercise with the intention that it should positively affect every aspect of a person's life—from movement to interpersonal relationships to heightened performance of daily tasks—leading the way to a state of total well-being. He believed that widespread practice of his system would eliminate many diseases and social ills. The Pilates method is more than a series of exercises; it is an approach to life, a philosophy. It dictates that we be aware of the changes that occur daily on every level of our being. These changes can be positive (such as rejuvenation and increased energy) or negative (such as rising stress and ailments). To benefit from the full potency of Pilates, you should make it an integrated part of your life—one that enriches every day. To practice Pilates is to strive to achieve balance and maximize the potential of the body, mind, and spirit.

The key to the positive effects of Pilates lies in its principles, not only in its exercises and equipment. It is a mind–body system that, unlike many other forms of physical fitness, addresses far more than easily measurable aspects of fitness such as strength, flexibility, and endurance. It encompasses awareness, balance, breath, concentration, center, control, efficiency, function, precision, harmony, and the far-reaching effects that these have on the body and the mind. Stabilization is developed, posture and alignment are refined, mechanics and efficiency of movement are improved, muscle recruitment patterns are reeducated, and function and well-being are reinforced—the ultimate goal of any good conditioning program. Pilates can and will improve every facet of your life.

> To achieve the highest accomplishments within the scope of our capabilities in all walks of life we must constantly strive to acquire strong, healthy bodies and develop our minds to the limit of our ability.
>
> —Joseph H. Pilates, *Return to Life Through Contrology*

Three Higher Principles

Return to Life Through Contrology opens with these words: "Physical fitness is the first requisite of happiness." Although this bold statement could seem judgmental, the book quickly makes clear that Joseph Pilates recognized that each person has different capabilities. What his opening statement means is that the mind and body are intricately linked: The condition of the body influences the state of the mind and vice versa. He continuously reinforces this premise in his writing and teachings, reiterating that physical condition relates not only to happiness but also to many other mental states (positive or negative, depending on the body's condition), such as relaxation, pleasure, anxiety, and depression. He claimed that by reawakening thousands of dormant muscle cells, we also awaken thousands of dormant brain cells—essentially a case of the muscles building the brain.

The way we define certain elements of the work and describe the movements may change as new research is conducted and modern terminology is created, but often these are only words and definitions, the glossary of the system. The philosophy encompassed in the higher principles never changes; it is the essence, the DNA, of the system itself. Despite the vastness, complexity, and scope of the Pilates method, three themes remain constant to help us navigate the lifelong exploration of Pilates. I call these the *higher principles*:

1. ***Completely coordinate the body, mind, and spirit***. This goal is the method's driving force—integrating into each exercise the balance of body, mind, and spirit. As Pilates wrote in *Return to Life Through Contrology*, achieving this balance "results in perfect posture." Although the relationship between the body, mind, and spirit is in a constant state of flux, these components are present throughout our lives. With the practice of Pilates, we become aware of them, and finding the balance between them is a lifelong quest.
2. ***Achieve the natural inner rhythm associated with all subconscious activities.*** The highest level of motor learning we can achieve is when an action is practiced to the point of becoming subconscious. This does not mean that we do it without concentration or awareness; instead, as the movement pattern becomes imprinted in the muscle memory, it becomes intuitive, and we can focus on fine-tuning, as opposed to being consumed with learning the action or skill itself. Mastery cannot be achieved in a short time; it is the reward of consistent training over a long period of time, sometimes years. In his book *Outliers*, Malcolm Gladwell discusses the "10,000-hour principle," which states that a person needs this many hours of practice to master a skill—any skill. Such practice requires discipline and commitment on every level as well as patience and endurance. This is the type of dedication to the practice of Pilates that leads to mastery of the system and ultimately to well-being. As Pilates wrote in *Return to Life Through Contrology*, "Correctly executed and mastered to the point of subconscious reaction, these exercises will reflect grace and balance in your routine activities" (p. 63).
3. ***Apply the laws of nature to everyday living.*** Pilates greatly admired nature and the animal kingdom. He often wrote about the graceful and efficient movements of animals, and he considered them far more evolved than humans in terms of movement and muscular development. Pilates wrote in *Your Health*, "Man has, in the race for material progress and perfection, entirely overlooked the most complex and marvelous of all Creations—Man himself!" Many of today's human ills and ailments are a result of sitting at computers for many hours a day, watching television for many more, eating far in excess of our needs (often unhealthy food), and driving more often than walking. We can learn a great deal from observing animals: their movements, their instincts, and their habits. For example, I have learned much from watching Shiloh, my little Jack Russell terrier. He stretches his spine hundreds of times a day, usually doing what Pilates practitioners call an Up Stretch (Down Dog in yoga terms), and he definitely knows how to relax, despite his very spirited nature.

The 10 Movement Principles

If the higher principles are the soul of the system, the 10 movement principles are its personality and character. I have identified these principles through my personal experience in this work and the writings of Joseph Pilates. They evolved from the three higher principles and are closely linked to their underlying philosophy.

Pilates practitioners should be mindful of these movement principles at all times, during both the teaching of the movements and the execution of the exercises. Each movement principle applies to every exercise in this book and should be integrated into your practice. They are the foundation of this mind–body system, a road map that serves to guide teachers and students toward understanding, mastery, and well-being.

The pursuit of awareness is endless—it is what makes Pilates so interesting, intriguing, and, ultimately, rewarding.

Principle 1: Become Aware

The first step into the wonderful world of Pilates, and every step that follows, should be filled with *awareness*. Be present in the movement with mind and body. In some forms of physical fitness and conditioning, everything about the environment seems designed to separate the mind from the body: loud music, television screens, computers mounted on exercise equipment, and myriad other distractions. Pilates is practiced in an environment that is conducive to stimulating and fortifying the mind–body connection, beginning with an awareness of one's own body.

No one can address the process of realigning the body without awareness of its structure and how it moves. Often I will say to a client whose leg is not straight, "Please straighten your leg all the way." He will answer, "But it is straight!" At other times I will adjust a client's head so that it sits on the centerline of the body, and the response is, "That feels very lopsided." Over time we become accustomed to misalignments, and the less aware a person is, the more severe these misalignments become, until an off-center body part feels centered or a bent limb feels straight. Bringing awareness to the body and the intricacies of movement establishes a foundation for change. Without awareness, little can be achieved.

Balance is the internal scale of life, dynamic and ever-changing. Pilates offers the path to equilibrium.

Principle 2: Achieve Balance

The term *balance* can mean many things. It can relate to components of fitness such as strength and flexibility, to the act of standing on one leg, or to the symmetry of the body. It can also describe a well-designed Pilates program, in which the exercises are proportionately distributed to work the different parts of the body in a session (an important consideration). Due to the method's focus on the abdominal region, Pilates programs are often excessively weighted toward abdominal work, particularly in forward flexion. This is a mistake. Work on the various muscle groups as well as the different planes of motion should be balanced. The word *balance* may also refer to the well-being of the whole individual: a balance of body, mind, and spirit. You should strive to achieve balance in every sense of the word and make it an integral part of your Pilates practice.

Joseph Pilates often mentioned the importance of a uniformly developed musculature, stating that only when the muscles are developed in such a way can body function be unhindered, true flexibility be present, and well-being be achieved. This idea touches on several issues, including muscular development, ease of function, and the mind–body relationship. Symmetrically and proportionately developed musculature allows the spine to properly support the body and assist in movement, ranging from fine, intervertebral articulation to large, powerful actions of the trunk.

Patterns of muscular imbalance may occur for multiple reasons. Some patterns are associated with dominance on one side (referred to as *handedness*), some with postural deviations such as scoliosis and kyphosis, and others with lack of flexibility or excessive flexibility. Imbalances that affect body alignment or result from misalignment are important factors in many painful postural conditions. At times muscles react to protect the body from harm or to reduce pain, with the result that certain muscles become overactive while others are inhibited. Muscle imbalance may also result from occupational or recreational activities that involve skills or movement patterns in which certain muscles are used persistently while the opposing muscles are recruited far less, or possibly not at all. Examples include habitually holding the phone to the ear on the same side, resulting in a chronic tilt of the head; standing with the weight shifted onto one leg, resulting in a perpetual tilt of the pelvis; and playing a one-side-dominant sport such as tennis, golf, or volleyball, resulting in asymmetrical muscular development.

Each person has different needs in terms of imbalances and how to alleviate them. Identifying and addressing these needs is the first step on the path to achieving balance. As we practice and teach Pilates, we act as "movement detectives," constantly making observations about our own bodies and those of our students. I provide some basic tools later in the book, such as the Mat: Roll-Down exercise in chapter 2, that help assess alignment and identify imbalances. In fact, I view all the exercises in this book as tools of analysis that can reveal a wealth of information about the intricacies of the body.

Principle 3: Breathe Correctly

As Pilates wrote in *Return to Life Through Contrology*, "Breathing is the first act of life, and the last . . . above all, learn how to breathe correctly." Breathing is synonymous with life and with movement. It is the all-encompassing link between body, mind, and spirit. Breathing is immensely important and powerful, yet it is so often ignored. One deep breath can promote relaxation, release tension, and make you smile.

Breathing is the inner shower that cleanses the body, guides the mind, and rejuvenates the spirit; it promotes natural movement and is the first step to educating the neuromuscular system. Breathing is also a vehicle for the achievement of an inner focus and an inner rhythm, a path to relaxing the mind and calming the spirit. It is the engine that drives all movement, and it lies at the heart of the Pilates method.

Certain muscle groups are recruited during the breath cycle to assist in respiration and therefore should be considered when determining a breathing pattern for a given exercise. For instance, it is theorized that exhaling during abdominal work maximizes abdominal recruitment because of the known participation of these muscles in exhalation. Conversely, it is theorized that because the trunk extensors assist in inhalation, inhaling during trunk extension maximizes their recruitment. Note that both of these muscle groups can be recruited during inhalation and exhalation, but muscle contraction may be more prominent when it corresponds with the breath cycle. Although scientific proof for these assertions is lacking, my experience as a practitioner and a teacher has convinced me of their relevance. I initially teach a specific breath pattern as a way of disciplining the mind and body. I believe that learning a set pattern is helpful in multiple ways. However, a breath pattern should not induce tension, which is exactly the opposite of what we are aiming for. Just as there is choreography for the movement, there is choreography for the breath, and both may take time to learn. The choreography of the breath (breath pattern) can and should be changed in the same fashion that we change the movement to expand our movement vocabulary.

Normal breathing is a complex process that involves many joints and muscles and is responsive to both voluntary and involuntary control. Basic understanding of this process is important because it offers insight into exercise and movement in general. A crucial muscle to cite when discussing breathing is the diaphragm, a dome-shaped muscle that forms a canopy underlying the rib cage. The diaphragm plays an important role in breathing and in creating the "muscular corset," the internal support system that is addressed throughout this book.

During diaphragmatic breathing, 75 percent of the respiratory effort comes from the diaphragm. When this muscle contracts during inhalation, it flattens, increasing the vertical dimension of the thorax (figure 1.1*a*). In addition, the external intercostal muscles also contract, pulling the lower ribs upward. Because of the orientation of the ribs and their joints (the lower part of the rib cage is wider than the upper part), the lower region of the thorax expands laterally as the diaphragm

Breathing

- Oxygenates the blood and nourishes the body on a cellular level
- Expels toxins from the body
- Improves circulation
- Improves skin tone
- Calms the mind and the body
- Encourages concentration
- Provides a rhythm for movement
- Assists in activating target muscles

Breath is the fuel for what Joseph Pilates called the *powerhouse*, the engine that drives the movement.

contracts, increasing the lateral dimension of the rib cage. In contrast, as the upper ribs rise, they increase the anterior-to-posterior dimension of the thorax, with the sternum moving forward (figure 1.1*b*). The overall effect is an increase in thoracic volume, a decrease in intrapulmonary pressure, and air flowing into the lungs—in other words, inhalation.

When the diaphragm relaxes, the abdominals and the organs in the abdominal cavity push it upward into its dome shape, thus decreasing the vertical dimension of the thorax. Additionally, the elasticity (recoil) of the lungs and chest wall create decreased thoracic volume and increased intrapulmonary pressure, resulting in air flowing out of the lungs, or exhalation.

When practicing Pilates, abdominal contraction typically accompanies most of the movements, which can be particularly challenging during inhalation. Therefore, in Pilates, we emphasize the lateral and posterior expansion of the rib cage during inhalation (called *lateral* or *costal breathing*). Besides assisting in drawing air into the lungs, this mode of breathing facilitates the maintenance of abdominal contraction throughout the exercise, which in turn assists in dynamic stabilization of the trunk (as opposed to the relaxation of the abdominal muscles that typically accompanies the contraction of the diaphragm during inhalation).

This by no means implies that diaphragmatic breathing is undesirable; it is the form of breathing primarily used in daily life. However, lateral breathing is the preferred mode of breathing during some forms of physical activity, including Pilates. An important point to stress is that practicing different breathing techniques should not cause tension; it should be viewed as expanding the breathing vocabulary so that the appropriate technique can be employed for a given task. This can be equated to the different breathing techniques used to play the various wind instruments, from the trombone to the flute to the didgeridoo. None are wrong; each merely requires a different breathing technique, and so it is with different physical activities.

During the exhalation phase of Pilates exercises, the abdominals contract to assist the diaphragm and intercostals in expelling air. (Imagine a process of milking the lungs and wringing the air out.) This in turn promotes deeper inhalation on the part of the primary respiratory muscles and the auxiliary muscles (including the back extensors), bringing in a healthy quantity of oxygen-filled air to nourish and rejuvenate the body.

Many people have commented to me over the years that they have found learning and practicing the technique of lateral breathing to be immensely beneficial. Those who have made such remarks have included sing-

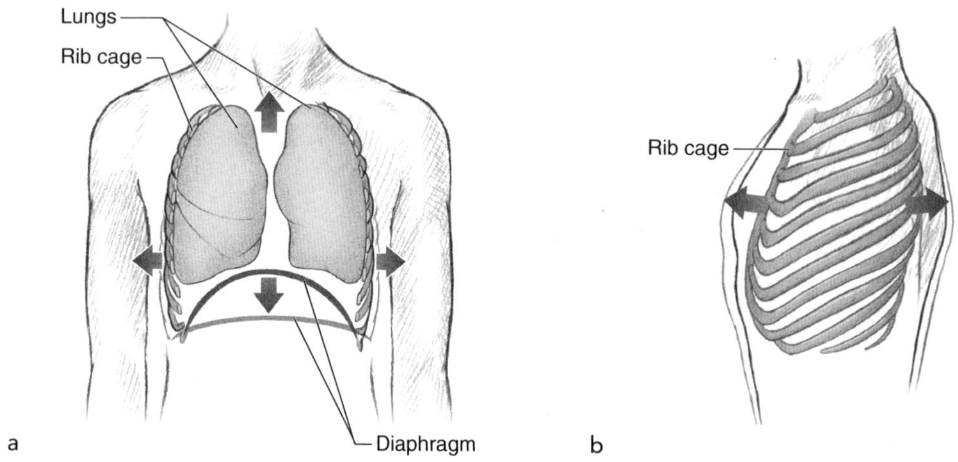

FIGURE 1.1 The diaphragm works with the abdominals to deepen inhalation and expand the thorax.

ers, musicians, and yogis, who are accustomed to using very specific breathing techniques. Focus and training in various modes of breathing promotes breath control.

Breathing can be practiced anywhere and at any time. I find two exercises particularly helpful in mastering lateral breathing. The first is to wrap a 3-foot (0.9 meter) length of rubber exercise band around your chest, holding the ends of the band in your hands, and expanding your chest against the resistance of the band to amplify the contraction of the intercostals. The other involves lying supine on a mat in a comfortable neutral spine position, knees bent, legs parallel, and arms by the sides of the body. With each breath, visualize the chest expanding and spreading laterally across the mat in both directions like two swells rising in the ocean and then gently falling back. This is an excellent form of meditation and good practice for breathing. You may also imagine the breath moving like a river of energy to either side of the chest, or to any part of the body that may need to be activated or relaxed. This is particularly helpful if an imbalance is present and the musculature on one side of the thorax is not as active as the other (often the case when scoliosis is present and one side becomes relatively compressed).

Principle 4: Concentrate Deeply

I view *concentration* as the bridge between awareness and movement. As you establish the start position for each movement, I encourage you to go through a checklist of important data: which muscles you need to recruit, how you should align your body, and which is your chosen breath pattern. Simply by concentrating on a particular muscle prior to the action, you can activate it more accurately and intensely than if you do not think about it. Concentrating on your body alignment will help you recruit the correct muscles and avoid unnecessary strain on the body. Concentrating on the breath pattern will help you maintain a good rhythm for the movement and keep your mind focused. However, keep in mind that concentration can be so intense that it may morph into tension. This can lead to a tightening of the musculature, a restriction in breathing, and halting movements rather than flowing ones. This is clearly not the intention and should be avoided.

Although awareness and concentration are closely related, I regard awareness as a state of mind—being mindful and feeling the movement—and concentration the cognitive process of understanding the movement. When combined with awareness, concentration not only promises precise movement but also gives the work a meditative quality. Being meditative does not imply that the work will lack vibrancy, challenge, physical demand, or intensity; it means ensuring a deep focus on the work that allows you to block out unnecessary disturbances and perform each movement to the maximum of your ability, tapping into the full potential of Pilates.

Pilates is meditation in motion—a physical, mental, and spiritual process.

Principle 5: Center Yourself

Centering yourself can be defined in purely physical terms—finding where your center of gravity lies. Differences in anatomy result in different weight distribution—men tend to be top-heavy and women tend to carry their weight in the pelvic region—so discovering and experiencing your body's center of gravity is important. It affects each exercise you do. This is also the region of the powerhouse. The concept of the powerhouse—that all movement emanates from this core—is a common thread in the practice of Pilates and is addressed in more detail in chapter 2. In Pilates, centering yourself means more than finding your center of gravity; it means uniting body, mind, and spirit.

The concept of centering is not new. In Eastern practices we learn of *ki* in aikido, *chi* in tai chi, *tan tien* in chi gong, and *chakra* in yoga—all refer, in general terms, to the life force that lies within us like a bottomless well of energy. Interestingly, in all these practices this life force is located in approximately the same area of the body. Martha Graham focused on this area in her modern dance technique and altered the way dancers approached dance and movement; the *contraction* (flexion of the spine), involving deep abdominal activation, became the foundation of her technique. The feeling

A strong center enhances performance, be it in everyday activities or athletic pursuits.

of being centered relates not only to the support provided by the area's strong intrinsic muscles but also to the energy emanating from this nucleus and a person's ability to make full use of this physical and metaphysical support system. It is not uncommon to hear a dancer speak of feeling centered or, conversely, uncentered. As you delve into Pilates and open yourself to finding and moving from your center, you will experience this most gratifying and elevating of sensations.

When control becomes innate, you have reached the point of mastery.

Principle 6: Gain Control

Gaining *control* is an amalgamation of all the preceding principles. When watching people move, particularly during complex movements, it is immediately evident whether they have a high level of control—or lack control. Few things are as beautiful and inspiring as viewing athletes, dancers, gymnasts, or figure skaters who have immaculate control over their movement. Similarly, watching a lion walk, a cheetah run, or a gazelle leap can evoke a feeling of awe. Kathy Stanford Grant, a student of Joseph Pilates who became a great teacher of his work, used to send me phenomenal pictures of animals in balance or in motion, pointing out to me their grace, effortless power, and unencumbered movement. These qualities are lofty goals for us humans, but worthy of aspiration, nevertheless.

Initially, achieving control of movement is a conscious process. It occurs through practice, practice, and more practice. Ideally, a teacher who has achieved control should guide you in this process. As you continue to practice and integrate the work into your life your own movement control becomes intuitive—like that of an animal—and a part of your being.

Watching effortless movement is awe-inspiring—and performing it is even more so. Efficiency is the first step to achieving effortlessness.

Principle 7: Be Efficient

Who does not want to conserve energy? Waste has become a by-product of our society in every way. Striving for *efficiency* teaches us to direct our movements like a laser beam: focused and precise. When performing Pilates, we do not grimace during effort or grunt as the movements become difficult and demanding. We focus the work where it is needed, exerting the required amount of energy, no more and no less. The rest of the body remains calm and relaxed. I have an internal agreement with myself when performing the work: The more difficult the movements are, the more consciously relaxed I strive to be.

Achieving efficiency applies not only to athletic feats but also to everyday movements. An important phase in the process of learning Pilates is transferring and integrating information learned in the Pilates session into everyday activities. A session lasts approximately 1 hour and is often supervised by an instructor. What of the remaining 23 hours of the day? We must actively and consciously direct our attention to how we move. I recommend creating mental reminders to help you practice this transfer (to keep your head and spine aligned, to use your powerhouse, to relax, and ultimately to move effortlessly).

Principle 8: Create Flow

Like all the principles, *flow* manifests itself both physically and mentally. It is present within each movement as well as within the Pilates session as a whole. Flow can be described as the unobstructed channeling and translation of energy into movement. It is also the seamless connection of one movement to the next, creating what appears to be a continuous stream of motion. Despite the fact that teachers offer correction and input to students and may need to stop the class periodically to do so, the overall sense of each individual movement and of the session as a whole should be one of continuum.

If you observe athletes like climber Alex Honnold, swimmer Michael Phelps, surfer extraordinaire Kelly Slater, brilliant dancer Mikhail Baryshnikov, and (my favorite) all-around waterman Kai Lenny, you will note a common quality: an apparent effortless flow in their movements. You can experience the same quality of flow through the practice of Pilates. Of all the principles, the quality of flow may be the most intriguing: It is intangible, difficult to describe, and impossible to achieve without full presence in the moment and complete integration of body, mind, and spirit.

Flow can be understood physiologically as the immaculate timing of muscle recruitment and movement through the joints. In each movement there is an optimum sequence in which the muscles should be activated, called a *muscle-recruitment pattern* or *muscle-firing pattern*. When muscle recruitment is timed down to the millisecond and combined with the inner rhythm of unobstructed breath and full immersion of the mind, the result is flow. Viewing two people performing an identical movement can be fascinating—even though the physical action is the same, they might look quite different from one another. Flow, or lack thereof, is frequently the reason for this difference. Of course, beauty is in the eye of the beholder, and flow is subjective and visceral, both to the person performing the movement and the person observing it.

I cannot identify the genesis of my fascination with the concept of flow, but I know it goes back to my early days as a swimmer. Later, I practiced Ashtanga yoga for many years, which possesses a unique quality of flow. As I started dancing, flow was a quality that I loved watching in others and sought to achieve in my own movement. Also, my deep interest and limited experience in the martial arts inevitably furthered my attraction to the quality of flow, which is intrinsic to the martial arts.

The concept of flow is as old as the ages. It is found, for instance, in yoga, martial arts, Zen, and Daoism. It is often described in these disciplines as a state of oneness (wholeness) of the universe, of mind and body, of self and the world. In the last 50 years or so there has been a resurgence of interest in the study of flow and mindfulness. The well-known psychologist Mihály Csíkszentmihályi has done much to promote the discussion and the research around this topic. His popular book *Flow* takes a deep dive into exploring the mental state of operation in which an individual is completely immersed in a particular activity—or "in the zone." The person experiences what may be described as energized focus, full involvement, and a sense of success in performing the activity.

In his book *Flow*, Csíkszentmihályi promotes his theory that people are most happy when they are in a state of flow. All of us have likely experienced this sensation, and many of us spend a lifetime chasing it. The feelings of freedom, joy, fulfillment, success, and loss of ego have a powerful draw. This draw morphs into motivation to seek more flow in our lives. It is certainly the fuel that drives my daily Pilates practice as well as my search for the perfect wave, ideal snow, consistent wind—when skill, mindset, conditions, and timing come together. That, for me, is the epitome of flow! Do I always achieve the state of flow? No. Do I continue to seek it? A resounding yes!

As teachers, we become guides for our students to reach a state of flow. A requisite of flow is that there needs to be a balance between the challenge of the task and the skill of the performer. If the task is not challenging enough, the student will not be fully engaged or immersed. If the task is too challenging, the student will likely become frustrated. To achieve the state of flow, a perfect balance must be struck.

Movement with flow, starting from the breath and leading to the recruitment of the muscles, focus of the mind, and full involvement of the entire being, becomes an inner quality, which is simultaneously calming and rejuvenating.

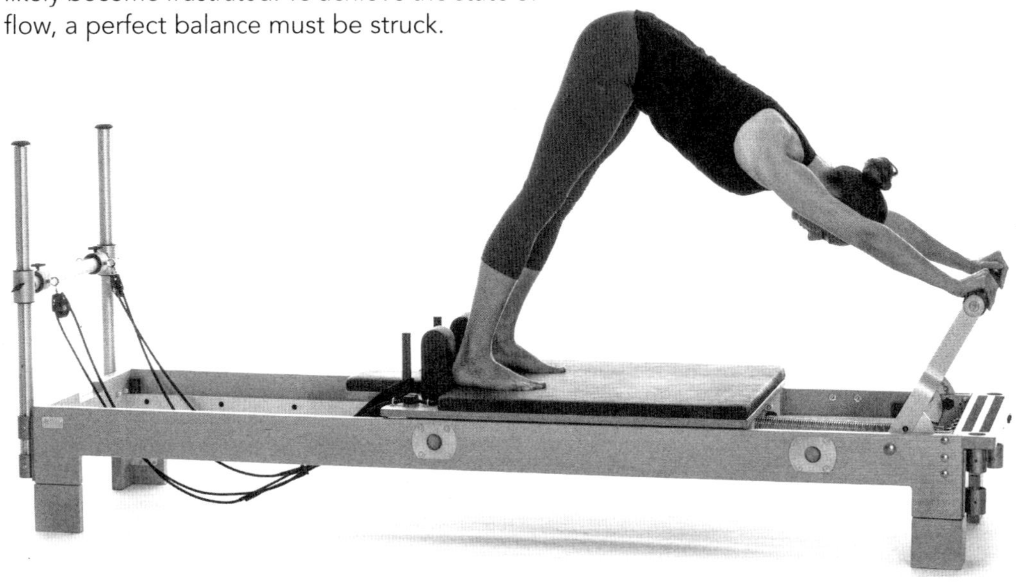

Precision is a fundamental ingredient in the practice of Pilates and a milestone on the path to mastery.

Principle 9: Be Precise

Without *precision*, Pilates becomes almost meaningless. It is popular in the fitness industry to speak of isolating muscles during a particular movement. Isolation depends entirely on precision. Yet those who claim to isolate muscles are often doing anything but. Either they lack precision in isolating an area, or they rely on external means to achieve this goal. For instance, someone who performs a biceps curl using a preacher curl bench is demonstrating nonfunctional isolation—although he is engaging the biceps, he is totally reliant on the bench. In life we cannot walk around with this type of support. Isolation is only meaningful when you can stabilize your own body and support the isolated movement independently. This is a mindful process that takes us back to the first movement principle, awareness, followed by concentration and control. As you gain more insight into your body, you will be able to achieve increasingly fine muscle isolation. I strive for the day that I am able to isolate and control every muscle fiber in my body. Of course this is impossible, but it is a goal that I strive for that keeps me motivated, grounded, and humble!

Precision requires complete integration of the body's musculature, which may then be followed by the isolation of certain muscles or muscle groups. You will feel the work more profoundly when you perform every movement with precision down to the finest detail. Precision is the basis of the corrective approach to working the body. We continuously strive to reach ideal balance and alignment. Students often comment that they feel an exercise more profoundly than ever, despite having done it many times before. Often it's a matter of adjusting the body one or two degrees this way or that—and suddenly the flame ignites. That is precision. Pilates demands a great deal of precision in the activation of each muscle and in the execution of each movement.

Moving through life in harmony with all that is around us and all that is within us is the ultimate achievement of the practice of Pilates.

Principle 10: Seek Harmony

Harmony is the whole, the culmination of all the preceding principles—efficient movement coupled with flow and precision. It is the ultimate reward for commitment and hard work. Harmony means walking out of a session and feeling completely rejuvenated, being aware of each muscle, and sensing the depth of each breath. It means being focused, centered, and in control. To feel all of these qualities is to be in harmony with oneself and with the environment.

Few forms of conditioning can boast the profound outcomes that Pilates can, as millions are now experiencing. The greatness of human potential is realized when the infinite power of the mind is combined with the immaculate engineering of the human body. The principles described in this chapter, individually and together, offer a path to harnessing this potential. However, the movements in Pilates, as beautiful and wonderful as they are, are only movements. The underlying principles and philosophy are what make them unique and able to transform lives. When correcting alignment and teaching positive movement patterns, you need to address more than just the physiological components, such as muscle strength and flexibility. You must also consider the principles behind the movements, which will guide your students through the internal process of transformation that leads to well-being.

The practice of Pilates opens the path to new discovery each day. Although I have done thousands of sessions and taught thousands more, I can honestly say that I have never done a personal workout or taught a session without learning something new. Of course, your body, mind, and spirit must be open to such learning in order to benefit from it. If they are, the possibilities are infinite.

2

Alignment, Posture, and Movement

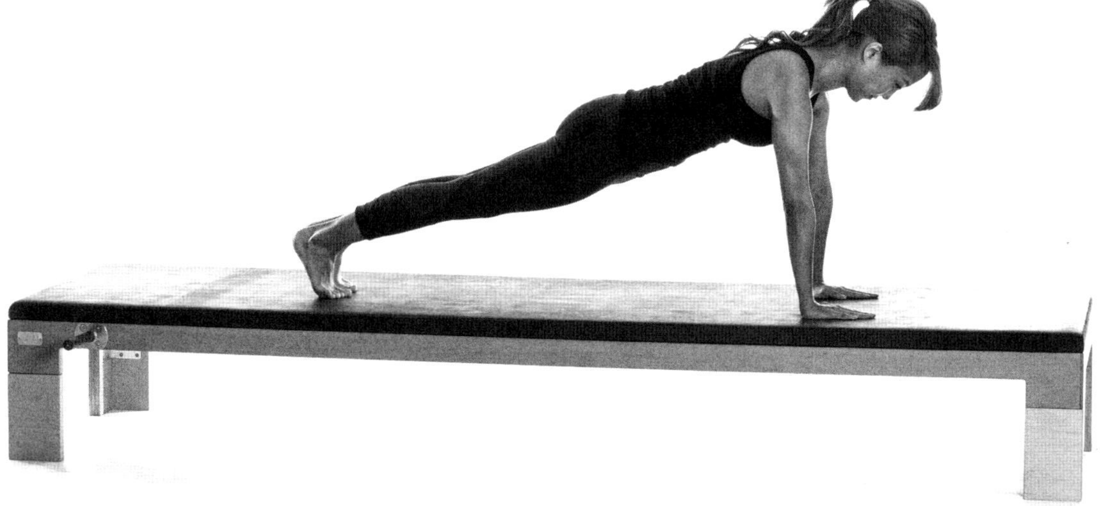

The previous chapter laid the foundation for understanding Pilates—its philosophy, principles, and potential. In the following chapters I discuss concepts that pertain to the science of human movement and their relationship to the Pilates method.

The human body is a complex instrument that can be likened, in its mechanical functioning, to a chain with multiple links—the kinetic chain. Exploring the kinetic chain is a fascinating study. Even though all bodies share predictable patterns of movement and muscle development, each body is different. As a movement occurs, the muscles are activated in a certain order, or pattern. If this pattern is faulty, the movement will likely lack efficiency and could potentially lead to injury.

The Pilates method addresses the kinetic chain in its entirety, recognizing the influence that one region of the body can have on another. Through a process of refinement, Pilates can bring about profound changes, which enhance the body's performance and lay a path to well-being.

Musculoskeletal Structure

The human body is the most masterful feat of engineering imaginable. Let us view the body from the inside out. The skeleton is the body's infrastructure, on which all else is built (figure 2.1*a*). Layered onto this well-structured and balanced frame are the muscles, which provide support and movement (figure 2.1*b*). The bones act as levers and the muscles as cables that move the body parts in the desired direction. Because of this ingenious structure, the musculature is able to work effectively. However, if the frame is out of alignment, it affects the entire structure, resulting in inefficient muscle action, stress, fatigue, and possible ailments.

The relationship between the skeletal structure and the muscular system is interesting and unique; it is the basis of all movement analysis. Often when exercising we place so much emphasis on the muscles that we ignore the skeletal structure. To achieve effective and efficient movement, we must consider both the skeletal and muscular systems (these categories are used in the broadest sense possible, including all bone and soft tissue—muscle, tendon, ligament, cartilage, and fascia). Pilates offers a path to discovering and utilizing the full potential of these systems.

Two well-known first-generation Pilates teachers, Eve Gentry and Bruce King,

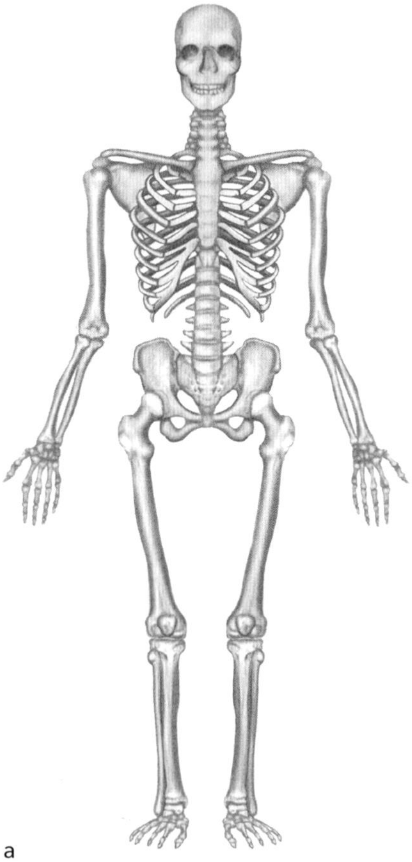

a

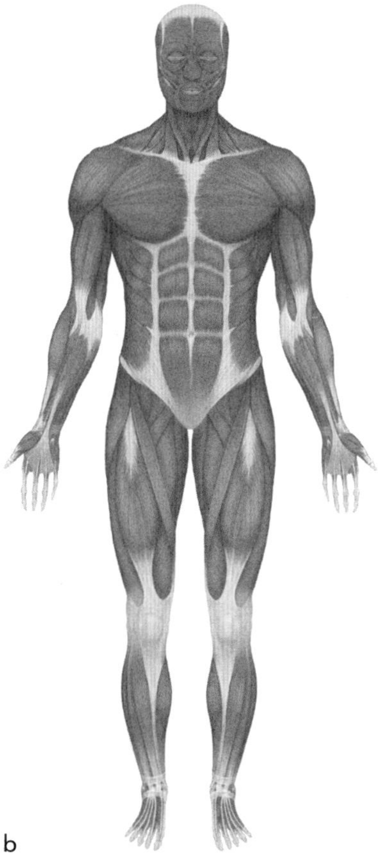

b

FIGURE 2.1 Proper skeletal alignment combines with good muscle mechanics to produce effortless and efficient movement.

often described Pilates movements in terms of the bones moving, as opposed to the muscles moving the bones. Using this imagery can help facilitate effortless motion, devoid of tension or excessive force (and the inevitable grimacing and groaning!). It's as if the bones move as a result of an intangible internal force. Focusing on the skeletal structure also draws more attention to alignment. Correct alignment is the first step toward a positive outcome and success in achieving the desired goals.

Spine

One of the most fascinating parts of the skeleton is the spine (figure 2.2). Made up of 24 moving vertebrae and 9 that are fused (this number can vary slightly), the spine can be extremely mobile, allowing multidirectional movement of the trunk. At the same time, it can be very stable, serving as a solid platform to support movement of the limbs. In fact, each individual vertebral joint moves very little, yet they combine to form a highly mobile mechanism. Distributing the work through the spine and maximizing the movement of all the vertebral joints is preferable to stressing one or two vertebral joints, which can result in shearing forces and excessive load in a specific area. The pelvis and lower spine are of particular interest in Pilates, because herein lies the powerhouse, the core, from which all movement emanates.

Pelvic Bowl

The pelvic bowl holds the essence of our being, the eternal spring of life. Here, where the body's center of gravity lies, is the meeting point of human anatomy with the metaphysical; the confluence of the musculoskeletal system with life force. This concept forms the basis of Pilates as well as other Eastern and Western practices, such as yoga, tai chi, aikido, and certain styles of dance. The pelvis is indeed the powerhouse!

Dr. Arnold Kegel, innovator of the much-advocated exercises that bear his name (which involve contracting, holding, and releasing the muscles of the pelvic floor), recognized the importance of the pelvic floor muscles and their development, particularly for women before, during, and after pregnancy. He furthered the premise that training the pelvic floor muscles can help to prevent and cure urinary incontinence and improve sexual function and satisfaction. I am sure he would delight in the attention the pelvic floor is receiving today. A

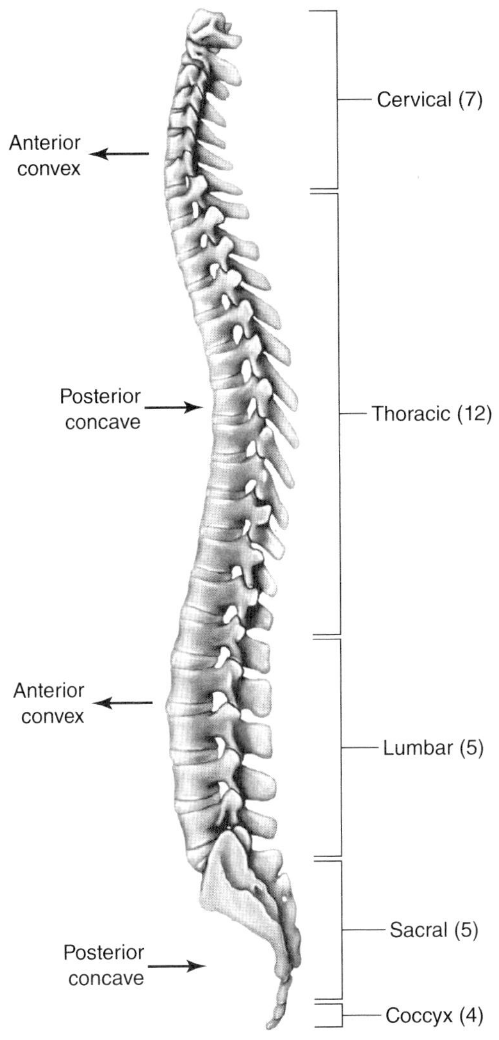

FIGURE 2.2 This side view of the spine illustrates the natural curves of the spine and proper spinal alignment.

healthy pelvic floor—strong and flexible, able to adapt to changes in internal pressure—is an integral part of the powerhouse, and one of the keys to well-being for both women and men.

Men are often surprised to learn that they even have a pelvic floor! Both genders need well-conditioned pelvic floor muscles (coccygeus, iliococcygeus, and pubococcygeus) for optimum function, and recruitment of these muscles should be integrated into every comprehensive exercise program. When the transversus abdominis muscle is contracted (as it is encouraged to be throughout much of a Pilates session), the pelvic floor muscles also contract. A similar correlation seems to exist between contraction of the hip adductors, another muscle group that is activated frequently in Pilates, and the pelvic floor muscles. In addition, stopping the flow of urine activates the pelvic floor muscles, so, by nature's design, the pelvic floor is regularly exercised throughout daily life.

However, heightening awareness and control of this muscle group is extremely beneficial. A well-conditioned pelvic floor supports the internal organs and provides added support during pregnancy. In addition, it assists in preventing or overcoming urinary incontinence and contributes to heightened sexual function and satisfaction. Actively working the pelvic floor, particularly the coccygeus, influences positioning of the sacrum and may help relieve or prevent lower back pain. Much recent literature and research indicate that the pelvic floor is fundamental to healthy functioning of the core (in terms of strength, support, and stabilization), primarily due to its role in enhancing intra-abdominal pressure.

Dr. Noelani Prietto, a specialist in gynecology based in Irvine, California, pointed out to me the uniqueness of the pelvic floor muscles: Like the diaphragm, they sit within a bony structure (in fact, the pelvic floor is sometimes referred to as the pelvic diaphragm); this is in contrast to most of the skeletal muscles, which attach outside the bony structure. The pelvic muscles work symbiotically—that is, they work cooperatively in order to adapt to the constant changes of internal abdominal and thoracic pressure. This mechanism of intra-abdominal pressure is thought to "un-weight" the spine and play a significant role in lumbopelvic stabilization (used synonymously in this context with the term *core*).

The pelvis serves as a bridge between the upper and lower body and is made up of three bones—the ischium, ilium, and pubis—bound together by cartilage (figure 2.3). Most people agree (myself included) that these cartilaginous joints allow varying degrees of very subtle movement. I must stress that the movement is miniscule. I often hear people referring to the movement of the sacroiliac joint as if it glides around like the scapulae. That is clearly not the case. At the same time, if these joints become immobile, undue strain is likely to be placed on the pelvis and spine. The reasons for either hyper- or hypomobility can vary, but for our purposes, simply being aware of the potential imbalances that can occur in the pelvis, addressing the imbalances, and seeking medical advice if a harmful condition prevails will suffice.

I like to visualize the pelvis as being made up of two rotating discs sitting on their sides facing each other. The degree of rotation of each disc is quite limited in either direction; however, a small amount of rotation is essential for healthy function of the pelvis and the body

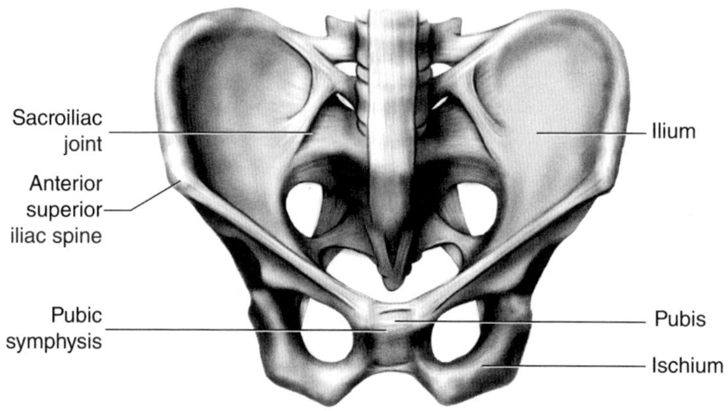

FIGURE 2.3 This front view of the pelvis clearly shows its structure and the joints that bind the parts together.

as a whole. This pattern of rotation of the two sides of the pelvis (innominate bones) is present during many basic activities, such as walking and running; as one innominate rotates in one direction, the other rotates in the opposite direction.

We need to consider the joints around, as well as within, the pelvis when discussing its function. The influence of the surrounding joints on the pelvis is profound and vice versa. In fact, the function of the pelvis can be best understood by viewing the movement of the surrounding joints. If the pelvis is misaligned, it adversely affects the function of body segments up and down the kinetic chain, resulting in inefficient movement, muscular imbalances, and stress on the structure of the body. Balanced development of the muscles around the pelvis is fundamental to achieving a well-aligned pelvis and ideal posture. Detecting imbalances is the first step toward understanding the body's movement. Remedying them is the next step, and this is where Pilates can play a crucial role in reeducating the neuromuscular system. Correct pelvic alignment is of paramount importance, whether you are doing Pilates, performing daily activities, or sitting at a desk.

One way to view the pelvis is as a suspension bridge with cables (the muscles) holding it from above, below, from the sides, and, very importantly, from within. As long as all the cables are tensioned correctly and proportionately, little strain is placed on any one cable and the bridge will be stable and level. However, the moment the balance of tension on the cables changes or the bridge is not level, excessive strain is placed on certain cables whereas others are underused. The result is that the entire bridge shows strain. Although the pelvis will not typically collapse under stress, as a bridge might, muscles that encounter excessive tension may become strained or even tear. Simply put, if the pelvis is out of alignment, the body is out of alignment.

To understand the bridge analogy and the impact the pelvis has on the entire body, we need only look at the list of some of the muscles that act on the pelvic complex—the pelvic floor muscles; spinal flexors, lateral flexors, rotators, and extensors; hip flexors and extensors; hip adductors and abductors; and hip external and internal rotators. This list doesn't even include the tendons, ligaments, and joints that also add support and provide mobility to this intricate structure. The pelvis is the bridge between the lower and upper body, the all-powerful lower limbs and the trunk. It is no wonder that the source of much of our movement emanates from this region. Pilates provides a path to discovering the powerhouse and unleashing the power of the pelvis. Keep in mind that working with precision when exercising the lumbopelvic region is imperative, possibly more so than with any other area of the body.

Muscles of the Powerhouse

In order to achieve good alignment and correct movement mechanics, the body must have the tools to do so; a well-balanced musculoskeletal system is the first step in this quest. Strength is obviously an important aspect of posture, yet other elements, such as habitual muscle activation patterns, genetics, and flexibility are also key components. In many instances, a lack of flexibility inhibits ideal alignment and recruitment of the correct muscles. Hypermobility, on the other hand, although not restrictive by nature, demands a great deal of body awareness and muscular control to maintain good alignment. In Pilates we strive to develop strong, flexible muscles that are effective in their function and adaptability.

Certain muscles play a crucial role in providing a stable and pliable core, without which good alignment and efficient function are not possible. These are the deep muscles of the pelvis and trunk. The superficial muscles are sometimes overdeveloped and overemphasized in comparison to the deep muscles, often at the expense of a strong, effective, efficiently functioning core. Being large does not necessarily translate into being functional. I regard muscle bulk that is not functional as extra baggage to carry around; ultimately,

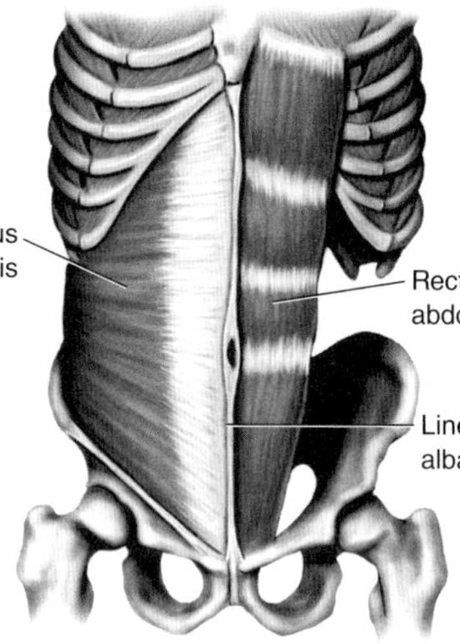

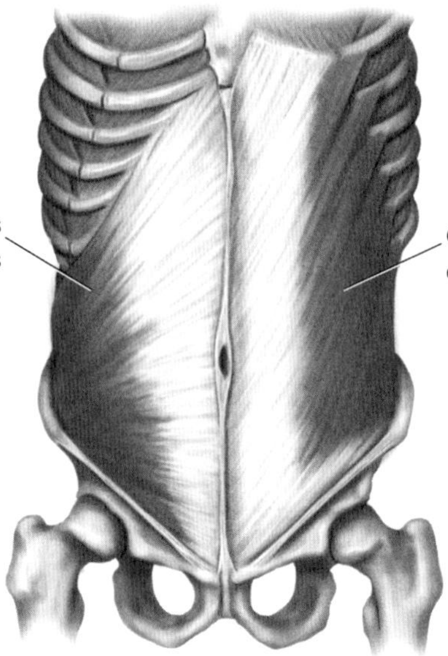

FIGURE 2.4 Major muscles of the abdominal muscle group.

it can burden the body. As with a tree, the deeper layers, not the bark, provide the support for it to stand upright and the flexibility to bend with the wind.

The back extensors and abdominals are key in providing the form and function of the trunk. They share a symbiotic relationship and there should be constant interplay between them. Both the abdominals and back extensors are made up of layers of muscle, and it is the deepest layers that are most prominent in providing stabilization and support to the spine. The abdominal group is made up of the rectus abdominis, external oblique, internal oblique, and transversus abdominis (figure 2.4). In the back, the large superficial group (erector spinae) runs longitudinally along the spine, whereas the deep posterior spinal group (which includes the multifidus), the intervertebral muscles that connect between the vertebrae of the spine, lie deeper (figure 2.5). The back also serves as the attachment for many dual-purpose muscles, such as those connecting to the neck and head, the upper limbs, and the pelvis. Within these two major muscle groups, the abdominals and back extensors, two muscles have been identified as having a particularly profound effect on stabilization and, in turn, function: the transversus abdominis and the multifidus.

The abdominals and back muscles, together with the diaphragm and the pelvic floor, create a cylinder of muscular support in the center of the body. I call this the *internal support system* (ISS). It is congruent with the powerhouse in Pilates, or the core in other forms of training. It is gratifying that scientific research is now substantiating much of what Joseph Pilates advocated so many years ago with regard to the importance of a strong, powerful, and functional core. During the practice of Pilates, you are encouraged to recruit the muscles of the ISS throughout. Movement is possible without activating the ISS; however, internal support, protection of the spine, and efficient function are likely to be diminished.

Another component that is important to consider in any discussion relating to the pelvis and the spine is the psoas. There are two psoas muscles, psoas major and psoas minor. Psoas major combines with the iliacus to form the iliopsoas (figure 2.6). Besides being powerful hip flexors, these muscles are believed to substantially influence spinal stabilization and alignment. Because the psoas is close to the axis of movement when performing flexion, lateral flexion, and extension of the lumbar spine, it compensates for imbalance between the anterior abdominal muscles and posterior spinal extensor muscles to help stabilize the lumbar spine. Some practitioners believe that most dysfunction of the spine and the hip joint can be attributed to a disturbance of function of the psoas and iliopsoas. They postulate that tight or weak psoas muscles are associated with abnormal pelvic tilt, exaggerated lumbar lordosis, lower back pain, sacroiliac dysfunction, degenerative disc disease, scoliosis, and misaligned posture, among other conditions. With extended sitting, a common by-product of the modern lifestyle, the hip flexors become tight and weak. The psoas and iliopsoas should be addressed in all exercise programs, if possible.

The psoas muscles and the abdominal muscles are agonists and antagonists as well as synergists—they can oppose one another's actions and work cooperatively. The psoas, and hip flexors in general, play an important role in much of the abdominal work in Pilates, particularly in the exercises in which the legs are held up off the ground. Typically, great emphasis is placed on recruitment of the abdominals, whereas the role of the hip flexors is often minimized or overlooked altogether. I believe that more focus should be placed on controlling and using the hip flexors correctly. They are vital to the successful execution of many Pilates exercises as well as to efficient function and general well-being.

Interestingly, all the muscles of the ISS are what I call "mind muscles"—activating them requires mental focus and a high degree of body awareness and concentration. Controlling the muscles of the ISS demands different skills than those used for controlling superficial skeletal muscles, such as the biceps or quadriceps, which are easily accessed and whose activation is readily apparent. It appears that nature intended that the journey toward the mastery of movement and attainment of fitness would incorporate mind–body exploration. As Joseph Pilates wrote in *Return to Life Through Contrology*, "exercises that produce a harmonious structure we term 'physical fitness,' reflecting itself in a coordinated and balanced tri-part unity of body, mind, and spirit" (pp. 32-33).

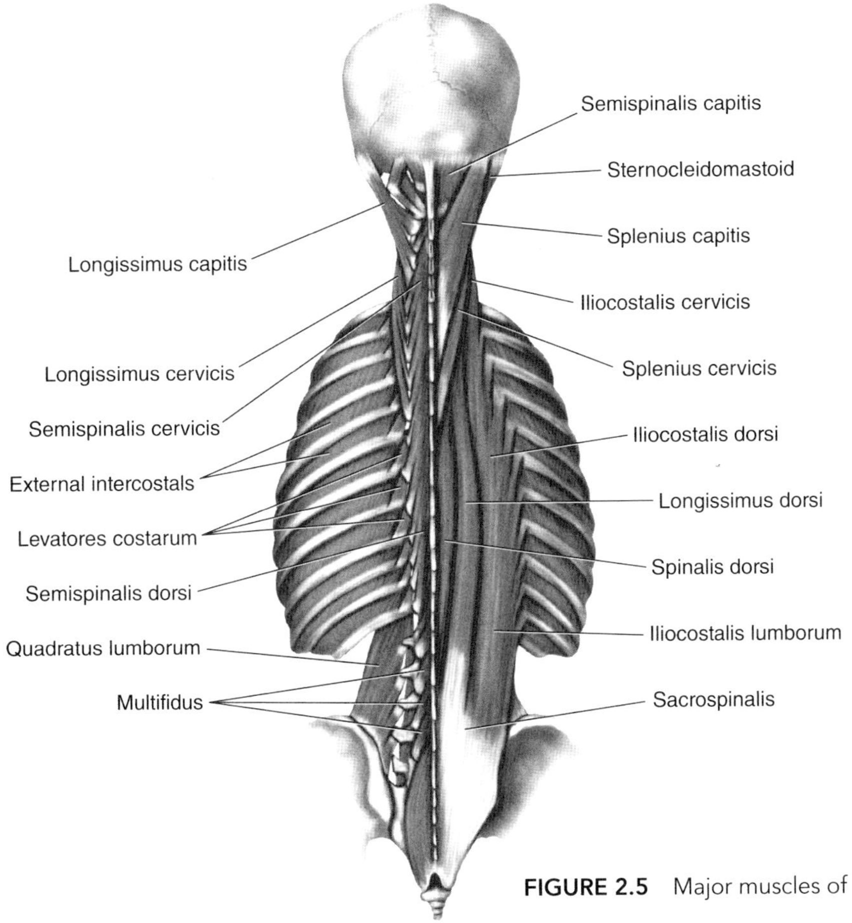

FIGURE 2.5 Major muscles of the back.

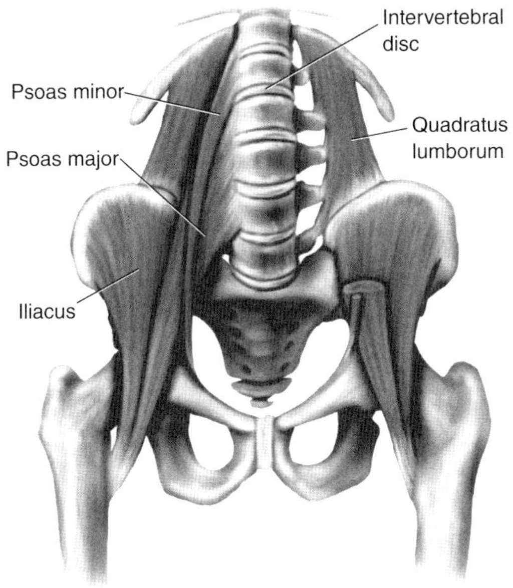

FIGURE 2.6 Major muscles of the pelvis.

RIPPLE EFFECT

All movement emanates from the center, both anatomically and energetically. The path of movement is like the ripple effect that occurs when a pebble is dropped into still water, creating a circular ripple that in turn creates many more ripples moving outward in progressively larger circles. Each movement starts from the inner core (the first circle of energy) and moves outward; the trunk is the second circle of energy, followed by the limbs and finally the periphery, the hands and feet. But don't think of the energy stopping at the fourth circle; it should continue outward, as if the movement is infinite. This is called the follow-through, and it has immeasurable value in terms of function and aesthetics. It is a concept promoted in all athletic activities, from jumping to throwing a ball to the elongated appearance of a ballerina.

Principles of Alignment and Posture

People often adopt a simplistic view when assessing posture and alignment; for example, they measure only strength and flexibility and ignore the complexity of the other factors involved. Strengthening a certain muscle group or stretching another to improve posture and alignment is not enough. Correcting alignment is a process of neuromuscular reeducation that requires enormous commitment, patience, and, preferably, the scrutinizing eye and astute cueing of a good teacher.

Posture can be assessed in terms of the alignment of the joints and bony landmarks and understood in terms of muscle balance and function. Alignment is often described relative to a plumb line—a straight line that runs vertically through the body. Figure 2.7 shows ideal posture viewed from the side. By viewing the body from the side in relation to the plumb line, deviations in an anterior–posterior direction (in the sagittal plane), such as hyperkyphosis and hyperlordosis, become apparent. The following landmarks of the body should line up vertically on the plumb line: the lobe of the ear, center of the cervical vertebrae, shoulder joint, midpoint of the trunk, greater trochanter of the femur, and a point slightly anterior to the midline of the knee and slightly anterior to the lateral malleolus (ankle). Posture should also be viewed from the front and back, focusing on the symmetry of the body and deviations from the midline in a sideways (lateral) direction (in the coronal plane), such as scoliosis. The space between the arms and the trunk, which I call windows of opportunity, should also be observed because they offer much information regarding alignment of the pelvis, spine, and the upper girdle.

Please note that ideal posture is an ideal, a goal that one strives for but may never achieve. Each individual is different in body type, center of gravity, habitual movement patterns, mental state, and genes; it is inconceivable to think that one posture will fit all. However, the concept of ideal posture serves as a guideline and a reference by which we can detect deviations and gauge changes.

Posture affects every movement, exercise, cue, and decision in an exercise program. Consider, for instance, a person who has fatigue posture, which is characterized by a rounded thoracic spine and the pelvis being forward of the plumb line in a posterior tilt. Although correction is complex, it generally involves strengthening the upper back extensors, strengthening the iliopsoas, and stretching the abdominal external obliques. Bringing the shoulders into ideal alignment over the pelvis is also often helpful. On the other hand, if a person has lumbar hyperlordosis, which involves an increased lumbar curve of the spine accompanied by an anterior tilt of the pelvis, correction generally focuses on strengthening the abdominals and stretching the hip flexors and lower back extensors. Clearly, these two people will receive different exercise programs, emphasizing different muscle groups, with the selection of exercises and the cueing being appropriate for their particular posture.

Alignment of the Spine

Good alignment translates into less stress on the spine and more economical muscular activity. When the spine is aligned with gravity, we are not fighting against gravity; in fact, gravity is assisting us. The body is working in harmony with the laws of nature. The moment the body is imbalanced and out of alignment, certain muscles become overworked and others become weak, resulting in stress and inefficient posture and movement. Maintaining the natural curves of the spine is important because they act as shock absorbers, protecting the body during impact, whether landing from a jump, running, or carrying a heavy load. We therefore always strive to attain ideal alignment and develop the musculature to support it.

Although much of our attention focuses on the musculature as it relates to posture and alignment, ideal alignment of the spine also facilitates efficient functioning of the internal organs. For instance, I have taught people who have scoliosis and who, with Pilates practice, begin to feel that they can finally breathe better. This is quite typical with scoliosis, because the muscles on one side of the thorax become tight, causing the rib cage to compress on that side and limit the function of the corresponding lung. Similarly, with kyphosis (increased thoracic curve of the spine) the rib cage becomes compressed and impairs respiration. Other body systems can also be affected; for example, a posture with exaggerated forward flexion places constant pressure on the digestive system, hindering its function.

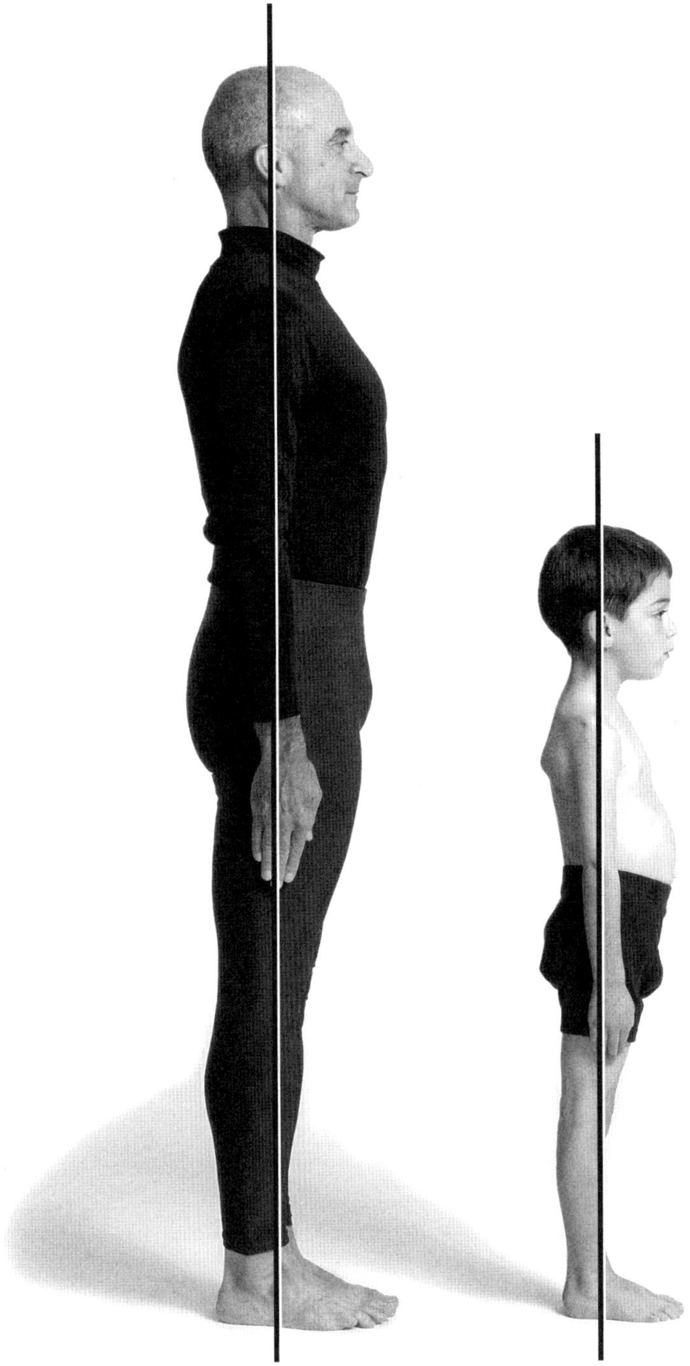

FIGURE 2.7 Good observation points and landmarks for assessing posture include the ears, shoulders, pelvis, knees, and ankles.

Placement of the Head

I like to think of the head as a ball balancing on a pin, or a large sunflower on a long, straight stem. None of the muscles of the neck should be strained; instead they should all act as cables connecting to the head to keep it balanced. None of the cables should have to overwork, but rather they should continuously make micro-adjustments to maintain balance. Adjusting the position of the head and the direction of the gaze of the eyes are among the most common and important corrections I give when I teach. I view the head as simply a large vertebra (or a large ball encompassing the first vertebra), an integral part of the spine, and as such it should follow the line of the spine. Deviations from this alignment, particularly because of the head's relatively heavy weight, inevitably result in neck tension and strain and can be aesthetically unpleasing. This situation tends to progressively deteriorate with time and age. It is even more pronounced when a person has a long neck, which essentially acts as an extended lever arm. For instance, if someone has forward head posture (the head is carried anterior to the plumb line), the neck extensors will become tight and overworked and the flexors relatively weak and inactive. The head weighs 12-14 pounds (approximately 5 kilograms), so shifting it away from the base of support has a significant effect on the musculature, an effect that grows exponentially as the head moves farther away from the plumb line with a longer lever (neck).

During abdominal exercises using forward flexion such as the Mat: Chest Lift, the trunk lifts up and forward, and the spine, including the head, must follow the natural curve (often referred to as the chest lift position). When forward flexion is inadequate, the head lies farther from the body's center of gravity, creating a longer lever. The result is often neck strain and tension. This inevitably happens when weak abdominals, tight lower back muscles, or both restrict the forward flexion of the trunk, and is often exacerbated by attempts to maintain a neutral pelvis when the body is inadequately prepared or able to do so (discussed in the next section). Contrary to this, people sometimes pull on the neck with the hands and push the chin to the chest. This also creates pressure on the neck and promotes excessive use of the neck flexors. To understand correct positioning, visualize the body in forward flexion with the sun shining directly overhead. The shoulder girdle would cast a shadow on the ground below, slightly larger than the actual size of the shoulder girdle. This shadow marks the base of support of the upper girdle; the head should be held within this area. Establishing a good position of the head and spine in this exercise is extremely important and lays the foundation for many of the abdominal exercises that follow, both on the mat and on the apparatus (figure 2.8*a*).

The Mat: Roll-Up offers a good illustration of spine and head alignment and a perfect example of how the art and science of human movement merge. In the sitting phase of this exercise, many people place the head down between the arms. I prefer that the head follow the natural C curve of the spine and be held above the arms, with the arms remaining parallel to the floor (figure 2.8*b*). Not only does this present a longer, more continuous line, which is visually pleasing, but it also encourages better placement of the head, shoulders, and scapulae, and a balanced interplay between the spinal flexors and extensors—leaving the body devoid of tension and lessening the load on the spine.

Neutral Pelvis and Neutral Spine

Neutral pelvis is defined as a position in which the anterior superior iliac spines (ASIS) and the pubic symphysis (PS) are in the same coronal plane (on a horizontal line when supine) and the two ASIS are in the same transverse plane. The term *neutral spine* emanates from a neutral pelvis and indicates that the natural curves of the spine are present (figure 2.9*a*). If the PS is higher than the ASIS, the pelvis is in a posterior tilt and the lumbar spine flattens (figure 2.9*b*); if the ASIS are higher than the PS, the pelvis is in an anterior tilt and the lumbar spine arches (figure 2.9*c*).

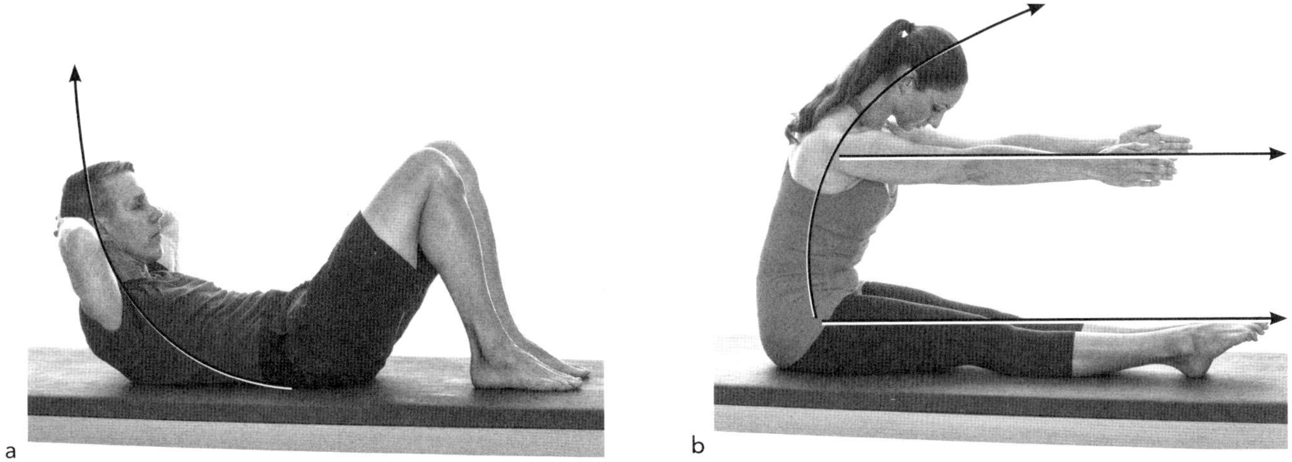

FIGURE 2.8 The head and spine align naturally, the line reaching upward out of the crown of the head in *(a)* Mat: Chest Lift and up and forward into a C curve in *(b)* Mat: Roll-Up.

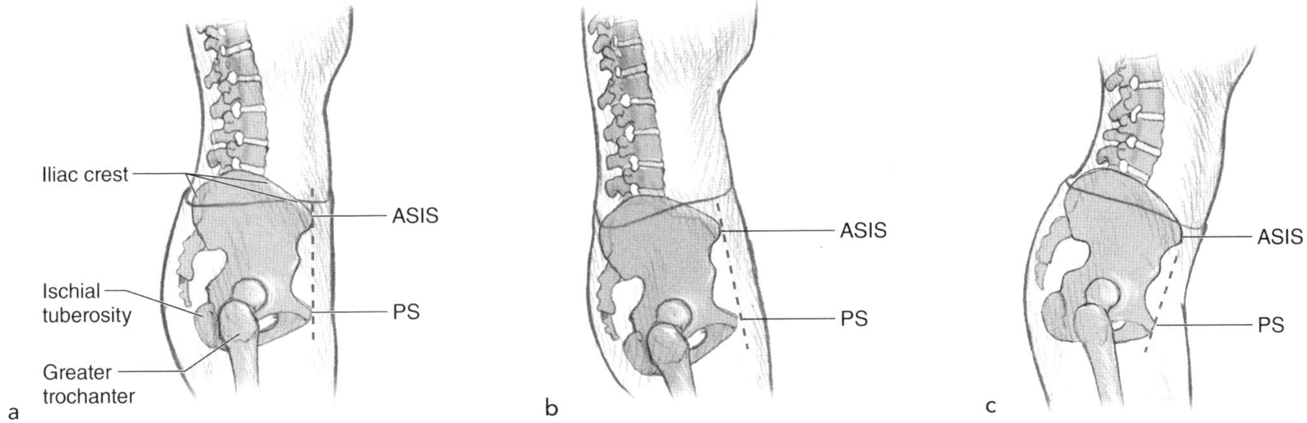

FIGURE 2.9 *(a)* Neutral pelvis, *(b)* posterior tilt, and *(c)* anterior tilt.

The neutral position of the pelvis and spine is a reference against which to compare and describe all other positions of your body during your Pilates practice and other activities. This is not to say that we never deviate from it; we frequently do. However, neutral is the foundation, and from this neutral alignment all other positions and movements are born. When the spine is in a neutral position, the pelvis by definition must also be neutral; however, instances do occur in which the pelvis is neutral and the spine is not, such as during the Mat: Single-Leg Stretch (figure 2.10) and many other abdominal exercises. Although discussion of the neutral pelvis arises predominantly in relation to abdominal exercises in forward flexion, the concept of neutral pelvis is also relevant during lateral flexion, rotation, and back extension.

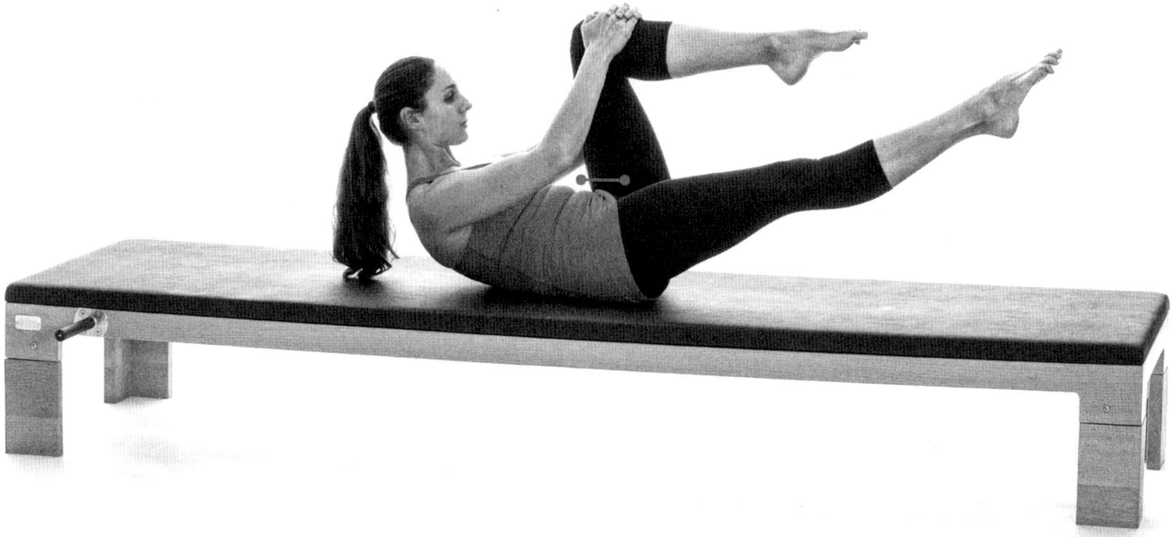

FIGURE 2.10 The Mat: Single-Leg Stretch is one of many exercises in which the pelvis is in neutral position while the upper spine is lifted.

Performing exercises in the neutral pelvic position yields several benefits. It encourages balanced muscular development of the pelvic complex and correct muscle recruitment. It teaches and reinforces efficient posture and ideal alignment, which is particularly important when upright. It can also assist in unloading the pelvis of undue stresses. However, keep in mind that the pelvis is dynamic and constantly adjusts to the body's movements and its ability, or inability, to perform a movement. At times, maintaining a neutral pelvis could prove counterproductive and lead to negative results. Appropriate positioning of the spine and pelvis should be assessed on a case-by-case basis. This is particularly pertinent during abdominal exercises. A neutral pelvis is the ideal, but it may be necessary at first to work with a slight posterior pelvic tilt in order to elongate (and at times relax) the back muscles of the lumbar region and strengthen the abdominals. As long as the back extensors are tight (or are contracting) they have a tendency to inhibit the recruitment of the abdominals and limit the degree of forward flexion. Once both flexibility of the lower back and strength of the abdominals have been achieved, the position of the pelvis can be adjusted from posterior to neutral.

It is important to recognize, as stated previously, that neutral pelvis and neutral spine do not always occur simultaneously, and they have different implications. When in a neutral position, the natural curves of the spine must be present; in forward flexion the natural curves cannot be present. I sometimes encounter students who claim to be attempting to work in a neutral spine position during abdominal exercises in forward flexion. Clearly, they are not (nor should they be). Once the head and trunk lift into forward flexion, the spine is no longer in a neutral position. However, maintaining a neutral pelvis during abdominal work in forward flexion is quite possible and, in many instances, desirable.

When teaching the Mat: Chest Lift, I instruct students to lift into forward flexion. Some lift only their heads off the mat, and not the entire upper girdle, in a misguided attempt to maintain a neutral spine. By performing neck flexion rather than trunk flexion, they are missing the point of the exercise, which is abdominal work. As a result, they are not working the abdominals effectively and are probably acquiring more neck and lower back tension than abdominal strength. I have witnessed similar scenarios with abdominal oblique work entailing rotation of the trunk, such as in the Mat: Criss-Cross. In an attempt to maintain a neutral spine in such exercises, students exhibit a great deal of neck flexion but little or no trunk flexion and rotation. In this instance, the lumbar spine sometimes lifts off the mat, placing excessive strain on the lower back.

I do advocate maintaining a neutral pelvic position during many of the abdominal exercises, but not at all costs. For example, if you have hyperlordosis and a tight lower back, performing abdominal exercises while maintaining a neutral pelvis could result in excessive contracture of the lower back muscles. This translates into insufficient forward flexion of the trunk, ineffective abdominal recruitment, and possibly excessive hip flexor activation (particularly when the legs are held off the mat), plus stress on the lower back and probably the neck. In an endeavor to work with a neutral pelvis, people sometimes compromise the outcome of the exercise and reinforce negative movement patterns, coming away with neck pain, back pain, and, to make it worse, weak abdominals.

A series of actions allow the lumbar spine to imprint (press) into the mat during forward flexion in a supine position: the abdominals contract, intra-abdominal pressure is increased, the back extensors elongate, and the lumbar vertebrae flatten out. This does not mean that the pelvis should be forcefully thrust into a posterior tilt (commonly called a tuck) in order to imprint the back into the mat. Rather, the trunk is lifted into maximum forward flexion while maintaining a neutral pelvis. At this point, if there is inadequate forward flexion and the lower back is not imprinted into the mat, the pelvis should then be progressively tilted posteriorly. This will help to achieve more lift of the trunk, increase abdominal activation, elongate the lower back extensors, and imprint the lower back into the mat. Continue modifying the position of the pelvis until you have addressed the limiting factors. Ultimately, as the strength of the abdominals increases, you will be able to perform the abdominal exercises with integrity and a positive outcome, free from excessive tension and (hopefully) in a neutral pelvic position.

Assessing Alignment

Over the years I have found it important to develop convenient methods of assessing posture. Very sophisticated systems of assessment are available, yet most are impractical to use at home or during a Pilates session. I recommend the Mat: Roll-Down as a simple but effective tool for assessing posture and alignment. It offers valuable information regarding structure, muscular development, and compensations. At the same time, it allows one to gently mobilize the spine and coordinate the breathing with the movement. Teachers who are assessing a student's alignment should observe the Mat: Roll-Down from the back, front, and side, because certain postural deviations are more apparent from a coronal (front and back) view and others from a sagittal (side) view. When using this exercise as a self-assessment tool, stand on a firm, level surface in front of a mirror if possible. Self-assessment demands heightened inner awareness and observation skills that should be honed constantly.

Roll-Down

Muscle Focus

- Abdominals
- Back extensors

Objectives

- To develop spinal articulation
- To improve back extensor flexibility
- To improve abdominal and back extensor control
- To improve body alignment and mental focus

I encourage the use of this exercise at the beginning and end of a session; however, it is not appropriate for everyone and should not be performed in certain instances, such as when lower back problems are present. If you have any reservations about yourself or a student doing this movement, substitute it with a modification by leaning the back against a wall, placing the feet hip width apart, 1-2 feet (30-60 centimeters) from the wall, and bending the knees. Doing the exercise in this position exerts less stress on the lower back. It allows the wall, rather than the spine, to bear much of the weight of the body and provides tactile feedback on the articulation of the spine.

During the movement, become internally aware of weight shifts within the body. Notice asymmetries and imbalances, and take note of deviations from the plumb line. Use the Mat: Roll-Down not only as a tool for assessment but also as a means of focusing the mind and tuning the body, just as you would tune a musical instrument before playing it.

Imagery

Imagine your back pressing against a pole that is keeping you upright and aligned. The head fills with water and becomes very heavy. It rolls forward, pulling the body away from the pole one tiny segment at a time. At the bottom, the water runs out the top of the head and the body becomes light again so that the spine rolls back up the pole, one segment at a time.

- ○ Establish ideal alignment in relation to the plumb line from the outset.
- ○ Keep the movement relaxed and avoid forcing a stretch of the hamstrings at the end range.
- ○ Maintain scapular stabilization with the palms facing the sides of the body and the fingers reaching down toward the floor.

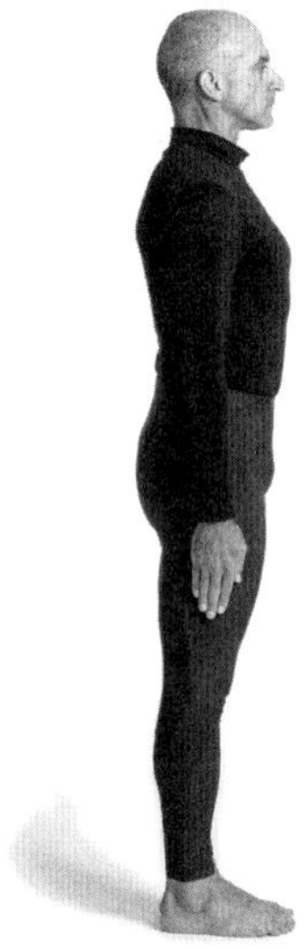

Setup. Stand upright in ideal alignment with the feet hip width apart and parallel. Prepare for the movement by going through a mental checklist of ideal alignment.

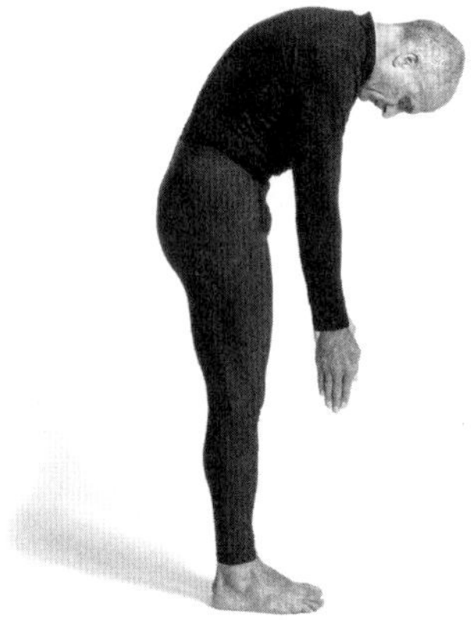

Exhale. Roll down through the spine, beginning with the head and articulating through each vertebra. It is optional to bend the knees as you roll down to alleviate any pressure on the lower back. This is particularly important if you have tight back extensors and hamstrings. Maintain a neutral position of the scapulae; avoid allowing them to glide up toward the head as the crown of the head reaches down toward the floor. Keep the palms facing each other and the arms hanging down directly from the shoulders, perpendicular to the floor. At the bottom of the movement, inhale, expanding the chest laterally and feeling the back expand, releasing all tension. Maintain active forward flexion (not slumped) with the back extensors moderately engaged. Relax the neck and allow the head to follow the line of the spine.

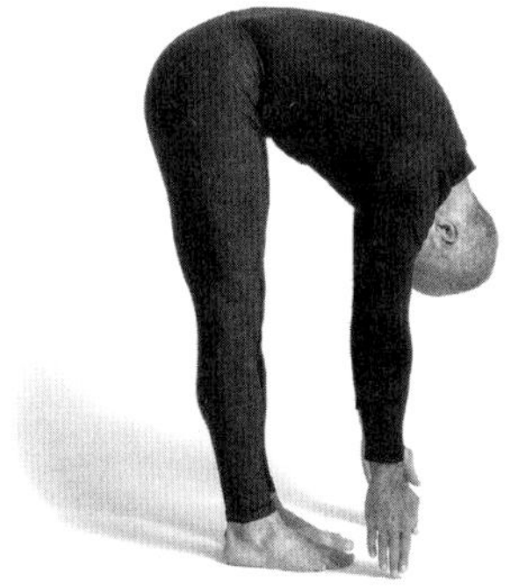

Exhale. Roll back up, first establishing the neutral position of the pelvis, and then continuing to articulate up through the spine, placing each vertebra back on the plumb line like building blocks until you have established ideal alignment. Return to the start position.

Foot Alignment

The feet are the foundation of the body when upright: standing, walking, running, and jumping. Any misalignment of the feet, in a static position or in motion, results in postural deviations and compensations all the way up the kinetic chain. The foot is a complex structure, made up of many joints, and identifying any one joint or aspect of the foot as particularly vulnerable is difficult. However, I will single out the subtalar joint (often mistaken for the ankle joint) due to its importance in relation to foot alignment. The subtalar joint controls the inward and outward motion (supination and pronation) of the foot and is vital to achieving correct foot alignment. A good guide when assisting someone to achieve neutral alignment of the foot while standing is to observe the Achilles tendon from the back (figure 2.11). The tendon should be perpendicular to the floor, and fine adjustments of the subtalar joint can be made to achieve this alignment. Becoming acquainted with neutral alignment is particularly helpful during the foot work on the Pilates apparatus.

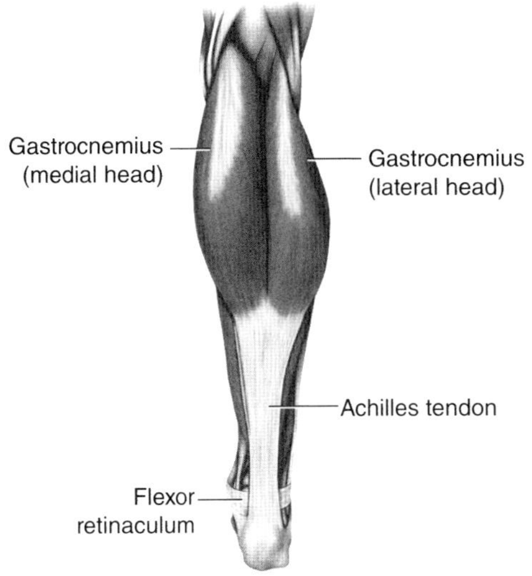

FIGURE 2.11 Alignment of the Achilles tendon.

EFFECTS OF CENTER OF GRAVITY

The body's center of gravity (COG) is important for both alignment and understanding the mechanics of exercises. Weight distribution can make exercises easier or more difficult, depending on the person's body type. Sometimes, difficulty executing an exercise successfully has little to do with lack of strength and much to do with physical build (body type)—specifically, the weight distribution of the body. For instance, a man with broad shoulders, a well-developed upper body, and short legs may find the Mat: Roll-Up extremely challenging, whereas a woman with a petite torso, substantial hips, and long legs will find the exercise relatively easy. The man is not necessarily weaker—in fact, he may well have far stronger abdominals—but he is top-heavy, whereas the woman has a lower COG. In other exercises, such as the Wunda Chair: Pike—Forward and the Reformer: Long Stretch, this man would have an advantage.

Given that each person's COG is slightly different, the way each person performs an exercise is also different. Understanding this fact is important in order to cue effectively, make exercises easier or more difficult, and, most importantly, make them safe. Considering Joseph Pilates had a very muscular build, like that of a gymnast, it is not surprising that many of the exercises he created require a strong, well-developed upper girdle. (This in no way implies that women cannot perform the repertoire very beautifully and successfully.) Understanding the mechanics of the body and the exercises will allow you to overcome obstacles for yourself and your students.

Let's take, for example, the Mat: Roll-Up. If a person is struggling with this exercise and the reason appears to be body type rather than weak abdominals or tight lower back and hamstrings, an excellent solution is to drape a light (2.2 pounds, or 1 kilogram) ankle weight over the ankles. This does not allow the person to rely on the ankle weight to pull the body up, as would be the case if the feet were placed under a secure foot strap; it simply changes the weight distribution, adding weight (or, in effect, length) to the legs and lowering the COG toward the pelvis. The individual essentially grew longer legs for the sake of the exercise. At other times, being top-heavy or shorter may prove an advantage. Regardless of body type, everyone faces different challenges and obstacles that can often be overcome with committed and dedicated practice . . . so enjoy your body and relish the journey!

3

Powerful Pilates Practice

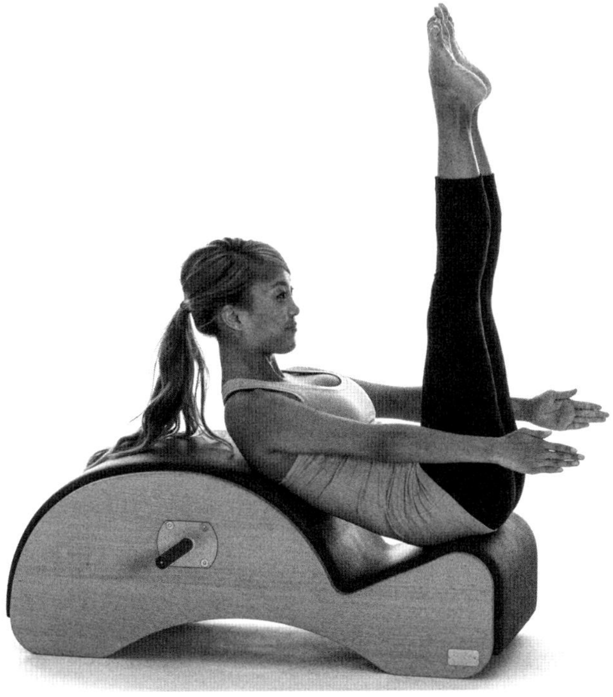

The foundation of the Pilates method as Joseph Pilates intended it, and as I approach it, views conditioning with the *whole* in mind. The body is the most intricate of instruments, and imbalance in one area will inevitably cause imbalances in other areas. Therefore, all Pilates programs should be comprehensive, regardless of age, fitness level, or ability. In some cases, you may certainly direct more attention toward a particular area of the body, but you should always keep in mind the intricate patterning of human movement. An injury, compensation, or any other restriction that adversely affects the body's ability to function can be regarded as a weak link in a chain. For the chain to function as a complete unit, you must address the weak link without losing sight of the fact that the goal is the efficient functioning of the chain as a whole.

Structure and creativity may seem to be diametrically opposed, yet one cannot exist without the other. Both are essential components of an effective Pilates program. Having a structure allows you to be creative and to adapt to personal and specific needs without compromising the concept of the whole. If you view Pilates as *only* exercise—particularly as exercise for only one part of the body—you risk sacrificing the essence of the system itself. Adhering to a structure allows you to compile an effective, comprehensive program. It also allows teachers to maintain the flow in a studio when teaching several people at the same time while still offering each an individualized program and personal attention. I liken the process to a conductor leading an orchestra—the conductor always knows what each section of the orchestra is playing while still maintaining an overall view of the piece. Maintaining flow within each person's individual session simultaneously while keeping a view of the entire studio can only be achieved with a clear and well-learned structure.

Over the years I have witnessed Pilates classes that lack structure, direction, and the concept of the *whole*. I always come away feeling that these sessions are missing the point; without a logical progression and a structure that addresses the whole, they lack the elements that make Pilates so valuable and its effects so profound. I sometimes see this happening in clinical environments: A therapist might take a patient through a few exercises on the reformer and then move on to another modality of treatment. Using a Pilates exercise here and there is not Pilates—it does not embody the system's philosophy and approach. Similarly, many Pilates studios and gym environments emphasize sweat, intensity, and "the burn" over mindfulness. I cannot say this is wrong; I can only say it is not the system that Joseph Pilates created and therefore is unlikely to achieve the outcomes that he described. (Of course many therapists, fitness trainers, and coaches have studied Pilates in depth and have integrated it successfully and with integrity into their practices as part of a complete system.)

Structuring Your Practice: The BASI Block System

My quest to find a useful structure for the practice of Pilates led me to develop the BASI (Body Arts and Science International) block system. Derived from many years of practicing and teaching the method and directing programs around the world, the BASI block system is the nucleus of my approach to Pilates. It is solidly grounded in the Pilates method while adhering to contemporary knowledge and principles of exercise physiology. The structure of the BASI block system ensures that practitioners address the whole body, providing a framework and clear guidelines for individual development while facilitating adaptability and creativity.

The BASI block system organizes the vast Pilates repertoire into blocks. It can be likened to a family tree; all the exercises emanate from the same roots and are related to each other, some more closely than others. Familiarity with the intricacies of the whole tree is essential in order to implement the BASI block system successfully, and this knowledge can be used to compile programs that are individualized according to level, personal needs, restrictions, and goals.

Without such a system, the hundreds of Pilates exercises become just that—exercises, like words without context. They are valuable in and of themselves, but they convey a message only when put together. The teacher compiles the session using exercises from each block, which are like chapters in a book; together, they create the whole story. Each movement takes on more meaning when it is placed within a well-conceived structure and sequence of movements—like poetry in motion. The more finely crafted the sentences, the more profound the message. This is where the art and the science of human movement unite. At this level, mind and body work as one; the work becomes deeper, yet more effortless. This is the level we strive for, where the greatest and most profound changes take place.

Fully grasping the many levels of the BASI block system can take years. However, even in its most simple form, the system provides a way to categorize the vast repertoire, maximize work time, and use the session to its full potential. It is essentially a filing system encompassing hundreds, if not thousands of Pilates movements. Because it is a standardized system, it allows trained practitioners to communicate and collaborate in a seamless and meaningful fashion, wherever they may be in the world. I am always filled with pride when I see how successfully the BASI block system has been implemented in different cultures and many countries around the globe.

All exercises in this book are laid out according to the BASI block system, which means that you can learn each exercise and its place in the overall structure concurrently. Each block is comprised of individual exercises or series of exercises. For example, the exercises that focus on the upper girdle fall into the *arm work block*, a pool of upper body exercises of varying levels of difficulty from which to choose. A series is a compilation of several exercises, performed in sequence, that complement each other to create a complete, integrated *exercise unit* for a particular area of the body. Finally, the term *group* of exercises refers to multiple exercises that share a common denominator, such as being performed on the long box placed atop the reformer. In contrast to a series, the exercises in a group are not typically all performed together in one session or practiced in any set sequence.

Two different and distinct BASI block systems have evolved over the years. The *comprehensive block system* is used for a typical Pilates session that utilizes the full complement of apparatus. The *mat block system* is used for a Pilates session that includes only exercises from the mat repertoire. The blocks that make up the comprehensive block system (figure 3.1) are as follows:

1. *Warm-up.* This block prepares the body for the work, both physically and mentally. It is typically a selection of mat work exercises.
2. *Foot work.* The foot work is performed on the reformer, cadillac, and wunda chair. With the innovation of a resistance mechanism added to the spine corrector—the F2 spine corrector—and the redesign of the arm chair—the F2 chair (F2 stands for form and function)—foot work can also now be done on these unique pieces of apparatus. The focus is on the entire lower limb complex: foot, ankle, knee, and hip. There is also great emphasis on lumbopelvic stabilization and establishing a neutral pelvis–neutral spine position. This block is regarded as part warm-up and part specific training for the lower limbs. (Use of the name *foot work* is to differentiate from *leg work* later in the session.)
3. *Abdominal work.* This selection of exercises is focused on developing the abdominals. Although the abdominals are engaged throughout the Pilates session, these exercises are specifically aimed at this region and address all the abdominal muscles as both movers and stabilizers.

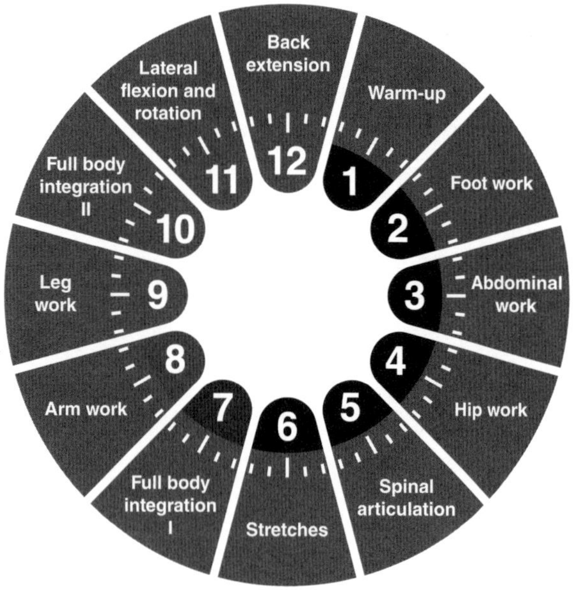

FIGURE 3.1 Comprehensive block system.

4. *Hip work.* This section demands work and control of the hip joint and is typically performed with the feet in the straps on the reformer or using the leg springs on the cadillac or other apparatus, such as the F2 wunda chair, F2 chair, and F2 spine corrector. Focus on control of the lumbopelvic region is key because of the close relationship of the pelvis to the hip joint.
5. *Spinal articulation.* This block is devoted to spinal mobility and developing control of the trunk muscles, particularly the deeper-lying muscles. Spinal articulation exercises can be found on almost all the apparatus, including the mat.
6. *Stretches.* Selections from this block can be performed on or off the apparatus and typically include stretches for the hip flexors and hamstrings. The selection of exercises depends on the needs and ability of each individual.
7. *Full body integration (FBI) I.* Although all Pilates exercises work the entire body, these exercises defy categorization by muscle group or area of the body and are specifically geared to full body motion. The exercises in FBI I are fundamental and intermediate level.
8. *Arm work.* This block is devoted to the upper girdle of the body. I have compiled several series consisting of exercises that work the various muscle groups of the arms and shoulders. Typically, a complete series is practiced to ensure a comprehensive workout for the upper body.
9. *Leg work.* These are exercises for the lower body to supplement the foot work. They typically emphasize the hip abductors and hip adductors. However, the BASI block system provides flexibility in options so that this section may be used for general conditioning of this region; specific skill training, such as when working with dancers, skiers, and runners; or for corrective and therapeutic work of the lower limbs.
10. *Full body integration (FBI) II.* As with FBI I, the exercises in FBI II work the entire body and cannot be categorized by one region. However, the exercises in FBI II are advanced and master level.
11. *Lateral flexion and rotation.* This block refers to exercises that work the lateral flexors and rotators of the trunk, with an emphasis on the abdominal obliques. These muscles are vital to healthy functional movement and support of the spine. Imbalances often exist between the muscles on either side of the body, for reasons ranging from scoliosis to the practice of certain athletic or occupation-related activities. I recommend always working toward balance and symmetry of the two sides of the body.
12. *Back extension.* This block is devoted to exercises for the spinal extensors. These muscles lie along the spine and span the back in layers. The superficial muscles are long, large muscles that are responsible for gross movement. The deeper

intrinsic muscles are intervertebral muscles that control fine, intricate movement of the spine. As with the abdominals, it is the deeper layers that are largely responsible for stabilization. This block should *not* be minimized or eliminated, if at all possible.

The mat exercises focus predominantly on the powerhouse—the spinal flexors (abdominals), lateral flexors and rotators, and back extensors. The blocks in the mat block system are intentionally very general and follow the layout and delineation of the chapters in *Pilates Anatomy* (Human Kinetics). These provide a necessary structure for the mat work and ensure that the entire body is addressed in a mat session. The description of each of these blocks appears in the comprehensive block system and applies to both block systems. The only blocks that are unique to the mat block system are *foundation* and *bridging and full body integration*. *Foundation* is synonymous with *warm-up* in the comprehensive block system. Bridging refers to exercises in which the pelvis is lifted off the mat, so the trunk forms a bridge shape while the limbs provide support for the bridge. The bridge can either be facing up, using primarily the extensors of the limbs and trunk, or facing down, in which case the flexors of the limbs and trunk will be predominant. The term full body integration is described in the comprehensive block system. For the purposes of the mat block system, these terms are synonymous and both terms can be applied equally to each exercise. The blocks that make up the mat block system are as follows (figure 3.2):

1. Foundation
2. Abdominal work
3. Spinal articulation
4. Bridging and full body integration
5. Lateral flexion and rotation
6. Back extension

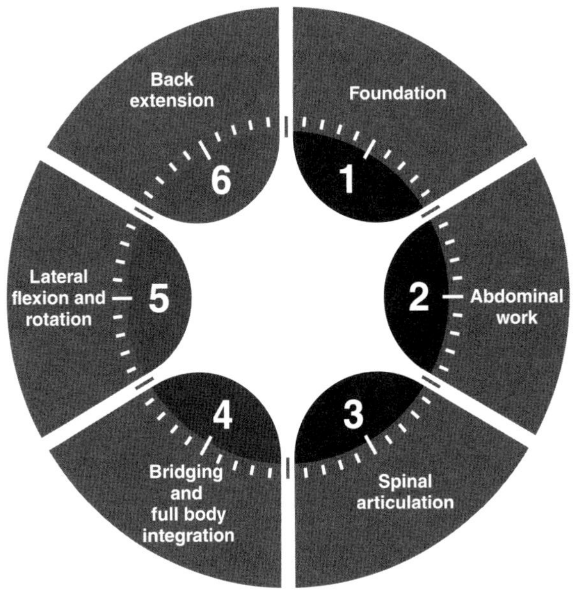

FIGURE 3.2 Mat block system.

Because of their versatility and transitional qualities, the mat exercises lend themselves more naturally to organization according to progression and flow. The *mat block system* is addressed further in chapter 4.

I sometimes hear an unjustified criticism of Pilates as having inadequate rotation and extension exercises. This is not accurate: There are myriad options in the Pilates repertoire for both spinal rotation and extension, which are important components of any comprehensive exercise program. Spinal extension becomes particularly important in an exercise program as we age. Over time, gravity tends to pull us forward into flexion. This tendency is exacerbated by the ravages of our modern lifestyle—hours spent sitting in front of computers, driving cars, checking smartphones, and taking part in recreational activities that involve forward flexion. The result is bleak, with a high incidence of round-shoulder syndrome and other shoulder problems, lower back pain, and neck tension. If Pilates or any other fitness regimen is performed in a way that focuses excessively on

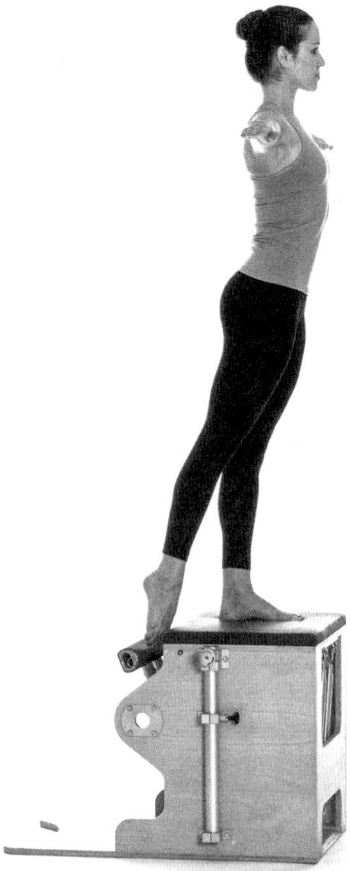

working the abdominals, with most of the exercises performed in trunk flexion, the picture gets even bleaker. Effective abdominal work is important, but it must be complemented with proportional work on other areas of the body, specifically the lateral flexors, rotators, and extensors of the spine. Proportional muscle development is a key component in achieving good alignment, balance, efficient movement, and general well-being.

I often look to babies and young children for guidance. Seldom do you see toddlers with bad alignment; they have strong backs and straight spines. I recall a wonderful incident when Lolita San Miguel, one of the Pilates "elders" and first-generation teachers, and someone I am honored to call a dear friend, was visiting my family in our home. My son Elan, who was about two years of age, was taking a bath and Lolita and I were sitting in the bathroom looking on. Together we marveled at the amazing musculature and posture of this little rambunctious ball of energy as he stood, sat, jumped, splashed, and showed off his athletic skills to his guest. As we age, we should not lose sight of the tendency toward deterioration of certain muscle groups—notably the hip flexors, hip abductors, and back extensors—and the importance of keeping them strong and flexible.

Exercise Descriptions

In order to apply an exercise or movement at the right time and in the most appropriate manner to achieve the desired outcome, it should first be analyzed. This analysis opens the door to understanding, as well as learning and teaching the movement. It is also invaluable in compiling exercise programs. In the following sections I explain the categories used for each of the exercises presented in chapters 4 through 11. These categories not only describe the exercise but also serve as a means of analysis.

I present each exercise by name, apparatus, block, level of difficulty, and the amount of resistance to use (if applicable). This information also includes a discussion about the exercise, its muscle focus, its objectives, and the cues I suggest using to achieve optimum results. The cues rely on imagery, a very powerful and personal teaching tool. Specific imagery may work in a given situation and with certain students, whereas for others, it may not. At the very least, I hope the imagery I offer sparks your imagination to create your own imagery and cues. I also include a checklist of key points you should observe. These too relate closely to effective cueing and ensuring a successful outcome. Finally, photographs illustrate the movement, accompanied by a description of the movement according to the breath pattern.

Classifying the Movement

The blocks are used to classify the exercises into categories. Each is also defined by its level of difficulty—fundamental, intermediate, advanced, and master. (Master-level exercises, as the name implies, take years to study and master. I offer only a couple, because that realm of the repertoire exceeds the scope of this book.) Classifying movements by level is a somewhat subjective process; what is difficult for one person may be relatively easy for another. Contrary, for example, to weight training, where progression may be based solely on increasing resistance, progression in Pilates is far more intricate and nuanced. Therefore, I allocate levels according to the complexity of the movement—the more complex the movement, the higher the level of difficulty.

I must emphasize that this system is not one in which you no longer practice fundamental or intermediate movements once you have learned an advanced movement. Each exercise becomes part of your movement vocabulary, to be used and enjoyed. When I construct programs for advanced students, I select exercises from all levels, not only the advanced repertoire. Including a wide range of exercises in a program is important, both physically and mentally. Ultimately, the goal of each movement is to assist in the pursuit of well-being.

I see as much value in the Mat: Pelvic Curl, one of the most fundamental exercises, as I do in the Reformer:

High Bridge (not included in this book), one of the most advanced movements in the repertoire. This example highlights two exercises that are closely related and illustrates the relationship between fundamental and advanced work, which should be established early on in the practice of Pilates. This allows you to prepare methodically as you move through each level, growing and maturing within the system.

I have spent much of my career working to master the most difficult movements in this method, and I certainly enjoy the exhilaration of performing the master-level work. With commitment, however, people can reap similar benefits from Pilates at any level of practice. The benefits do not only depend on the movements performed, but also on their quality and the integration of the Pilates principles into one's practice and one's life. Too often, I see the master-level repertoire becoming the sole focus of a person's practice, at times being performed by people who have little experience in this work. A talented gymnast or dancer could probably perform all the master-level work almost immediately. Does this mean they know Pilates? No. It means that they can learn choreography and perform it—exactly what they are trained to do.

Some people try to learn the repertoire as quickly as possible, steering away from the fundamental exercises, preferring to move on to the more difficult work. But every movement has infinite layers, regardless of the level. I encourage you to delight in the process of becoming intimately familiar with each exercise rather than rushing. You can do an exercise thousands of times and always find new meaning in it. I do not believe that any movement is easy or simple, nor should it become boring or mundane. The development of familiarity and understanding, not the ability to perform an advanced exercise, reflects true learning.

Resistance

Pilates is unique in its ingenious use of both gravity and springs for resistance. The pull of gravity will always be consistent, although its relative effect on the body depends on a variety of factors such as body type, center of gravity, placement of the body on the apparatus, and apparatus settings. Therefore the impact of gravity has not been noted specifically for each exercise in this book. However, for exercises that use springs for resistance (as do the majority of exercises on the apparatus), the appropriate amount of resistance is noted. In some instances, there is an effect from both the springs and gravity, and an understanding of the mechanics of the apparatus and the exercise is essential. Springs provide *progressive (variable) resistance*, meaning that the resistance increases as the spring is tensioned. This differs from *constant (non-variable) resistance*, in which the resistance does not change—for example, when using weights. Take into account that when working with resistance, whether progressive or constant, the effect on the muscle changes through the range of motion because of the mechanical advantage or disadvantage at certain angles of the joint.

Much debate surrounds the question of which type of resistance is preferable. This cannot be answered or resolved simply, and I think the points made in favor of each are valid. Ultimately, it comes down to personal preference. I personally favor working with springs because they can be easily adapted to simulate multiple activities and skills, and they appear to be more functional in their effect. They also feel alive with energy, a sensation that I enjoy.

You can change the intensity and outcome of an exercise significantly by increasing or decreasing the tension of the springs. Settings vary from one piece of apparatus to another, and even the same piece of apparatus can vary depending on the manufacturer. Unfortunately, no universal standard for spring tension exists. Adding to the complexity is the fact that the spring setting for an exercise will depend on a person's fitness level, Pilates level, body type, gender, experience, and restrictions. Even the age of the springs can become a factor when choosing a spring setting.

Pilates is not the performance of choreography; it is the never-ending process of learning about the body, controlling movement, and striving for well-being.

A distinction must also be drawn between absolute and relative resistance. *Absolute resistance* means, for instance, that two springs are always two springs. *Relative resistance*, on the other hand, refers to how heavy or light the tension feels for a particular exercise. For example, two springs would typically be regarded as very light for foot work but would be extremely heavy for most arm work exercises.

With all these factors in mind, Pilates professionals must become familiar with the resistance settings for every exercise on each piece of apparatus. As an example, when doing foot work on the reformer, *heavy* might mean four springs; on the cadillac, the equivalent might be two heavy springs; and on the wunda chair this might mean two heavy springs on the top setting. The only way to learn how to determine spring settings and their effect on an exercise is through practice and experience—doing each movement many times and experimenting with different settings. There will always be a logical range within which to execute an exercise, but determining your exact setting within that range requires practice, knowledge, and experience.

For these reasons, I have not included an actual spring setting for each exercise. Instead I offer an absolute resistance range, which translates to a limited number of spring setting options. You must then make micro-adjustments according to your individual needs.

The following are BASI guidelines for resistance and spring settings on the reformer. The same concept can be applied to the other apparatus, although the number of springs will change. Through experience you can establish the setting for each resistance category on the respective piece of apparatus.

Extra-light	→	0.25-0.5 spring (light spring)
Light	→	1-1.5 springs
Medium	→	2-3 springs
Heavy	→	3.5-4 springs
Extra-heavy	→	4.5-5 springs

Muscle Focus

The muscle focus identifies which muscle or group of muscles are targeted by the exercise. Although it is often one muscle or muscle group, there may be more depending on the complexity of the exercise and positional changes. Identifying the muscle focus assists you in achieving the desired goal of the exercise. Note that in many instances, increasing or decreasing the resistance or adjusting the body position even slightly will change the muscle focus. Therefore, precision is vitally important.

You are encouraged to recruit the internal support system (ISS)—the transversus abdominis, pelvic floor, diaphragm, and the multifidus—throughout the session. Therefore, these muscles are not mentioned in each exercise as target muscles unless the exercise is specifically for one or more of these core muscles.

Objectives

Objectives relate to the broader context of an exercise or action. In contrast to the muscle focus, which is very specific, the objectives describe the action of all the muscles involved. An exercise may have only one muscle focus, but it can have several objectives, which may not necessarily relate only to the area of the muscle focus. For example, in the case of the Mat: Hundred (chapter 4), a signature Pilates abdominal exercise, the muscle focus is the abdominals and hip flexors, whereas the objectives are to improve abdominal strength, improve hip flexor control, and develop lumbopelvic stabilization. The objectives for many Pilates exercises relate to increasing control, strength, flexibility, stabilization, mobilization, disassociation, or isolation.

Strength Versus Control

In describing the objectives and effect of an exercise, I use the words *strength* and *control* in a very specific manner. The term *strength* is often used too liberally and broadly in Pilates. In order to strengthen a muscle, certain criteria need to be met, one being *overload*. If insufficient load is placed on a muscle, it will not increase significantly in strength. That is not to say the muscle is not being activated, which in itself has value in terms of neuromuscular patterning and body awareness. Thus, I use the term *control* when a muscle is being recruited but not overloaded sufficiently for significant strength gains to be realized.

Stabilization

Developing stabilization in a particular area of the body is a common objective in Pilates. Each exercise can be broken down into muscles that stabilize movement (stabilizers) and muscles that produce movement (movers). Both are important in maintaining the integrity of the exercise. There is also a third category, synergists. These are recruited to neutralize undesired muscle actions and assist in achieving the correct movement, which help ensure the desired outcome. For instance, in the Reformer: Chest Expansion—Kneeling (chapter 5), a shoulder extensor exercise, the following sequence of events should occur.

The stabilizers are recruited first—initially the stabilizers of the trunk (local stabilizers), then those of the scapula and elbow (global stabilizers). The movers, in this case the shoulder extensors, come next. Prominent among these is the latissimus dorsi, a shoulder extensor, shoulder adductor, and shoulder internal rotator. In this exercise, we encourage the first two actions but do not want shoulder internal rotation. Therefore, we must recruit the shoulder *external* rotators to prevent the shoulder from internally rotating. The shoulder external rotators function as synergists to keep the shoulder in the desired neutral position and assist the prime mover in performing the desired action, ultimately maintaining the integrity of the exercise.

In any exercise, I encourage first focusing on the stabilizers, because without correct stabilization efficient movement cannot be achieved. Once correct stabilization has been established, focus on the initiator, which can be described as the primary focus or initial cue of the movement. This is a crucial link between the stabilization and the mobilization in any movement. Finally, focus on the movers. I call this the *SIM (stabilize–initiate–move) formula*. After this process has been learned and practiced many times, it becomes second nature.

Most traditional forms of movement analysis address the stabilizers and movers but not the initiator. This is understandable, because the initiator is in fact either a stabilizer or a mover and therefore falls into one of these categories. However, using the concept of the initiator encourages mental focus, concentration, body awareness, and control, all of which in turn contribute to successful performance and allow you to derive maximum effect from the exercise.

Besides highlighting the importance of stabilization, Pilates also focuses on ranges of motion of the joints and different types of muscle contraction. The stabilizers work isometrically to a large extent, meaning that the muscles contract with no change in their length or in the angle of the joints on which they are acting. Note that this is a dynamic process of agonist and antagonist muscles working in a symbiotic relationship, continuously making micro-adjustments to the changes occurring in the body. Although from the outside it may seem like a static process, it is anything but. The movers work isotonically (dynamically), both concentrically (decrease in muscle length and joint angle) and eccentrically (increase in muscle length and joint angle).

Pilates encourages the development of both agonist and antagonist muscles and highlights the relationship that exists between them; as one muscle or group of muscles contracts concentrically, the other contracts eccentrically. In certain instances they both contract isometrically to stabilize a joint or area (co-contraction). It is important to strive for a good balance between agonist and antagonist muscle groups in terms of strength, flexibility, and control.

Stabilizing the Trunk and Pelvis The term *trunk stabilization* describes a stable position of the spine and in this context is synonymous with *spinal stabilization*, *core stabilization*, *torso stabilization*, and *lumbopelvic stabilization*. It is important to recognize, as noted earlier, that stabilization is dynamic and that the stabilizers are continuously adapting to a changing environment.

I typically use the term *trunk stabilization* when the trunk is stable and the upper girdle is being mobilized, because of the close relationship between the two regions. The movement of the arms has a direct influence on the thoracic spine and, conversely, certain muscles of the thoracic region play an important role in correct mechanics of the shoulder girdle. Furthermore, achieving good head alignment and shoulder function is impossible without correct alignment of the trunk. Similarly, I use the term *lumbopelvic stabilization* when the lower limbs are being mobilized due to the close relationship between the lower limbs and the pelvis. If the pelvis is out of alignment or unstable, it will directly affect the function of the limbs as well as the alignment and function of the spine. Essentially, the pelvis acts as a bridge between the lower limbs and the spine. The position of the spine and the direction of the pull of gravity or resistance determine which muscles are recruited and to what extent.

Maintaining a stable position of the trunk and pelvis is fundamental to the success of many Pilates exercises. In order to achieve trunk stabilization, the ISS must be recruited. Depending on the position of the trunk—flexion, neutral, or extension—certain muscles are activated more than others. It is the intricate interplay between the agonists and antagonists that create and maintain the position (shape). For instance, in Mat: Rolling Like a Ball, the abdominals draw the spine into forward flexion; however, the back extensors play an important role in moderating the degree of flexion and creating the gradual curve of the back. In Mat: Front Support, the abdominals, together with the hip flexors, play a vital role in stabilizing the trunk and avoiding collapse through the center. In the Mat: Back Support, on the other hand, although the abdominals are recruited to add support to the structure, it is primarily the back extensors, together with the hip extensors and shoulder extensors, that hold the structure up. Further insight into this topic is found in the individual exercise descriptions.

In a standing position, the gravitational pull is equal in the front and back of the body (ideally). In this case the abdominals and back extensors work in a state of co-contraction to stabilize the trunk. The back extensors hold the body upright and prevent it from folding forward. At the same time, the abdominals play an important role in creating a girdle of support around the midsection, preventing excessive stress on the lower spine and, in effect, functioning as a second spine.

Note that the abdominals tend to decondition more rapidly than the back extensors, and the back extensors tend to respond to conditioning more readily than the abdominals. Add to this the fact that the back extensors are used most of the time to keep us upright, and the result is that they are typically better conditioned than the abdominals. However, the almost constant use of the large back extensors, particularly the erector spinae, can in itself create a problem. These superficial muscles may become hypertonic (overused) and very tight. "Dimming" (inhibiting) them, or in some cases "switching them off" to allow the deep posterior spinal extensors and abdominals to fully engage, is a crucial first step in creating balance in the trunk and achieving healthy trunk and lumbopelvic stabilization.

To stay well conditioned, the muscles of the trunk should be worked in all ranges of motion: flexion, extension, lateral flexion, and rotation. Individual needs vary, but a safe guideline is to allocate 50 percent of the time spent working core muscles to the spinal flexors, 25 percent to the lateral flexors and rotators of the spine, and 25 percent to the spinal extensors. Of course, Pilates exercises often include the combined activity of many muscle groups in various ranges of motion, so this percentage allocation should only serve as a general guideline and not a steadfast rule. It is interesting to note that exercises geared toward endurance, as opposed to strength, appear to have a more prominent effect on enhancing spinal stability. This is not surprising considering they need to function for extended periods of time during our daily activities. The BASI block system helps ensure that all these factors are addressed in a well-rounded Pilates session.

Stabilizing the Scapulae We tend to think of the shoulder as only the glenohumeral joint, a ball-and-socket joint that facilitates movement of the arm in every direction. But the shoulder is in fact an intricate structure that involves precise interplay of various bones, joints, and muscles. The humerus, scapula, and clavicle form the shoulder complex, which is directly connected to the axial skeleton (skull, spine, and ribs) only at the tiny sternoclavicular joint. The scapulae articulate with the ribs, connected only by muscles. Because of the lack of bony and ligamentous support, the shoulder is *muscle dependent*—it relies heavily on the musculature for its function and stability. Although the terms *shoulder stabilization* and *scapular stabilization* are often used interchangeably, *scapular stabilization* may be a more precise term because the stabilization mechanism of the shoulder typically emanates from the scapula (in the same way hip movement emanates from the pelvis and we refer to *lumbopelvic stabilization*). Scapular stabilization does not necessarily mean keeping the scapulae still, but rather preventing them from moving excessively in an undesired direction. For instance, in many exercises the scapulae tend to elevate and adduct, requiring that they be depressed and abducted to maintain the integrity of the movement. In this book I use *scapular stabilization* to refer to keeping the scapulae in the correct, desired position—most often a neutral position.

The shoulder complex is of great personal interest to me, having been born with a hooked acromion process. Throughout my life I have participated in activities with a high level of shoulder activity and my supraspinatus eventually tore and retracted on both sides. After extensive open rotator cuff surgery, I began a personal journey of exploration to find solutions within Pilates that would help bring me back to 100 percent functionality. I learned a tremendous amount, including how difficult and painful rehabilitation can be. But probably the most important lessons I learned were how intricate the mechanics of the shoulder are, how few people use their shoulders correctly, and how far-reaching the implications of incorrect use are. Clearly, there is a universal need to address the shoulder complex.

The back extensors, particularly those of the mid-back, play an important role in correct shoulder mechanics, not only because of their direct participation in the positioning of the scapulae but also because of their importance in alignment and posture (figure 3.3). As mentioned previously, our modern lifestyle exacerbates certain postural deviations, such as round-shoulder syndrome, and typically leads to other related problems. These include weak back extensors and shoulder external rotators; tight pectorals, hip flexors, hamstrings, and shoulder internal rotators; and, often, overactive levator scapulae and upper trapezius. Throw in some

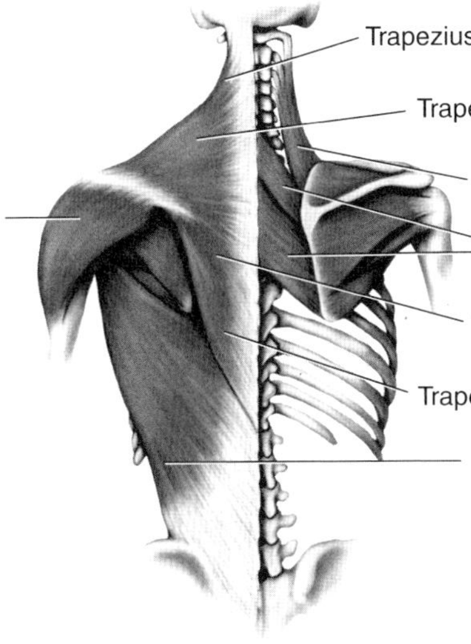

FIGURE 3.3 The muscles of the shoulder complex and the mid-back contribute greatly to the mechanical function of the shoulder joint and to shoulder stabilization.

mental tension and you have a recipe for the type of neck, shoulder, and lower back problems that are so prevalent in our society.

So where do we start? We start with the muscles that hold us up: the back extensors, supported by the ISS. As long as the body is in good alignment, as close to the plumb line as possible, achieving good shoulder mechanics is possible. Conversely, without proper alignment and posture, good shoulder function is unlikely—and faulty shoulder mechanics will probably result in shoulder problems. Rounded shoulders can lead to impingement; impingement can lead to rotator cuff inflammation; inflammation to tearing and, potentially, incapacitation and surgery. This downward spiral begins with habitual movement patterns that in turn cause incorrect posture and muscular imbalance.

Disassociation

Disassociation—in which one area of the body remains stable while a connecting part moves freely—requires the synthesis of two of the pillars of human motion: stabilization and mobilization. The more stable the foundation, the more precise and efficient the movement. The value of disassociation can be described thus: *Effective stabilization equates to efficient movement, and efficient movement equates to safer movement.* Conversely, ineffective stabilization translates to an unstable base of support, wear and tear on the body, and possible injury. Ineffective movement lacks efficiency and fluidity, and typically relies on muscle-substitution patterns (compensations) to perform the motion.

Muscle Isolation

Although muscle isolation and muscle integration may appear to be diametrically opposed concepts, attaining *functional* muscle isolation relies heavily on muscle integration in order to maintain a stable body while moving only one region. It's true to say that *effective integration equates to heightened isolation.* Much of the conventional fitness equipment found in gyms is designed to support the body from every angle, thus facilitating the isolation of a muscle group without necessarily requiring integration. I do not consider this functional isolation because the support is being provided by extrinsic rather than intrinsic means. Intrinsic stabilization, provided by the body itself, demands heightened body awareness and control and involves the recruitment of well-conditioned muscles and well-coordinated muscle activation. Pilates offers a road map to mastering both integration and isolation.

Imagery

Imagery is a key tool in the exercise chapters that follow. This effective and artful means of understanding movement is commonly used in the practice and teaching of Pilates. Explanations involving an abundance of technical information can at times be confusing and counterproductive, if not almost impossible to accurately describe. For example, if you want the movement to flow, how would you describe it anatomically? Yet, simply the word "flow" accompanied by an illustrative gesture or calming tone of voice will most likely produce the desired effect.

Imagery should be used with insight to avoid misunderstandings and breakdowns in communication. The image should be suited to the client's life experience and image vocabulary. If not, the image may seem meaningless or even ludicrous. Common expressions such as "inner pillar of support," "internal reinforcement," and "bracing the center" are examples of imagery that refer to the action of engaging the ISS. Teaching the recruitment of the ISS (and use of the powerhouse) is challenging because of the high level of awareness, concentration, and control required. Appropriate imagery is often the key.

Effectively cueing an exercise (for yourself or others) by means of imagery requires good understanding of the movement, of human science, and of the person being cued. Cueing is an art that comes in different forms—tactile, verbal, and visual—that can be delivered in different ways. Succinct cueing is equivalent to good communication, and good communication leads to better understanding and positive outcomes. Deeper understanding is the basis of quality practice. Consistent, high-quality practice is the path to mastery and success.

A key component in developing and improving cueing skills is experience: There is simply no shortcut. Just as a student cannot learn all the nuances of an exercise in one session, so a teacher cannot learn all the cues from the pages of a book. Knowledge, practice, experience, intuition, compassion, understanding, and life experience are all ingredients that make for good cueing and effective teaching. It is also the reason cueing is so personal. Cues for an exercise may change from person to person and day to day, illustrating the reason cueing is truly an ever-changing, lifelong exploration and the essence of teaching itself.

Following are brief explanations of some of the terms that I often use in my imagery when teaching and therefore often appear in the imagery descriptions in this book.

Lengthening

The term *lengthen* is frequently used in Pilates. This is a complex directive that can mean different things to different people. Working full ranges of motion can encourage lengthening. It is also helpful to think of the co-contraction of the muscles of all the joints along a kinetic chain (such as a limb) working symbiotically to create the desired shape. This can give the appearance and feeling that the whole kinetic chain is functioning as one long segment (reaching out in space) rather than as short individual links.

When using imagery, it is important to stress the difference between concept and physiological fact and to not confuse the two. For example, commands such as, "Lift the leg forward from the back [the hamstrings]," "Lengthen out of the hip joint," "Draw the legs in with the abdominals," and "Reach the arm up from underneath" use imagery to achieve a physical result but are anatomically imprecise. This is not to say these images cannot and should not be used—they can often be used very effectively and successfully—but teachers and students should always be aware of the line between fact and poetic license.

A related point of discussion is the question: How straight is straight? Because of the often-heard instruction to avoid locking the knees or elbows, many people no longer straighten their limbs completely. This results in inefficient movement, incomplete use of the joint, an unstable joint, inadequate muscle recruitment, and even the possible onset of problems such as patellofemoral syndrome (often caused by a weak quadricep muscle, particularly the vastus medialis oblique, leading to misaligned tracking of the patella). *Locking* refers to hyperextension of the joint, which should be avoided when doing Pilates. However, it does not mean that you should not completely straighten the joint; it means reaching the straightest line possible without going beyond the straight line. This is achieved by becoming aware of what *straight* is. First, create an imaginary straight line across the joint. Then activate both the agonist and antagonist muscle groups (co-contraction). In the case of the knee, the hamstrings and quadriceps should be in a state of co-contraction with the knee joint fully extended. In this position the joint is well supported, the correct muscles are perfectly activated, and a long line is achieved.

Remember, a straight limb is longer than a hyperextended or slightly bent one. This is easy to feel on the reformer when doing the foot work (chapter 5). As long as the carriage is traveling away from the footbar, the leg is still straightening. Once the leg is completely straight, the carriage will no longer move in that direction, and it is time to bend the knee and return. If the knee continues extending past the straight line into hyperextension, the carriage will actually start returning toward the footbar—a slight but distinct movement.

Ultimately, creating length is both anatomical and an inner quality and is conveyed through relaxed, rather than tension-filled, movement. A wonderful dance teacher once showed me how a straight arm can look short, or by contrast, appear infinite in length. It was difficult to identify exactly what the difference was, but it was clearly apparent and I have never forgotten that lesson. I try to re-create that quality in every move I do.

Relaxing the Ribs

In discussing imagery, we need to pay particular attention to the lower rib cage, which tends to be thrust forward when standing upright or lifted off the mat when lying supine. This is typically a result of overusing the back extensors, particularly those of the lower back. I like to think of the lower ribs as being connected to the pubic symphysis with two rubber bands, one from each side of the bottom of the rib cage, which allow the ribs to glide up and down the front of the body but remain controlled and not thrust forward. This image encourages the muscles of the lower back to elongate and the abdominals to activate. You will often hear Pilates teachers say, "Drop your ribs" or "Relax your ribs." What is being implied in physiological terms is to engage the abdominals (without overengaging them and going into spinal flexion) and decrease the intensity of contraction of the spinal extensors, resulting in ideal alignment with appropriate co-contraction of the abdominals and back extensors. Breathing can play a valuable role in this process. Often one deep exhalation achieves the desired result. Try it right now—inhale and exhale fully!

Imprinting

Credit for the concept of *imprinting* must be given to Eve Gentry, one of the great first-generation Pilates teachers. It was a central motif of her teaching and the powerful imagery she used with great success. I had the pleasure of experiencing Eve's teaching firsthand, and what a tremendous honor it was.

Lying on a mat, visualize the body sinking into soft sand, making an imprint. In this form of work, the focus on the individual muscles is minimized while attention is shifted to the motion of the body part, as if moving only the bones. Ideally, this results in movement that is fluid and void of tension. For example, when performing the Mat: Pelvic Curl, you may imagine an imprint of the spine in the sand. Note that the spine still maintains its natural curves; the very reason the image of soft sand works well is that it conforms to the shape of the body. The pelvis and each vertebra are lifted out of their imprint and then returned to the same place in the sand. The result is sequential articulation of the spine without excessive muscle activity (or at least without the tension associated with trying too hard). You can apply this concept to any part of the body in any position. It allows the body to move with graceful correctness without being bogged down with information.

In conclusion, effective learning and teaching strategies may vary according to the movement, the student, and the instructor. Some people learn better when presented with a picture or a demonstration of the movement, which they then emulate and practice. Others learn better by breaking the exercise down into small movements. Still others prefer a verbal explanation or the use of touch. In most cases, a combination of approaches is best, using every angle to improve performance and heighten understanding.

The following general guidelines will prove helpful in achieving a positive outcome:

- Go through a mental full body scan to make sure the positioning is correct.
- Precede the movement with the breath and eliminate tension.
- Set up the exercise before moving (engage the ISS).
- Concentrate on the muscle focus (initiator).
- Keep the head aligned with the spine.
- Direct the eyes forward, in line with the head.
- Breathe throughout the exercise (even if it is not the set breathing pattern).

- Keep the shoulders and neck relaxed.
- Create long lines with the movements.
- Move with efficiency, flow, precision, and harmony.

Movement Description

Each exercise in the following chapters includes a description of the movement, with step-by-step instructions for correct execution. Although the words *exercise* and *movement* are used interchangeably in this book, I often refer to *movement* rather than *exercise* to differentiate the Pilates approach from the notion that an exercise is merely a physical action. Even the most basic movement has many layers of information, with the physical motion being only one of them (and the most superficial one at that). This is not meant to devalue the physical aspect of an exercise but to bring attention to the underlying approach, in which the movements are a vehicle for reaching a higher purpose—well-being.

Before starting an exercise, it is important to set up the body to perform the movement correctly. I often say to students that the *setup* is 100 percent of the exercise, because without a good, precise setup, the movement has little to no chance of being correct and producing the desired results. The setup allows the mind and body to work together to achieve optimum alignment and muscle recruitment.

The setup may demand 5 seconds or 30 seconds—take the time you need to align the body, engage the ISS, and establish a connection with the muscle focus of the exercise. Mentally review the breath pattern and do a scan to make sure that each body part is in place. Go through a checklist of the nuances of the movement. If you are working alone, cue yourself and make corrections to the movement before the mistakes or deviations ever occur. The better you know your body and recognize your own habits and compensations, the more refined this process becomes. In essence the

REPETITION IN PILATES

Being mindful in each exercise and each repetition is the goal. Joseph Pilates spoke of *mindless repetition*; I like that term because I believe that a high rate of repetition invariably becomes mindless and produces diminishing returns. You can practice an exercise routine that is based on a high number of repetitions with no real focus or control, and it becomes mindless as opposed to mindful. In order to achieve mindfulness, both physically and mentally, I recommend a limited number of repetitions, usually 5-10, depending on the intensity and complexity of the movement. The more complex and demanding the movement, the fewer the repetitions required. Use the low end of the scale for the very difficult and complex repertoire and the high end (still relatively low compared to many typical endurance-based workouts) for the fundamental work or instances where muscle endurance is an objective.

One reason profound effects are achieved from so few repetitions is the precision with which Pilates movements are executed and the resulting recruitment of the appropriate muscles. When many repetitions are done, compensations often creep in; other muscles (usually the larger, superficial ones) take over, and the effect on the desired muscles is minimal at best. Other negative effects of doing excessive repetitions are fatigue, wear and tear on the joints, boredom, and, in some instances, injury. Pilates encapsulates the concept of *less is more* (quality versus quantity), which holds the key to deeper work, enhanced performance, and in many cases, better results.

exercise begins long before movement is apparent. I can often be heard saying, "The exercise begins with the intention, not the movement." The process of setting up gives each exercise, and the session as a whole, a deep focus and a meditative quality.

Achieving Symmetry

Is symmetry attainable? Is it desirable? My wife, Adelle, likes to remind me that in nature there is no absolute symmetry—close, but not absolute. I have also worked with athletes who have questioned whether it is advisable to tamper with the physical asymmetries that have developed as a result of their many years and thousands of hours of training, and are serving them well. This is particularly noticeable in sports such as tennis, volleyball, golf, and others that are asymmetrical by nature. Athletes can still strive for core strength and enhanced performance without altering the balance (or imbalance) in their bodies. So should we strive for symmetry in our bodies? It is certainly a legitimate question. Personally, I like to promote symmetry as an ideal, a reference point to which we strive and one that can be used to measure improvement and change. Symmetry can also serve as a guideline for cueing. I believe that training toward symmetry ultimately enhances performance and function in both everyday and skill-specific activities; it prevents undue stresses on particular areas of the body and possibly the eventual deterioration of the body as a whole.

Furthermore, when practicing movement on one side of the body, a transfer of information to the other side occurs. That means that if one side is injured, exercising the non-injured side has a positive effect on the injured side. This transfer applies not only to injuries but also to all motor skills, including athletic activities.

Training toward symmetry is complex; therefore a conservative approach is the most prudent one. Do not rush to make drastic changes. I use the following steps when dealing with imbalances. Note that I use the first and second steps in a well-rounded session for several months before proceeding (only if necessary) to steps 3 and 4.

1. Work bilaterally, raising awareness of asymmetrical muscular activity and development.
2. Work unilaterally, using the same number of repetitions and resistance on both sides.
3. Work unilaterally, loading the weaker, less dominant side more than the other.
4. Work unilaterally, working only the weaker, less dominant side.

Moving With the Energy Lines

As a dancer, I was taught to think of movement in terms of energy lines or energy paths; this is a concept that adapts well to Pilates. Energy paths can be straight, circular, or spiral shaped. Fundamental movements such as the Mat: Pelvic Curl or Mat: Chest Lift have only one or two energy lines (figure 3.4*a*). More complex movements have more energy lines, because various parts of the body extend in different and often opposing directions. For example, the Mat: Spine Twist—Sitting has vertical, horizontal, and spiral energy lines (figure 3.4*b*). The vertical line, which travels up and down the spine and continues into space, keeps the trunk straight. The horizontal line, running across the shoulders and traveling outward through the arms and fingers in both directions, anchors the movement and keeps the arms, shoulders, and back as broad as possible on one plane. We add to this a spiral, which travels up the trunk, illustrating the rotation that occurs in the spine. The energy moves in all these directions at the same time, making this movement relatively complex.

Think of energy lines as a diagram of the energy in each exercise. Understanding these lines will bring clarity and simplicity to the exercises and result in precise movement. You can utilize this principle in every exercise. Once you understand the energy lines

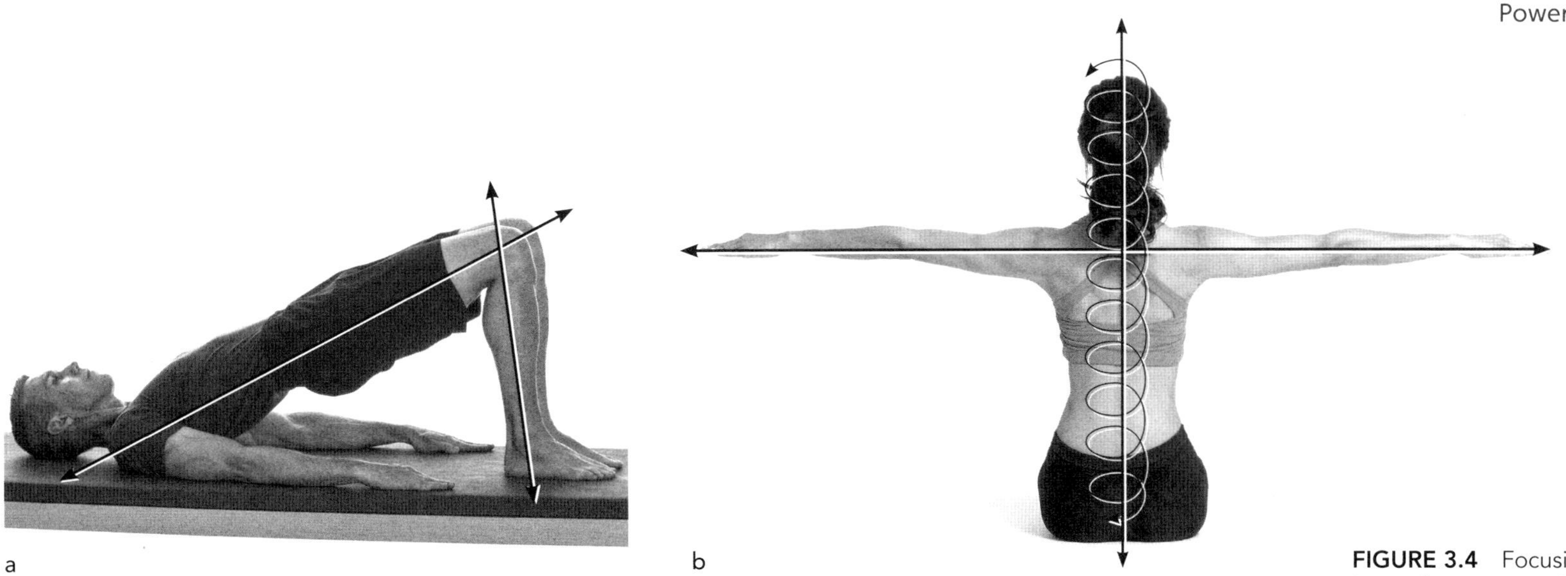

FIGURE 3.4 Focusing on the energy lines of exercises will guide you along the correct movement paths. The energy in the *(a)* Mat: Pelvic Curl moves along two simple lines, whereas the energy in the more complex *(b)* Mat: Spine Twist—Sitting moves in multiple directions simultaneously.

of an exercise, the choreography becomes clear and the correct muscles will likely be activated in the most effective manner.

Adapting Exercises

It is important to view Joseph Pilates' original body of work in the context of the time and place it was created: the early part of the 20th century in Europe and New York. The habits, occupations, and lifestyles of society at that time and those places were very different from those seen today. Computers were nonexistent, cars were scarce, air travel was a dream, the Internet was decades away, and recreational activities were simple and low-tech. The evolution of this system and its adaptation to the needs of people today is justified and should be celebrated.

But as we progress, we must not lose sight of the value of Joseph Pilates' work. I've seen people create variations of Pilates exercises simply to be different or to avoid boredom. Others choreograph variations because they are unfamiliar with the original exercises. I do not support changing an exercise for any of these reasons. The essence of the exercise should not be lost in a mass of choreography, ceasing to have any resemblance to the original exercise or its intention. Rather, it should be refined according to advances in scientific knowledge and the needs of the individual—but always build on the foundation of the original work. The goal is to promote growth, keep the system alive and contemporary, and to adapt the work to individual and societal needs while still preserving the legacy of Pilates.

Modifying exercises is necessary at times in order to achieve the desired objectives while avoiding negative movement patterns, compensations, and contraindications. However, maintaining the essence of the exercise is critical, which means that one must know the original movement and understand the intention and mechanics of the exercise and its possible contraindications. Creating necessary modifications is an integral part of being a creative, innovative, and interactive teacher.

This approach to modifications also applies to *assists*. Assists are external aids such as springs, rubber bands, cushions, balls, or adjustments to the apparatus that help achieve the goal. Again, complete understanding of the exercise and the exerciser is essential, as well as being well informed about the many choices of apparatus and which would be best suited for each scenario. In short, intimate familiarity with the Pilates repertoire, the human body and its movement, and the myriad choreographic and apparatus options available make this work an ever-evolving process.

In the first edition of *Pilates* I intentionally abstained from offering modifications and assists. Too much information and too many variations can lead to confusion and I wanted people to gain knowledge and understanding of and experience in the original repertoire. In the second edition of *Pilates*, following the requests of students and readers, I included variations for many of the exercises. Now, in this third edition, I have created three distinct categories of exercise variations:

1. A *modification* changes the choreography with the goal of making the exercise more accessible (easier).
2. A *variation* changes the choreography of an exercise without meaningfully changing the level of difficulty; it simply offers variety.
3. A *progression* changes the choreography with the goal of making the exercise more challenging.

An assist (small apparatus) can be employed in any of the three categories.

By offering modifications, variations, or progressions for most of the exercises in the book, I hope to spark ideas for alternative choreography while never losing sight of the original exercises and their intentions. I stress that each person is an individual with unique needs, restrictions, and personal goals that must be considered when selecting or creating a modification, variation, or progression of an exercise. In addition, body type, suitability of apparatus, and desired outcome are also important factors. Finally, safety must always be at the forefront of every decision. Choose or create movements that will allow you and your student to perform the work safely and enjoy years of Pilates practice.

4

Mat Work

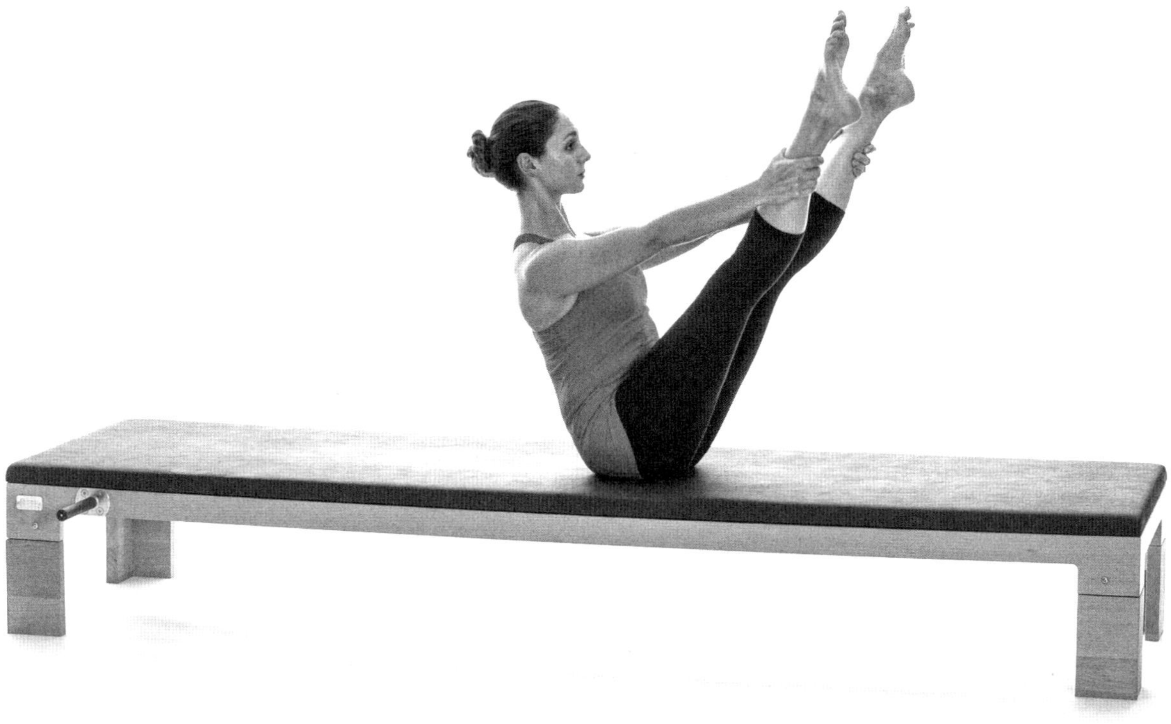

Mat work is the foundation of the Pilates method; most, if not all exercises in the Pilates repertoire can be traced back to the mat work. The mat work never ceases to challenge even the most seasoned of practitioners. Without an intricate familiarity with mat work, you will inevitably lack a fundamental component in your Pilates practice.

Mat work can be practiced anywhere and everywhere, with no special apparatus other than a mat. You can practice it at any time of the day and at any level of challenge. You can structure it to meet multiple goals—for instance, as a warm-up for a Pilates class on the apparatus or for other athletic activities, as part of a daily conditioning program, as a means of improving general body awareness, or as a pre- and postnatal fitness routine.

The block designations provided in this chapter will assist you in structuring mat work sessions. As noted in chapter 3, the *mat block system* differs from the *comprehensive block system* used to structure a session that uses all the apparatus. Most mat exercises focus on developing the core, and therefore the mat work blocks relate primarily to the conditioning of the core and the movements of the pelvis and spine.

The exercises in this chapter are presented with both progression and flow in mind. Mat work embodies the principle of flow more fully than the work on any of the other Pilates apparatus. I have created what I call *flow sequences*, which offer a unique way to practice traditional mat work. These sequences, which appear in chapter 12 and vary in duration, incorporate the original movements arranged according to block and level of challenge such that each exercise flows seamlessly into the next.

I typically conclude a mat work session with a few minutes of relaxation and focus. Whether it involves performing slow movements, sitting still in a comfortable position and listening to calming words or music, or going through a short, guided meditation, this relaxation period serves as a cool-down for the body and a chance to mentally and spiritually integrate the work that you have just done. This is possibly the most valuable part of the session.

Don't view the mat work as the underdog in the Pilates system; it is the crown jewel. Enjoy!

Foundation

The foundation block focuses on exercises that are typically performed at the beginning of the mat session and serve as an introduction to the session or a warm-up for other activities. These exercises lay the foundation to all that follows on the mat and on the apparatus. They place great emphasis on the *powerhouse*, and they increase physical and mental awareness of the core.

Although these exercises are not as complex as some of the movements that follow later in the book, they should be performed with concentration, control, and precision. Foundation exercises should be performed slowly, providing a perfect opportunity to pay attention to the finer details of the movements and internal aspects of doing the work correctly.

The essential muscle actions of this block are the recruitment of the pelvic floor muscles, the activation of the abdominals (in particular the transversus abdominis), the co-contraction of the abdominals and back extensors (particularly the deep-lying muscles), and the positioning and movement of the pelvis by the hip flexors and hamstrings. Both stabilization and movement are pivotal aspects of the work, as is unobstructed articulation of the spine.

Another concept that is important to grasp early on is the establishment of certain body shapes. Think of yourself as a sculptor creating shapes with your own body. The shapes can be equated to learning basic musical scales without which you could not learn more complex compositions. These shapes include the neutral spine position, the C curve of the trunk, and the tabletop position of the legs, all of which will be applied later to more advanced and demanding movements.

Pelvic Curl

The Mat: Pelvic Curl has myriad benefits. Not only does it mobilize the spine and prepare it for exercises to come, but it also teaches recruitment of the internal support system (ISS). The Mat: Pelvic Curl develops body awareness and draws focus to the powerhouse. This exercise promotes mobility and stability in the pelvic region and spine and potentially releases both physical and mental tension in the process. No matter how many times I do this exercise—and I have done it thousands of times—it simply feels good!

Imagery

Imagine a string of large pearls being lifted off beach sand, one pearl at a time, and then slowly and deliberately being placed back into each individual imprint in the sand. Allow the feeling of gentle resistance and fine articulation of the spine to be central to the exercise.

- ○ Begin and complete the movement in a neutral spine position.
- ○ Maintain a slight posterior tilt of the pelvis when at the top, contracting the abdominals and hamstrings and stretching the hip flexors.
- ○ Keep the shoulders and neck relaxed and uninvolved.

PROGRESSION

Perform this same exercise with a single leg while holding the lifted leg in a tabletop position (right angles at the knee and hip joints) from the outset. The angle in the hip joint will change as the body is lifted and lowered, but keep the right angle in the knee constant throughout, with the shin parallel to the mat and the thigh perpendicular to the mat. This progression adds exponential challenge in terms of lumbopelvic stabilization and hip extensor control. Repeat 5 times before switching to the other leg.

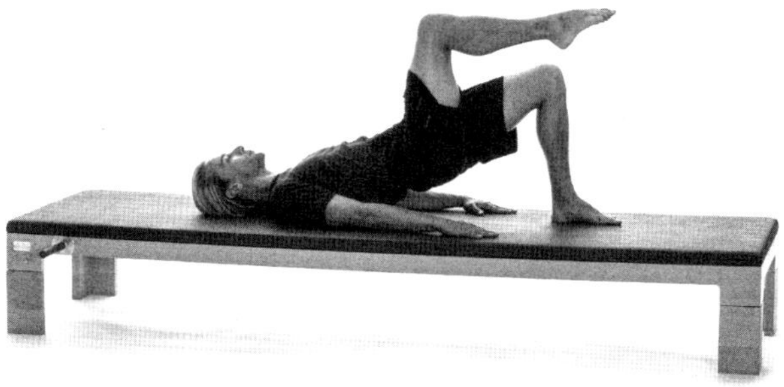

MAT

Foundation

FUNDAMENTAL

Muscle Focus

- Abdominals
- Hamstrings

Objectives

- To develop spinal articulation
- To develop lumbopelvic stabilization
- To improve abdominal and hamstring control

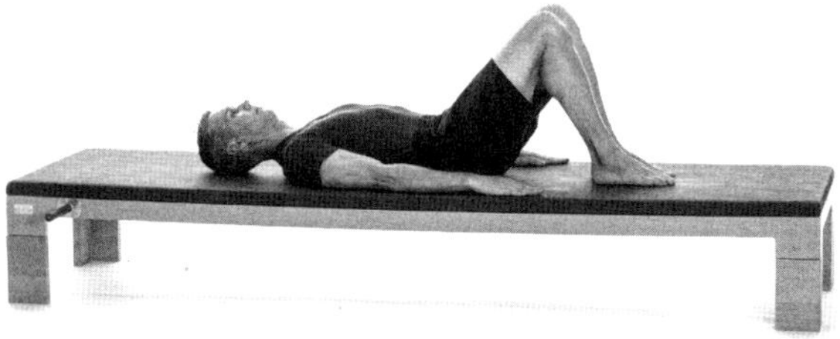

Setup. Lie supine with the spine in a neutral position, keeping the entire body relaxed. Bend the knees and place the feet hip width apart. Sense the elongation through the spine while keeping the scapulae in a neutral position, the arms straight by the sides, and the fingers reaching toward the feet. Make sure the neck is relaxed and the chin is tilted slightly toward the chest.

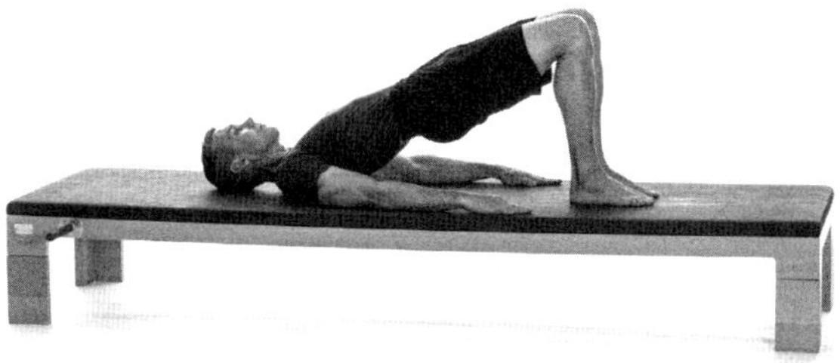

Exhale. Draw in the abdominals. Begin to curl the pelvis, lifting the sacrum and lumbar spine vertebra by vertebra off the mat. Midway through the motion, recruit the hamstrings to lift the pelvis and trunk higher, continuing to articulate the spine one vertebra at a time.

Inhale. Keep the body still and the legs parallel, maximizing the hip flexor stretch. Engage the shoulder extensors to accentuate the extension of the upper back.

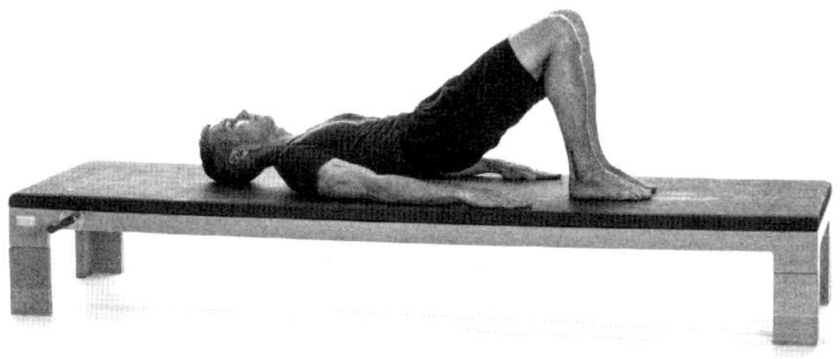

Exhale. Articulate the spine in reverse order from the top of the spine, vertebra by vertebra, accentuating the flexion through the lumbar region. Return to the start position. Repeat 5-10 times.

Spine Twist—Supine

Muscle Focus

- Abdominal obliques
- Hip flexors

Objectives

- To improve abdominal control
- To improve hip flexor control
- To develop spinal rotation
- To develop lumbopelvic stabilization

This exercise prepares the body (specifically the spine) for rotational movements. It also activates and brings awareness to the abdominal obliques. The degree of rotation should be dictated by your flexibility and abdominal control. Maintain strong lumbopelvic support, avoiding hyperlordosis throughout the movement. This is particularly pertinent when in rotation, because the tendency to exceed the controllable range of motion often results in the back arching excessively.

Imagery

Imagine the pelvis turning like a doorknob, with the pelvis, legs, and feet rotating from side to side fluidly while the door itself (the shoulders) remains stable.

- ○ Keep the shoulder girdle and neck relaxed and still.
- ○ Visualize the movement occurring in the waist area (although anatomically the rotation is distributed throughout the spine, with the majority of the rotation taking place in the thoracic spine).
- ○ Keep the knees and feet together, avoiding any gliding back and forth.
- ○ Maintain a long line across the chest, from the fingertips of one hand to the fingertips of the other.

MODIFICATION

Perform the same movement pattern, but instead of placing the legs in a tabletop position to begin, bend the knees and place the feet flat on the mat. The pelvis and legs move as one unit; as the pelvis and legs move to the right, the left foot rises off the mat and the outside of the right foot rests on the mat. Bring the pelvis and legs back to the start position. Rotate to the opposite side.

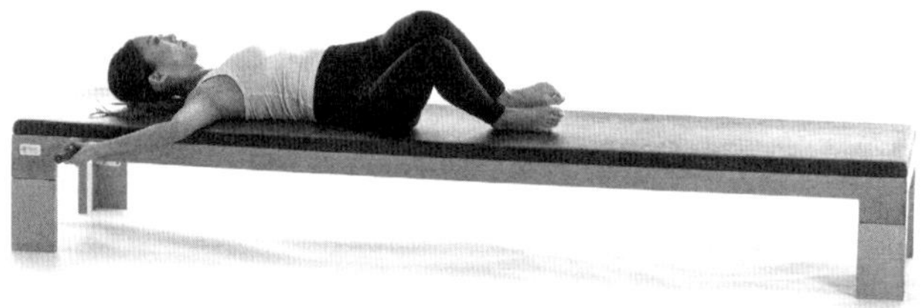

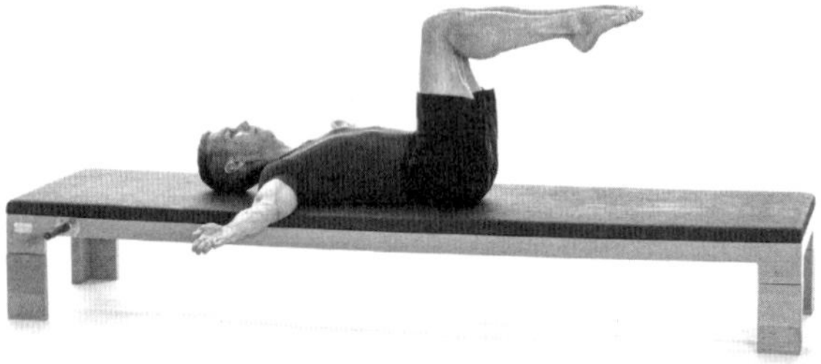

Setup. Lie supine with the arms in the T position, palms facing upward. Draw the lumbar spine into the mat, maintaining a slight posterior pelvic tilt. (You can also begin this exercise from a neutral pelvic position, although greater control is required to avoid hyperlordosis and excessive stress on the lower back.) Hold the legs in a tabletop position (legs together, right angles at the knee and hip joints).

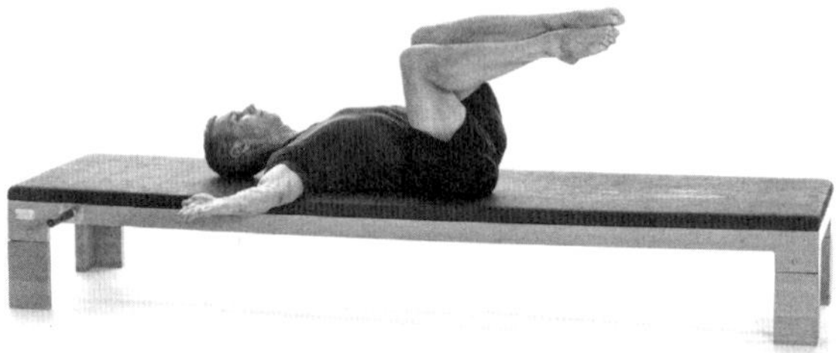

Inhale. Rotate the spine, moving the pelvis and the legs as one unit to one side, keeping the knees together. Move in the transverse plane, with the shoulder girdle providing a stable base around which the movement occurs.

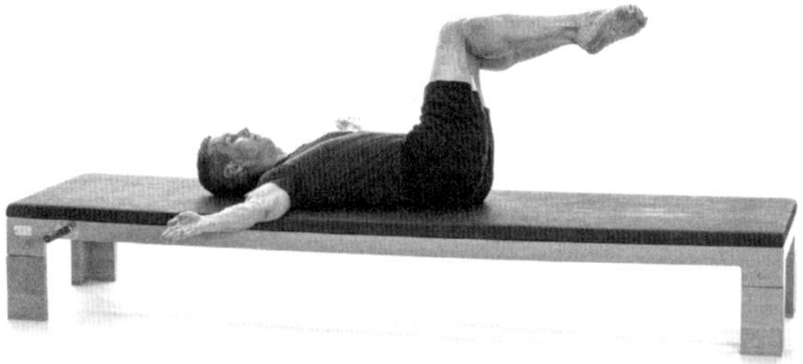

Exhale. Draw the pelvis and legs as one unit back to the center.

Inhale. Rotate to the opposite side. Repeat 5 times to each side.

Chest Lift

This exercise strengthens the abdominals, teaches correct recruitment of the ISS, and lays the foundation for much of the abdominal work that follows. Although it resembles the infamous crunch, it is a completely different exercise. Most notably, the pace is much slower, which minimizes momentum and encourages the abdominals to facilitate the movement. The positioning of the spine and pelvis are also different: The crunch is typically done with the pelvis in posterior tilt and the spine pressing into the mat from the outset, whereas the Mat: Chest Lift begins in a neutral spine and neutral pelvic position and the neutral pelvis is maintained throughout, although the spine does imprint into the mat when in the lifted position. The Mat: Chest Lift should be challenging, regardless of your fitness level. Remember: Exercises do not get easier (as we get stronger), they get better (as we perform them more accurately and feel them more intensely!).

Imagery

Imagine the spine being a strip of spring metal, flexible and strong. One end is riveted down onto a stable surface; the other end is free to be lifted. As you begin to lift the free end of the metal strip, it curves; as you continue, the curve is distributed evenly throughout the movable portion, while the riveted end of the strip remains absolutely stable.

- ○ Avoid pulling on the neck.
- ○ Lift the head first, followed by the shoulders and upper trunk.
- ○ Maintain a neutral pelvis, or as close as possible.

PROGRESSION

After lifting the upper spine, vertebra by vertebra, bringing the scapulae off the mat, inhale while placing the hands behind the thighs. Exhale; lift the trunk slightly higher, assisting with the arms. Inhale; place the hands back behind the head while maintaining the same height of the trunk. Exhale and slowly lower the trunk.

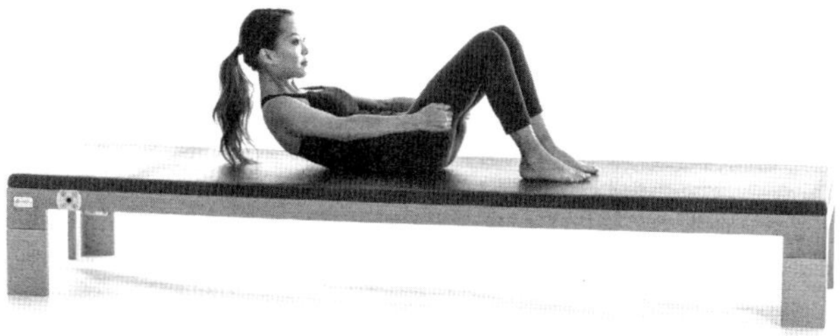

Muscle Focus

- Abdominals

Objectives

- To improve abdominal strength
- To develop pelvic stabilization and control

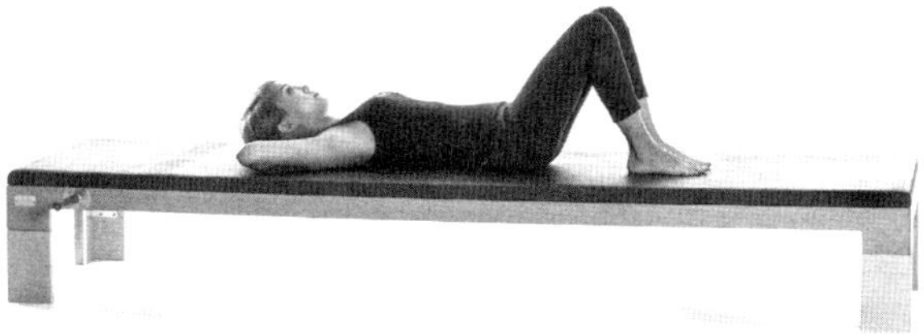

Setup. Lie supine with the pelvis and spine in a neutral position, the knees bent, and the feet hip width apart. Feel a sense of elongation through the spine. Interlace the fingers and cradle the head in the hands. Make sure the neck is relaxed, with the chin tilted slightly toward the chest. Engage the ISS, highlighting awareness of the abdominal region.

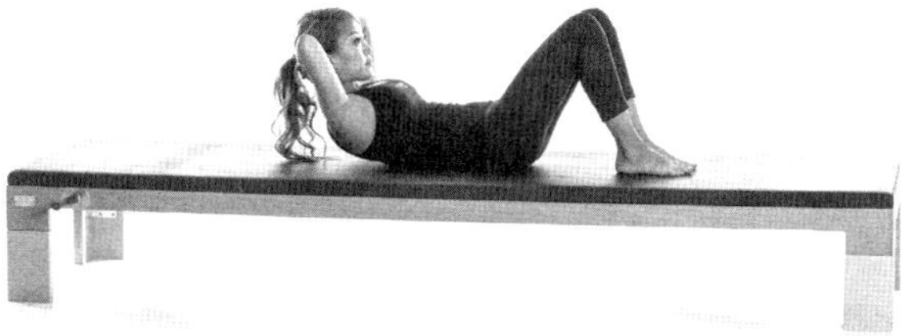

Exhale. While contracting the abdominals, lift the upper spine and shoulder girdle, beginning with the top of the head, and allow the lumbar spine to sink into the mat. Sense a hinging action just under the sternum and maintain stability of the body below this point. Continue lifting the upper spine, vertebra by vertebra, until the scapulae have lifted off the mat.

Inhale. Maintain the maximum height you can achieve with the upper trunk. Contract the abdominals further and focus on the neutral position of the pelvis.

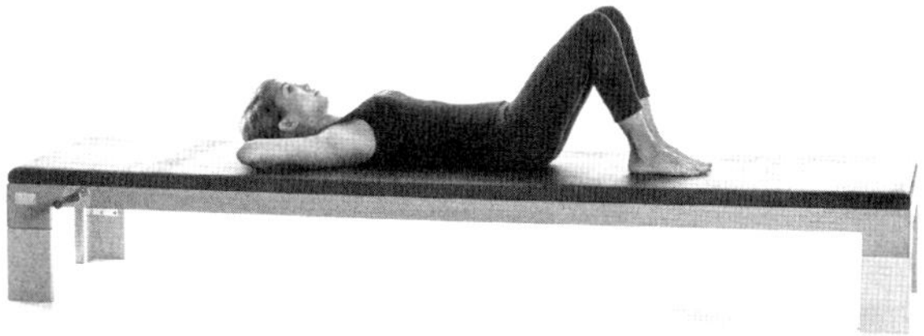

Exhale. Lower the spine without releasing the contraction of the abdominals. Return to the start position. Repeat 5-10 times.

Chest Lift With Rotation

Muscle Focus

- Abdominal obliques

Objectives

- To improve abdominal strength with emphasis on the obliques
- To develop pelvic stabilization

This exercise is an extension of the Mat: Chest Lift. It adds the element of rotation and further challenges the abdominals by loading the obliques in a bilateral pattern. This lays the foundation for more challenging rotational abdominal exercises, such as the Mat: Criss-Cross, and prepares the body for the many rotational activities that everyday life and athletic activities demand.

Imagery

A good image for this exercise is a combination of the doorknob turning described in the Mat: Spine Twist—Supine and the spring metal strip described in the Mat: Chest Lift.

- Move the head, arms, and upper trunk as one unit during rotation.
- Avoid pulling on the neck and moving the elbows forward.
- Maintain consistent forward flexion as you transition from side to side.

PROGRESSION

Perform the exact same movement pattern as the Mat: Chest Lift With Rotation. However, when rotating to the right, lift the right knee toward the chest. Return to center and place the foot back on the mat. Rotate to the opposite side, lifting the left knee toward the chest. Repeat 5 times to each side. On the final repetition, rotate back to the center, contracting the abdominals further before returning to the supine position. This progression amplifies the rotation of the trunk while keeping the pelvis stable. It is also an excellent preparation for the Mat: Criss-Cross and similar challenging abdominal rotation exercises.

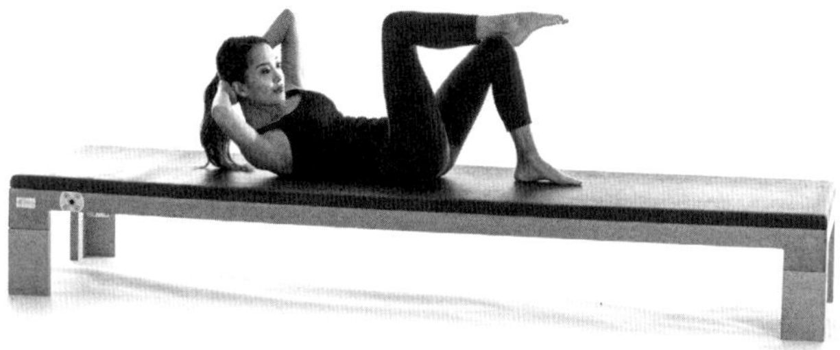

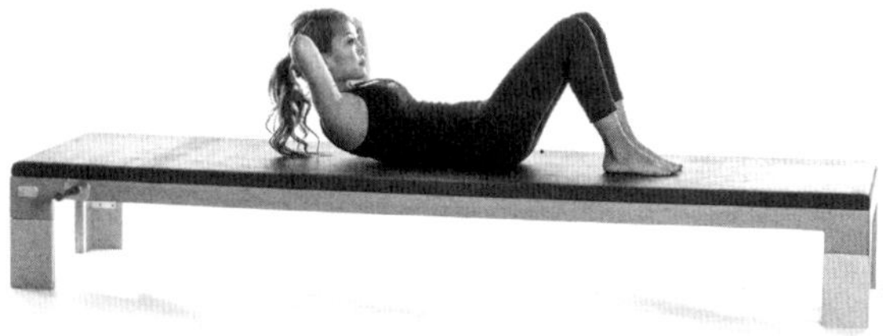

Setup. Lie supine with the pelvis and spine in a neutral position, the knees bent, and the feet hip width apart. Interlace the fingers and cradle the head in the hands. Engage the ISS, draw in the abdominals, and lift the upper spine and shoulder girdle, beginning with the top of the head, and allow the lumbar spine to sink into the mat.

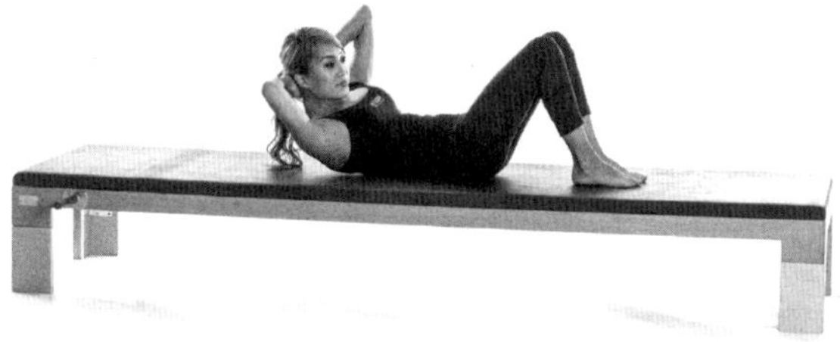

Exhale. Rotate the upper girdle to one side. Focus on contracting the abdominals and moving from above the pelvis, maximizing flexion and rotation of the trunk while avoiding lateral flexion. Maintain stability of the pelvis.

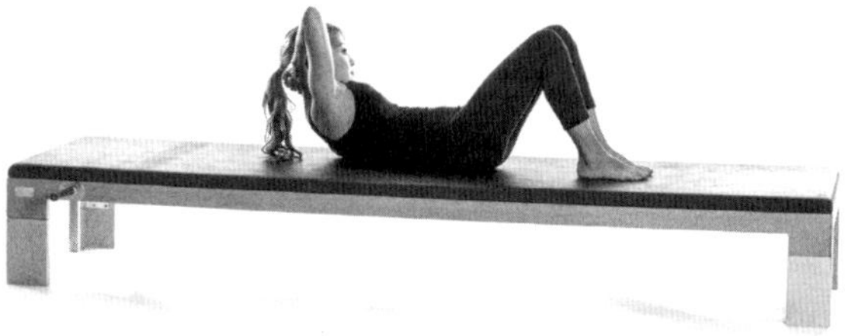

Inhale. Rotate the upper girdle back to the center without lowering the trunk.

Exhale. Rotate the upper girdle to the opposite side.

Inhale. Return to the center without lowering the trunk. Repeat 5 times to each side. On the final repetition, rotate back to the center, contracting the abdominals further, and lower the trunk. Return to the start position.

Single-Leg Lift

This exercise uses the abdominals as stabilizers rather than as movers. It is particularly useful when pelvic stabilization is lacking or abdominal strength is insufficient to lift the trunk into forward flexion. By keeping the entire body still, particularly the lumbopelvic region, and moving only one leg up and down, you learn to bring awareness to the powerhouse and stability to the pelvis.

Imagery

The pelvis should be as stable as a rock and the leg as light as a feather, floating up and down without affecting the pelvis. These opposing images help create the correct sensation in the body.

- Avoid tension in the lower back and possible hyperlordosis when lifting the leg.
- Move the leg as one unit, maintaining a right angle at the knee.
- Minimize the weight shift onto the supporting leg when lifting the opposite side.

PROGRESSION

To raise the level of difficulty and challenge, work both legs at the same time. Lift one leg into tabletop position, and as you lower that leg to touch the mat with the tip of the toes, lift the other leg into tabletop position. Continue changing legs simultaneously, performing the same number of repetitions on each leg.

To add even more challenge, pass the perpendicular position of the thigh and continue flexing the hip, moving the knee toward the chest. This adds range of motion to the hip movement, amplifies the hip flexor activation, and potentially provides a mild stretch to the hamstrings. This can be done with both the Mat: Single-Leg Lift and the progression.

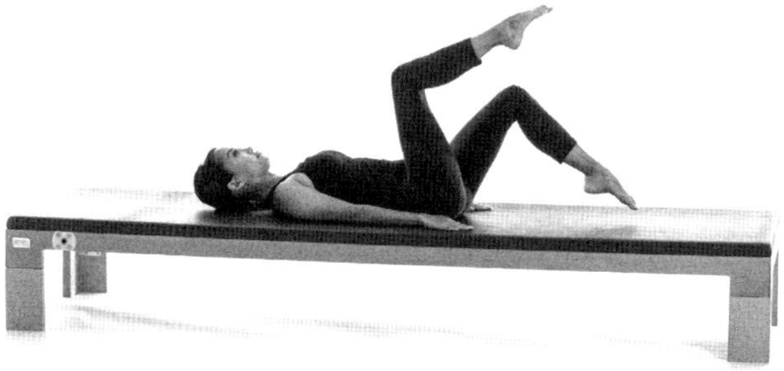

Muscle Focus

- Abdominals
- Hip flexors

Objectives

- To develop lumbopelvic stabilization
- To develop hip disassociation
- To improve abdominal and hip flexor control

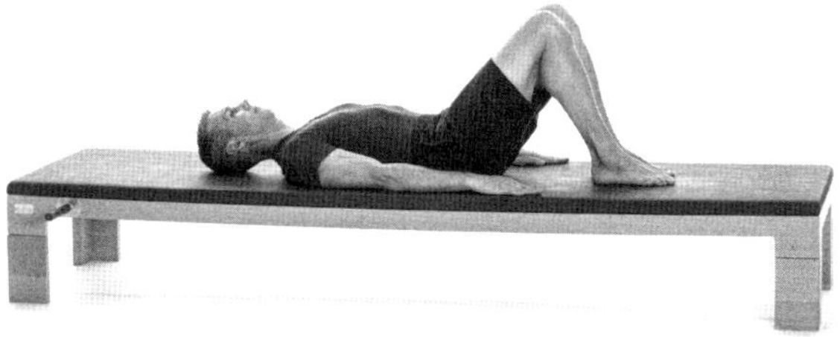

Setup. Lie supine with the spine in a neutral position, bend the knees, and place the feet hip width apart. Hold the arms straight by the sides, with the fingers reaching toward the feet, the neck relaxed, and the chin tilted slightly toward the chest. Emphasize lumbopelvic stabilization and an even distribution of weight on the feet.

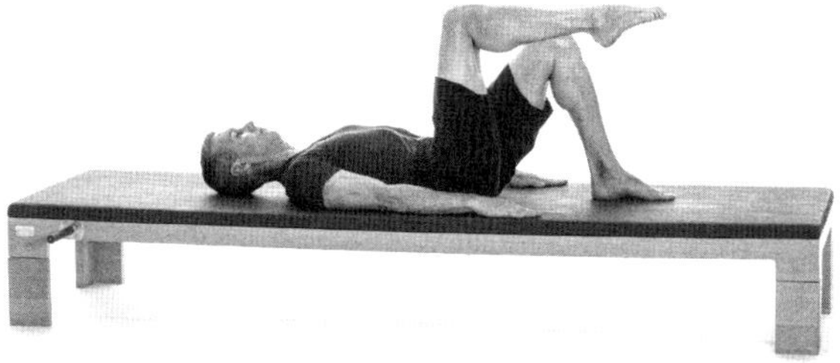

Exhale. Lift one leg, focusing the movement in the hip joint only and maintaining a perfect right angle in the knee throughout the full range of motion. Continue the movement until the hip joint reaches a right angle and the thigh is perpendicular to the floor (tabletop position).

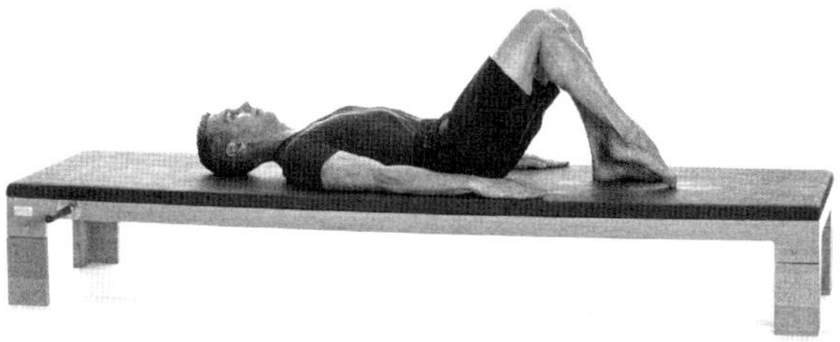

Inhale. Keep the knee at a right angle and lower the leg gently, touching the floor with the tip of the toes without placing any pressure on the foot. Repeat 5-10 times before switching to the other leg.

Leg Circle

Muscle Focus

- Abdominals
- Hip flexors

Objectives

- To develop lumbopelvic stabilization
- To develop hip disassociation
- To improve hip flexor control

This exercise is an excellent example of how coordinated stabilization and mobilization produces disassociation. While the pelvis remains anchored and the spine remains stable, the hip joint fluidly rotates and the leg circles effortlessly. Hip mobilization and disassociation, a pattern often found in Pilates exercises, is a requisite for many activities, such as cycling, running, and certain dance and gymnastic movements. When executed correctly, this movement may also help release hip and lower back tension and assist in remedying sacroiliac dysfunction.

Imagery

Imagine the leg as a big spoon that is stirring thick syrup in a large pot. The motion should be gentle and smooth, with a continuous flow. Thinking of a fall-and-retrieve action, like a yo-yo rolling down and then up, may also be helpful.

- ○ Maintain a neutral pelvis and spine.
- ○ Keep the movement in the hip joint unrestricted and fluid.
- ○ Keep the neck, shoulders, and chest relaxed.

MODIFICATION

This exercise can be performed with a rubber exercise band draped over the foot of the lifted leg, with the hands holding each end of the band and the elbows firmly planted on the mat by the sides of the body. This version allows the hip flexors to relax and assists in achieving the desired fluidity of movement in the joint as the leg rotates—it is a very helpful option when the hamstrings are tight.

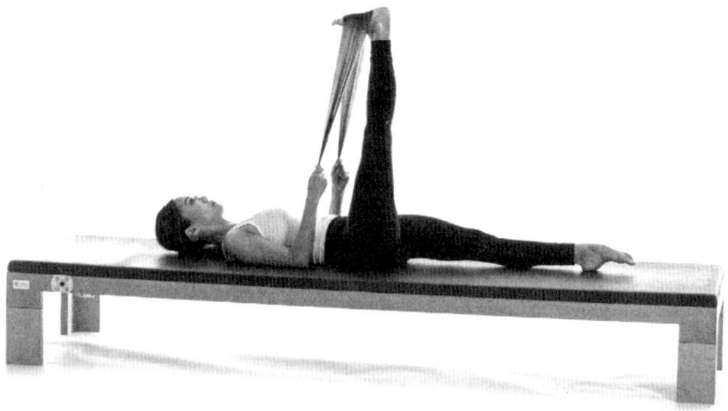

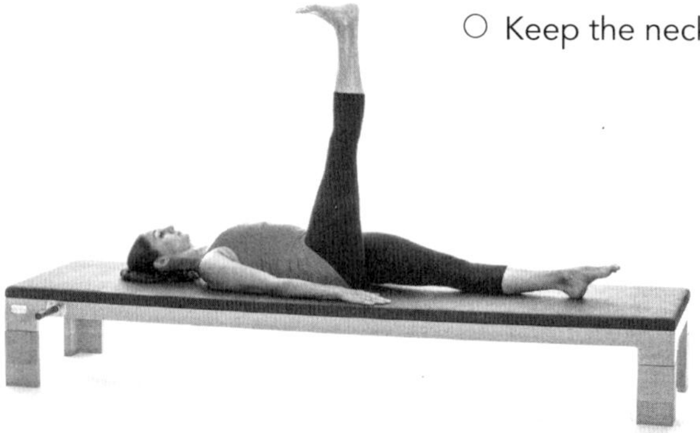

Setup. Lie supine and place the arms by the sides of the body or in a T position with palms facing up. Keep the legs straight and together, with the feet gently pointed. Bend one leg toward the chest.

Straighten the leg upward to form a 90-degree angle in the hip joint, holding the leg perpendicular to the floor, and dorsiflex the foot. Keep the other leg straight and actively engaged on the mat, with the foot plantarflexed.

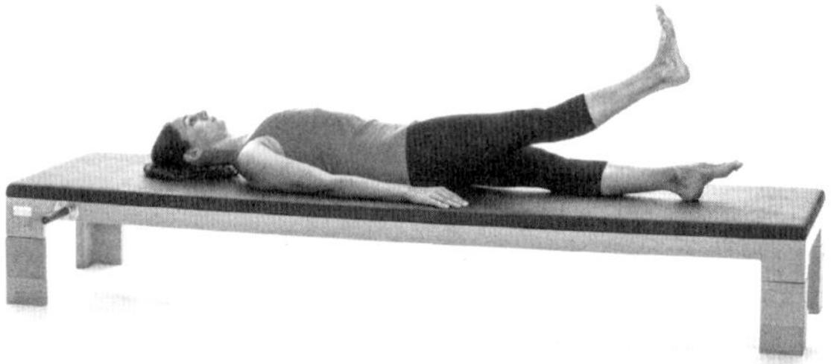

Inhale. Circle the raised leg inward, bringing it slightly across the centerline of the body, then down and around. The range of motion of the circle is dictated by your ability to stabilize the pelvis. The larger the circle, the more difficult it is to stabilize.

Exhale. Repeat the movement, alternating the breathing on each circle and pausing slightly (suspending the movement) each time the leg reaches the perpendicular position. Repeat 5-10 breath cycles (inhale and exhale).

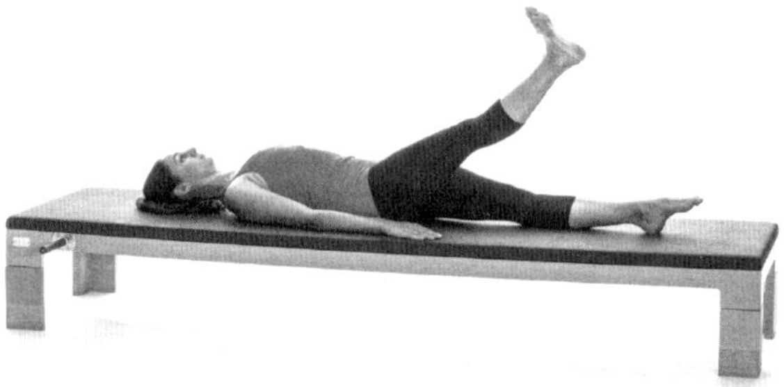

Reverse the circle and repeat the breath pattern, completing one circle of the leg on each breath. Start at the centerline and circle the leg outward and downward before coming back up the center. Emphasize lumbopelvic stabilization and the free-flowing movement of the hip joint. Repeat 5-10 breath cycles (inhale and exhale), returning to the perpendicular position after the final repetition. Plantarflex the foot, bend the leg to the chest, and straighten it on the mat. Return to the start position. Repeat on the other side.

Abdominal Work

Despite the fact that the abdominals are engaged to some extent in every exercise in Pilates because they are integral to the concept of the powerhouse, this block is devoted specifically to their development. The abdominals are also a key element in the concept of core strength and spinal stability, which is increasingly popular in the areas of general fitness, rehabilitation, and athletic performance. In addition, well-conditioned abdominals play a vital role in ensuring healthy functioning of the back as well as protection from undue stress and injury.

The exercises in this block focus particularly on strengthening the abdominals in their action of spinal flexion and on recruiting the abdominals for lumbopelvic and trunk stabilization. As previously mentioned, these terms are synonymous in the context of this book. However, using these respective terms helps draw attention to the area in discussion. When the stability is focused in the lower spine, namely the lumbopelvic region—typically when the hips and legs are involved in the exercise—I have referred to this as *lumbopelvic stabilization* (stability). When the stability is focused more on the thoracic region, such as when the upper body is involved, I have referred to it as *trunk stabilization* (stability).

As always, precision in activating the correct muscles and in the execution of the movement is crucial to achieving a positive outcome. If done poorly, not only will the exercise fall short of its goal, but it may actually result in injury or compound an existing problem.

It is important to note that Pilates is not a one-size-fits-all method of conditioning. Often, modifications need to be made in order to achieve the desired objectives, particularly when working the abdominals. It is imperative to work at an appropriate level and increase the challenge incrementally. Ultimately, well-conditioned abdominals contribute positively to many activities of daily living and to athletic pursuits.

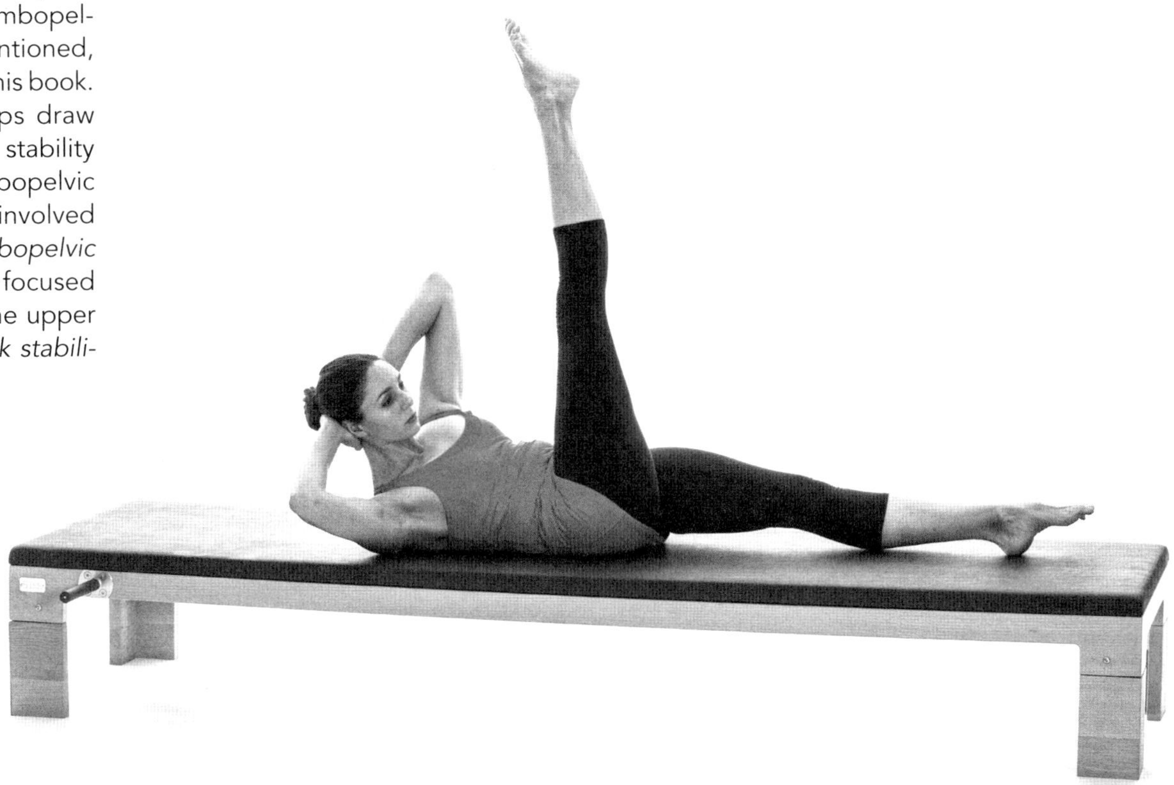

Hundred

Muscle Focus

- Abdominals
- Hip flexors

Objectives

- To improve abdominal strength
- To improve hip flexor control
- To develop lumbopelvic stabilization

This exercise is one of the signature abdominal exercises of the Pilates method, highlighting the powerhouse. The name of the exercise is derived from the breath pattern—each inhalation and exhalation is a single breath cycle and should last for 10 counts (5 counts for the inhalation and 5 counts for the exhalation). This breath pattern is repeated 10 times, totaling 100 counts. This does not mean taking 100 breaths!

I often use *active breathing* during this exercise, in which the work of the respiratory muscles is accentuated by dynamically contracting the muscles involved in exhalation and inhalation. Ron Fletcher, a wonderful first-generation teacher and pioneer of Pilates, whom I am honored to have called a friend, coined the term *percussive breathing.* The percussive quality of the breath going in and out as well as the arm movement makes both the breath and movement more active and dynamic—this is a good strategy if done well. However, if it induces tension, a more relaxed approach should be adopted. The active breathing together with the brisk motion of the arms will increase the heart rate, stimulate circulation, and elevate the body temperature, which was supposedly one of Joseph Pilates' goals for this exercise.

The Mat: Hundred can be counterproductive if certain elements are not in place, including strong abdominals and the ability to lift the trunk into adequate spinal flexion. I encourage you to practice preparation exercises to build up to this exercise (see Modification). When doing the Mat: Hundred, keep the legs at a height that your abdominal strength and control can support—legs perpendicular to the floor is less challenging; legs lowered toward the floor is more challenging. Ultimately, the lower back must not lift off the mat. The classic version of the exercise, as Joseph Pilates performed it, is with the feet at eye level. However, keeping the legs at this height demands a great deal of strength, control, and practice.

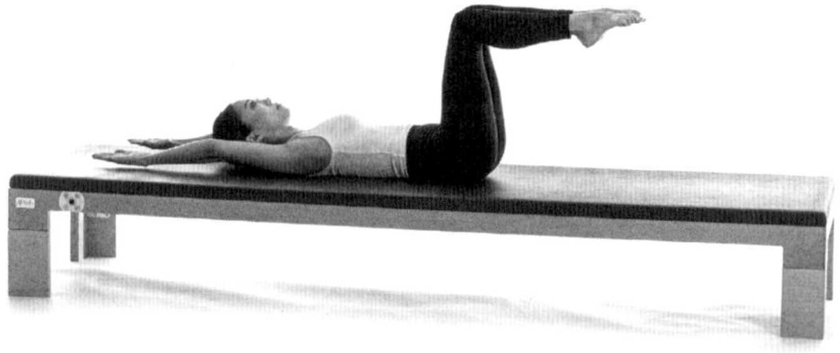

Setup. Lie supine with the legs in a tabletop position. Hold the arms straight, directly overhead and shoulder width apart, with the palms facing up.

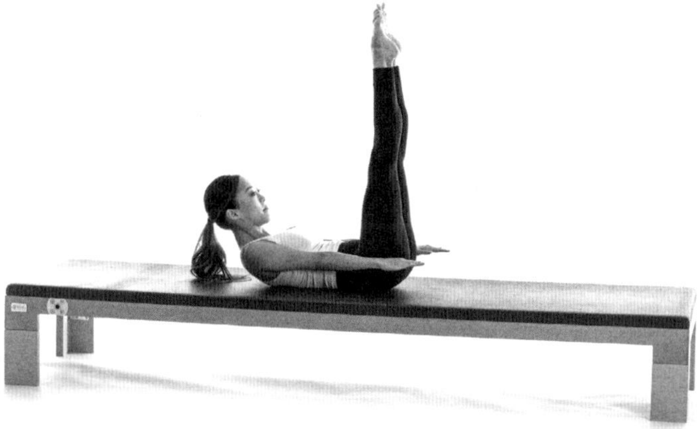

Exhale. Lift the trunk into the Mat: Chest Lift position by drawing in the abdominals, lifting the upper spine, and lowering the arms to the sides of the body until they are parallel to the floor. Allow the lumbar spine to sink into the mat when lifting the upper spine, vertebra by vertebra, until the scapulae have lifted off the mat. Simultaneously straighten the legs to the appropriate height for you (the lower the legs are held, the more challenging the exercise becomes).

Inhale. Maintain consistent height of the upper trunk while keeping the legs stable and focusing on the contraction of the abdominals. Prepare to begin pumping the arms for 5 counts.

Imagery

Visualize the movement of the arms generating energy like a generator; this energy helps keep the trunk stable, the abdominals active, and the legs supported.

- Contract the abdominals, imprinting the lower back into the mat.
- Relax the neck and shoulders.
- Keep the pumping motion smooth, small, and free of tension.

MODIFICATION

To make this exercise easier while building up the required skills, keep the feet on the floor or the legs bent in tabletop position, thereby decreasing the load on the hip flexors and lower back, and in turn lowering the demand on the abdominals.

Furthermore, if you have tight hamstrings, I recommend bending the knees during this exercise. Tight hamstrings will make it difficult to straighten the legs while keeping them in a perpendicular position (if your abdominals are not yet strong enough to hold them opposite the eyes). The result is that the legs will be forced to be held low, making the exercise excessively challenging for the abdominals.

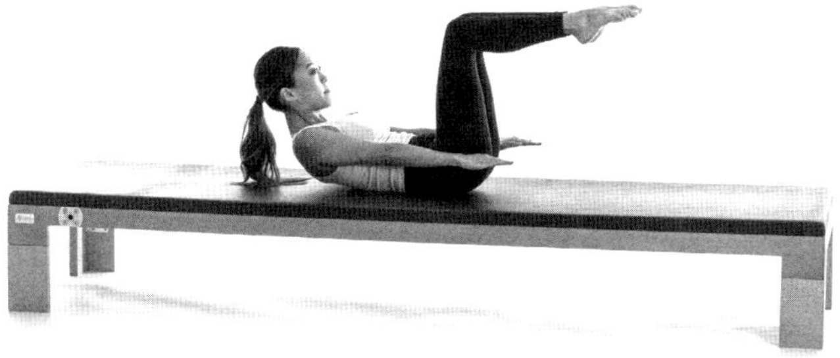

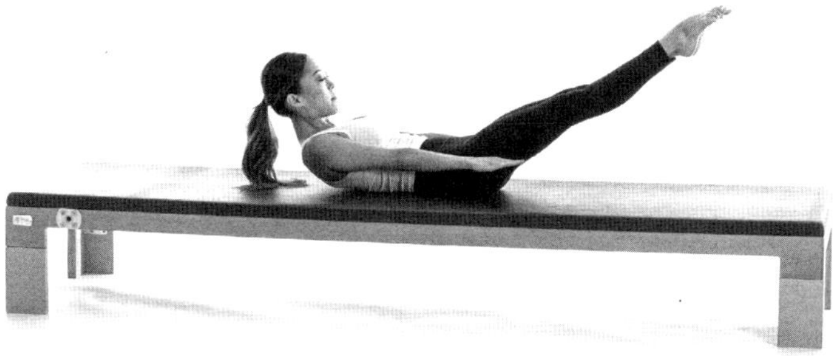

Exhale. Pump the arms up and down with a small pulsing movement for the duration of 5 counts. Legs on a diagonal with the feet opposite the eyes is the optimum position.

Inhale. Continue to pump the arms for the duration of 5 counts. Keep the arms close to the sides of the body. Repeat the breath cycle (exhale and inhale) 10 times.

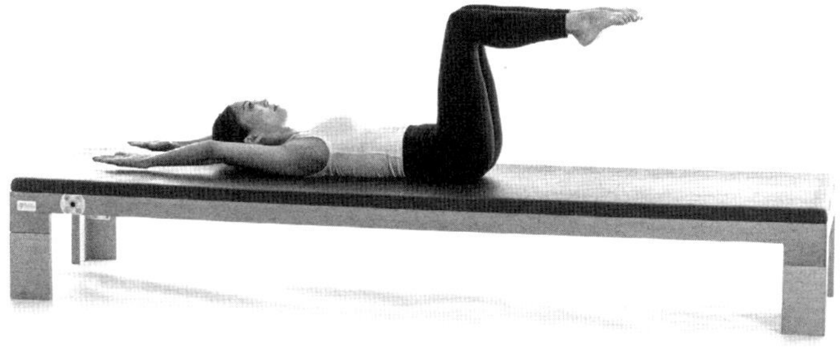

Exhale. Bend the legs to tabletop position and lower the spine, taking the arms overhead. Return to the start position.

Roll-Up

Muscle Focus

- Abdominals
- Hip flexors

Objectives

- To improve abdominal strength
- To improve hip flexor control
- To improve lower back flexibility
- To develop spinal mobility and stability

The Mat: Roll-Up activates the abdominals as both movers and stabilizers. In the initial phase, the abdominals are recruited to move the body into spinal flexion. Next, the hip flexors are introduced to lift the trunk and pelvis off the mat, flexing the body at the hip joint while the abdominals (with assistance from the back extensors) stabilize the trunk and maintain the desired C curve of the spine. In the sitting position, with the shoulders directly above the hip joints, concentrate on further engaging the abdominals, remaining in the C curve and elongating the muscles of the back (particularly the lower back).

I have made several choreographic changes to this exercise from the classic form. The first is that I advocate pausing in the sitting position with the shoulders above the hips, rather than reaching all the way forward with the trunk over the legs. The reason for this change is to avoid stretching the hamstrings excessively too early in the session, when they may not yet be ready to be stretched. The objective is to gently warm up the back muscles and the abdominals while providing a very light stretch for the hamstrings.

The second change is the positioning of the head. In the classic form, the head is lowered and placed between the arms when in the sitting phase of the exercise. I prefer that the head follow the natural line of the spine, in which case it is held higher up so that the neck and face can be clearly observed from the side, with the arms parallel to the floor.

Finally, in the classic form the feet are dorsiflexed. I prefer the feet to be plantarflexed, with the legs straight, or slightly bent if the hamstrings are tight. When the feet are dorsiflexed, there is a strong tendency to overuse the quadriceps, including the rectus femoris (a two-joint hip flexor). I prefer to downplay the activity of the hip flexors in this exercise because they have a tendency to overshadow the work of the abdominals, making it difficult to maintain the C curve when lifting off the mat. That said, the hip flexors clearly play an important role, particularly when the pelvis, together with the trunk, is lifted off the mat. This version of the roll-up accentuates the long lines of the arms, legs, and spine and is aesthetically very appealing. In addition, by adopting a large

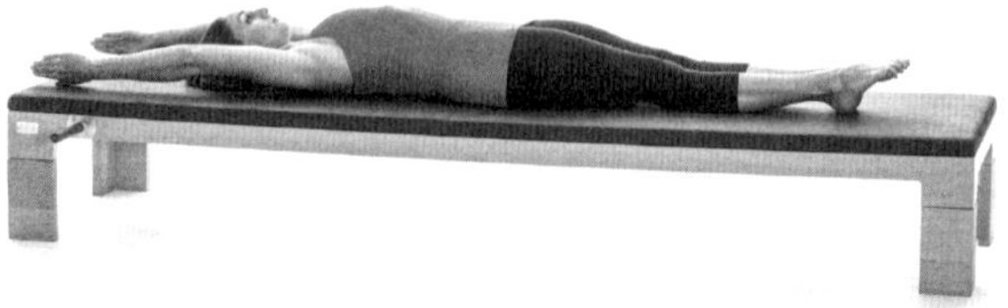

Setup. Lie in a supine position with the arms overhead, palms facing each other, legs straight and together, and feet plantarflexed. Draw the ribs down and together while accentuating the overhead reach of the arms. Keep the arms shoulder width apart.

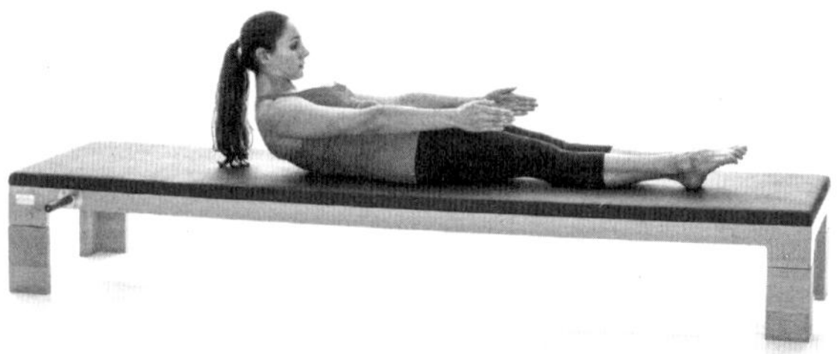

Inhale. Engage the abdominals and begin the movement with the arms, following with the head and upper spine. Pause in the chest lift position, further engaging the abdominals and imprinting the lower back into the mat. Prepare to lift forward off the mat to a sitting position by activating the hip flexors.

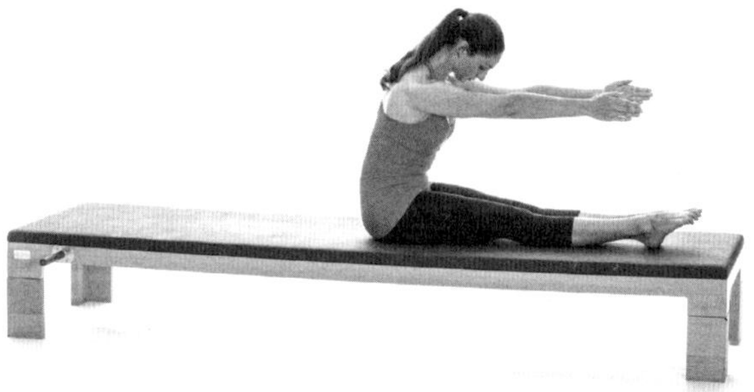

Exhale. Maintain stability of the trunk with the abdominals, assisted by the back extensors, as you peel the spine off the mat, vertebra by vertebra, keeping the C curve shape of the trunk. Pause when the shoulders are above the hips. The curve should extend from the top of the head and the fingertips through the spine to the tips of the toes—hollow and deep.

C curve as opposed to a small C curve (found in the classic form), the back muscles are activated, which in turn assist to unload and protect the spine—the perfect blend of aesthetic appeal and scientific rationale.

Imagery

As you roll up, visualize holding the reins of a horse and being gently raised off the mat and then lowered back down. The movement should appear effortless and the gentle C curve of the body should remain consistent and stable when lifting and lowering the trunk.

- When supine, do not allow the ribs to thrust upward as the arms reach overhead.
- Maintain a C curve of the trunk when lifting off the mat and lowering back down, as well as when in the sitting position.
- Keep the head aligned with the spine.

MODIFICATION

If the regular Mat: Roll-Up proves too difficult because of tight lower back muscles, tight hamstrings, or insufficient abdominal strength, start the exercise with the knees bent. Inhale; lift the arms, head, and upper spine. Exhale; roll up, simultaneously straightening the legs. Inhale while maintaining the C curve in the sitting position. Exhale and roll down, simultaneously bending the knees. Return to the start position. Straightening the legs at the most challenging point in the exercise, when the trunk and pelvis are lifted off the ground, assists in overcoming this obstacle.

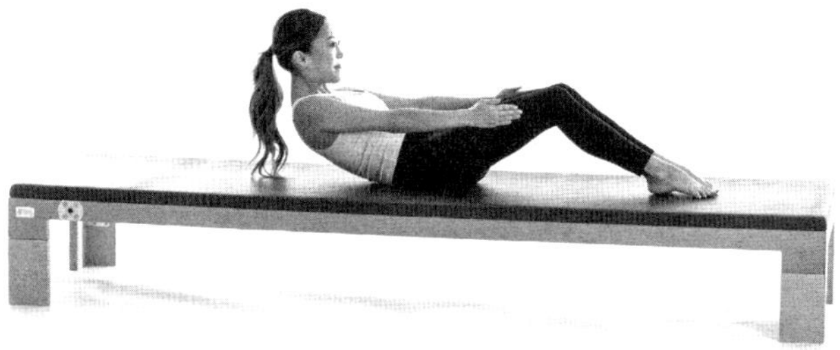

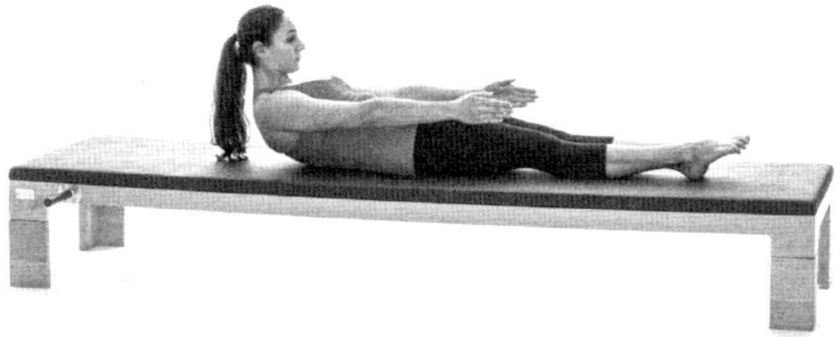

Inhale. Maintain this stable position with the trunk, emphasizing the stretch in the lumbar spine. Hold the arms at shoulder height (parallel to the floor) and accentuate the elongated neck position, keeping the neck and shoulders relaxed.

Exhale. Roll down, vertebra by vertebra, through the spine. Avoid burying the head between the arms. Pause momentarily when the lower back is imprinted into the mat, before lowering the trunk fully and taking the arms overhead. Return to the start position (neutral spine). Repeat 5-10 times.

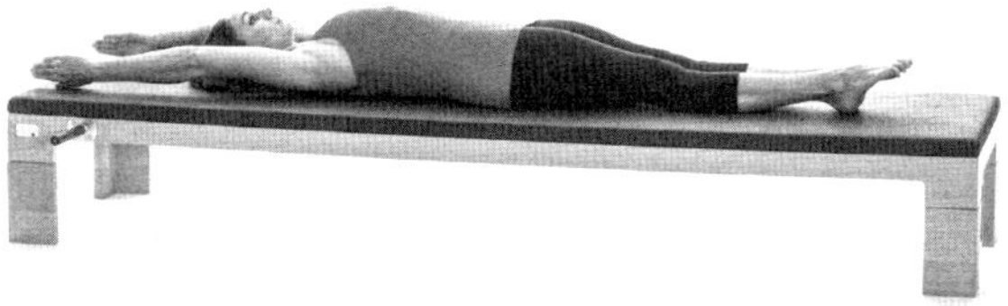

Establish a stable core with the abdominals, controlling the tendency to thrust the ribs forward and hyperextend the lumbar spine when taking the arms overhead.

Neck Pull

Muscle Focus

- Abdominals
- Hip flexors
- Back extensors

Objectives

- To improve abdominal strength
- To improve hip flexor control
- To improve back extensor control
- To improve hamstring flexibility
- To develop spinal mobility and stability

Contrary to what the name implies, pulling on the neck is the one thing to avoid in this exercise. Tackle this exercise only after having achieved proficiency in the Mat: Roll-Up. Placing the hands behind the head (as opposed to the arm movement in the Mat: Roll-Up) alters the center of gravity and the levers of the movement, making the Mat: Neck Pull more difficult than its "cousin." In addition, reaching forward over the legs with the trunk demands more flexibility than is required in the Mat: Roll-Up. Extending the spine in a sitting position and establishing upright alignment of the trunk necessitates core strength and well-conditioned trunk stabilizers, particularly back extensors, as well as adequate hamstring flexibility.

From the sitting position, hinge the trunk backward as one unit, keeping the back straight, before rolling down. Due to the demands of this exercise, it should be performed later in a session and not as part of a warm-up.

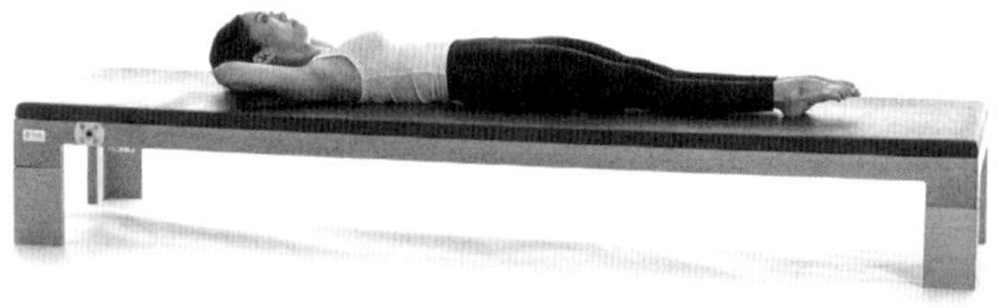

Setup. Lie supine with the legs straight and together, feet plantarflexed. Interlace the fingers behind the head and keep the elbows wide.

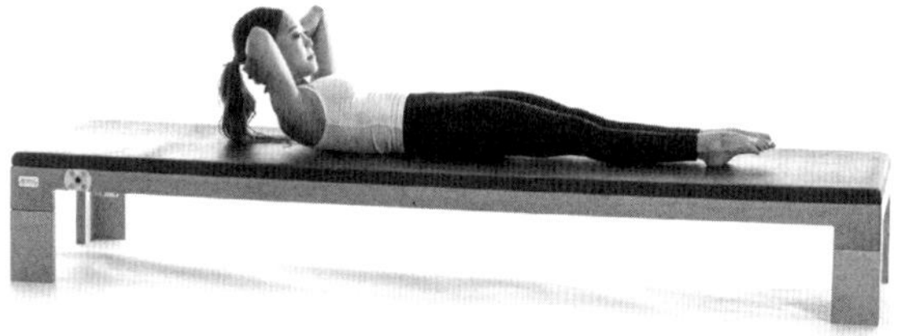

Inhale. Lift the upper spine and shoulder girdle, beginning with the top of the head, and allow the lumbar spine to sink into the mat.

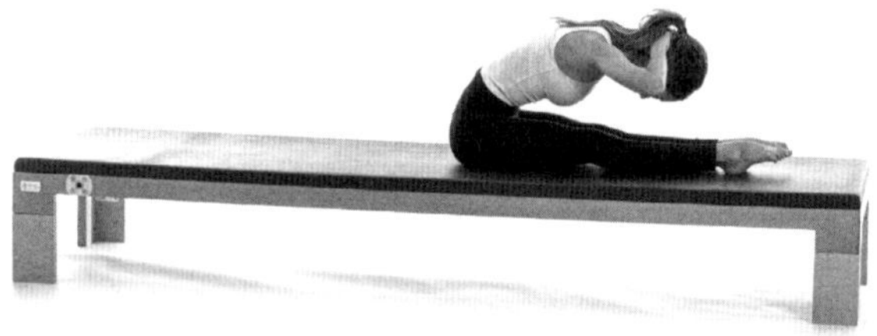

Exhale. Roll up, continuing the movement forward until the trunk is over the legs.

Imagery

The smooth, rolling motion that is desired in this exercise is similar to that of a carpet rolling up. The second phase, the move from forward flexion into the upright sitting position, can be likened to pulling over a young, green tree and then allowing it to slowly spring back. Another image I often use is rolling up with the back against a wall.

- Keep the elbows wide.
- Avoid pulling on the neck and thrusting the head forward during the roll-up phase.
- Hinge back with a straight and stable trunk before rolling down through the spine.

MODIFICATION

A less challenging version may be used until adequate control has been achieved to perform the original exercise. Once the head and shoulders have been lifted off the mat, reach the arms forward toward the feet as in the Mat: Roll-Up. Roll up, and when the chest is over the legs, place the hand back behind the head. When returning to the supine position, rather than hinging back, roll the spine down from the upright perpendicular position, vertebra by vertebra, starting from the sacrum.

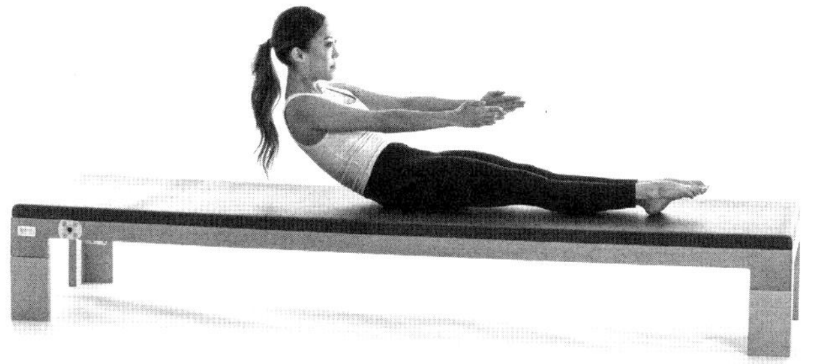

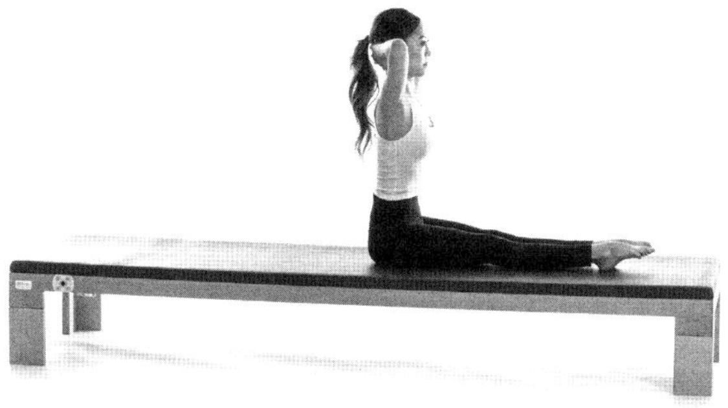

Inhale. Roll the spine up to a sitting upright position, articulating each vertebra on the longitudinal axis.

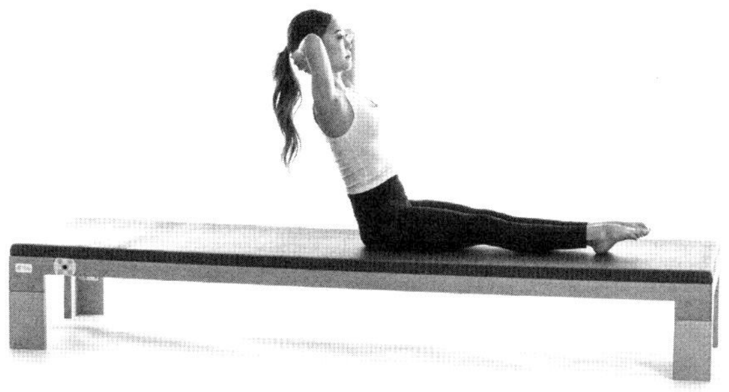

Exhale. Hinge back, keeping the trunk straight on a diagonal line.

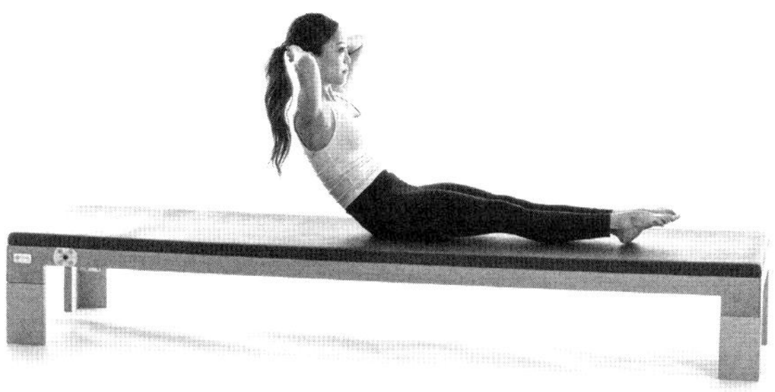

Roll down to the supine position, articulating through each vertebra. Return to the start position. Repeat 5-10 times.

MAT

Abdominal Work

INTERMEDIATE

Muscle Focus

- Abdominals
- Hip flexors

Objectives

- To improve abdominal strength
- To improve hip flexor control
- To develop lumbopelvic stabilization

Single-Leg Stretch

This exercise belongs to a relatively large group of abdominal exercises that develops abdominal strength in a stabilizing mode (isometric contraction), meaning the trunk and the pelvis are absolutely stable as the limbs move. It is important to pay attention to the positioning of the head, which should be aligned with the spine, supported, and held as still as possible. The pumping action of the legs, which amplifies the abdominal work, should not affect the stability of the pelvis, trunk, or head. With each repetition, press firmly into the shin just below the knee and bear down as if driving the hip into the mat. This helps to accentuate the contraction of the abdominals as well as assist in keeping the trunk lifted.

This exercise is an excellent preparation for the Mat: Double-Leg Stretch, in which both arms reach overhead as both legs straighten forward, making stabilization of the pelvis and trunk much more challenging. In the case of the Mat: Single-Leg Stretch, only one leg straightens at a time while the other offers support for the trunk as the hands hold on to it.

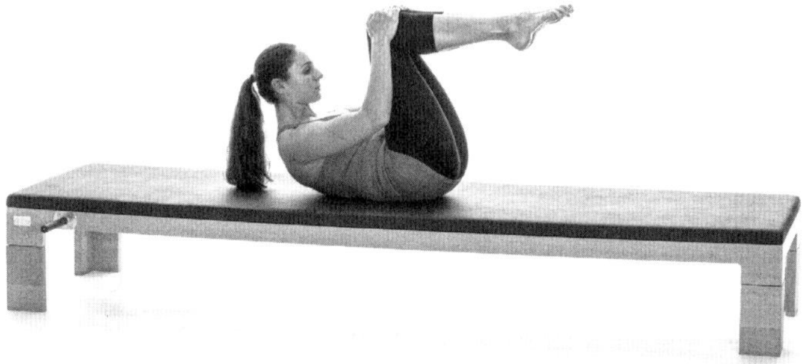

Setup. Lie supine and draw the knees toward the chest to approximately 100 degrees of hip flexion (10 degrees beyond perpendicular) and the shins parallel to the floor. Simultaneously lift the trunk into forward flexion with the scapulae off the mat and allow the lumbar spine to sink into the mat. Place the hands on the shins just below the knees.

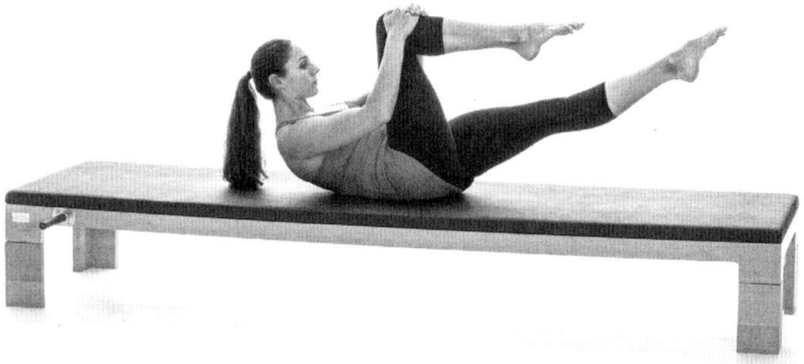

Exhale. Straighten one leg and place the hands firmly on the shin of the opposite leg just below the knee. Hold the bent knee slightly closer to the chest than in a typical tabletop position; however, keep the shin parallel to the floor.

Imagery

The in-and-out movement of the legs conjures up the image of the pistons of an engine as they fire, moving with absolute precision. The powerhouse serves as the engine that drives the pistons.

- Keep the trunk stable.
- Keep both feet at approximately eye level as they alternate in and out.
- Make sure the shin of the bent leg is parallel to the floor and do not bring the knee in too close to the chest (the angle of the thigh should be approximately 10 degrees beyond the perpendicular).

PROGRESSION

After the basic version of the exercise has been mastered, an alternate arm pattern can be used to accompany the movement of the legs. The hand on the opposite side as the bent knee is placed on the shin just below the knee, pressing down to amplify the abdominal work. The other hand reaches toward or actually holds the heel of the bent leg (depending on arm length); this encourages keeping the trunk lifted in forward flexion and introduces an additional element of coordination.

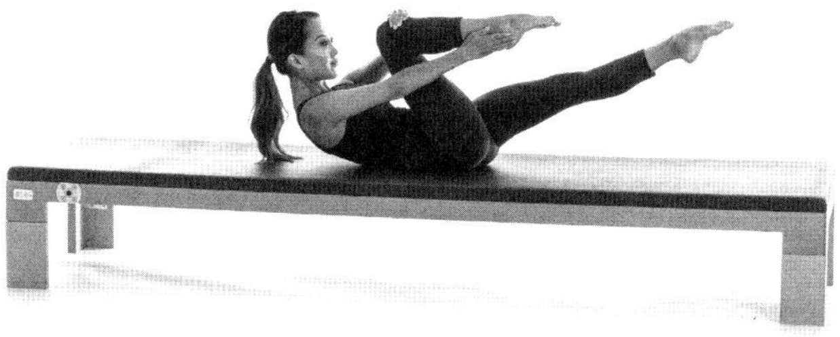

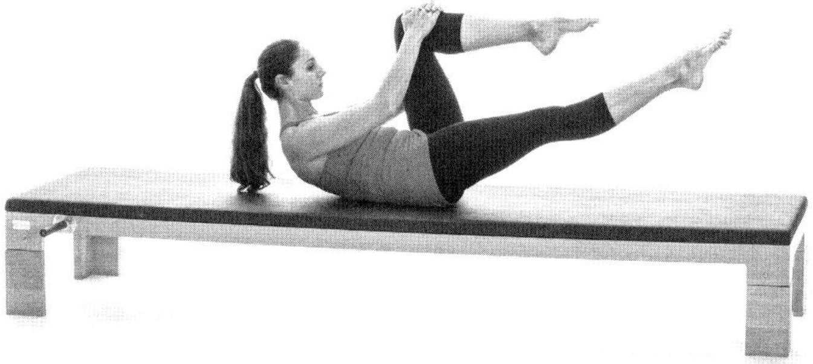

Inhale. Let go of the shin and simultaneously change legs, keeping the feet on the same horizontal plane and the legs close to the centerline of the body as you do so.

Exhale. Straighten the opposite leg fully and transfer the hands to the bent knee. Repeat the breath cycle (exhale and inhale) 10 times.

Criss-Cross

Muscle Focus

- Abdominal obliques
- Hip flexors

Objectives

- To improve abdominal strength with emphasis on the obliques
- To improve hip flexor control
- To develop pelvic stabilization and trunk rotation

The action of the lower body in this exercise is identical to that of the Mat: Single-Leg Stretch. It is a pumping motion, keeping the feet at the same level (horizontal line) and creating a sense of internal resistance for the hip flexors as you draw the knee of the straight leg toward the chest.

The rotation of the trunk is key because it emphasizes the work of the abdominal obliques. There is a tendency to laterally flex the trunk and flare the ribs on the side of the bent leg during the rotation, resulting in a swivel-type motion as opposed to a true rotation. You can prevent this by contracting the internal obliques on the bent-knee side, drawing the lower ribs toward the pelvic crest. In addition, as fatigue sets in, the height of the trunk sometimes begins to decrease and the lower back starts to lift off the mat into hyperlordosis. If this occurs, immediately pause and reestablish the proper position, lifting into forward flexion, before continuing. Forward flexion is the foundation with rotation layered on top of it. It is preferable to stop rather than to compromise good form. Practicing incorrect form, even with the best of intentions, is counterproductive and can lead to

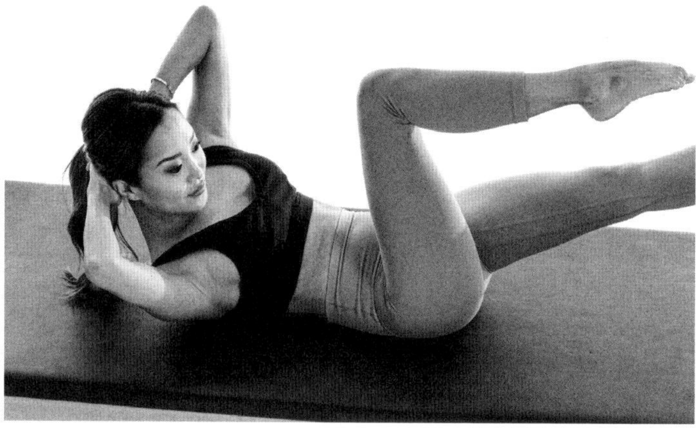

This close-up illustrates the rotation of the trunk and the stability of the pelvis, resulting in strong abdominal oblique activation.

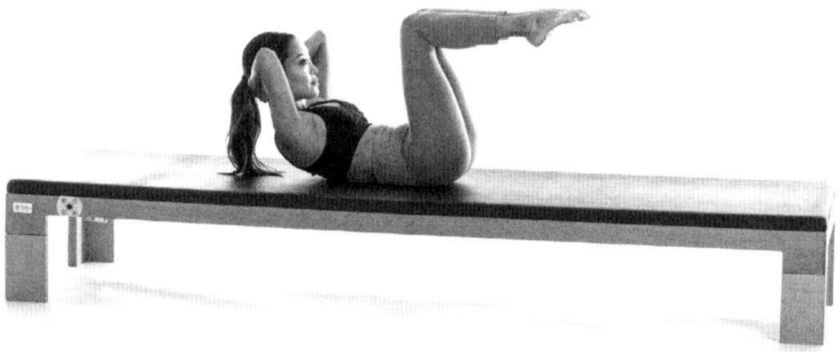

Setup. Lie supine and draw the knees to the chest. Interlace the fingers behind the head and hold the elbows wide. Lift the trunk into forward flexion with the scapulae off the mat, the thighs at approximately 100 degrees of hip flexion, and the shins parallel to the floor.

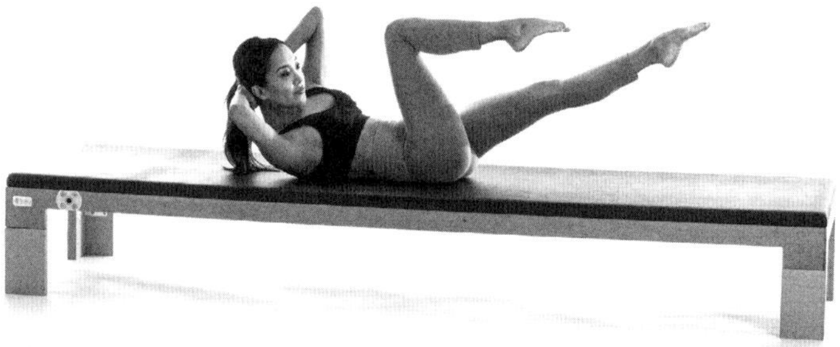

Exhale. Rotate the trunk toward one bent knee, straightening the other leg.

habitually negative movement patterns and possible physical ailments. If the fatigue is excessive, choose an exercise that is similar but easier such as Mat: Chest Lift With Rotation, or cease working the abdominals and move on to the next block.

One other common mistake is flapping the elbows back and forth in an attempt to reach for the knee, with minimal or no rotation of the trunk. This is completely counterproductive. The upper body, including the head and arms, must move as one unit. Keeping the elbows opposite the ears is typically a good, comfortable position.

Imagery

The piston imagery describing the precise leg movements in the Mat: Single-Leg Stretch applies here. The feeling in the waist should be like a rotating disc with the lower section (the pelvis) held absolutely stable and the top section (the trunk) rotating on an axis. Another image might be a chicken turning on a skewer that runs longitudinally through its body.

- Keep the elbows wide and stable.
- Imagine rotating from the waist, avoiding lateral flexion.

MODIFICATION

To assist in achieving correct form during rotation, place the upper hand on the opposite knee (when rotating to the right, place the left hand on the right knee, and vice versa) and use the arm to help lift the trunk into an optimum position. Hold the position of the trunk stable as the hand is placed back behind the head before transitioning to the opposite side and changing legs. Repeat the same on the opposite side.

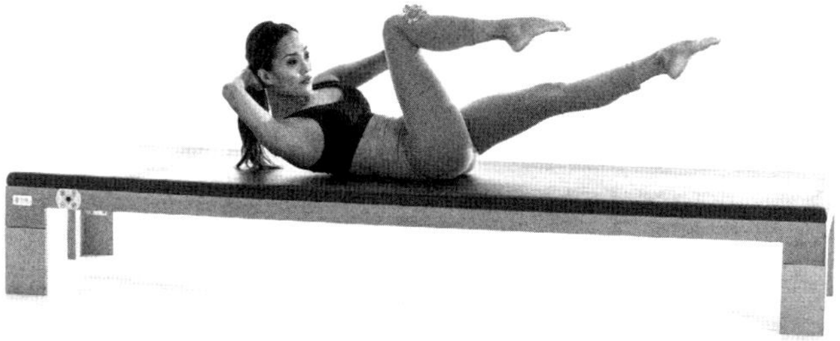

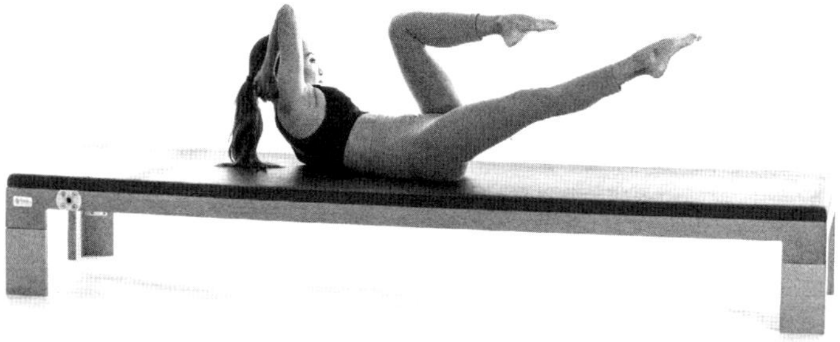

Inhale. Rotate the trunk back to center as it transitions to rotation on the opposite side, and simultaneously begin changing legs, bending the straight one and straightening the bent one.

Exhale. Complete the rotation of the trunk to the opposite side, straightening one leg and bending the other.

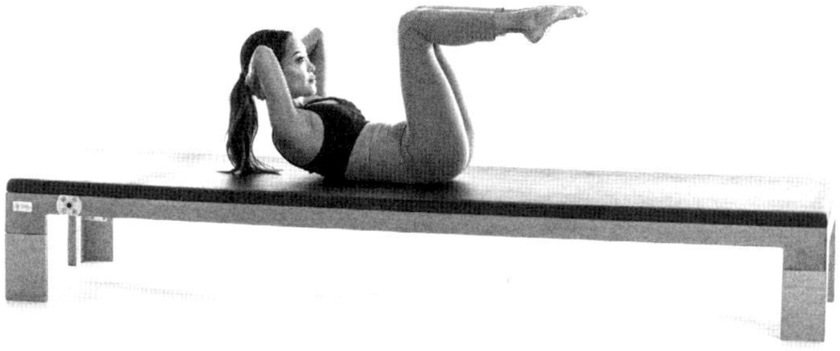

Inhale. Return to the start position. Repeat 5-10 times to each side.

Double-Leg Stretch

Muscle Focus

- Abdominals
- Hip flexors

Objectives

- To improve abdominal strength
- To improve hip flexor control
- To develop lumbopelvic and trunk stabilization

The Mat: Double-Leg Stretch is a very challenging abdominal exercise that emphasizes lumbopelvic and trunk stabilization. The lower back remains firmly anchored on the mat as the arms and legs stretch away from the center of the body and then are drawn back toward the center. Keep the eyes focused forward, the head stable, and the neck and shoulders relaxed. The abdominals provide support and stability as the hip flexors draw the legs in toward the chest and the arms circle around. As the hips reach approximately 100 degrees of hip flexion and the shins are parallel to the floor, place the hands firmly on the shins, press down, and deepen the abdominal contraction. The hip extensors and knee extensors then straighten the legs as the shoulder flexors take the arms overhead.

Imagery

Imagine a rubber band being stretched from both sides and then rebounding, just as the arms and legs are stretched out in opposite directions and are then pulled back to center. This recoiling quality provides the desired dynamic that is the essence of the exercise.

- ○ Maintain a stable spine from the top of the head to the tailbone, imprinting the lower back into the mat.
- ○ Reach the arms as far back overhead as possible, palms facing the ceiling and thumbs touching, without lowering the trunk or elevating the shoulders.
- ○ Keep the feet at eye level (if abdominal strength allows), or raise them if the back starts lifting from the mat.
- ○ Keep the eyes focused forward.

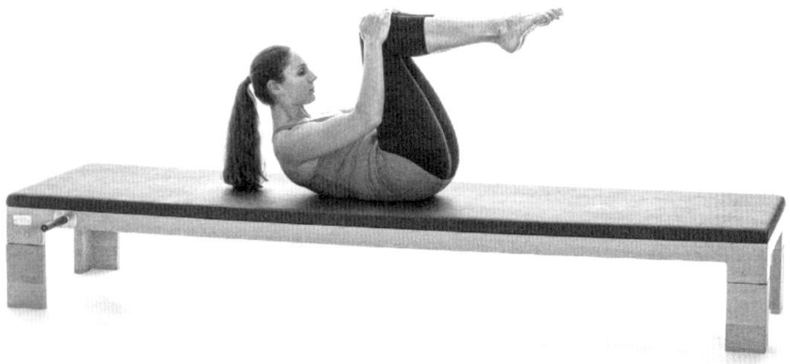

Setup. Lie supine and draw the knees toward the chest. Simultaneously lift the trunk into forward flexion with the scapulae off the mat, the thighs at approximately 100 degrees of hip flexion (10 degrees beyond perpendicular), and the shins parallel to the floor. Place the hands on the shins just below the knees.

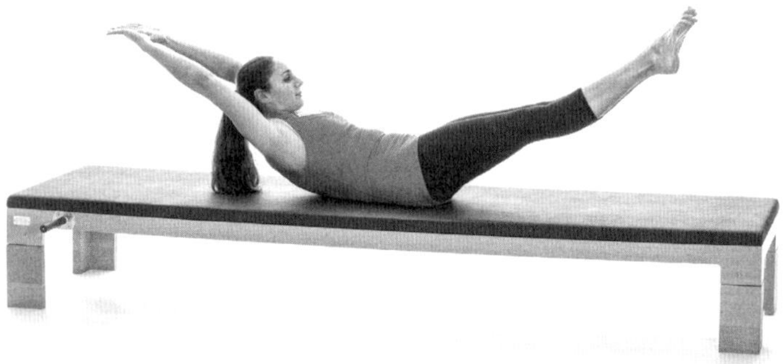

Inhale. Lift the arms overhead and simultaneously straighten the legs in the opposite direction, keeping the trunk stable and the feet at eye level. Recruiting the abdominals and imprinting the back into the mat are vital at this point.

VARIATION

This variation magnifies the concept of elongation and also focuses on the dynamic of a rubber band or spring being stretched and then rebounding. The initial movement of straightening the legs and reaching the arms overhead in the opposite direction is identical to the Mat: Double-Leg Stretch. However, instead of circling the arms around to place the hands back on the shins, the arms reverse the path and return in a straight line directly back to the knees. This variation is very helpful when giving a mat class and there is a lack of space, because the arms do not circle around.

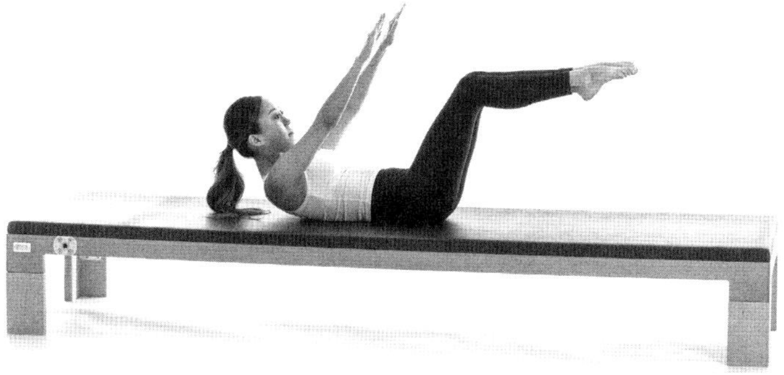

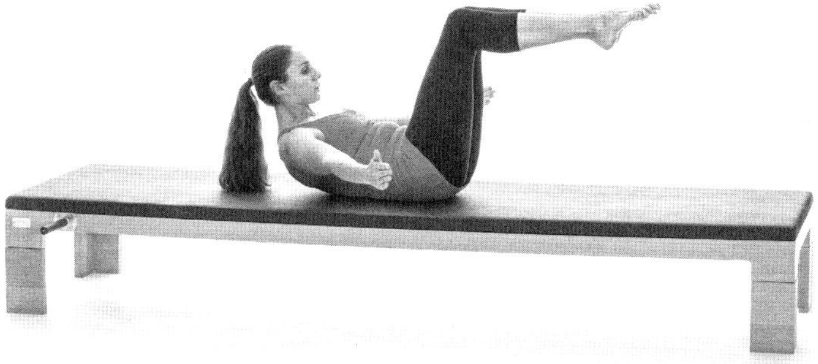

Exhale. Circle the arms out and around while still maintaining a stable trunk. Begin drawing the knees toward the chest.

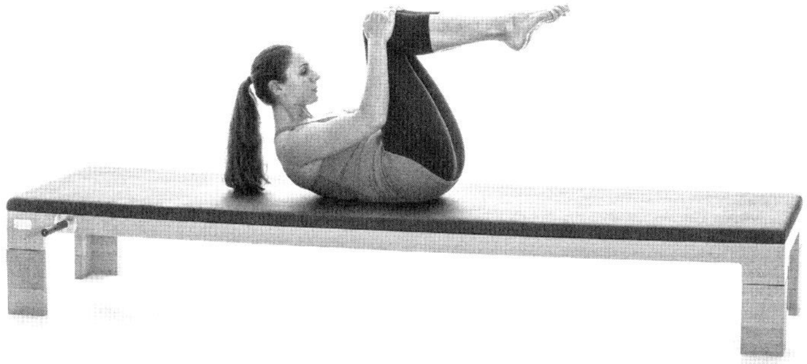

Draw the knees in toward the chest and firmly place the hands on the shins. Return to the start position. Repeat 10 times.

MAT

Abdominal Work

INTERMEDIATE

Hamstring Pull

Muscle Focus

- Abdominals
- Hip flexors
- Hip extensors

Objectives

- To improve abdominal strength
- To improve hip flexor control
- To improve hamstring and hip flexor flexibility
- To develop lumbopelvic stabilization

The Mat: Hamstring Pull prepares you for the high level of lumbopelvic stabilization and abdominal work needed for other intermediate-, advanced-, and master-level exercises. With each pulse of the leg toward the chest, you should focus on deepening the contraction of the abdominals as well as that of the hip flexors, specifically the psoas and iliopsoas, rather than pulling on the hamstrings as the name implies. The support for the position emanates from the abdominals, not from holding on to the leg. Although this exercise is often performed with the lower leg floating about 6 inches (15 centimeters) above the mat, anchoring the lower leg on the mat creates a stable base for stretching both the hamstrings of the lifted leg and the hip flexors of the lower leg. The movement of the legs should be disassociated from the pelvis and not affect its stability. Lift the leg only as high as your flexibility and pelvic control allow.

Imagery

A wonderful image for this movement is a handheld fan opening and swishing closed, then opening in the other direction. The legs move so swiftly that they create a blur of movement.

- Maintain lumbopelvic stabilization as you change legs.
- Maintain consistent trunk flexion.
- Cradle the lifted leg with the hands behind the calf (if flexibility allows).
- Keep the shoulders and neck relaxed.

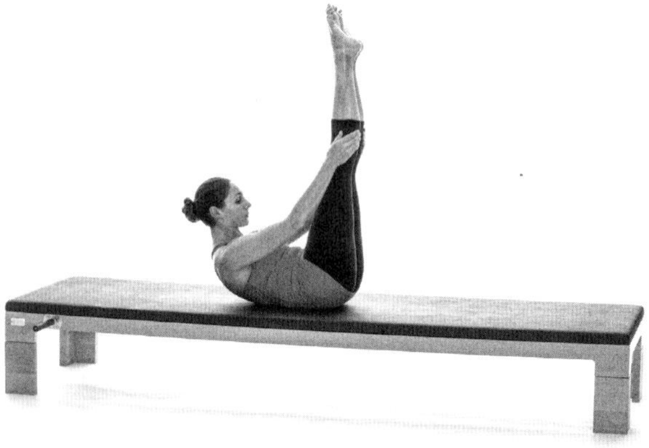

Setup. Lie supine and draw the knees toward the chest, simultaneously lifting the trunk into forward flexion with the scapulae off the mat. Straighten the legs toward the ceiling so they are perpendicular to the mat.

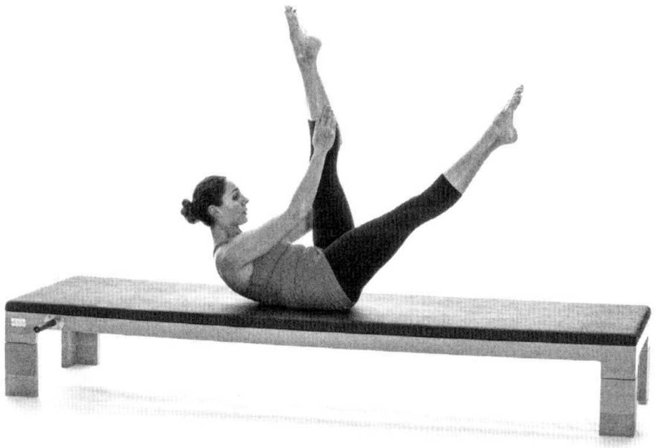

Inhale. Place the hands behind the calf of one leg, and lower the other leg to the mat and anchor it.

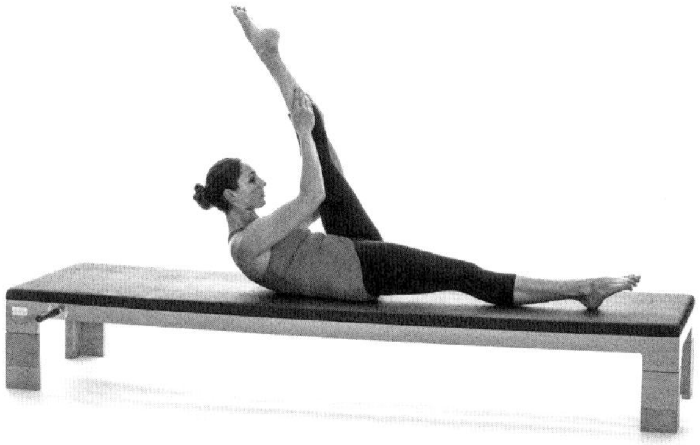

Exhale. Draw the lifted leg closer to the chest, deepening the abdominal contraction, and do two small pulses with the leg. Use percussive breathing, exhaling a puff of air with each pulse.

PROGRESSION

For additional challenge, place the hands behind the head with the fingers interlaced. To add even more challenge, rotate the trunk toward the lifted leg. The three versions (regular, hands behind the head, and trunk rotation) can be done in a sequence of 5-10 repetitions (breath cycles) of each.

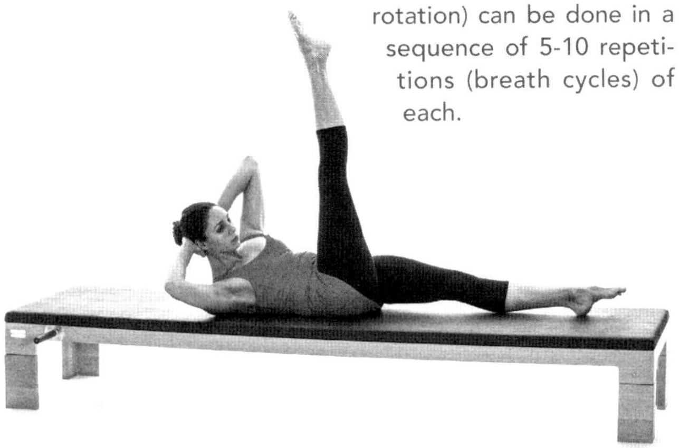

MODIFICATION

Following are several suggestions of modifications for different situations. People with tight hamstrings or hip flexors can bend the knees slightly to assist in achieving proper alignment and positioning of the pelvis. Those with weak abdominals can switch the legs one at a time rather than simultaneously. Use the perpendicular position of the legs as the start position. Holding on to one leg, lower the other to the mat and bring it back to the perpendicular position before lowering the other. As strength improves, the switch can be performed simultaneously.

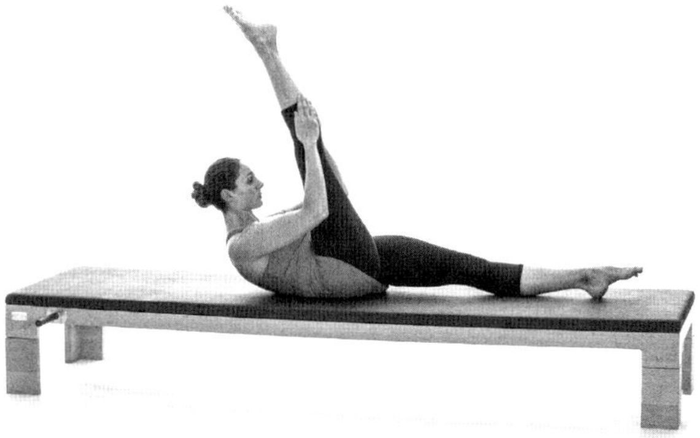

Inhale. Change the legs simultaneously, lowering the lifted leg to the mat and lifting the other toward the chest. The switch should be swift, with absolute stability in the pelvis and trunk. Continue the exercise, alternating legs with each repetition. Repeat the breath cycle (inhale and exhale) 10 times.

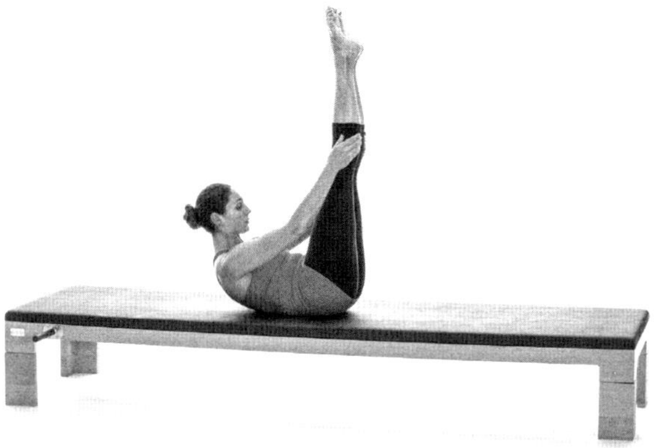

Finish the exercise in the start position, with both legs perpendicular to the floor. Bend the knees and lower the trunk. Return to the start position.

Teaser Prep

Muscle Focus

- Abdominals
- Back extensors
- Hip flexors

Objectives

- To improve abdominal and back extensor strength
- To improve hip flexor control

This exercise prepares you for advanced abdominal work, specifically the Mat: Teaser, and full body integration movements. Although typically categorized as an abdominal exercise, the Mat: Teaser Prep, Mat: Teaser, and their many variations fit comfortably in both the abdominal work block as well as the full body integration block. To view them as only abdominal exercises ignores their multifaceted nature. For the purposes of this book, I have decided to place these exercises in the abdominal work block. The Mat: Teaser Prep, like the Mat: Teaser to follow, incorporates the principles of several of the more fundamental mat work exercises, such as the Mat: Roll-Up, Mat: Rolling Like a Ball, and Mat: Open-Leg Rocker. However, this exercise is more difficult because it requires a high level of control and eliminates the support of the hands and the use of momentum. Find the point of equilibrium, using the back extensors supported by the abdominals and the hip flexors, to create a stable structure. Note that the legs should remain stable throughout, with the shins parallel to the floor. As with the earlier exercises, focus on articulation of the spine when transitioning from extension to flexion and vice versa.

Imagery

The image of a fishing line unwinding as the body rolls down and then being reeled in as the body rolls back up helps to give the feeling of continuous, seamless, and effortless movement, as if being controlled by an external force.

- ○ Articulate the spine when lowering and lifting the trunk.
- ○ Keep the legs stable with the shins parallel to the floor.
- ○ Use the back extensors to complete the movement.

MODIFICATION

Rather than reaching the arms forward, wrap each hand behind the respective thigh and use the arms for support. As you roll down, allow the arms to straighten while still supporting you. When you roll back up, bend the elbows to assist with the roll-up, particularly with the final phase of the back extension. The arms will help achieve the flat back we desire.

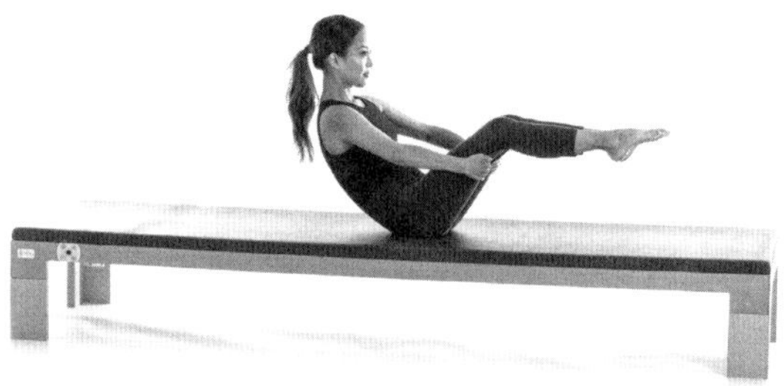

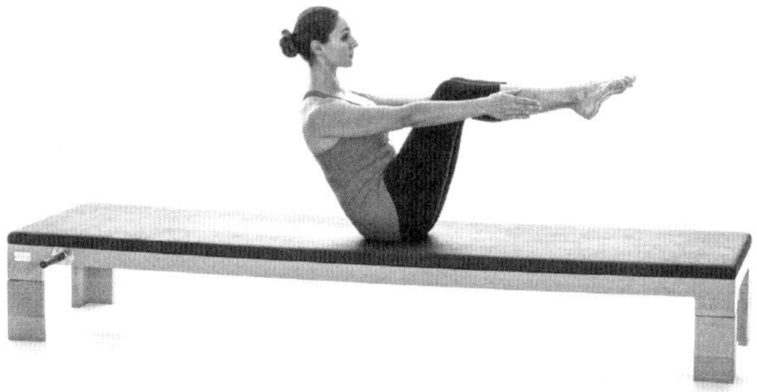

Setup. Sit upright, balancing on the base of the pelvis (sit bones), arms reaching forward in front of the shoulders. Bend the knees with the shins parallel to the floor.

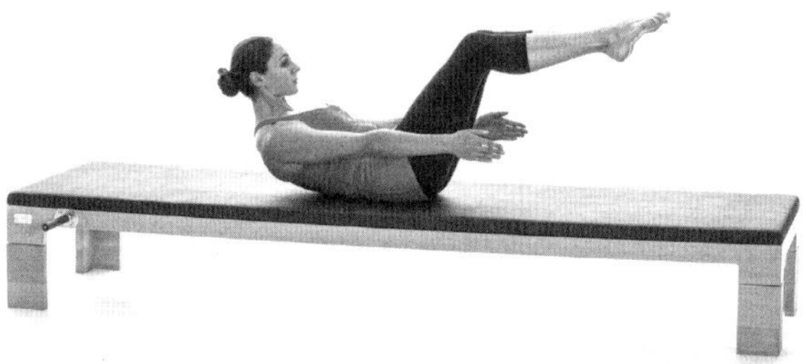

Exhale. Round the lower back and lower the spine to the floor. Go down only to the point where you can maintain complete control, no farther than the base of the scapulae.

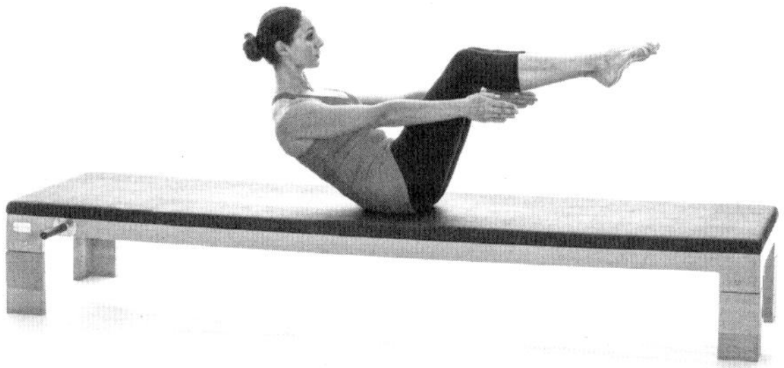

Inhale. Roll back up, maximizing the articulation of the spine.

Complete the movement by extending the back. Return to the start position. Repeat 5 times.

Teaser

This is a combination of several abdominal exercises, particularly the Mat: Teaser Prep and Roll-Up, and balancing exercises, specifically the Mat: Open-Leg Rocker. The start positions of the Mat: Teaser and Open-Leg Rocker are similar, except that in the Mat: Open-Leg Rocker the legs are separate and the hands are holding the legs, while in the Mat: Teaser the arms are overhead and the legs are together. Roll down the spine and reach the arms overhead, keeping the legs stable. Roll up as you would in the Mat: Roll-Up, except that in this exercise the legs are in the air and the movement is completed with the spine extended rather than in a C curve. Maintaining this leg position demands hip flexor control, which in turn demands strong abdominal engagement to prevent stress on the lower back and hyperlordosis. Although this full body exercise places great emphasis on the abdominals, the strength of the back extensors and hip flexors should not be overlooked. They play a prominent role in the success of the movement.

Imagery

Visualize holding the reins of a horse and being gently lowered down and then raised up off the mat. In addition, the image of an inflated tire rolling smoothly (used in the rolling exercises) will assist in making the movement smooth and uninterrupted.

- ○ Articulate the spine when rolling down and up.
- ○ Keep the legs at a consistent angle (whatever angle is appropriate).
- ○ Use the back extensors and lift of the arms overhead to complete the movement.

Muscle Focus

- Abdominals
- Back extensors
- Hip flexors

Objectives

- To improve abdominal and back extensor strength
- To improve hip flexor control
- To develop trunk and lumbopelvic stabilization

PROGRESSION

The Mat: Teaser is a signature Pilates exercise with many variations. I will offer two that can follow in sequence after the movement presented above. The first demands keeping the trunk and arms as stable as possible while the legs are lowered about 6 inches (15 centimeters) and then lifted. This version focuses on lumbopelvic and trunk stabilization, and very controlled activation of the hip flexors. For additional progression, begin from the start position of Mat: Teaser. Lower the trunk to the mat and reach the arms overhead. Simultaneously lower the legs (as low as abdominal strength permits without touching the mat). Then lift the trunk, arms, and legs, returning to the start position. Perform 5 repetitions of each version described.

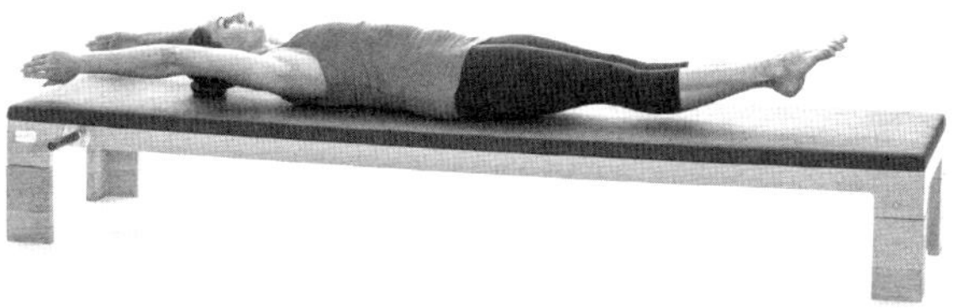

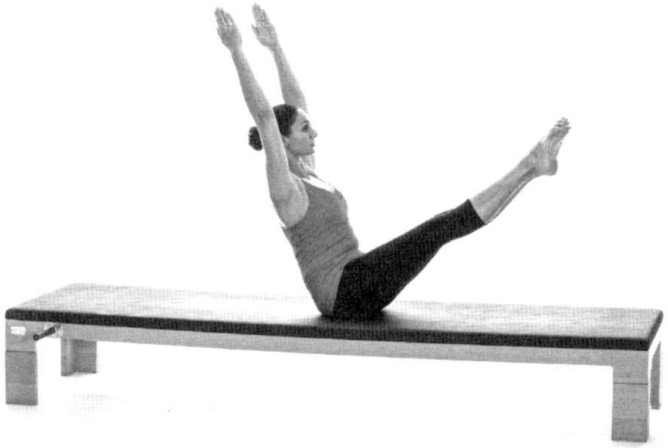

Setup. Sit upright, balancing on the base of the pelvis (sit bones), and straighten the legs at approximately 60 degrees to the floor, creating a V position with the body. Lift the arms overhead.

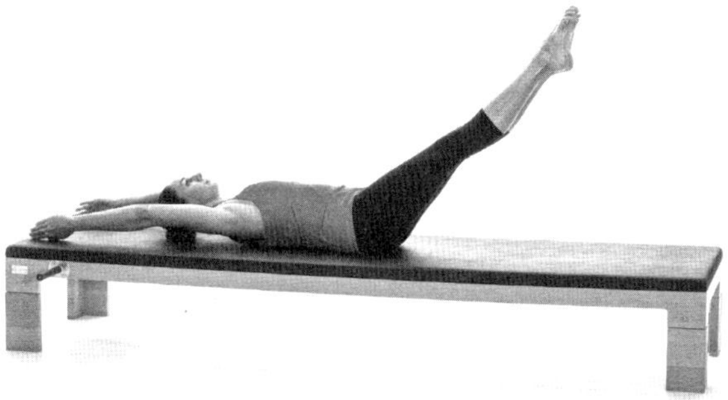

Exhale. Roll down, lowering the arms to shoulder height as you begin to articulate down through the spine, and then reach them overhead after rolling out the spine onto the mat. Keep the legs stable.

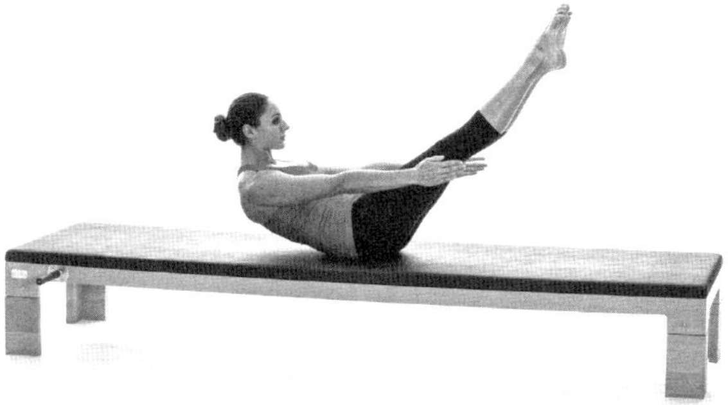

Inhale. Roll up, emphasizing the articulation through the spine.

Complete the movement with back extension and arms overhead. Return to the start position. Repeat 5 times.

Spinal Articulation

When functioning as a coordinated and integrated unit, the spine can move in many directions and ranges of motion with great flexibility. Yet each vertebral joint alone actually offers very little movement. *Spinal articulation* refers to the fine, precise, sequential movement of each vertebra of the spine relative to the next vertebra, as opposed to movement of the spine in rigid sections or even as one "fixed" unit. This concept of sequential spinal mobility was one that Joseph Pilates promoted tirelessly.

The focus of this block is fine articulation of the spine during spinal flexion. It is common for people to be very inflexible in their lower backs, particularly during spinal flexion, because of the lower back's natural orientation toward an arched shape (the opposite of flexion). The motions of spinal flexion and spinal articulation tend to stretch this area and can be very helpful in restoring healthy flexibility to the lower back. Even when individuals have adequate flexibility, they often lack the fine control of the spine required to perform spinal articulation.

Because the abdominals are the flexors of the spine, they are pivotal in the action of spinal articulation. Yet the back extensors should not be ignored. Spinal articulation is a delicate interplay of the flexors and extensors of the spine. In fact, the concept of spinal articulation can be applied to spinal extension as well, which will be discussed in a later chapter.

This chapter contains exercises that involve both extreme flexion of the spine and a degree of weight bearing on the neck and shoulders. It should be noted that both the flexion and weight bearing are controversial because of the potential risks involved. Therefore, extra caution should be adopted and decisions made on a case-by-case basis. When in doubt, seek advice from a medical professional.

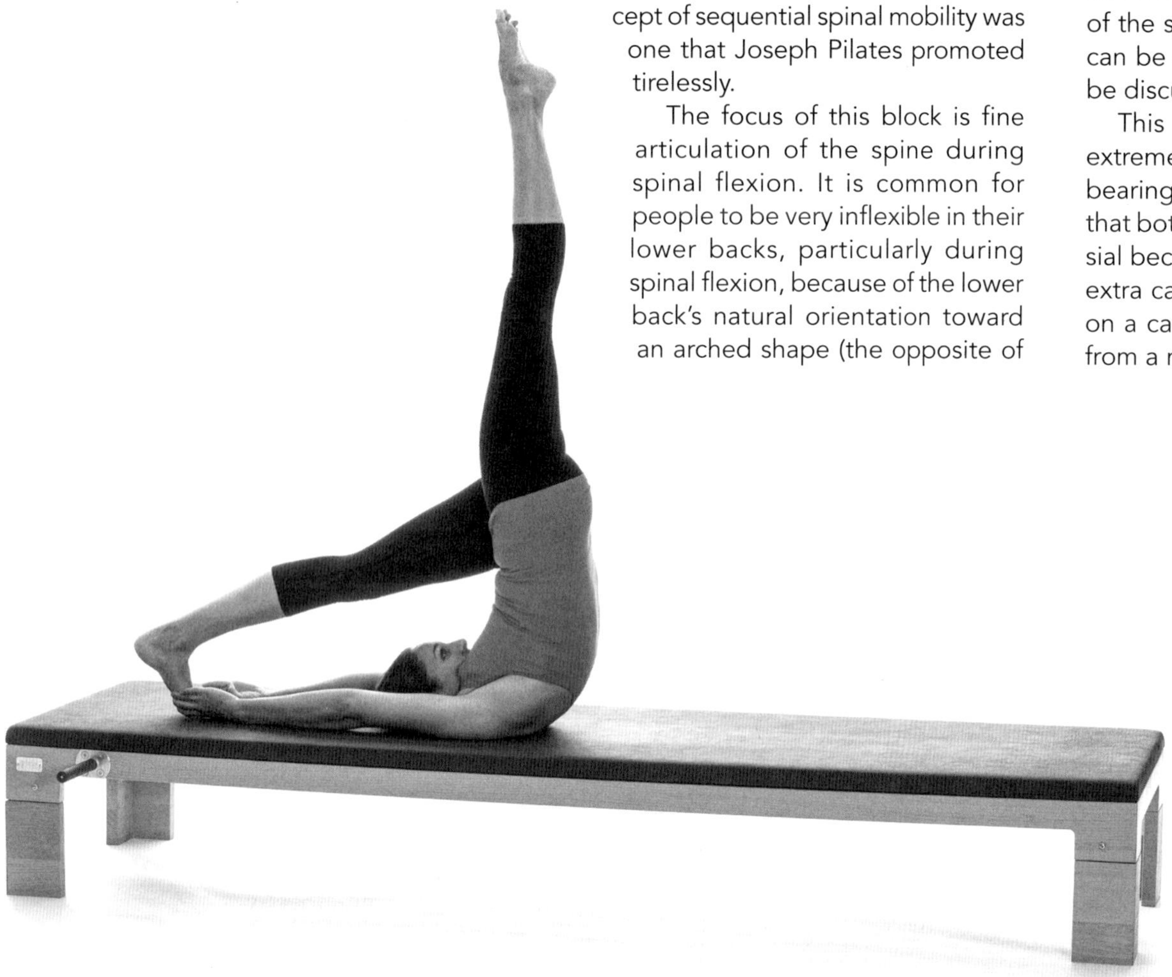

Spine Stretch

This exercise teaches articulation of the spine in a sitting rather than supine position. Emphasize rolling or "peeling" the spine off a wall, vertebra by vertebra, as the trunk moves into forward flexion. Once the spine has completed its range of motion and reached the sacrum, tip the pelvis forward to provide a stretch to the hamstrings. Then place the pelvis back into its upright position, and articulate through the vertebrae in reverse as the trunk moves back into the upright position along the plumb line. There are two distinct phases during the roll-down and roll-up: the articulation of the spine and tipping the pelvis forward and back. The prominent interplay between the spinal flexors and extensors in this exercise helps develop spinal mobility and stability and enhances core control. This exercise can help improve seated posture enormously.

As the upper body rolls forward and then back to the seated position, focus on keeping the legs slightly wider than shoulder width apart, the pelvis stable, and the feet dorsiflexed. Keep the toes facing the ceiling; this ensures that the legs remain in a neutral position (as opposed to internally or externally rotated).

Imagery

Visualize the motion of a young, green tree being pulled over by its top branches and then slowly being released to find its stable, upright position.

- Maximize articulation of the spine when moving from sitting to spinal flexion and when moving back through spinal extension to sitting.
- Keep the feet dorsiflexed, with the toes reaching toward the ceiling.
- Keep the shoulders relaxed.

Muscle Focus

- Abdominals
- Back extensors

Objectives

- To develop spinal articulation
- To develop trunk stabilization
- To improve hamstring flexibility

PROGRESSION

This challenging progression should only be done once you have mastered the original version. When in the forward flexion position over the legs, extend the spine by reaching forward and upward from the lower back through the trunk and head to create a diagonal line. Complete the movement with the arms in line with the trunk and opposite the ears before returning to forward flexion, restacking the pelvis, and rolling through the spine to the upright position.

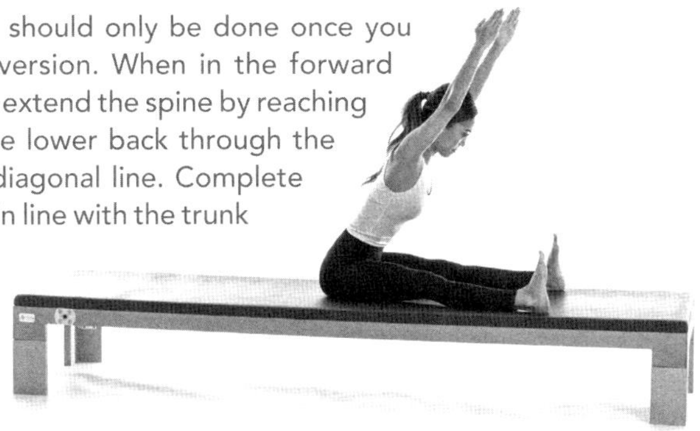

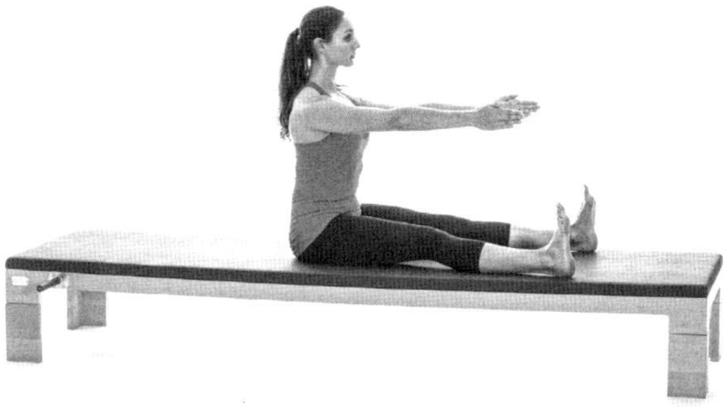

Setup. Sit with the trunk upright and the legs straight, slightly wider than shoulder width apart. Dorsiflex the feet and reach the arms forward, shoulder width apart and parallel to the floor, with palms facing each other.

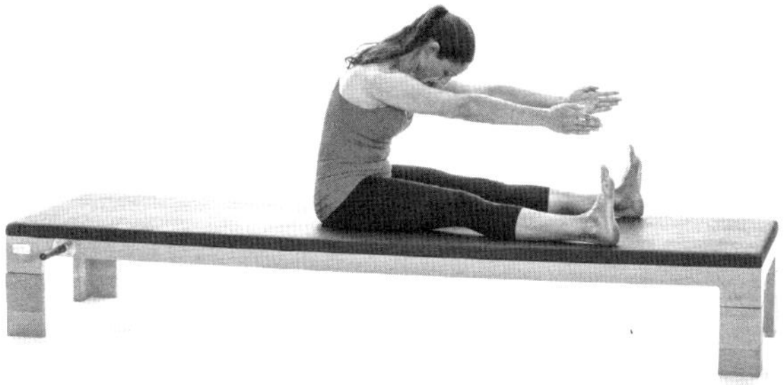

Exhale. Roll down and forward through the spine, starting from the head. Once the articulation of the spine is complete, tip the pelvis forward.

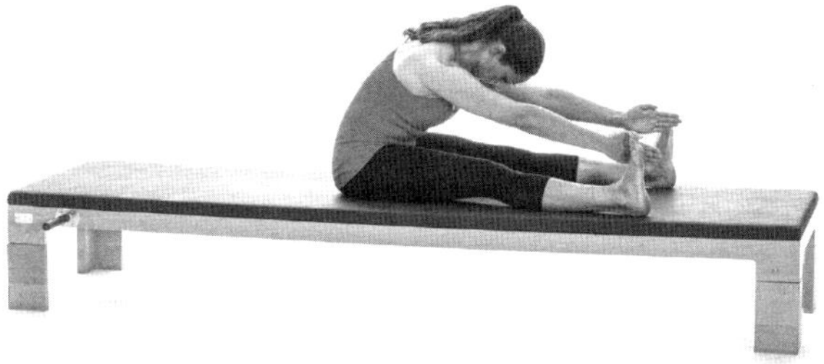

Inhale. Deepen the stretch of the lower back muscles and the hamstrings by drawing the spine further into forward flexion and reaching forward. Keep the shoulders relaxed and the neck elongated.

Exhale. Restack the pelvis and then roll the spine back up to an upright position. Return to the start position. Repeat 5 times.

Rolling Like a Ball

Muscle Focus

- Abdominals
- Back extensors

Objectives

- To develop trunk stabilization
- To develop efficient use of energy
- To develop balance
- To improve spinal flexibility and abdominal control

This exercise embodies the concepts of stabilization and internal flow of energy. The more stable the position is, the smoother the movement will be. It illustrates the controlled eccentric contraction of the back muscles (particularly those of the lower back), deep engagement of the abdominals, and the gentle and consistent rounding of the spine (C curve), which is necessary for the successful execution of much of the abdominal work in Pilates. It is worth noting that although the focus is placed on the abdominals, it is in fact a co-contraction of the back extensors together with the abdominals that creates the desired elongated C curve of the trunk. Once the shape has been established, both the abdominals and back extensors are contracting isometrically. This exercise also introduces balancing on the sit bones, a position that repeats itself in several increasingly challenging exercises. The key to the success of the exercise is keeping the ball shape of the body as consistent and stable as possible. Another muscle group that is significant in maintaining the C curve shape, although not the focus of the exercise, is the biceps. The biceps are activated to help keep the ball shape as contained and compact as possible, ideally with the thighs pressing against the chest and the shins pulled toward the body.

Imagery

Visualize an inflated wheel that rolls effortlessly and without obstruction. The more inflated it is, the more smoothly it rolls. When it is deflated, the rolling is interrupted and halting, just like this exercise appears when a consistent, smooth spinal curve is not maintained, usually due to a tight lower back or a lack of abdominal control.

- ○ Keep the trunk as still and stable as possible.
- ○ Maintain a consistent curve in the spine from the head to the tailbone.
- ○ Pause momentarily on the sit bones and on the shoulders, without the head touching the mat, in each repetition.

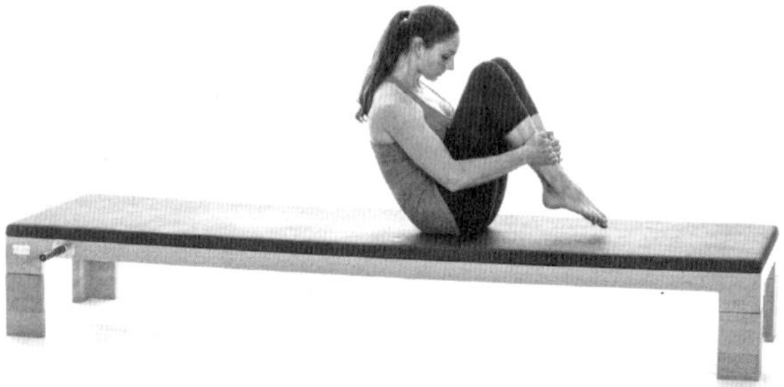

Setup. Sit on the mat with the legs pressed together, holding each leg just above the ankles. Draw the spine into an elongated C curve and lift the feet slightly off the mat, feet plantarflexed. Balancing on your sit bones, keep the head aligned with the natural curve of the spine. (Do not bury the head between the knees.) Deepen the C curve and solidify the position, holding on to the legs for support. Keep the heels as close to the back of the thighs as possible.

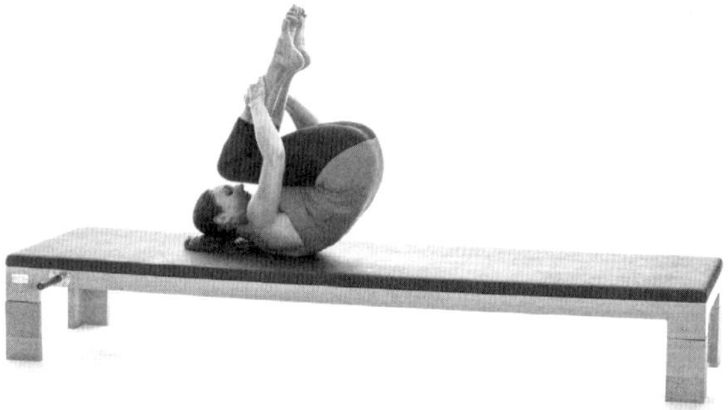

Inhale. Roll back, shifting the weight with as little disruption of the ball shape of the body as possible. Roll only as far as the shoulder girdle (avoid rolling onto the neck and head).

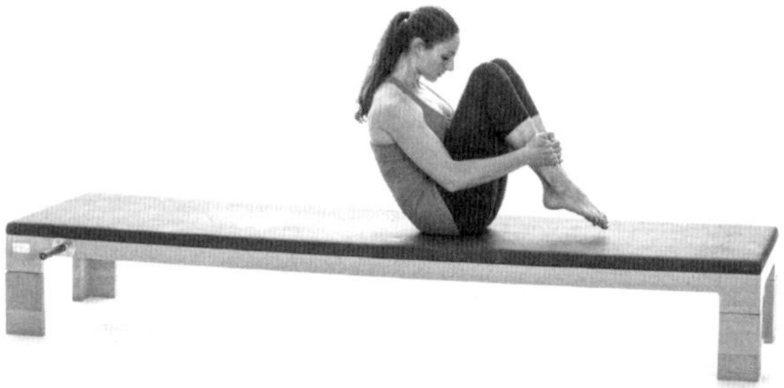

Exhale. Pause (but do not stop), and reverse the direction of the roll, transferring the weight forward. Continue holding the trunk in a stable C curve position, slightly increasing the activation of the biceps by pulling on the legs with the hands. Roll forward through the thoracic and lumbar vertebrae onto the sit bones. Return to the start position.

Pause on the sit bones momentarily before rolling back again. Focus on the internal work occurring in the body to maintain this dynamic, balanced position and keep the internal energy flowing. Repeat 5-10 times.

Seal Puppy

The Mat: Seal Puppy is often done at the end, or near the end, of a mat work routine as a form of stretching and relaxation. I encourage using this exercise to focus on the many movements that have been performed in the session and to allow the effort of the session to culminate in this moment of flow and balance.

This exercise stretches the muscles of the back, shoulders, and neck, particularly the upper trapezius, and also stretches the hip joints. As with the Mat: Rolling Like a Ball and Open-Leg Rocker, you should focus on the internal flow of energy and on balance. Clapping the feet when balanced on the sit bones and when the legs are overhead requires you to pause without stopping the flow of the energy within the body.

Imagery

The image for this exercise is the same as that of several of the rolling exercises, such as the Mat: Rolling Like a Ball—keeping the feeling of an inflated tire rolling back and forth without obstructions or jarring movements. In the balance position, I like to imagine I am balancing on a precipice or floating on a cloud, completely relaxed and void of tension. This is the position in which I often do some relaxation, inner focusing, and meditation.

- Maintain a constant C curve of the spine.
- Keep the head aligned with the spine, and relax the shoulders.
- Place the inside of the legs as high up on the arms (as close to the shoulders) as possible.

MODIFICATION

Lack of hip, shoulder, or back flexibility can often be a limiting factor in this exercise. As a modification, balance on your sit bones, holding on to the ankles with the feet together and the knees facing outward (hip joints in external rotation). Roll back and forth and clap the feet together in the exact same manner as described in the Mat: Seal Puppy. This less demanding position will make the exercise far more accessible.

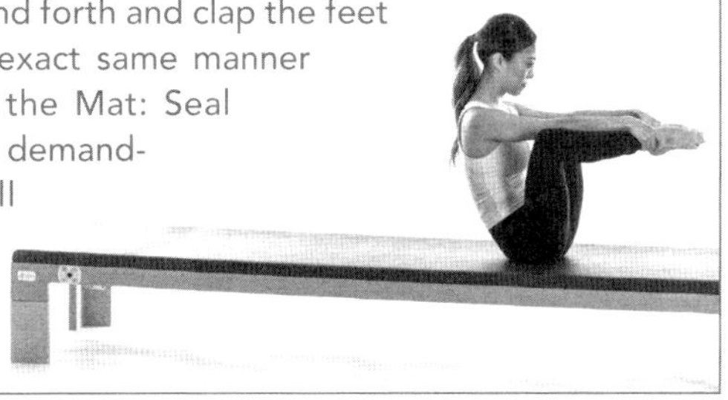

Muscle Focus

- Abdominals
- Back extensors

Objectives

- To develop trunk stabilization
- To develop balance
- To improve spinal flexibility and abdominal control
- To improve hip flexibility

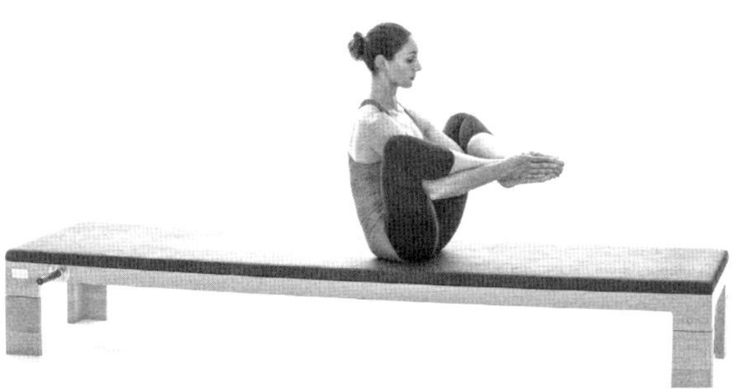

Setup. Sit with the knees open and feet together. Lift one leg and place it over the arm on the same side, as close to the shoulder as possible. Reach the arm under the leg and wrap it around the lower leg, placing the palm on top of the foot. While balancing on the sit bones, do the same with the other leg and arm. Balance in this position with the back rounded, the arms wrapped around the legs, and the hands resting on the feet. Moderately engage the back extensors to avoid excessively rounding the thoracic spine. It will also prove advantageous to slightly adduct the scapulae, because they tend to abduct in this position.

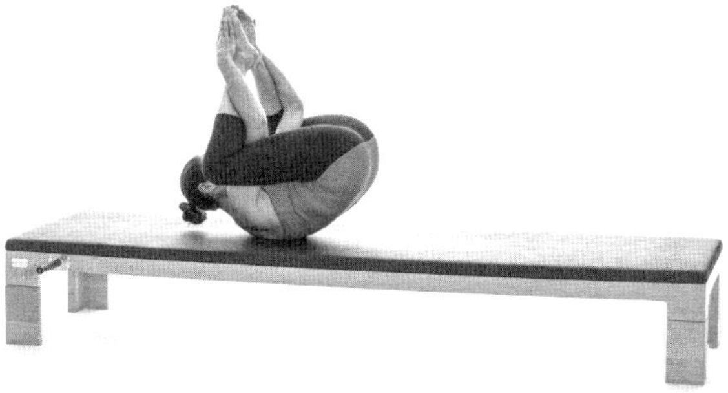

Inhale. Roll back onto the shoulders (avoid rolling onto the neck and head) and clap the feet together three times by moving the legs slightly in and out from the hip joints. Keep the feet relaxed.

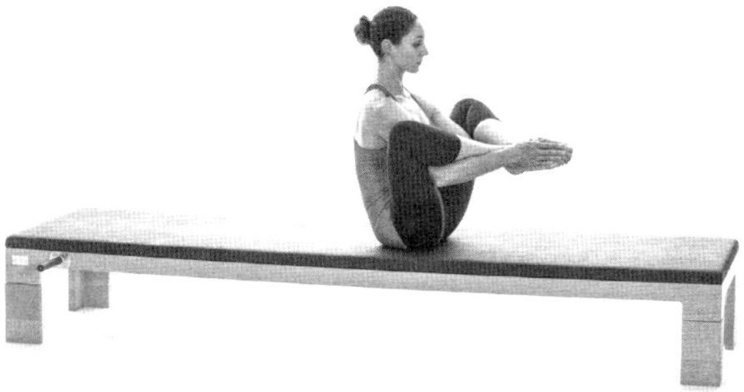

Exhale. Roll up to the balance position on the sit bones and again clap the feet together three times while balancing. Repeat 5-10 times.

After the final repetition, unwrap the legs and arms and roll the spine up to an upright position, holding on to the legs just above the ankles and using the arms to provide support for the trunk. This is a perfect way to complete a mat routine, if you so choose.

Open-Leg Rocker

Muscle Focus

- Abdominals
- Back extensors

Objectives

- To develop trunk stabilization
- To develop balance
- To improve spinal flexibility and abdominal control
- To improve hamstring flexibility

This exercise demonstrates the movement principles of Pilates clearly and profoundly. Not only does it integrate awareness, balance, breath, and control, but it also demands concentration, centering, efficient use of energy, precision, flow of movement, and ultimately, harmony. It demonstrates coordinated activation of the abdominals and the back extensors. Mastering the Mat: Open-Leg Rocker is an exceptional preparation for more advanced, full body exercises, such as the Mat: Teaser and its many variations, as well as similar exercises on the other apparatus.

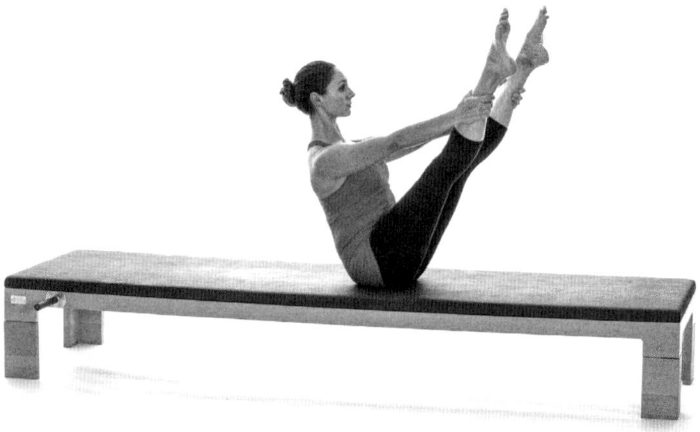

Setup. Sit balanced on the sit bones in a V position with the back and legs straight. Hold the ankles (or just above) firmly with the hands, keeping the legs shoulder width apart and focusing the eyes straight ahead.

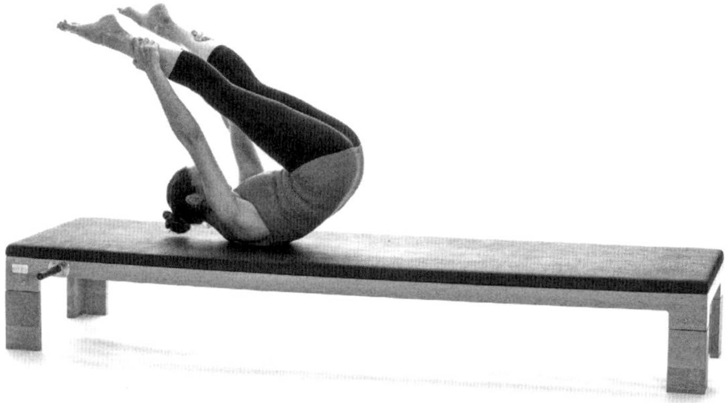

Inhale. Round the back, initiating the movement from the lumbar spine, and roll back to the shoulders (avoid rolling onto the neck and head).

Imagery

Visualize an inflated wheel that rolls effortlessly and without obstruction. Maintaining a consistent spinal curve when rolling back and forth keeps the wheel moving smoothly; conversely, a tight lower back or a lack of abdominal control deflates the wheel, causing the rolling to be interrupted and halting. Sitting on the sit bones in the V shape at the point of balance should be effortless. This pinnacle is where body, mind, and spirit unite; it is the culmination of every Pilates principle—the point of harmony.

- Use the back extensors to complete the movement.
- Keep the arms straight.
- Hold the legs firmly without pulling on them.

MODIFICATION

Perform the exercise with the legs bent and the hands holding the backs of the thighs. This version is particularly suited for people with tight hamstrings.

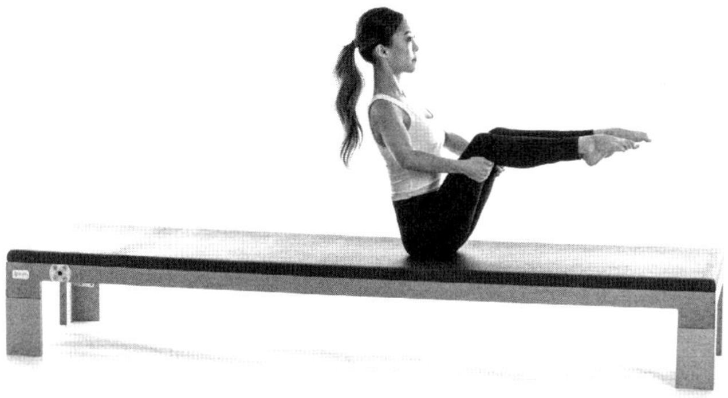

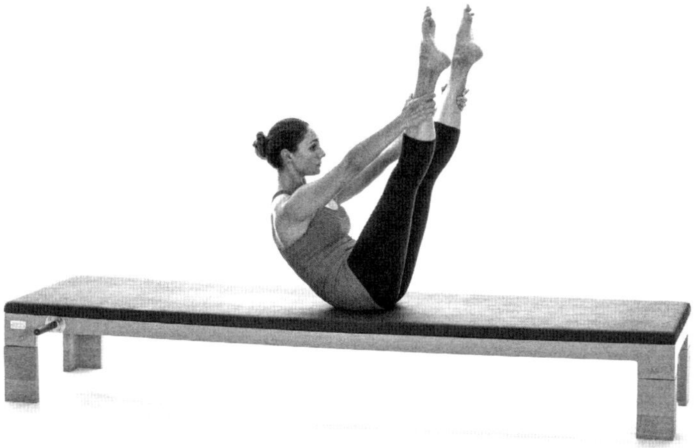

Exhale. Roll up, first keeping the spine round and then extending it. Return to the start position. Balance momentarily on the sit bones before rolling back again. Repeat 5-10 times.

Roll-Over

Muscle Focus

- Abdominals
- Hip flexors
- Hamstrings

Objectives

- To develop spinal articulation
- To improve abdominal control
- To improve lower back and hamstring flexibility

It is important to follow certain guidelines to make this exercise effective and meet its desired objectives. The roll-over motion should be facilitated by flexion of the spine, particularly the lower spine. This is achieved by contracting the abdominals. Avoid the tendency to use the momentum of the legs to roll over. Instead, once the legs are lifted to a 90-degree angle at the hip joint in the initial phase, maintain this angle and articulate the spine during the roll-over phase. This helps to maximize the abdominal work and the rolling of the spine sequentially off the mat. On the return, however, you can enhance the stretch of the hamstrings and the lower back by keeping the thighs close to the chest, creating a tight pike position.

People who have neck problems should be extremely cautious when doing this exercise; some individuals may need to avoid it completely (as with all other Pilates exercises that place weight on the cervical spine), even though most of the weight should be borne on the shoulder girdle rather than the neck.

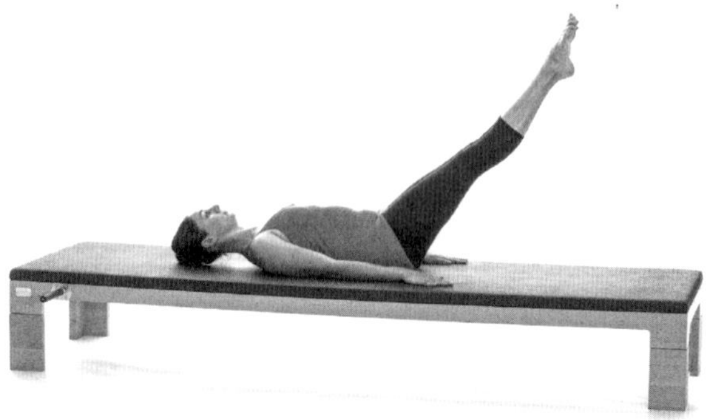

Setup. Lie supine with the arms by the sides and the legs straight. Bend the knees toward the chest and then straighten them at a 60-degree angle to the mat, legs together, feet plantarflexed.

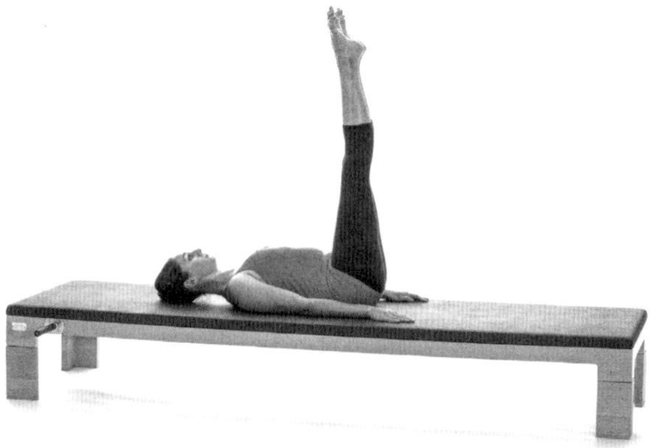

Inhale. Lift the legs to a 90-degree angle in the hip joint, so they are perpendicular to the floor.

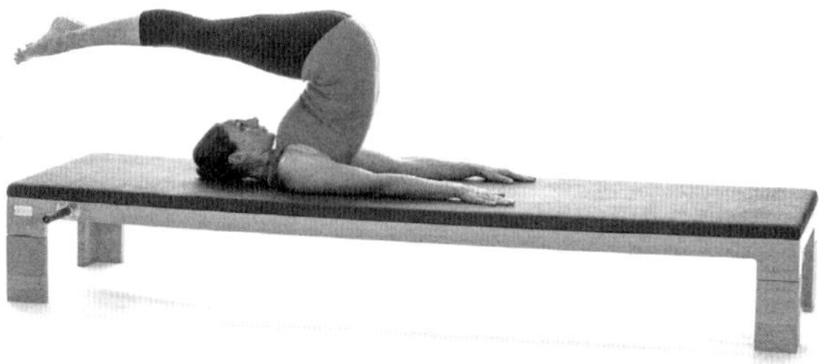

Exhale. Round the trunk and roll over, peeling the spine off the mat and bringing the legs overhead. Rest the weight on the shoulder girdle and keep the legs parallel to the mat.

Imagery

In the roll-over phase, when taking the legs overhead, visualize creating a ball out of the lower back (see also Mat: Rolling Like a Ball). On the way back, the feeling should be like spring metal being bent in half and then opening out to the start position.

- Avoid using momentum to roll over.
- Keep the hip joint at a consistent 90-degree angle during the roll-over phase.
- Deepen the abdominal contraction to achieve maximum lumbar flexion.
- Keep the thighs close to the chest in the roll-back phase.

VARIATION

The action of the legs can be reversed. Open the legs to hip width apart and lift them to a perpendicular position. Roll over with the legs separated. Dorsiflex the feet and bring them together when they are overhead and parallel to the mat. Lower them toward the floor and then roll back with the legs together and close to the chest. When the legs are perpendicular to the mat, plantarflex the feet, anchor the sacrum, and lower the legs to a 60-degree angle.

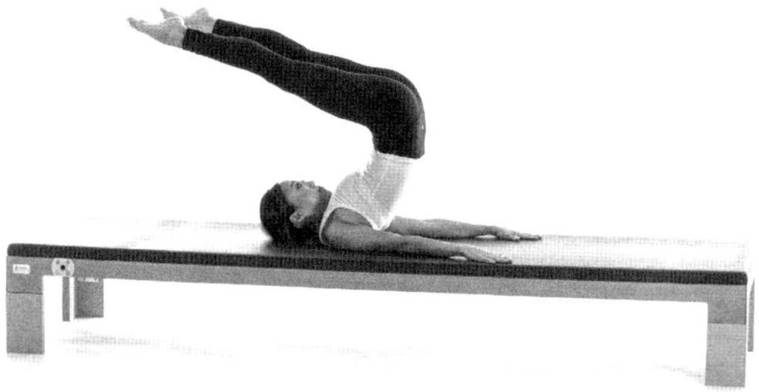

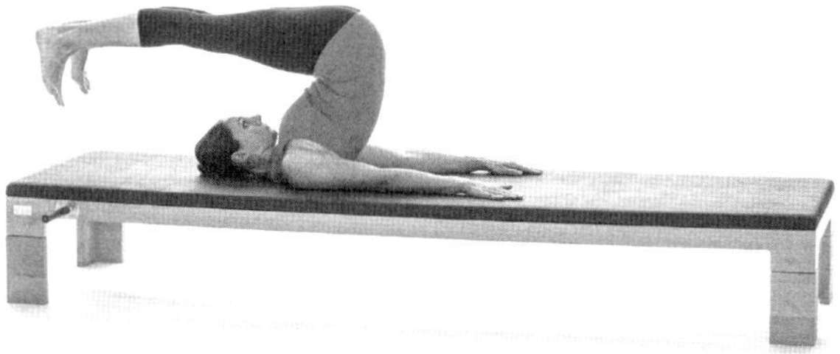

Inhale. Dorsiflex the feet and separate the legs to shoulder width.

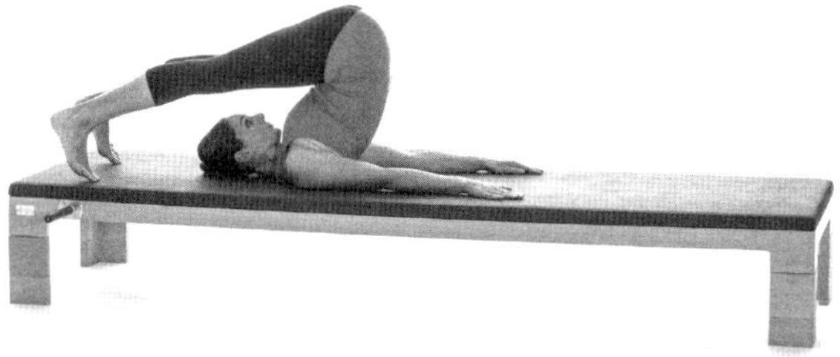

Continuing to inhale, lower the feet toward the floor above the head (touch the floor if flexibility allows).

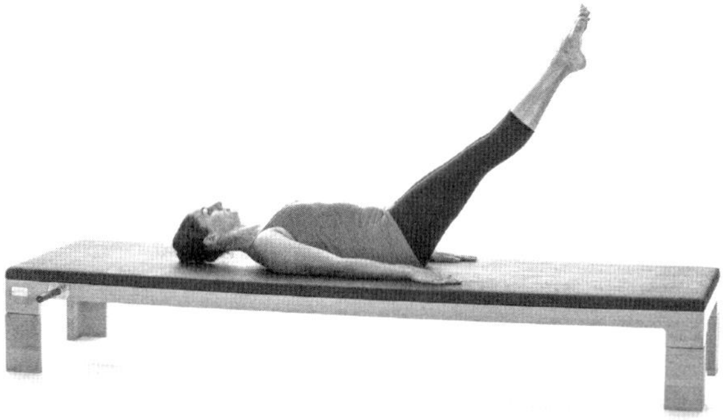

Exhale. Articulate the spine down to the mat, keeping the legs close to the chest. Anchor the pelvis on the mat and lift the legs. Plantarflex the feet when the legs are perpendicular to the floor. Continue to lower the legs to the 60-degree angle and bring them together. Return to the start position. Repeat 5 times.

Control Balance

Muscle Focus

- Hip extensors
- Hip flexors
- Abdominals
- Back extensors

Objectives

- To improve hip extensor strength
- To improve hip flexor flexibility
- To develop lumbopelvic stabilization

In addition to requiring a great deal of core control, this exercise relies greatly on hip flexor flexibility and hip extensor strength. The extensors, primarily those of the hip and back, facilitate the lifting of the leg perpendicular to the floor, creating a straight line through the trunk and up through the leg.

This exercise is a one-legged version of the Mat: Jackknife, and may serve as an excellent preparation for that exercise although many people find the Mat: Control Balance more difficult than the Mat: Jackknife. Both exercises place greater pressure on the cervical spine than does the Mat: Roll-Over, so I advise erring on the side of caution when performing them. They are absolutely contraindicated for anyone with neck problems, particularly those related to disc dysfunction.

Imagery

Visualize two energy lines: One runs from the shoulders through the trunk and the upright leg to the ceiling, and the other creates a stabilizing force by stretching from the hip joint down through the lower leg into the ground. With one foot anchored firmly on the ground, the other can reach higher toward the ceiling.

- ○ Keep the focal point of your weight on the shoulder girdle.
- ○ Keep the pelvis and trunk stable as the legs change.
- ○ Minimize weight bearing on the cervical spine.

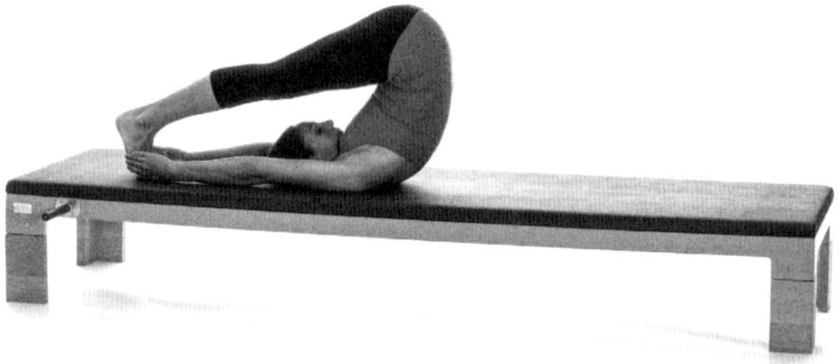

Setup. Lie supine with the arms by the sides and the legs straight. Bend the knees toward the chest and then straighten them at a 60-degree angle to the mat.

Inhale. Lift the legs to a 90-degree angle in the hip joint, so they are perpendicular to the floor.

Exhale. Round the lower back and roll over.

Inhale. Rest the weight on the shoulder girdle. Dorsiflex the feet and anchor them on the floor. Circle the arms overhead to hold on to the feet.

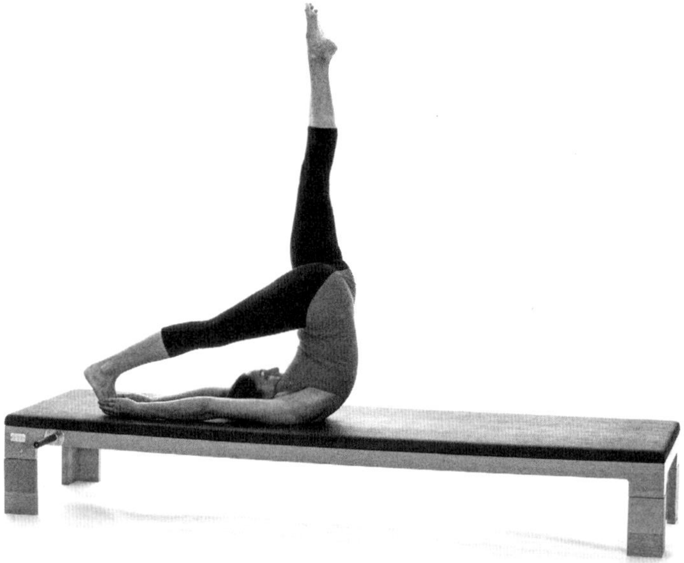

Exhale. Extend one leg up toward the ceiling. Perform two pulses with this leg when reaching maximum height (aiming to increase the hip extension with each pulse). Use percussive breathing, exhaling a puff of air with each pulse.

MODIFICATION

An alternative version, which places less weight on the cervical spine, is to do exactly the same movement pattern but roll onto the upper back and shoulders, as opposed to the shoulders and neck. In this version, which in fact is more closely aligned with the classical version, the leg switch will remain the same, but the lifting leg will not reach as high toward the ceiling. The work of the hip extensors and the stretch of the hip flexors is not quite as profound, but it is certainly an excellent exercise and minimizes the potential risks of placing weight on the cervical spine.

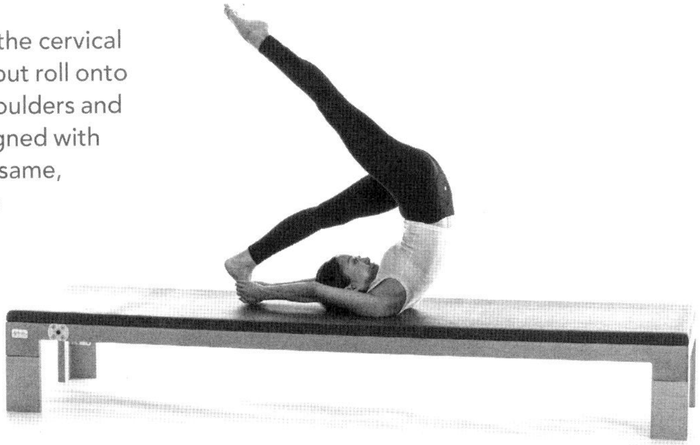

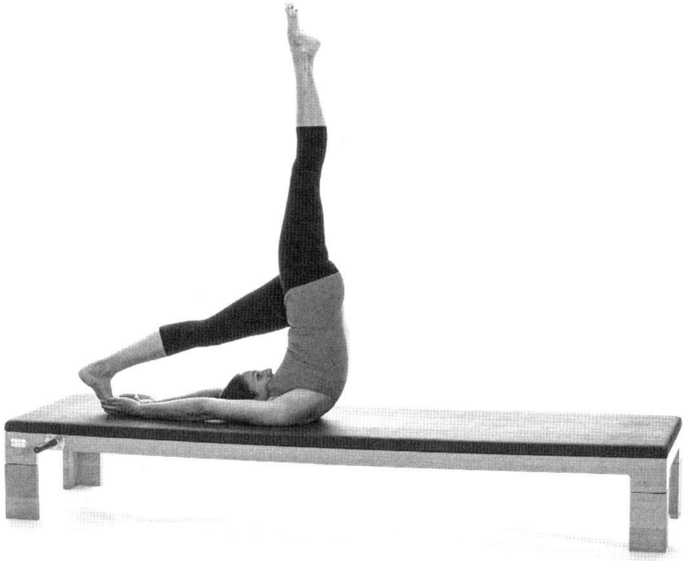

Inhale. Switch the legs simultaneously, keeping the pelvis and trunk as stable as possible. Repeat 5 times on each leg.

After the final repetition, bring the top leg back to a dorsiflexed position on the floor next to the other leg, and then roll down, keeping the thighs close to the chest. When the legs are perpendicular to the mat, plantarflex the feet, anchor the sacrum, and lower the legs to a 60-degree angle. At this point, bend the knees toward the chest, place the feet on the mat, and straighten the legs. Return to the start position.

Jackknife

Muscle Focus

- Hip, back, and shoulder extensors
- Abdominals

Objectives

- To improve hip extensor and shoulder extensor strength
- To improve back extensor control
- To develop spinal articulation
- To develop trunk stabilization

The Mat: Jackknife is an extension of the Mat: Roll-Over and should not be attempted until you have mastered that exercise. It also relates closely to Mat: Control Balance, some using it as preparation for the Mat: Jackknife and others finding it more difficult. Initially the feet reach overhead and are parallel to the floor, before dorsiflexing and being lowered to the floor as in the Mat: Roll-Over. At this point, however, rather than rolling down again, you recruit the hip extensors, shoulder extensors, and spinal extensors to swiftly reach the legs up toward the ceiling, creating a perpendicular line from the floor up through the shoulders, trunk, hips, legs, and feet. Recruiting the shoulder extensors is important to assist in keeping the structure stable and upright and alleviating pressure from the cervical spine. When rolling the spine down, vertebra by vertebra, keep the feet above the face until the pelvis reaches the floor, then lower the legs to the start position.

Because of the weight that this exercise places on the cervical spine, people with neck problems should avoid it. Although the weight is distributed between the shoulders and the arms, minimizing the pressure on the cervical spine, the neck still bears significant weight.

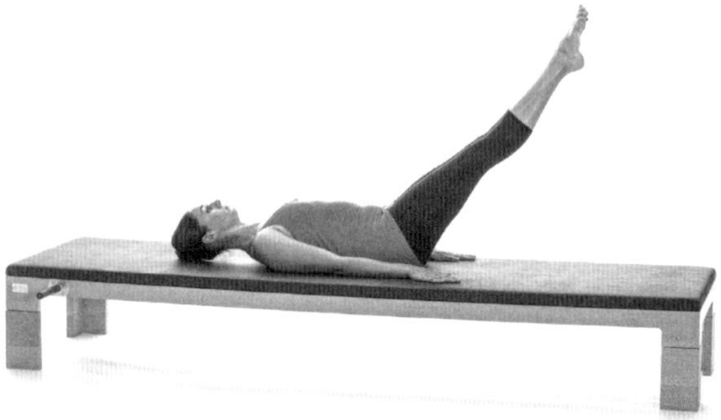

Setup. As with the Mat: Roll-Over, lie supine with the arms by the sides of the body and the legs straight at approximately a 60-degree angle to the floor.

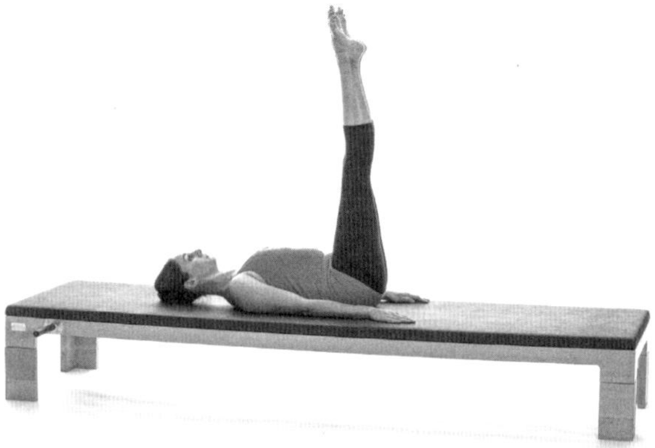

Inhale. Raise the legs to a 90-degree angle, anchoring the pelvis and continuing to sink the lower back into the mat.

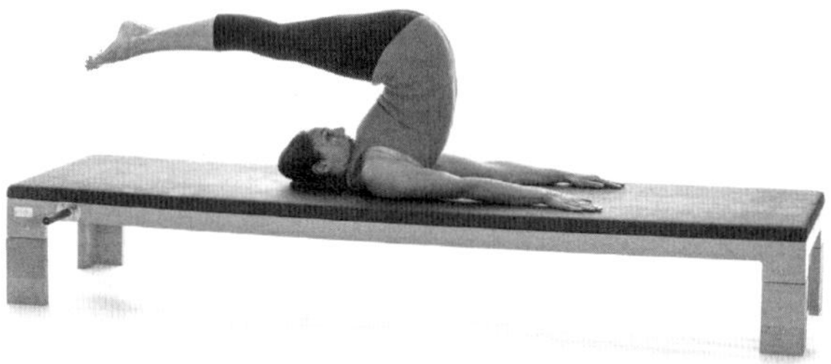

Exhale. Roll over, maximizing the flexion of the lumbar region and maintaining a 90-degree angle in the hip joint. Complete this phase with the legs parallel to the floor and the weight on the shoulders.

Imagery

As the name implies, the Mat: Jackknife should feel like a spring-loaded hinge or knife closing and opening (at the hip joint), with a swift movement of the legs into the air.

- Maximize flexion of the lumbar spine during the roll-over phase.
- Use the hip, shoulder, and back extensors to achieve maximum height of the legs and trunk.
- Roll down, hinging at the hip joint with the feet opposite the face.

PROGRESSION

The Mat: Jackknife is a very difficult exercise as is, so to add difficulty is not advised until the exercise has been mastered. In order to add intensity once mastery has been achieved, rather than hinging at the hip joints and rolling down with the feet opposite the face, try to keep the legs as close to perpendicular as possible as the spine rolls down until the pelvis reaches the mat. Anchor the pelvis and lower the legs to a 60-degree angle.

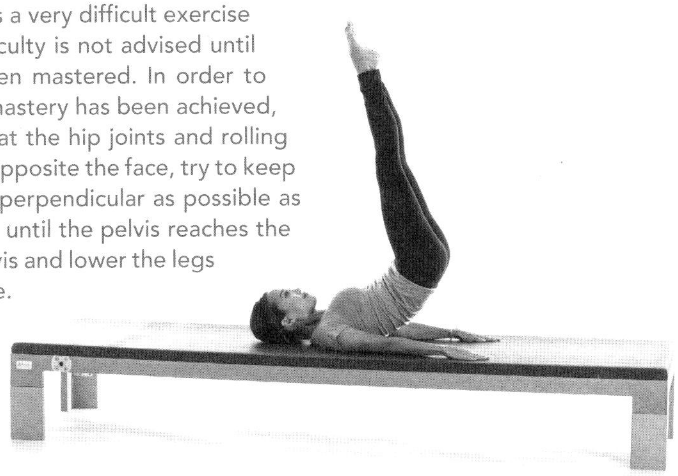

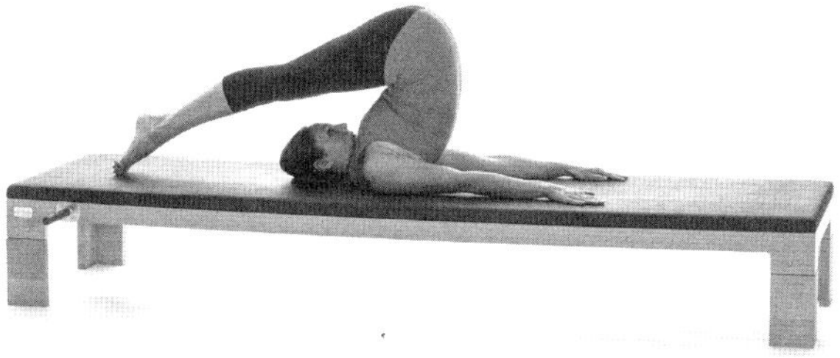

Inhale. Lower the legs toward the floor.

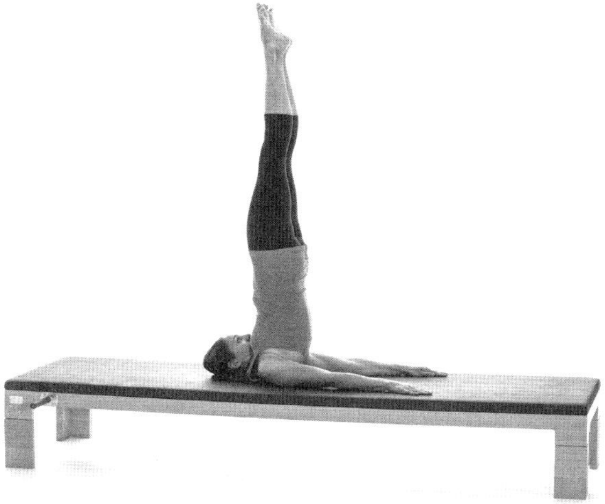

Continuing to inhale, lift the legs toward the ceiling. Move the pelvis forward and press the arms into the mat.

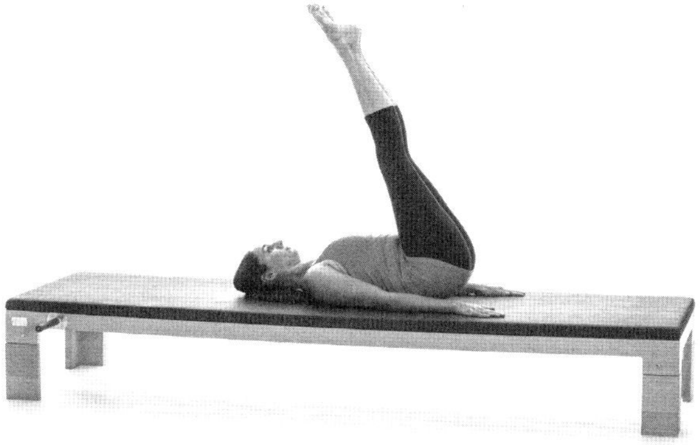

Exhale. Slowly roll down, articulating the spine and keeping the feet opposite the face. Bring the legs back to perpendicular to the mat, anchor the sacrum and lower the legs to a 60-degree angle. Return to the start position. Repeat 5 times.

Boomerang

Muscle Focus

- Abdominals
- Back extensors
- Hip flexors

Objectives

- To improve abdominal and back extensor strength
- To improve hip flexor control
- To improve thoracic flexibility
- To develop balance

This is a high-level exercise because of its complexity. It also demonstrates the progression of exercises in Pilates, the logical methodology of one exercise building on another. The Mat: Boomerang requires strength, flexibility, and, most importantly, coordination. It draws from the Mat: Roll-Over and Mat: Teaser, which should be mastered before embarking on this exercise. It also resembles the Reformer: Rowing Back 1 in its movement pattern, again displaying how Pilates exercises are related in one way or another. Understanding these connections and relationships is so important in both the teaching and practice of Pilates.

Imagery

It takes a while to understand why this exercise is called the Mat: Boomerang, but once you achieve precise positioning and flow, it becomes apparent. At the point where the body rolls down to the lumbar region, before the legs are taken overhead, the shape resembles a boomerang. In this position the body should feel firm, and the legs and trunk should be integrated so that you can rock back and forth like the base of a rocking chair. In fact, I often use the rocking in this difficult position as an exercise in and of itself because it demands tremendous core strength and control.

After the legs change position overhead, the body rolls back momentarily to the boomerang position before lifting

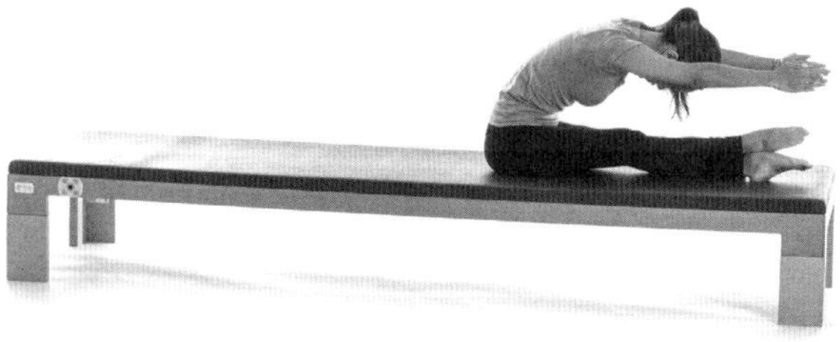

Setup. Sit with the legs straight and crossed, feet plantarflexed. Fold the trunk over the legs and reach the arms forward.

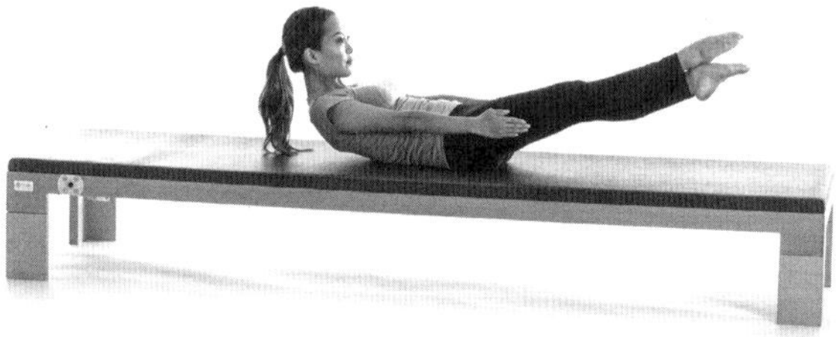

Inhale. Roll down while lifting the legs, feet opposite the eyes, and pause when you reach the lumbar region. Hold the trunk and legs stable in this boomerang position.

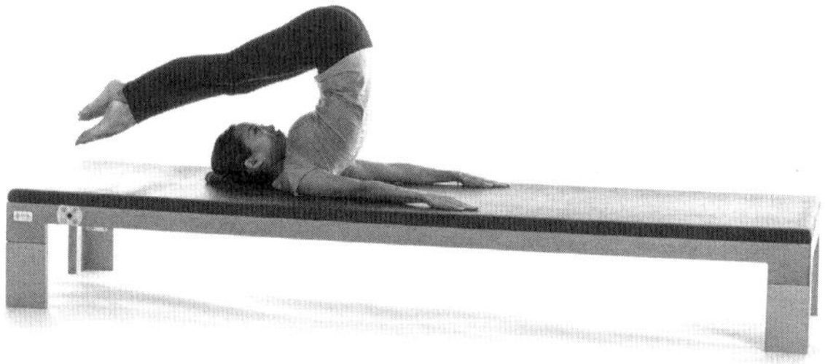

Exhale. Lower the chest and head and lift the legs so they are perpendicular to the floor. Round the lower back further and roll over. Lower the legs toward the mat, keeping the feet plantarflexed.

into the teaser position. This is the point where exceptional balance is needed. Holding the body stable in this balanced position, the arms reach back, and the fingers are interlaced to provide a significant stretch to the muscles of the shoulder and chest. The arms then circle around to the front as the legs are lowered and the trunk reaches over the legs for a stretch. Return to the start position—and there we have the boomerang!

- Keep the movement fluid.
- Stretch the muscles of the chest and shoulders as the arms reach back and the fingers are interlaced.
- Use trunk stabilization during the balance phase, keeping the legs as high as possible.

MODIFICATION

This modification can serve both as a preparation for the Mat: Boomerang and for the Mat: Crab. Start in the same position as Mat: Boomerang. Once in the boomerang position with the lower back on the mat and the legs and trunk lifted, bend the knees with the legs crossed. Hold each foot with the respective hand. Tuck the body into a ball shape and roll over onto the shoulders. In this position with the legs overhead, straighten the legs and switch them. Bend the knees and roll like a ball back to a balanced position. Place the feet on the mat, straighten the legs, and fold the trunk over the legs, reaching the arms forward.

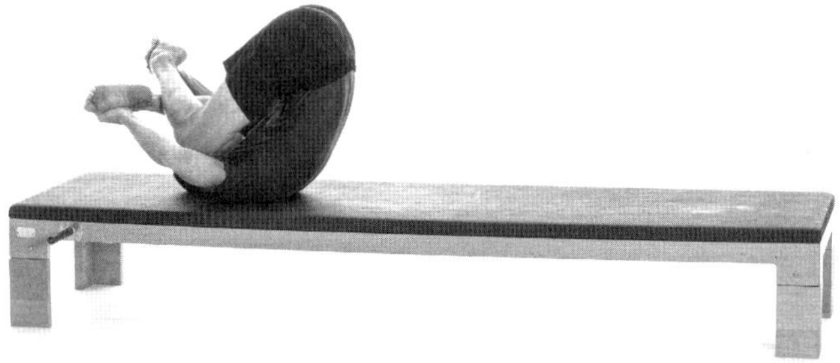

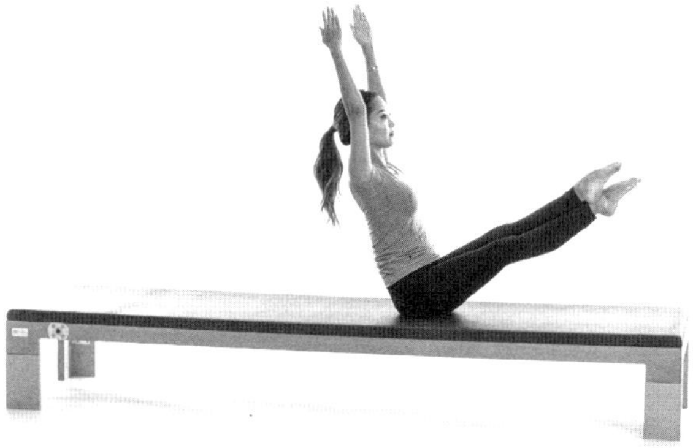

Inhale. Switch the legs.

Exhale. Take the legs back over to return toward the boomerang position, and then roll up into a teaser position.

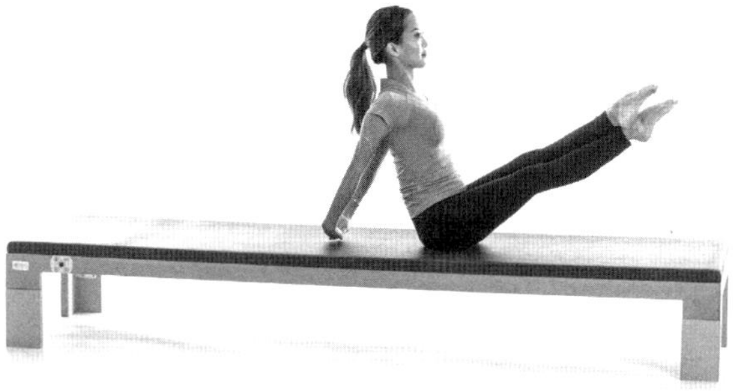

Inhale. Circle the arms around and interlace the fingers behind the back as you lift the chest and extend the trunk further.

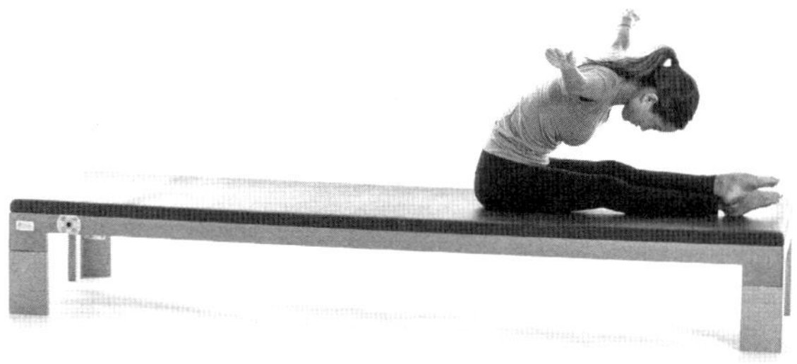

Exhale. Lower the legs and release the hands. Circle the arms around to the front, bringing the body forward over the legs. Return to the start position. Repeat 4-6 times.

Crab

Muscle Focus

- Abdominals
- Triceps

Objectives

- To improve neck and lower back flexibility
- To improve upper body strength
- To develop trunk stabilization

Although this exercise may visually appear uncomfortable and even dangerous because it involves leaning forward onto the head and seemingly transferring weight onto the neck, it is in fact enjoyable and beneficial if done correctly. The key point is that the body's full weight should never be placed on the neck. Instead, transfer the weight cautiously and with control onto the head, with most of the weight being supported by the upper body and legs. Other than the rolling onto the head, the rest of the exercise is very similar to the Mat: Rolling Like a Ball, Seal Puppy, and Boomerang, with elements of coordination and control added. In addition, because the legs are held close to the body by the arms in the cross-legged position, the possibility of straightening the legs and using them for momentum to roll over is diminished. The use of upper body strength during the final phase of transitioning over the folded legs, specifically the triceps, should not be minimized. The upper body plays a key role when transferring the weight over the legs onto the head.

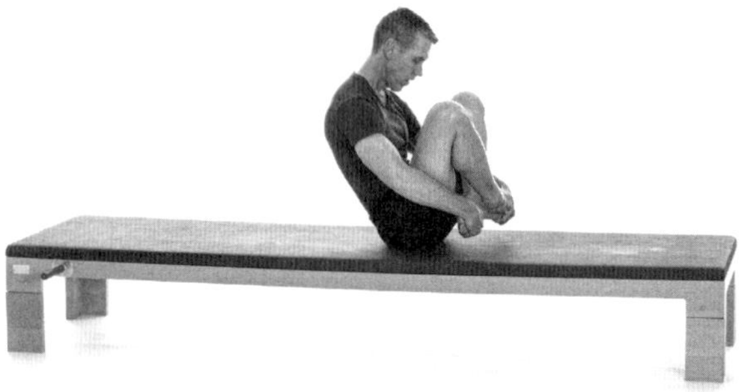

Setup. Sit in a balanced position on the sit bones with the body in a ball shape. Cross the legs, reach the arms around the legs from the outside, and hold the feet with the thumbs wrapped under the feet and the fingers on top. The left hand holds the right foot, and the right hand holds the left foot.

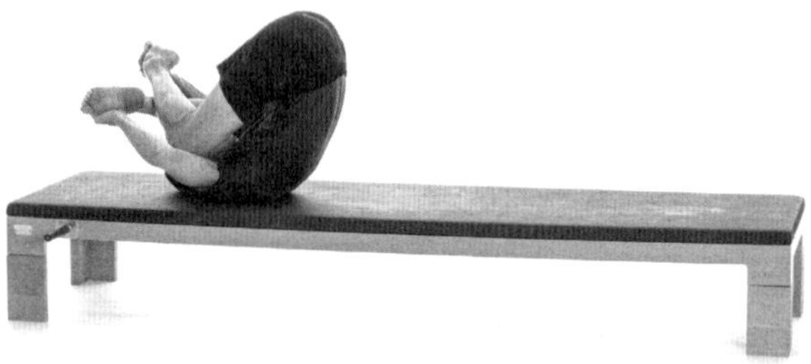

Exhale. Roll back onto the shoulders.

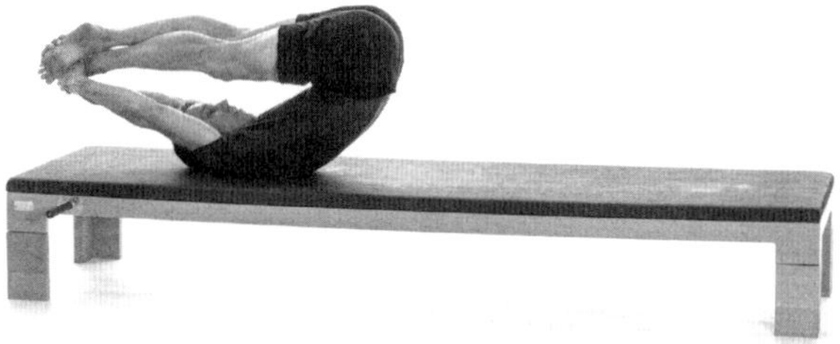

Inhale. Straighten the legs overhead and switch them, as in the Mat: Boomerang. Bend the knees and take hold of the feet again, tucking back into a ball shape.

Imagery

Although the cross-legged position does have some remote resemblance to the underside of a crab, I have never been able to relate this exercise to a crab—despite spending hours observing crabs run across many a beach! I find using the image of a rolling wheel, keeping a consistent shape of the trunk, and the never-ending internal flow of energy more beneficial.

- Transfer weight cautiously onto the head.
- Maximize lumbar flexion when rolling.
- Push into the hands, as if straightening the arms, when rolling over the legs.
- Keep the legs close to the body when rolling.

VARIATION

This variation is for those who cannot, or do not wish to, place any pressure on the head and neck. Instead of rolling over the legs and forward onto the head, roll over the legs but lift into an upright position, kneeling with the legs still crossed and arms overhead. This upright position is a welcome change after the deep spinal flexion that is maintained in this exercise. This position demands good balance and core strength. Employ as much control as possible as you lower the pelvis back down.

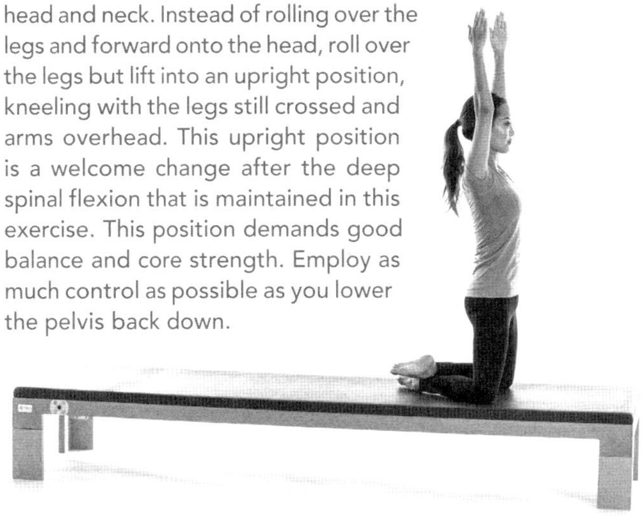

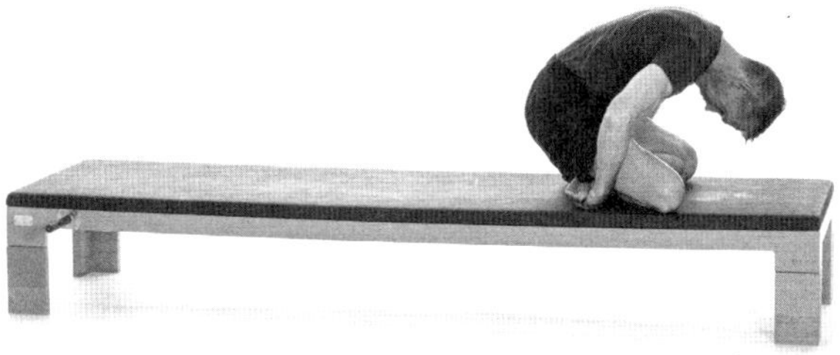

Exhale. Roll forward, transferring the weight over the legs. Use the arms to assist rolling over the legs by pressing the hands into the mat.

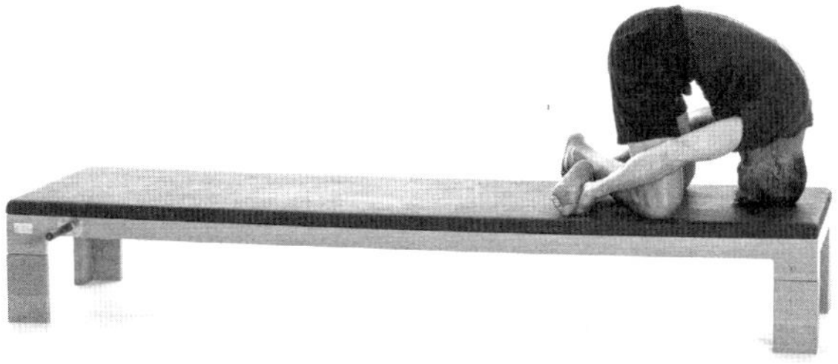

Inhale. Place the head on the floor and roll slowly over onto the head, cautiously transferring the weight toward the neck and stretching the neck extensors. Lower the pelvis back to the mat and balance on the sit bones. Return to the start position. Repeat 4-6 times.

Bridging and Full Body Integration

The "bridging" aspect of this block is unique to the mat block system, while full body integration is a very prominent part of both the mat and comprehensive block systems. The term *bridging* can have different connotations depending on the context in which it is used. Here it relates primarily to the shape of the body and not to muscle function—its name is derived from the bridge shape formed by the trunk of the body in these exercises, with the pelvis lifted off the mat and the limbs supporting the structure. Because bridging is closely related to, and requires, full body integration, I have elected to put them together in the same category.

The importance of abdominal strength and control in achieving spinal stabilization has been discussed in connection with other blocks. In contrast to the exercises in the abdominal work block and the spinal articulation block, which are performed in spinal flexion, the bridging exercises are performed with the pelvis and spine in a neutral position, or very close to one. Developing the muscles in this position is thought to be more functional than developing them in spinal flexion; however, I recommend practicing both. Each position has a role to play in achieving spinal stabilization.

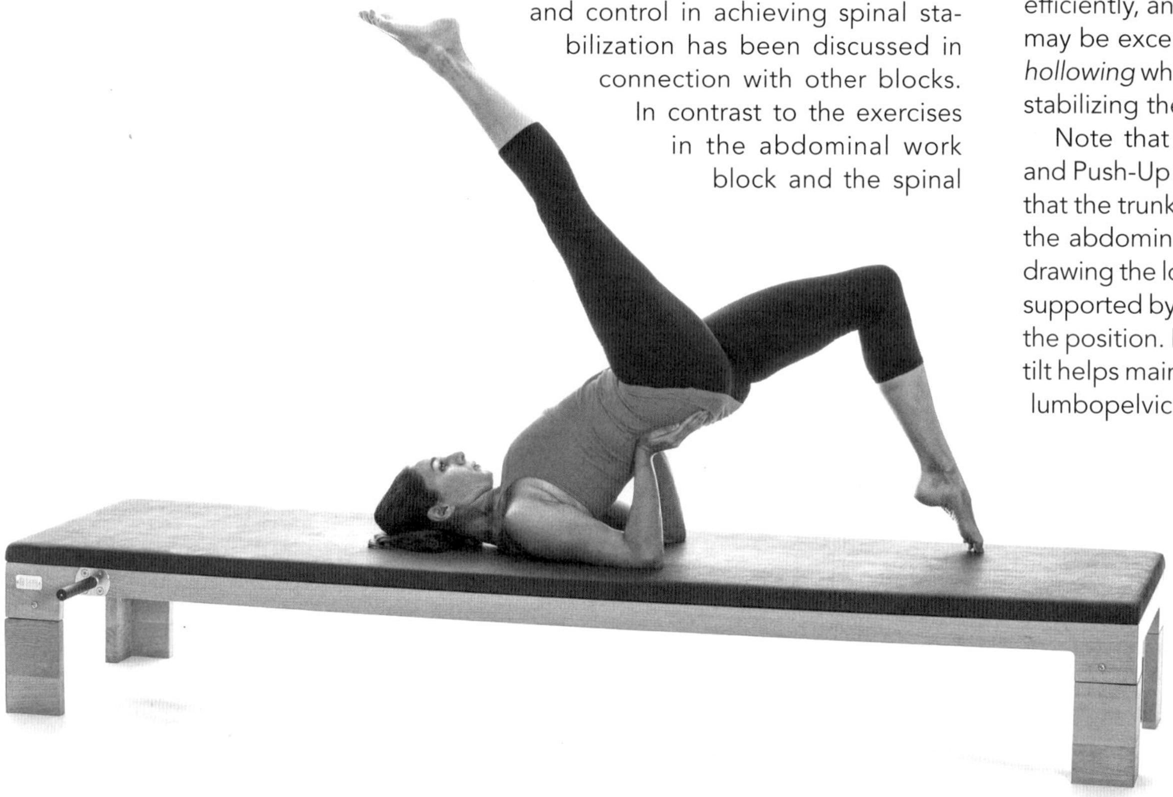

The term *bracing* is often used to describe the action of the muscles in stabilizing the pelvis and spine. This is different to the *scooping* or *hollowing* action of the abdominals often preferred in the abdominal work and spinal articulation blocks. Some argue that bracing is more effective in stabilizing and protecting the spine than hollowing. I believe that all forms of muscle control contribute to the vast movement vocabulary that allows us to enjoy life to its fullest and perform our daily activities and athletic endeavors effectively, efficiently, and safely. As a general rule (meaning there may be exceptions), I would advise using *scooping* or *hollowing* when articulating the spine and *bracing* when stabilizing the spine.

Note that the Mat: Front Support, Leg Pull Front, and Push-Up differ from the other bridging exercises in that the trunk is facing down versus up. In this position, the abdominals need to work to prevent gravity from drawing the lower back into an arch. The abdominals are supported by the hip flexors to maintain the integrity of the position. Biasing the pelvis toward a slight posterior tilt helps maintain abdominal engagement and achieve lumbopelvic stabilization.

Shoulder Bridge Prep

This exercise combines lumbopelvic stabilization with hip disassociation. It places the body in a challenging bridge position, starting from the up phase of the Mat: Pelvic Curl and continuing with the lifting of one leg. The hip extensors of the supporting leg are crucial to maintaining this challenging bridge position. The pelvic stabilization in this exercise relies greatly on the hamstrings and the abdominals, which together hold the pelvis stable with a bias toward a posterior tilt: the abdominals pulling the pubic symphysis upward and the hamstrings pulling the ischial tuberosity downward. The back and shoulder extensors also provide important support to the structure and should not be overlooked.

Imagery

Feel an energy line running diagonally through the body, outward and upward through the supporting knee and downward from the knee through the trunk and shoulders. Use this sense of oppositional forces to keep the body aligned and to balance the work of the flexors and extensors of the trunk, which are co-contracting. This stable position will facilitate the moving leg being lifted and lowered with a free, floating feeling. You may also visualize a suspension bridge on which a mechanical arm goes up and down without affecting the stability and strength of the bridge.

- ○ Keep a consistent 90-degree angle in the knee of the moving leg.
- ○ Initiate the movement from the hip joint.
- ○ Maintain hip extension in the supporting leg along with a stable pelvis.

MAT

Bridging and Full Body Integration

INTERMEDIATE

Muscle Focus

- Abdominals
- Back extensors
- Hamstrings
- Hip flexors

Objectives

- To improve hip extensor strength
- To improve back extensor and shoulder extensor control
- To improve hip flexor control
- To develop lumbopelvic stabilization
- To develop hip disassociation

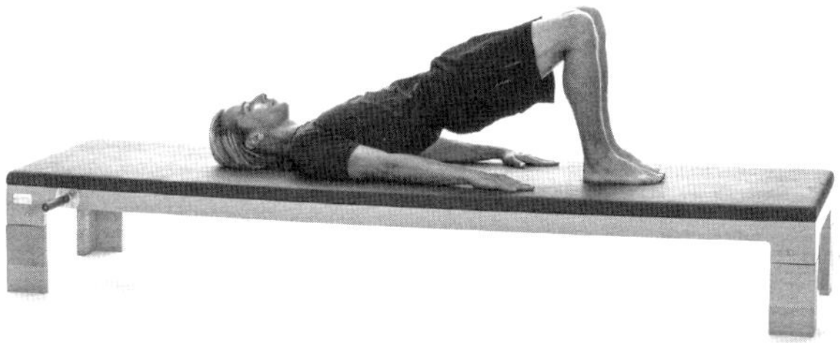

Setup. Lie supine with the spine in a neutral position. Bend the knees and place the feet hip width apart. Keep the scapulae in a neutral position, the arms straight by the sides, and the fingers reaching toward the feet.

Exhale. Draw in the abdominals and tilt the pelvis in a posterior direction. Lift the spine off the mat, one vertebra at a time, while extending the hips. Create a straight line from the shoulders to the knees.

Inhale. Hold this position, distributing the weight evenly on the feet and keeping the legs parallel. Elongate the hip flexors while engaging the shoulder extensors to support the structure and to accentuate the mid- and upper back work.

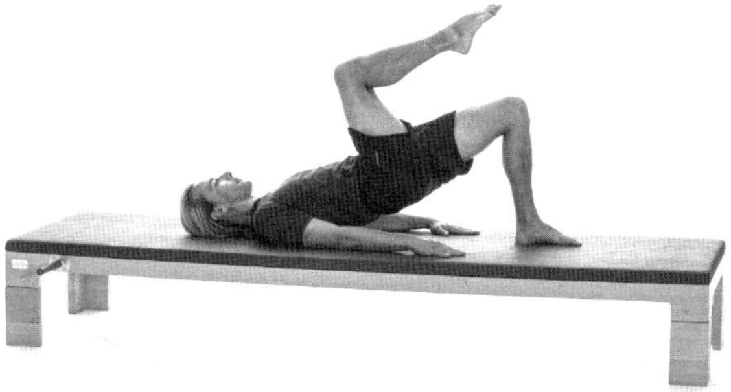

Exhale. Lift one leg from the hip joint, maintaining a 90-degree angle in the knee and plantarflex the foot. Keep the pelvis stable and level throughout, with minimal shifting of weight to the supporting leg.

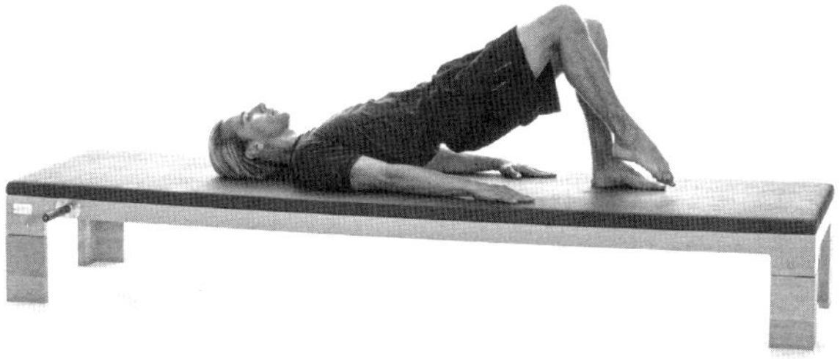

Inhale. Lower the lifted leg and touch the mat lightly with the toes.

Exhale. Lift the leg. Keep the hip extensors of the supporting leg working, and avoid lowering or tilting the pelvis. After 5-10 repetitions, place the foot on the mat and switch legs, again with minimal shifting of weight, and repeat the exercise with the other leg.

Inhale. Complete the exercise by placing both feet on the mat and exhaling while rolling down, vertebra by vertebra, from the top of the spine through the lumbar region to the sacrum.

Shoulder Bridge

Muscle Focus

- Abdominals
- Back extensors
- Hamstrings
- Hip flexors

Objectives

- To improve hip extensor strength and flexibility
- To improve hip flexor control and flexibility
- To improve back extensor and shoulder extensor control
- To develop lumbopelvic stabilization

This exercise builds on Mat: Shoulder Bridge Prep. The key is maintaining a stable pelvis throughout. Feel the hip flexors stretching as the leg swings down and the hamstrings stretching as the leg swings up. The hamstring stretch is enhanced by the dorsiflexion of the foot.

Orient the pelvis toward a posterior tilt to prevent hyperlordosis and pressure on the lower back, particularly when the leg is lowered.

Imagery

Visualize a ride at an amusement park featuring a carriage on the end of a girder that swings like a pendulum. The leg is the girder that swings in an arc shape, and the foot is the carriage. The body is the stable, solid structure that supports the swinging girder.

- ○ Maintain consistent height of the pelvis from the mat.
- ○ Avoid tipping the pelvis to one side.
- ○ Keep the pelvis neutral or in a slight posterior tilt.
- ○ Keep the swinging leg straight.

PROGRESSION

The primary objective of this progression is to challenge pelvic stabilization and hip extensor control of the supporting leg. After the final repetition, maintain dorsiflexion and keep the leg perpendicular. Take it out to the side without shifting the pelvis and return to center. Repeat 5 times. Plantarflex the foot, bend the knee, and place the foot on the floor. Switch to the other side.

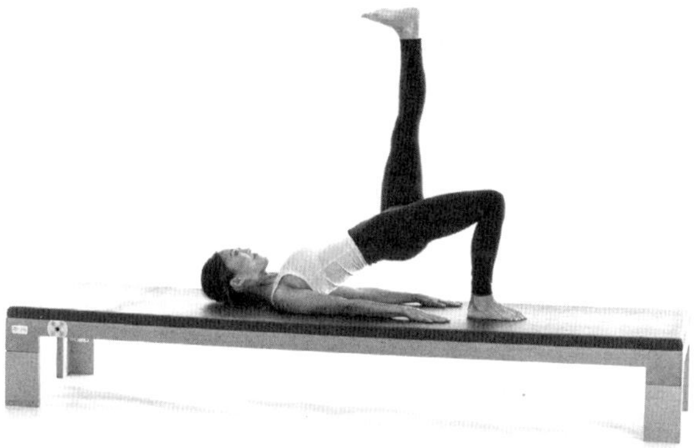

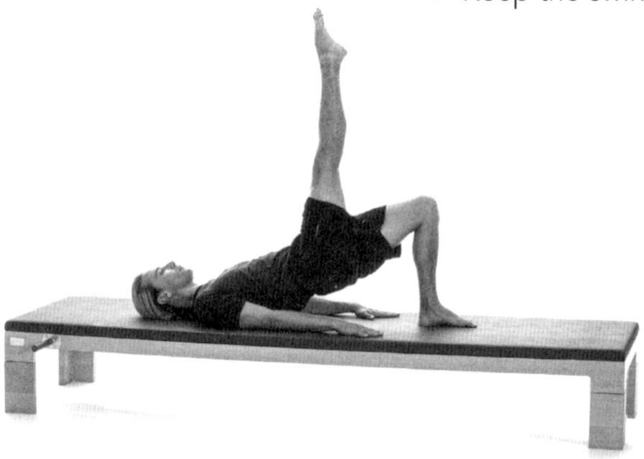

Setup. Lie supine with the knees bent and the feet firmly placed on the ground. Perform the Mat: Pelvic Curl, pausing in the top position (start position). Lift one foot off the ground, bending the knee toward the chest, and then straighten the leg upward, plantarflexing the foot and pointing the toes directly toward the ceiling.

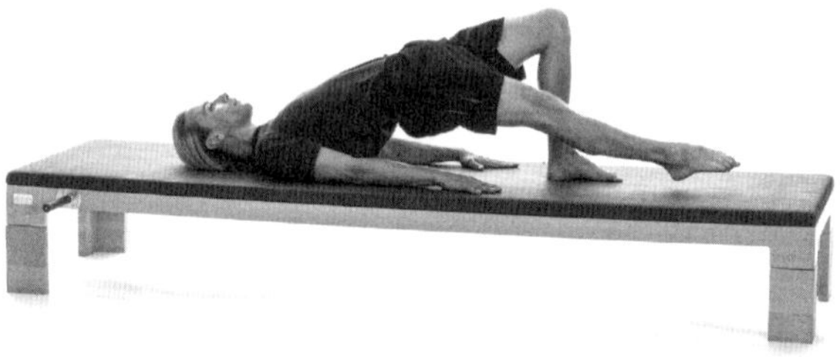

Exhale. Lower the straight leg toward the floor with the foot plantarflexed (touch the floor if possible).

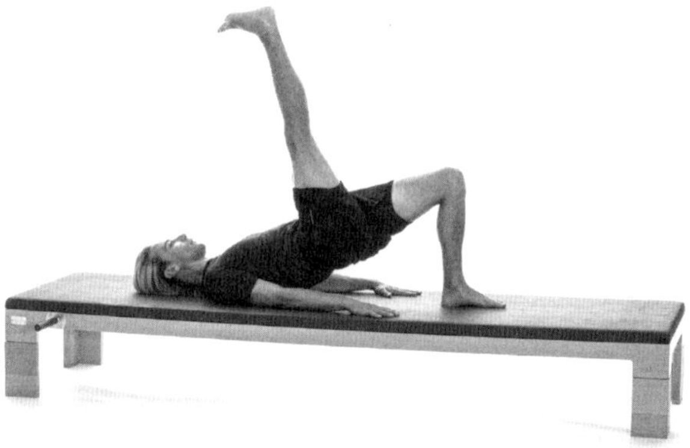

Inhale. Kick the straight leg upward, as high and close to the chest as possible, dorsiflexing the foot. After 5-10 repetitions, pause with the leg reaching toward the ceiling and plantarflex the foot. Bend the knee and place the foot on the floor. Return to the start position. Switch legs and repeat on the other side. Complete the exercise by placing both feet on the mat and rolling down to the mat.

Scissors

The Mat: Scissors is a challenging exercise, in large part because of the arched position of the lower back. This position feels precarious and demands a high level of lumbopelvic stabilization. The same position is used for the Step Barrel: Scissors, except that here the arms take the place of the barrel, making it far more challenging. The pelvis should be stable and anchored, serving as a foundation as the legs perform a scissors action, alternating as they pass through the centerline (the starting point) perpendicular to the floor.

Note that the elbows should be directly under the pelvis (or as close as possible); without their support, the pelvis would sink and the whole structure would begin to collapse. Keeping an equal degree of split in each leg creates the desired wide V position and an equal stretch of the hip flexors and hamstrings.

Imagery

Picturing the spine being supported by a rounded barrel is helpful. Imagine the legs opening wide like a handheld fan, then closing and opening to the other side. In addition, imagine the pelvis like a large bowl being firmly held in your hands.

- ○ Maintain an arc shape of the spine.
- ○ Keep the elbows parallel to each other (or as close as possible).
- ○ Cradle the pelvis in the hands.

Muscle Focus

- Hip extensors
- Hip flexors
- Abdominals

Objectives

- To improve hip flexor control and flexibility
- To improve hip extensor control and flexibility
- To develop scapular and lumbopelvic stabilization

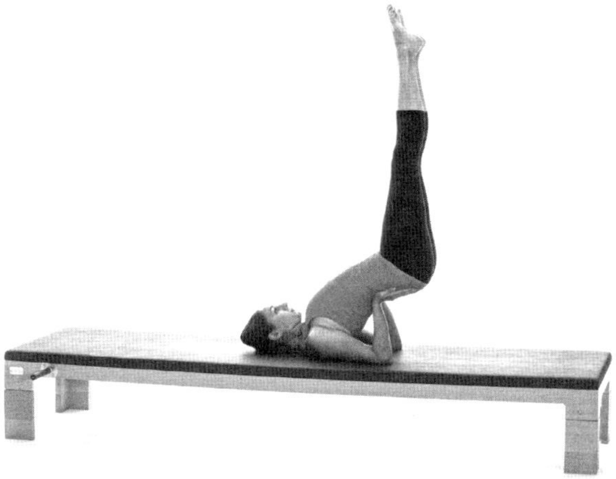

Setup. Begin by doing the Mat: Roll-Over. Bend the knees, creating a ball shape, and place the hands under the pelvis. Lower the pelvis into the hands as if holding a bowl and create an arc shape with the trunk. Straighten the legs up toward the ceiling, perpendicular to the floor.

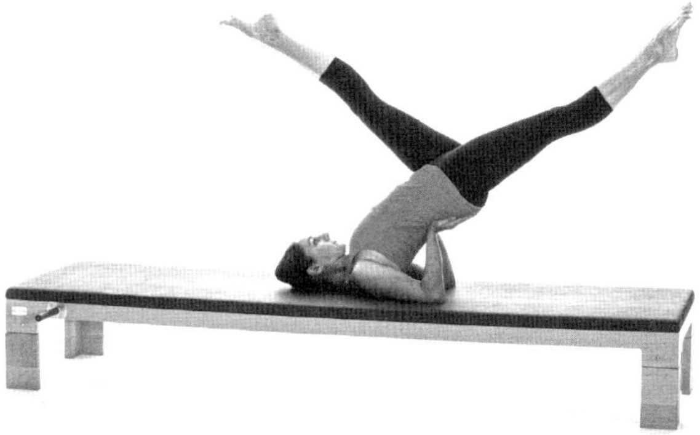

Exhale. Open the legs (one forward, one backward; equidistant from the centerline) into a wide V position. Pulse the legs twice in the open scissors position, reaching in opposite directions, exhaling on each pulse.

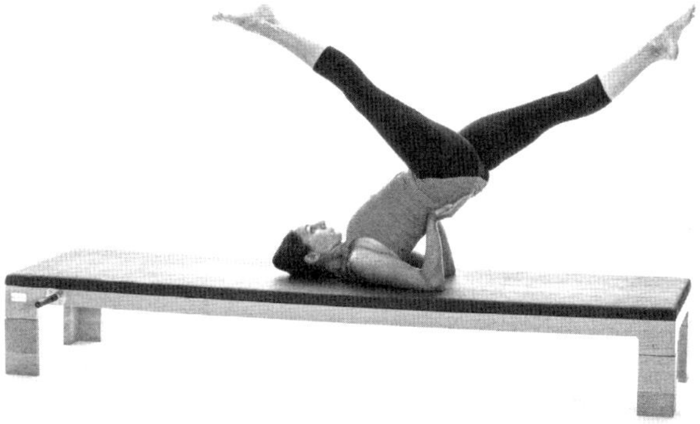

Inhale. Switch legs, passing through the start position (perpendicular), and repeat the pulses in the open V position on the opposite side, again exhaling on each pulse. Repeat 6-10 complete cycles (both legs).

Muscle Focus

- Hip extensors
- Hip flexors
- Abdominals

Objectives

- To improve hip flexor control and flexibility
- To improve hip extensor control and flexibility
- To develop scapular and lumbopelvic stabilization

Bicycle

The Mat: Bicycle is an extension of the Mat: Scissors, therefore proficiency in that exercise is a prerequisite. Although both legs perform a large cycling action (one bending and the other straightening simultaneously), at one point in each cycle they are in the straight-legged scissors position, which can be a reference point. Try to touch the floor with the toes of the back leg as the knee bends—a position that demands a high degree of spinal extension and hip flexor flexibility. However, avoid compromising lumbopelvic stabilization and arching the lower back excessively to achieve more range. This will invariably increase the pressure on the lower back and potentially cause discomfort and even injury. Focus should be placed on the abdominals to protect the lower back and achieve the heightened support needed for this exercise. Flexibility, awareness, and strength developed from practicing the Mat: Scissors will assist you in executing this very challenging exercise.

Imagery

The large, fluid, circular motion of the legs conjures up an image of cycling a penny-farthing (an old-fashioned bike with one large wheel in front and a small one in back).

- ○ Maintain an arc shape of the spine.
- ○ Perform elongated movements with maximum fluidity.
- ○ Keep the legs parallel, avoiding external rotation of the hip, particularly when bending the knee of the leg that is in hip extension.
- ○ Keep the elbows parallel to each other (or as close as possible).

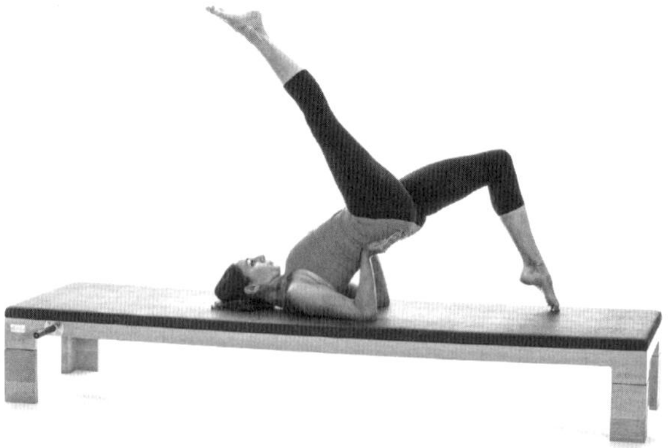

Setup. Lie in a supine position and draw the knees toward the chest. Create a ball shape with the body and roll over onto the shoulder girdle. Place the hands under the pelvis and lower the pelvis into the hands as if holding a bowl, and create an arc shape with the trunk. Now straighten the legs up toward the ceiling. Open the legs (one forward, one backward; equidistant from the centerline) into a wide V position.

Exhale. Extend the back leg (furthest from the face) toward the floor. Bend the knee and touch the floor with the toes (or as close as possible).

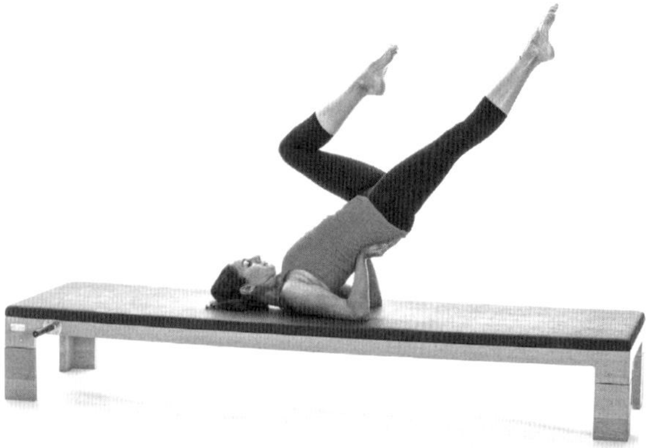

Inhale. Flex the hip and bring the bent leg toward the chest. At the same time, extend the hip of the straight leg, which now becomes the back leg.

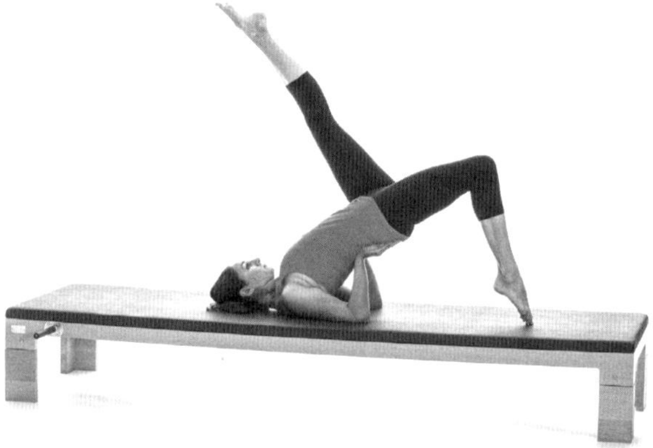

Begin straightening the bent leg in front of the face as the straight one starts bending to touch the floor with the toes. Continue this large cycling action. After 6-10 complete cycles (both legs), reverse the direction of the cycling. (Although more difficult to touch the floor with the toes of the back foot in this direction, continue striving to do so.)

Back Support

This exercise emphasizes the co-contraction of the trunk flexors and extensors to create a stable trunk. It directly strengthens the shoulder and hip extensors and develops back extensor control. At the same time, it addresses the need for flexibility and control of the opposing flexors, particularly the shoulder and hip.

The initial movement, once the setup position has been achieved, is hip extension supported by shoulder and back extension. During the hip extension, the hamstrings should engage before the gluteals. Deviating from this sequence of muscle recruitment (by recruiting the gluteals first) may lead to incorrect positioning of the pelvis (tucking) and lack of hamstring activation.

Finally, although articulation of the spine is often used in Pilates, in this case, strive to keep the spine in a stable, neutral position and hinge from the hip and shoulder joints, lifting the trunk as one stable unit.

Imagery

Think of the hips as the hinge of a door on its side, opening as the pelvis lifts and closing as the pelvis lowers. Alternatively, visualize two energy lines: one running from the head through the trunk to the hip joint, and the other running from the ankles through the knee to the hip joint. As the pelvis lifts, the two lines connect and become one. As the pelvis lowers, the joined line splits in two.

- Avoid flaring the ribs.
- Lift the pelvis from the hip joint in a hinging action, keeping the back and legs straight.
- Allow the head to follow the line of the spine.

Muscle Focus

- Shoulder extensors
- Hip extensors
- Back extensors

Objectives

- To improve shoulder extensor and hip extensor strength
- To improve back extensor control
- To develop trunk and scapular stabilization

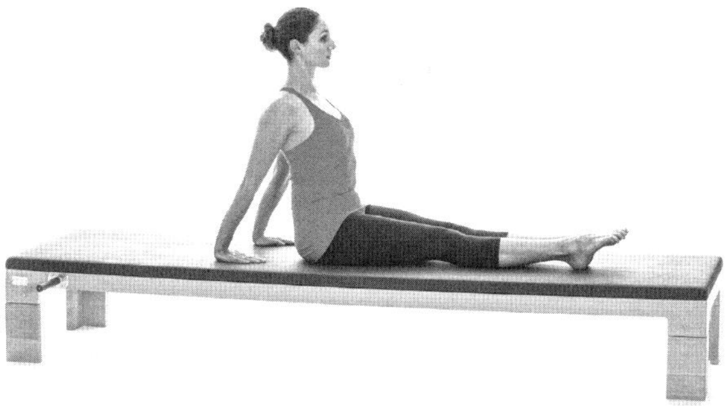

Setup. Sit with the hands approximately 12 inches (30 centimeters) behind the pelvis, fingers facing the pelvis. Straighten the legs out in front, hip width apart, and plantarflex the feet. Engage the back extensors and scapular stabilizers.

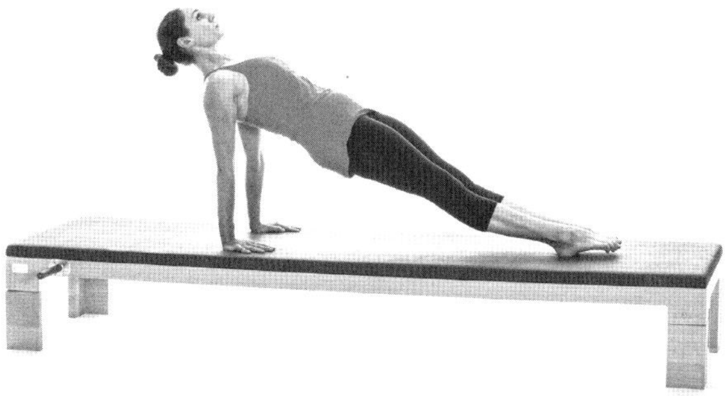

Exhale. Lift the pelvis off the mat, hinging at the hip and shoulder joints, until the body is in a straight line.

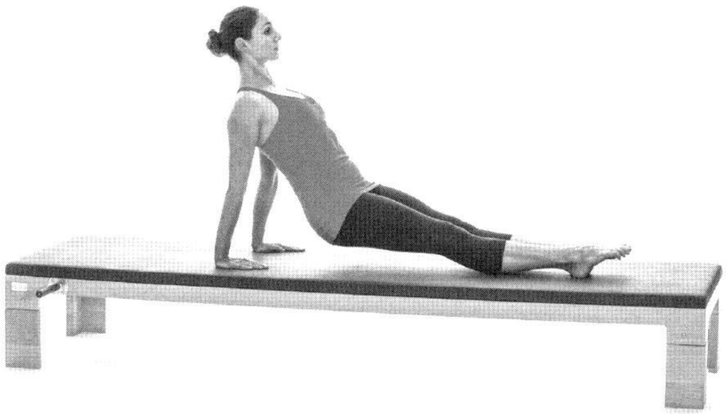

Inhale. Lower the body, hinging at the hip and shoulder joints without quite touching the mat. Repeat 5 times. After the final repetition place the pelvis on the mat. Return to the start position.

Leg Pull Back

Muscle Focus

- Hip, back, and shoulder extensors
- Hip flexors

Objectives

- To improve hip extensor and shoulder extensor strength
- To improve back extensor and hip flexor control
- To develop trunk and scapular stabilization

The Mat: Back Support is a prerequisite to learning and mastering this exercise. As with the Mat: Leg Pull Front, the key to the exercise is maintaining stability in the body, except for the leg that lifts and lowers.

Flexibility is a major factor in the success of this exercise. Without it, your ability to perform the exercise will be limited. The flexibility of the shoulders is already challenged by the back support position. As the leg lifts forward and up, hip flexor strength and hamstring flexibility play a vital role.

Imagery

Use the concept of the energy lines discussed in the Mat: Back Support. Keep the line from the head through the ankles stable and straight. Visualize the lifting leg as a second energy line attached to the side of the pelvis. The leg swings up and down without affecting the large, stable central line.

- Isolate the movement of the leg as you lift it and lower it.
- Keep the hip extensors of the supporting leg, the shoulder extensors, and the back extensors engaged.
- Align the head with the spine.

MODIFICATION

This exercise can be performed with the supporting leg bent, making this challenging exercise more accessible. This position helps alleviate pressure from the back of the supporting knee, which can be an obstacle for some, particularly if hyperextension is present. This version tends to stretch the front of the shoulders and chest more than the original, which may prove more difficult (but also very beneficial) for those with tight shoulders and kyphotic posture. At the start of the exercise, both legs are bent and the pelvis is lifted off the mat. Strive to achieve a long line stretching from the knees through the trunk, shoulders, and head. Maintain this position as one leg is straightened to the front with the foot plantarflexed. Kick the leg up toward the ceiling and then lower to touch the floor. Repeat 5 times before bending the knee, placing the foot on the mat, and returning to the start position. Switch to the other side.

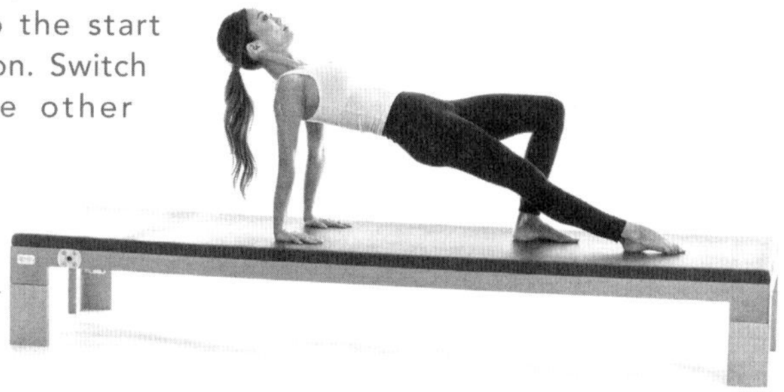

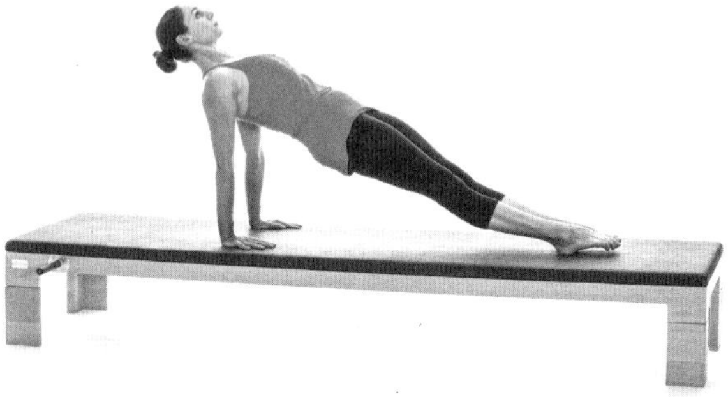

Setup. Sit with the hands approximately 12 inches (30 centimeters) behind the pelvis, fingers facing the pelvis. Straighten the legs out in front, hip width apart, and plantarflex the feet. Engage the back extensors and scapular stabilizers. Lift the pelvis off the mat, hinging at the hip and shoulder joints, until the body is in a straight line.

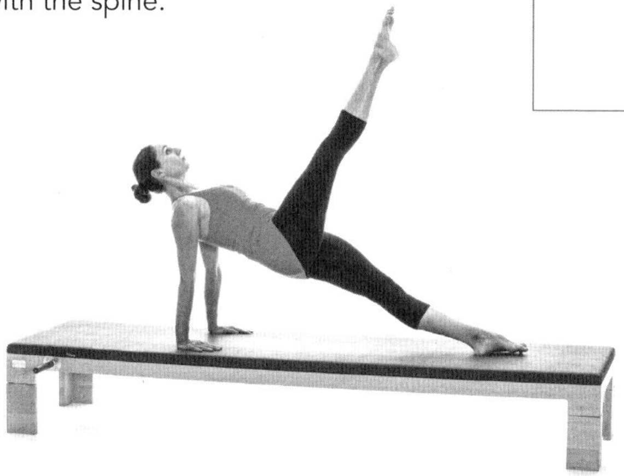

Exhale. Flex the hip, lifting one leg up toward the ceiling.

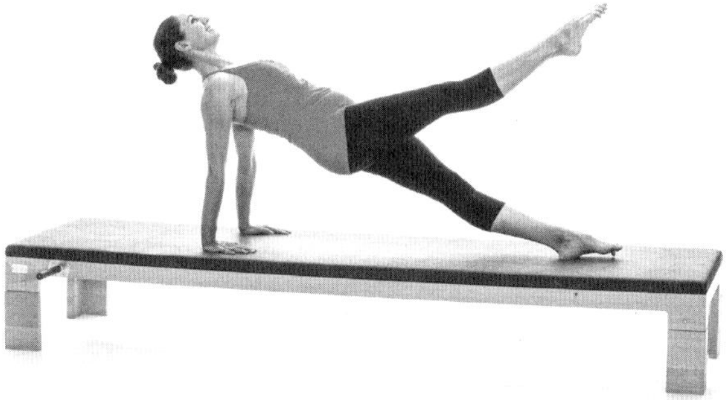

Inhale. Lower the leg, lightly touch the mat. Repeat 5 times before switching to the other side. Return to the start position.

Cat Stretch

This exceptional exercise achieves three important goals: spinal flexion (focusing on the abdominals), spinal extension (focusing on the back extensors), and trunk stabilization (focusing on the abdominals and back extensors co-contracting) in a quadruped position, laying the foundation for the Mat: Front Support and Leg Pull Front. It has the added benefit of stretching the muscles of the lower back during the flexion phase and improving lumbopelvic stabilization during extension. The Mat: Cat Stretch can prove particularly valuable for low-load abdominal and back work, like that required during pregnancy, rehabilitation, and for the older adult population.

This exercise is often performed with excessive rounding of the upper back during the flexion phase and hyperlordosis during the extension phase. The version offered in this book counters those tendencies by focusing the flexion on the lower back and the extension on the mid- and upper back. The pelvis is held in a neutral position (or as close as possible) during the extension, as opposed to an anterior tilt.

Imagery

Spinal flexion evokes an image of a ball of energy or a whirlpool that stirs up in the abdominal region, creating a firm, round shape. Spinal extension evokes a feeling of elevating the sternum to create the distinctive look of a sphinx, proud and determined. Also, as the name implies, the image of a cat awakening and taking a lengthy stretch is essential to the dynamic of this exercise. Visualize the cat's spine rounding and arching, displaying its phenomenal mobility and elasticity.

- ○ Keep the hips above the knees and the shoulders above the wrists.
- ○ The movement occurs in the trunk, between the hip joints and shoulder joints.
- ○ Maximize flexion in the lower back during the first phase and extension in the mid- and upper back during the second phase.
- ○ During the first phase, avoid rounding the upper back excessively, dropping the head too far between the arms, or tucking the pelvis aggressively.

Muscle Focus

- Abdominals
- Back extensors
- Scapular stabilizers

Objectives

- To improve mid- and upper back extensor strength
- To improve abdominal control
- To improve lower back flexibility
- To improve trunk and scapular stabilization

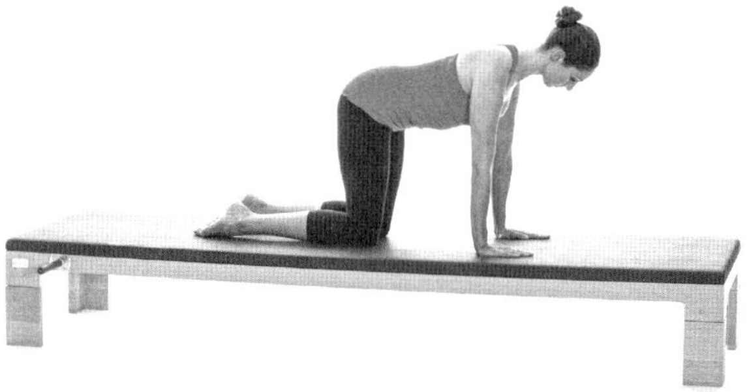

Setup. Kneel in a quadruped position, with the knees hip width apart directly under the hip joints, and the hands shoulder width apart, wrists directly under the shoulders. Establish a neutral position of the spine, weight evenly distributed between the upper and lower body. Sense the elongation and elasticity of the spine from the tailbone to the top of the head, drawing awareness to the ISS.

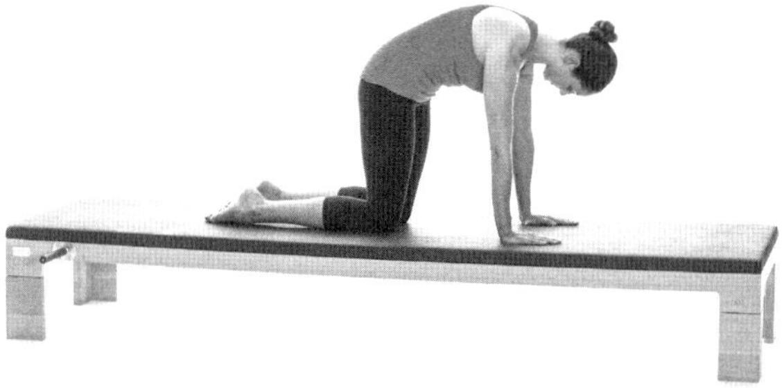

Exhale. Engage the abdominals and draw the spine into flexion while accentuating the curve in the lower back region, allowing the head and pelvis to respond and follow the natural line of the spine.

Inhale. Return to the neutral elongated spinal position (neutral spine). Do not release the abdominal or back muscles during this phase; they continue co-contracting to create a stable trunk.

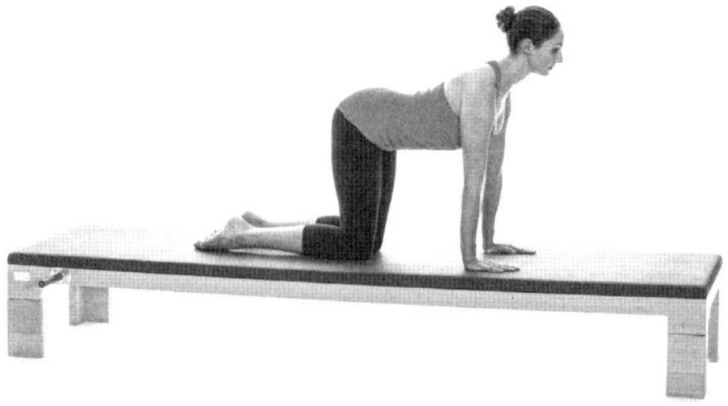

Exhale. Extend the back, accentuating the arch in the mid- and upper spine, while maintaining stability of the lumbopelvic region. Externally rotating the shoulders slightly helps to facilitate the upper back extension.

Inhale. Return to the neutral elongated spinal position (neutral spine), co-contracting the abdominals and back extensors to create a stable trunk. Repeat the complete cycle 5 times.

Front Support

Muscle Focus

- Abdominals
- Hip flexors
- Scapular stabilizers

Objectives

- To improve upper body strength
- To develop lumbopelvic and scapular stabilization

Also known as the plank or push-up position, the Mat: Front Support uses two critical areas of stabilization: the lumbopelvic region and the shoulder girdle. Strengthening these two areas and establishing good muscle activation provides efficient stabilization for subsequent and more challenging exercises on all the apparatus. It is very common to see push-ups being done incorrectly, with little attention devoted to the setup, and quantity overriding the importance of quality and precision. When good alignment and solid stabilization are lacking, the trunk and the shoulder region collapse, resulting in inefficient and sometimes harmful positions.

Imagery

Imagine the body as a strong, solid bridge or ramp that will not budge under immense weight.

- Keep the body in a straight line from head to toes.
- Maintain lumbopelvic and scapular stabilization.
- Keep the wrists directly under the shoulders.

PROGRESSION

To further challenge yourself in this front support position, exhale, and bend one leg in toward the chest (touching the knee down lightly if necessary). Inhale, and straighten the leg back to the front support position. Exhale, and bend the other leg. Inhale, and return to the front support position. Continue alternating legs.

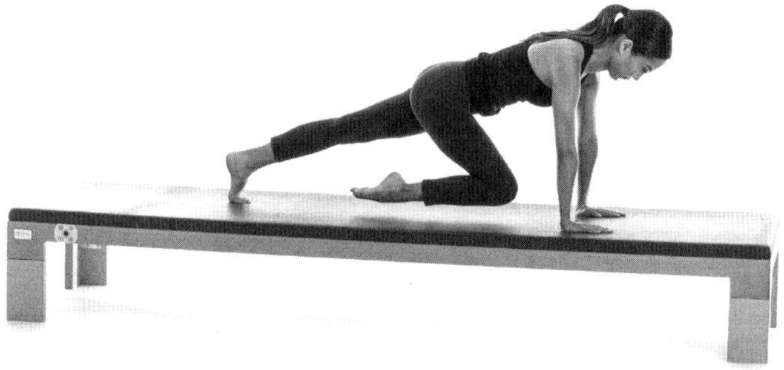

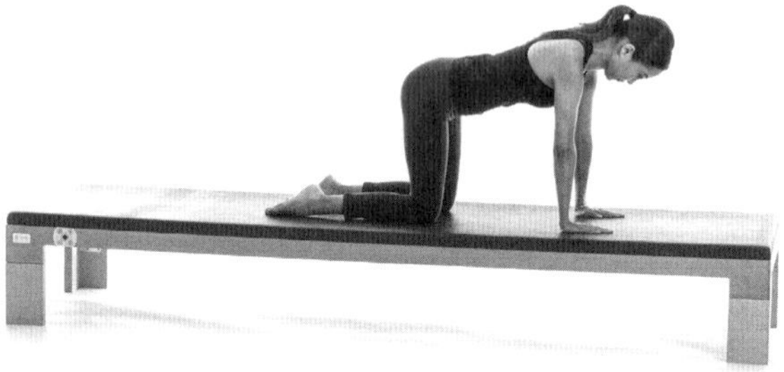

Setup. Kneel in a quadruped position, with the knees hip width apart directly under the hip joints and the hands shoulder width apart, wrists directly under the shoulders. Establish a neutral position of the spine, weight evenly distributed between the upper and lower body.

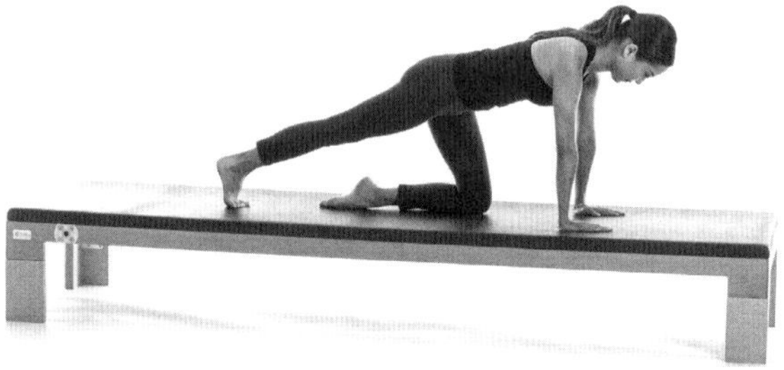

Exhale. Reach one leg back with minimal weight shift. Further stabilize the shoulder region.

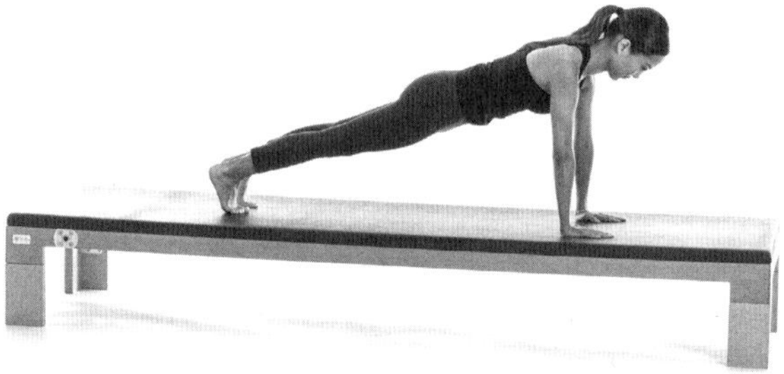

Inhale. Reach the other leg back into the front support position, with the arms and legs firm and straight, feet hip width apart. Hold this position for 30-60 seconds while further engaging the ISS, maintaining stability throughout the body. Bend one knee in and then the other. Return to the start position. Repeat 2-4 times. Alternate the starting leg.

Leg Pull Front

Mastering the Mat: Front Support before learning this exercise is imperative, because it is the foundation on which the Mat: Leg Pull Front is built.

The key to the exercise is maintaining stillness in the body, except for the leg that lifts and lowers. Using only one leg for support while moving the other makes this difficult position less stable and therefore more challenging. Note that when the leg lifts to the back, the pelvis remains stable. This means that the leg may extend no more than a few degrees (depending on hip flexor flexibility) before the pelvis starts tilting anteriorly. Stop before this happens. Dancers may be tempted to do a full arabesque, but I urge you to keep the pelvis neutral and maximize height without tilting the pelvis. This translates into pure hip extension. Then, when the pelvis is allowed to tilt anteriorly and rotate to maximize turnout and height, the leg will be higher and stronger than ever before.

Imagery

Imagine a drawbridge: One part of the bridge remains stable and still as the other section lifts to allow tall ships to pass under it. Another valuable image is that of an energy line running through the body from the feet to the crown of the head. A second energy line represents the moving leg that swings freely without disrupting the stable energy line.

- Maintain a plank position of the body.
- Keep the pelvis neutral with a bias toward a slight posterior tilt.
- Maintain scapular stabilization.

MODIFICATION

Start in a quadruped position. Straighten one leg back with the foot plantarflexed and toes touching the mat. Lift and lower the leg so the toes touch the mat lightly. Focus on hip disassociation, keeping the trunk and pelvis as stable and still as possible as the leg lifts and lowers. Repeat 5 times before switching to the other side.

Muscle Focus

- Abdominals
- Hip flexors
- Hip extensors
- Scapular stabilizers

Objectives

- To improve upper body strength
- To improve hip extensor control
- To develop lumbopelvic and scapular stabilization

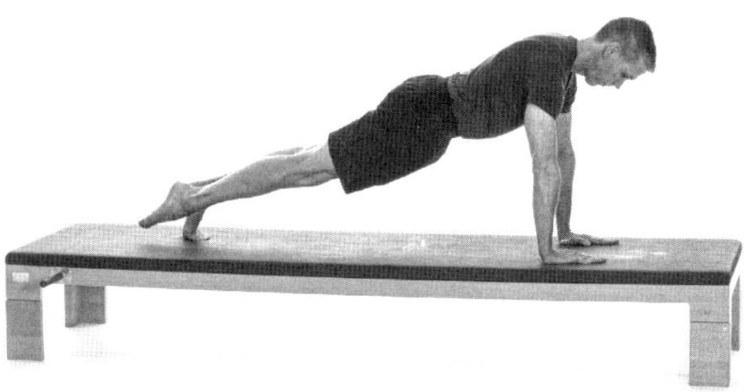

Setup. Kneel in a quadruped position, with the knees hip width apart directly under the hip joints and the hands shoulder width apart, wrists directly under the shoulders. Establish a neutral position of the spine, weight evenly distributed between the upper and lower body. Reach one leg back with minimal weight shift, and then extend the other leg back into the front support position, with the arms and legs firm and straight. Lift one leg slightly off the ground, plantarflexing the foot.

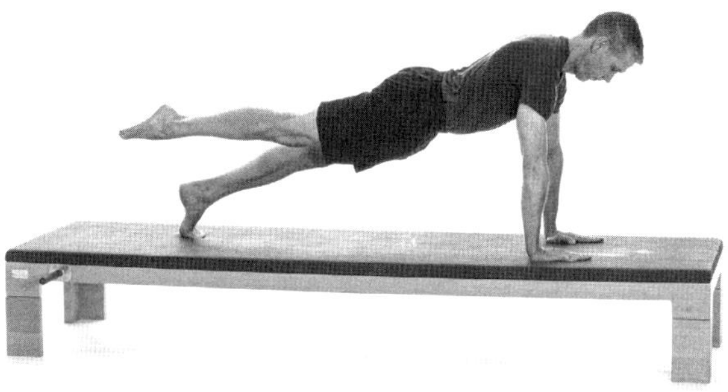

Exhale. Extend the hip, lifting the leg higher.

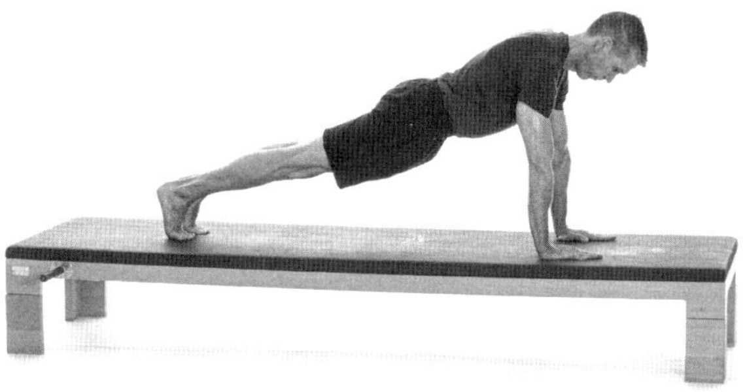

Inhale. Lower the leg so the toes touch the mat lightly, maintaining plantarflexion. Repeat 5 times before switching to the other side.

On the final repetition, dorsiflex the foot and place it on the ground, returning to the front support position.

Push-Up

Muscle Focus

- Elbow extensors
- Shoulder flexors
- Scapular stabilizers
- Abdominals

Objectives

- To improve elbow extensor and shoulder flexor strength
- To develop lumbopelvic and scapular stabilization
- To develop spinal articulation

Unlike a typical push-up, the Pilates version is a movement sequence that involves the entire body, shifting from the front support position, through a roll-up, to standing upright, and back again. Within this sequence are the actual push-ups, which, with the elbows kept close to the sides of the body, amplify the work of the triceps. Of primary importance is keeping the scapulae stable as the elbows bend and the body is lowered and then lifted back up. The level of scapular stabilization determines the depth of the elbow flexion—as soon as the scapulae start to elevate or adduct, lift the body back up and regroup before doing another repetition. It is important to not lose sight of the lumbopelvic stabilization throughout the exercise.

Few people are initially able to keep the scapulae stable in a neutral position. Many a "muscle man" has crumbled trying to do push-ups keeping the scapulae stable. During a large presentation in China in 2003, I asked for a volunteer to do no more than 10 push-ups correctly (I defined "correctly" as holding the trunk and scapulae absolutely stable and moving only the arms). A hulk of a man with muscles bulging everywhere came up. I must admit, I thought that I'd met my match and my experiment would fail. As he proceeded with the utmost confidence, I stopped him each time his scapulae began to move, both inward and upward. He did not get very far, and when I feared that the pool of sweat that had built up under him was about to drown us both, he collapsed and, with a slight smile, conceded that he needed to learn how to do push-ups again (after doing 500 a day for 20 years!). We gave each other a hug, and no words were necessary to express the understanding, camaraderie, and respect we felt for each other—and the work.

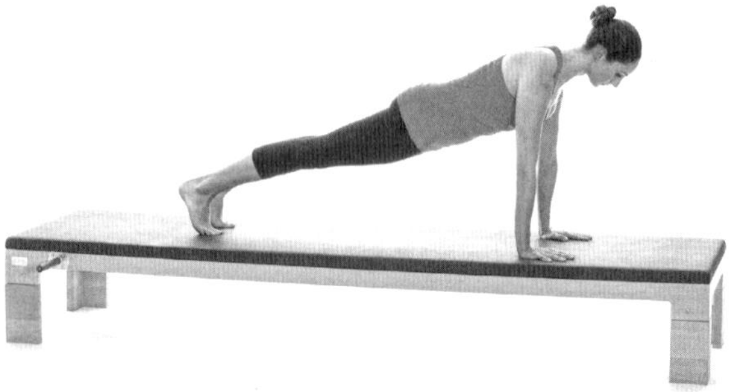

Setup. Kneel in a quadruped position, with the knees hip width apart directly under the hip joints and the hands shoulder width apart, wrists directly under the shoulders. Establish a neutral position of the spine, weight evenly distributed between the upper and lower body. Reach one leg back with minimal weight shift, and then extend the other leg back into the front support position, with the arms and legs firm and straight.

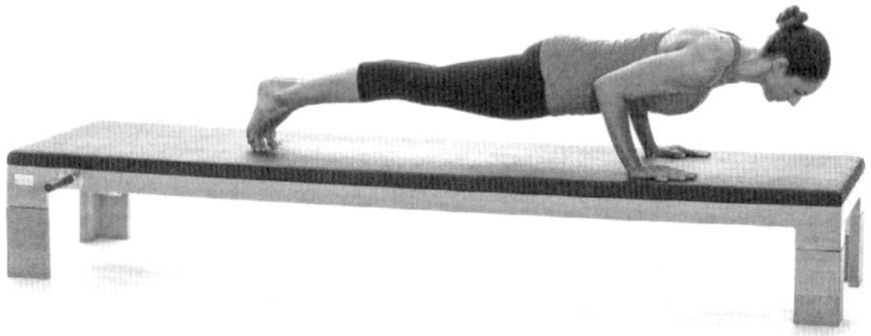

Inhale. Bend the elbows, keeping them close to the sides of the body (as in a push-up).

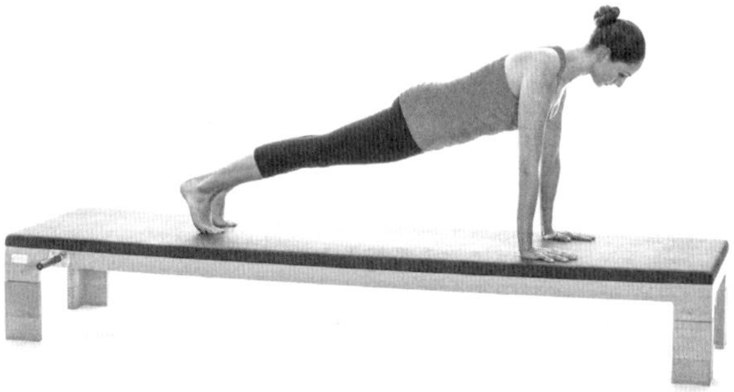

Exhale. Straighten the elbows, keeping them close to the sides of the body. Repeat the push-up twice.

Imagery

Imagine the body as a strong, solid bridge that will not budge under immense weight. When the pelvis is lifted prior to moving into an upright standing position, visualize the body as a pyramid, with the tailbone as the tip and the feet and hands as the base. When lifting into the roll-up, the sense should be of a band around the midsection of the body with an external force, like a crane, pulling you up from the back and then lowering you again following the upright standing position. The dynamic should be brisk and smooth.

- Engage the abdominals.
- Keep the elbows close to the sides of the body, particularly when bending and straightening.
- Do not allow the scapulae to adduct or elevate.

PROGRESSION

Once you have mastered moving from the front support position to standing and back again, gradually decrease the number of arm walks. Achieving two arm walks in each direction is challenging but achievable by most. An excellent goal is to strive to do the movement with no arm walking—just one swoop up and then a dive back to the front support position. This demands pushing off from the arms while simultaneously lifting the pelvis high into the air, transferring the weight to the feet, and then rolling up through the spine. Reverse this sequence to return to the front support position.

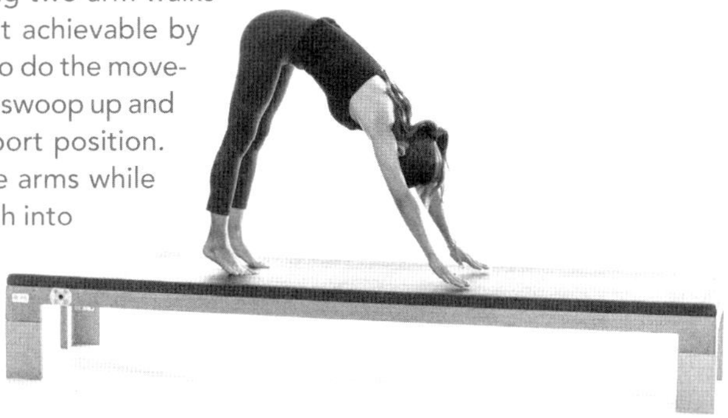

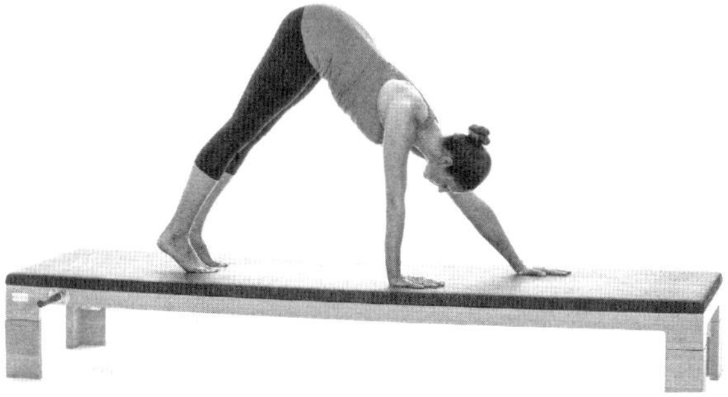

After the second repetition, lift the pelvis upward and walk the hands toward the feet, transferring the weight to the feet. Keep the elbows straight when walking the hands back.

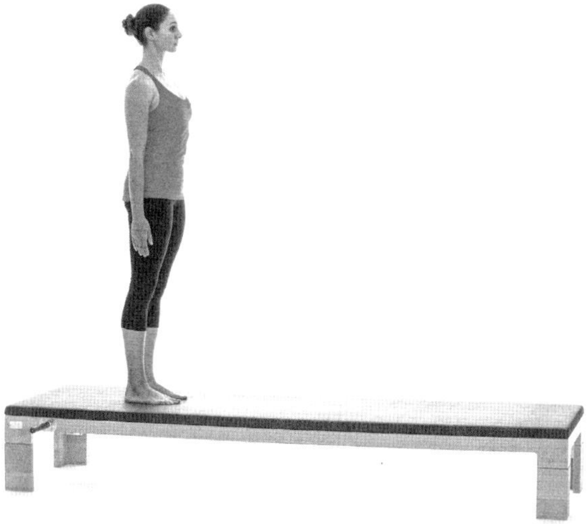

Roll up to a standing position.

Inhale. Establish good upright alignment.

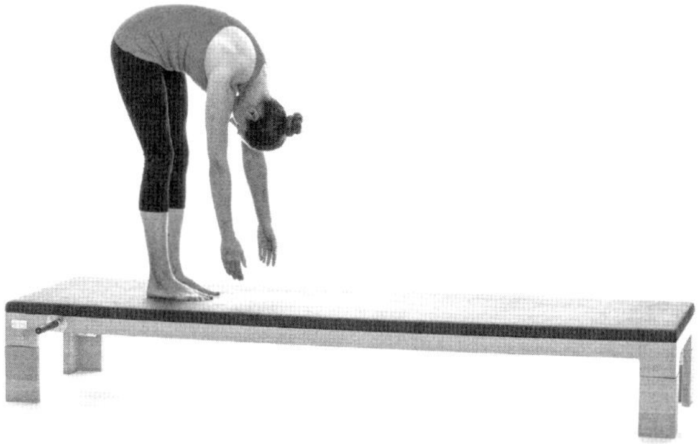

Exhale. Roll down and walk the hands forward to the front support position. Keep the elbows straight when walking the hands forward. Repeat the entire sequence 3-5 times.

Lateral Flexion and Rotation

The focus of the exercises in this block are movements that involve lateral flexion and rotation of the spine. These movements place greater emphasis on the abdominal obliques versus the rectus abdominis. The abdominal obliques (located toward the sides of the trunk versus the front), particularly the internal obliques, work with the transversus abdominis to stabilize the spine and protect the back from injury. Many athletic and recreational endeavors, such as swimming, kayaking, golf, throwing sports, and tennis, involve extensive use of the very powerful obliques. Greater strength and coordination in the obliques can enhance athletic performance.

The abdominal obliques are key lateral flexors of the spine; however, the quadratus lumborum and spinal extensors can also produce lateral flexion. Excessive contraction of the obliques combined with inadequate use of the spinal extensors causes the trunk to round forward (spinal flexion) as it flexes laterally. Conversely, excessive contraction of the spinal extensors causes the back to arch (spinal extension) as it flexes laterally. Therefore, finely coordinated contraction of the anterior and posterior muscles of the spine is required to achieve the desired position for lateral flexion. Exercising in this side position provides valuable practice for maintaining neutral alignment of the pelvis and spine during everyday activities, and learning to brace the muscles of the core allows you to support and protect the spine during those activities.

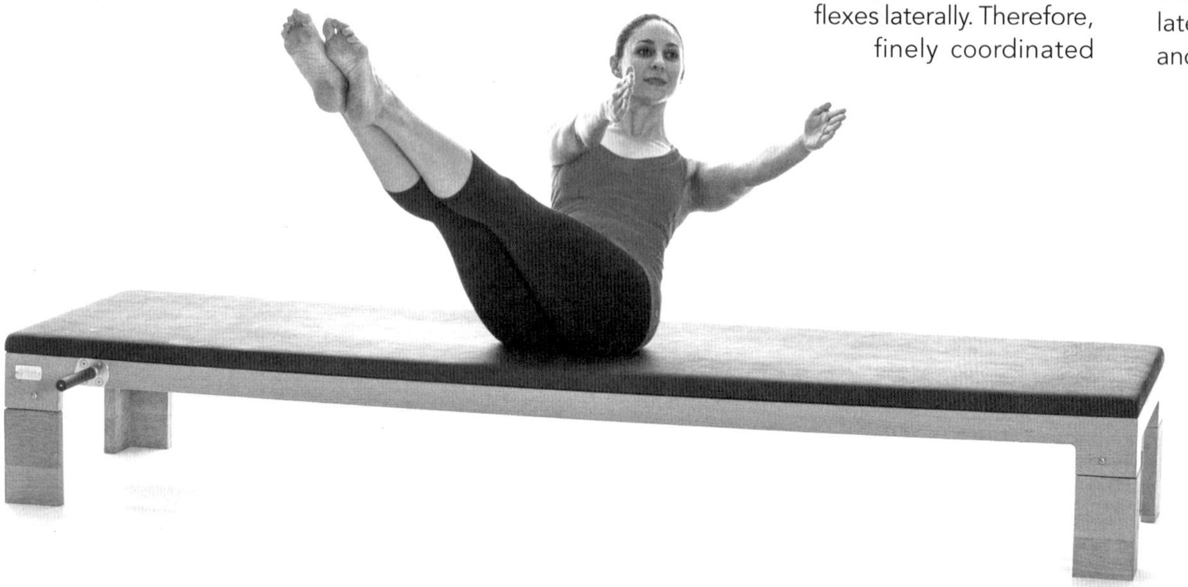

Certain exercises in this chapter use rotation of the spine in some form—some from a sitting position as in the Mat: Spine Twist—Sitting and the Mat: Saw, others from a supine position as in the Mat: Corkscrew, and even some from a side plank position as in the Mat: Twist. All the exercises emphasize the abdominal obliques, yet each is unique in its pattern of coordinated recruitment of the spinal flexors, lateral flexors, rotators, and extensors. The name of this block illustrates the close relationship that exists between the lateral flexors and rotators, plus many exercises incorporate both. However, for the sake of clarity, I have divided this block into two subsections: The first encompasses the exercises that focus on lateral flexion; the second highlights rotation. I have done this only for the mat work. On all other apparatus I have categorized exercises that use lateral flexion, rotation, or both into the lateral flexion and rotation block.

Side Leg Lift

Muscle Focus

- Abdominal obliques

Objectives

- To improve lateral flexor strength
- To improve hip adductor control
- To develop lumbopelvic stabilization

Every good, well-balanced exercise program should include lateral flexion of the trunk. The Mat: Side Leg Lift is a fundamental exercise that is relatively simple to execute and teach yet profound in its effect. Significant imbalances in strength and range of motion between the two sides of the trunk are common, and this imbalance should be addressed by working each side independently, which the Mat: Side Leg Lift achieves. This exercise also develops lumbopelvic stabilization.

The ideal alignment of the body in this exercise is a straight line, with the spine in a neutral position, the trunk flexors and extensors co-contracted, and the lateral flexors on both sides engaged. As the lateral flexors on the top contract concentrically and shorten, the lateral flexors on the underside contract eccentrically and elongate.

Imagery

Imagine a long energy line reaching from the top of the head through the trunk, legs, and feet. The body creates an elongated bow shape as the legs lift. Another helpful image is that of a fish on its side with its tail swooping upward.

- ○ Keep the abdominal obliques on both sides recruited.

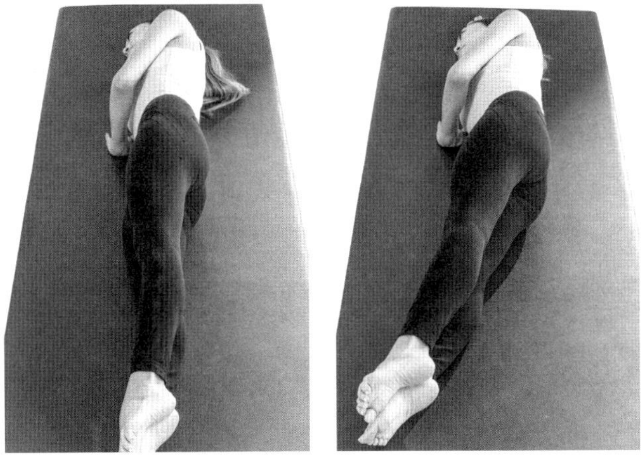

If the ideal plumb alignment cannot be achieved because of excessive back extensor activation, shift the legs slightly forward of the centerline, creating a banana shape. Do not allow the legs to move too far forward, however, which may result in undesired hip flexion.

- ○ Keep the adductors engaged, moving the legs and pelvis as one unit.
- ○ Maintain a sense of lengthening the lower leg, keeping it alongside the top leg.

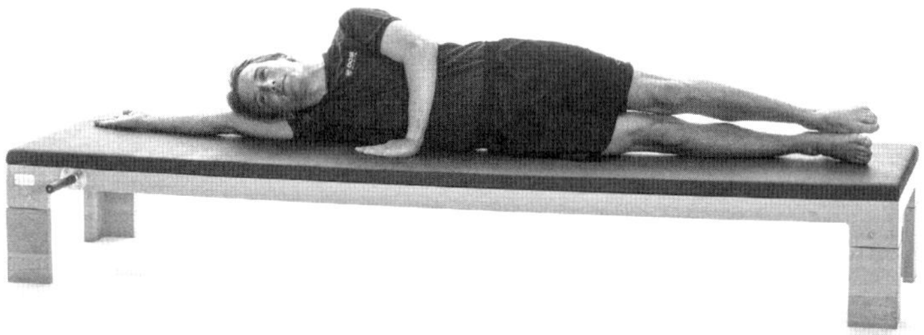

Setup. Lie on one side with the bottom arm straight in line with the body and the head resting on it. The pelvis is "stacked" perpendicular to the mat and the legs are pressing together. The top arm is either bent, with the palm down on the mat in front of the body, or straight, with the palm resting on the top thigh (more challenging).

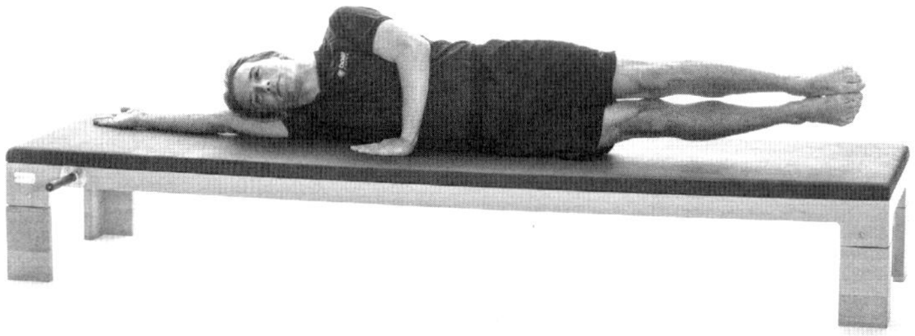

Exhale. Lift both legs by laterally flexing the trunk (tilting the pelvis), keeping the legs together and the body aligned.

Inhale. Lower the legs without allowing the feet to touch the mat. Repeat 10 times. Following the final repetition, lower the legs to the mat. Return to the start position. Switch to the other side.

Side Kick

Muscle Focus

- Hip abductors, flexors, and extensors
- Abdominals
- Back extensors
- Scapular stabilizers

Objectives

- To improve hip flexor and hip extensor control and flexibility
- To improve hip abductor control
- To develop trunk and lumbopelvic stabilization
- To develop hip disassociation

This exercise reinforces the concept of trunk and pelvic stabilization with hip disassociation. A side-lying position relies on a much smaller and narrower base of support than one that is supine or prone. Consequently, the level of difficulty is increased, and the lateral stabilizers of the body are activated significantly more. By focusing on scapular and trunk stabilization, you minimize the pressure on the elbow and maximize stability. As the leg swings back and forth, spinal flexors and extensors are in a state of balanced co-contraction, holding the trunk and pelvis stable. When the leg swings forward, the spinal extensors work to prevent spinal flexion; when it swings back, the abdominals work to prevent spinal hyperextension. These subtle internal adjustments are hardly visible, but their impact on the pelvis and spine is significant.

This exercise is an excellent example of how the body adapts to changes in the center of gravity. As the leg swings back and forth, the pelvis adapts by shifting slightly in the opposite direction of the leg. This small motion of the pelvis assists greatly in maintaining a balanced, stable position, both in this exercise and in everyday movements. However, this should be differentiated from a distinct anterior or posterior tilt of the pelvis, which is not desirable and would be regarded as a compensation.

Imagery

Imagine the swinging motion of a pendulum on its side. The motion of the leg should feel like a pendulum, swinging freely and effortlessly.

- ○ Minimize rocking of the trunk as the leg swings forward and backward.
- ○ Maximize the range of motion of the leg forward and backward (without tilting the pelvis posteriorly and anteriorly).
- ○ Maintain scapular stabilization with particular attention on the lower shoulder.
- ○ Keep the underside of the trunk lifted and avoid the ribs flaring.

MODIFICATION

Instead of resting on the lower elbow, which offers very little support and makes the structure unstable, place the entire forearm on the floor, fingers facing forward. This position offers more stability. The rest of the exercise is exactly the same as described.

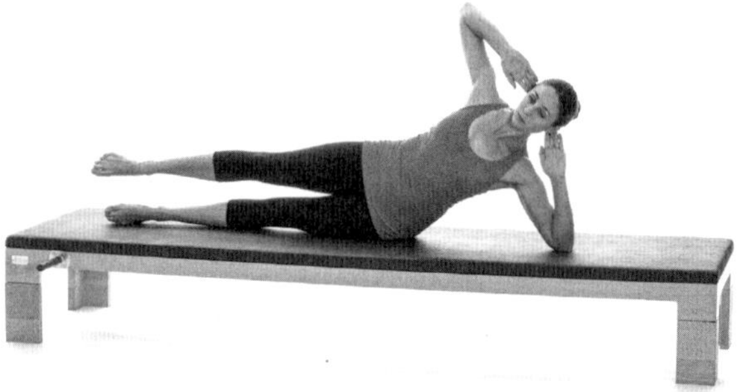

Setup. Lie on one side, leaning on the elbow of the lower arm with the hands behind the head. Engage the underside abdominal obliques and scapular stabilizers to support the trunk. Stabilize the bottom leg on the floor and hold the top leg at hip height, engaging the hip abductors.

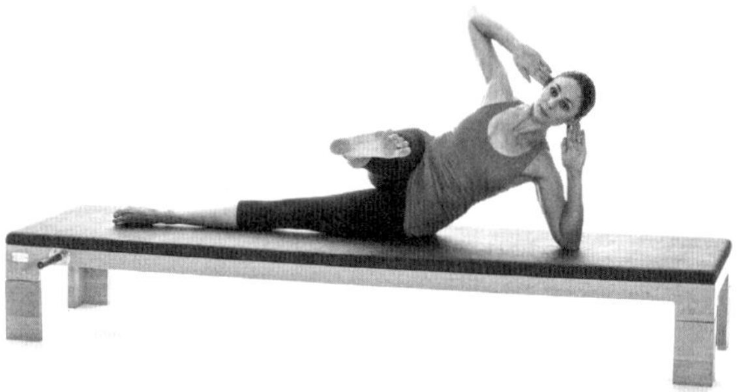

Exhale. Swing the top leg as far forward as possible, dorsiflexing the foot and pulsing twice (exhaling on each pulse) when the leg reaches maximum range. Maintain a neutral position of the pelvis (avoid posteriorly tilting the pelvis).

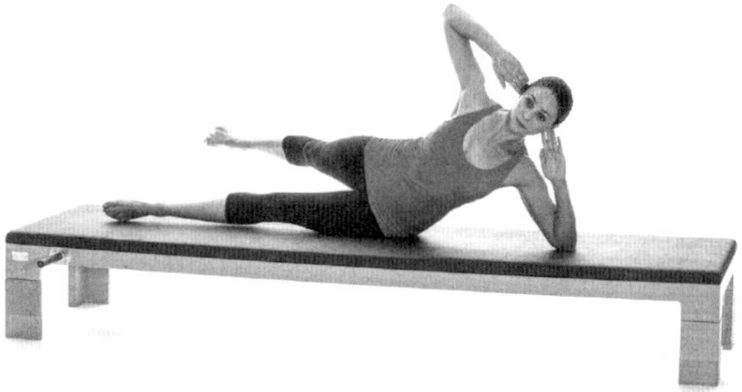

Inhale. Swing the leg back as far as possible, plantarflexing the foot and elongating the leg, pulsing twice (inhaling on each pulse) when the leg reaches maximum range. Maintain a neutral position of the pelvis (avoid anteriorly tilting the pelvis and hyperextending the back). Repeat the cycle 10 times, finishing in the backward swing position. Switch to the other side.

Side Kick—Kneeling

Muscle Focus

- Hip abductors, flexors, and extensors
- Abdominals
- Back extensors
- Scapular stabilizers

Objectives

- To improve hip flexor and hip extensor control and flexibility
- To improve hip abductor strength
- To develop trunk and lumbopelvic stabilization
- To develop hip disassociation

This exercise is an extension of the Mat: Side Kick, made more difficult by decreasing the base of support to one hand and the lower leg. The primary focus remains on lumbopelvic stabilization and hip flexion and extension. Keep the swinging leg at a consistent height (as high as possible) during the transition from front to back; this increases the hip abductor work exponentially. The head should be aligned with the spine throughout, which decreases the chance of neck tension.

Effective shoulder and trunk stabilization is fundamental to this exercise and helps moderate the weight bearing on the wrist.

Imagery

Use the imagery of a pendulum on its side described in the Mat: Side Kick. Add to this the feeling of being suspended like a bridge.

- ○ Minimize rocking of the trunk as the leg swings forward and backward.
- ○ Maximize the range of motion of the leg forward and backward while keeping the leg at hip height or above (as high as possible).
- ○ Maintain arm support and scapular stabilization with particular attention on the lower shoulder.
- ○ Keep the underside of the trunk lifted and avoid the ribs flaring.

VARIATION

One of the most common complaints about exercises in which one or both wrists bear the weight of the body is discomfort and even pain in the wrist. To decrease pressure on the wrist, make a fist with the supporting hand before placing it on the mat. This position decreases or eliminates excessive wrist extension by facilitating a neutral position of the wrist.

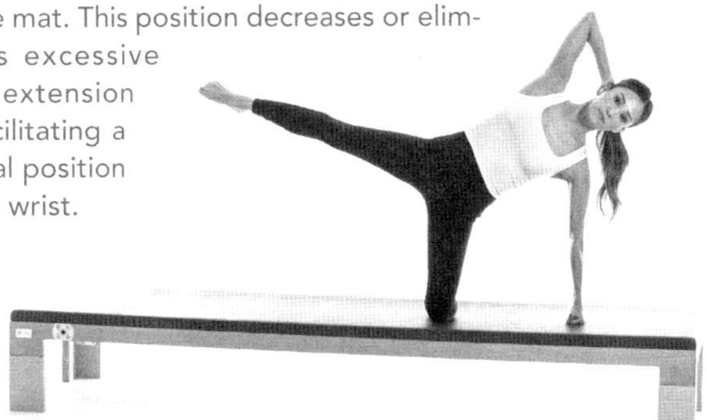

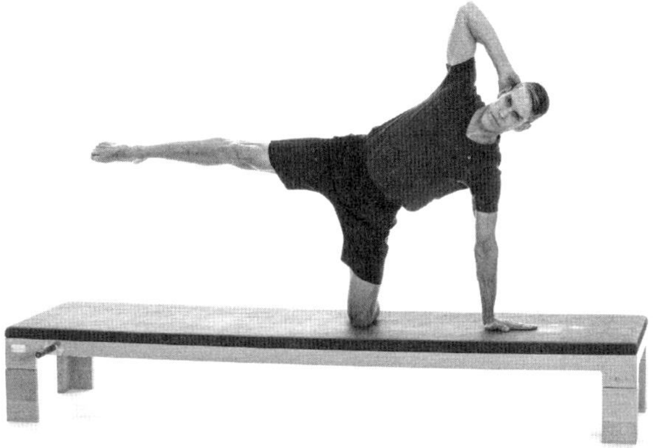

Setup. Kneeling, shift the weight to one knee with the lower leg reaching directly back. Place the supporting hand (same side of the body as the weighted knee) on the floor, wrist directly under the shoulder. The other leg is straight, foot plantarflexed. Lift the leg to hip height or higher if possible. Place the free hand behind the head.

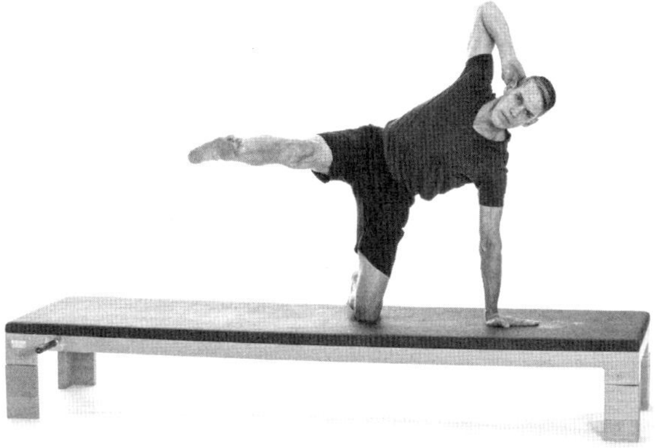

Exhale. Swing the top leg as far forward as possible and dorsiflex the foot (avoid posteriorly tilting the pelvis), pulsing twice (exhaling on each pulse) when the leg reaches maximum range.

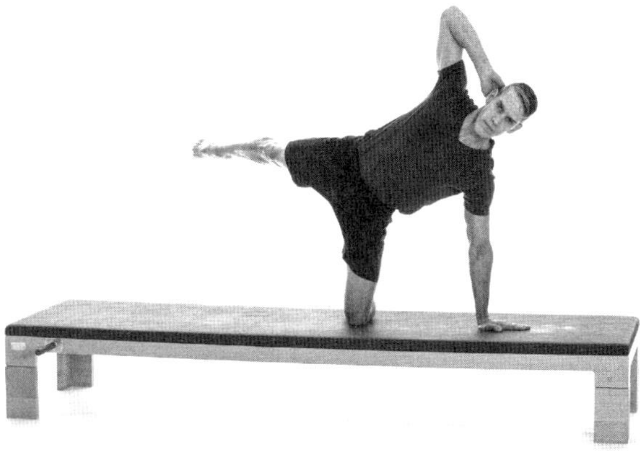

Inhale. Swing the leg back as far as possible and plantarflex the foot (avoid anteriorly tilting the pelvis and hyperextending the back), pulsing twice (inhaling on each pulse) when the leg reaches maximum range before swinging it forward again. End the exercise with the leg reaching back. Repeat the cycle 10 times before switching to the other side.

Side Bend

Muscle Focus

- Abdominal obliques
- Scapular stabilizers

Objectives

- To improve abdominal oblique strength and flexibility
- To improve shoulder strength
- To develop scapular and trunk stabilization

As you enter the realm of advanced-level work, the base of support becomes smaller and, in many cases, less stable. The Mat: Side Bend relies primarily on trunk and shoulder strength and stabilization. In this exercise, the pivot point around which much of the movement occurs is a single shoulder joint, which, by its nature, is very mobile and potentially unstable. Therefore, you must focus particular attention on correct function of the shoulder. As the body arcs at the top position, the pelvis should lift as high as possible while the free arm swoops over the body, accentuating the arc shape. The head must follow the line of the spine, focusing the gaze toward the hand on the floor. Resist the tendency to lift the head and look upward; doing so can result in neck tension.

The musculature should not relax between repetitions—you should keep a sense of continuous movement. Ideally, even in the bottom phase (the "resting" position) there should be room enough for a piece of paper to pass between the pelvis and the mat. Tremendous support must come from the underside, the lateral aspect of the trunk. The abdominal obliques are crucial to the success of this exercise.

Imagery

A wonderful image to aid in lifting and arcing the body is that of a dolphin leaping out of the water. This movement of course is on the side, but the action and grace of the movement is similar. Imagine that the movement is being performed between two panes of glass to accentuate the two-dimensional quality of the exercise.

- ○ Initiate the movement from the abdominal obliques; avoid relying on the legs to lift.
- ○ Maintain abdominal engagement.
- ○ Keep the scapular stabilizers engaged.

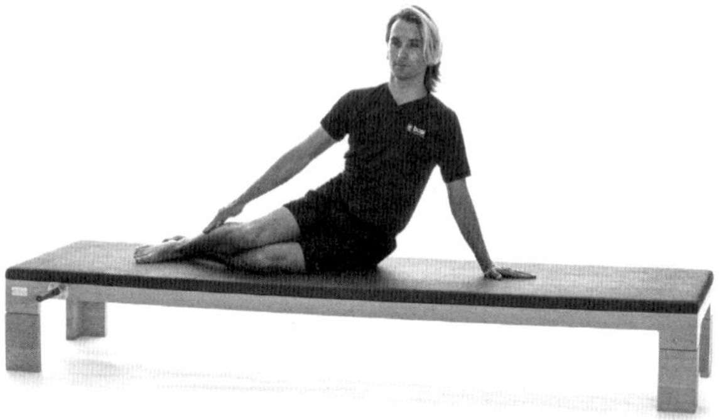

Setup. Sit sideways with the weight on one side of the pelvis. Bend the legs and place the top foot in front of the bottom one. Rest the upper body weight on the supporting arm while maintaining scapular stabilization and recruiting the abdominal obliques. Rest the other arm on the side of the legs.

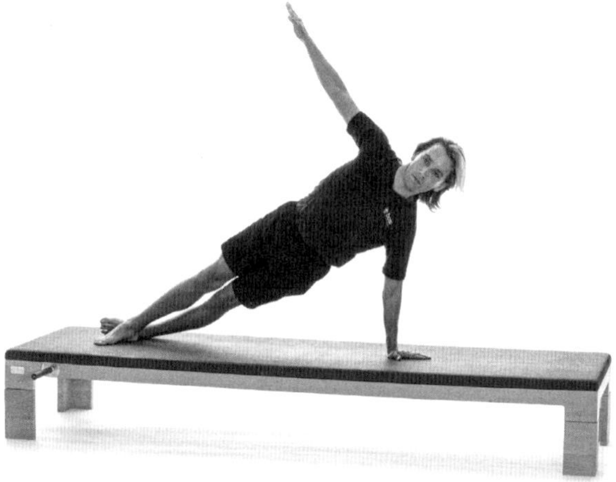

Inhale. Lift the pelvis away from the floor while straightening the legs, establishing a straight diagonal line with the body. Raise the upper arm to shoulder height, creating a 90-degree angle between the arm and the trunk, fingers directed diagonally toward the ceiling.

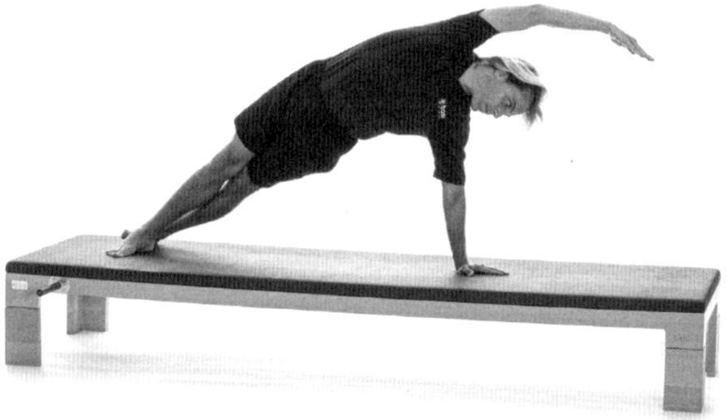

Exhale. Contract the lateral muscles of the underside of the trunk and lift the pelvis toward the ceiling, creating an arc shape with the body as the upper arm reaches overhead.

VARIATION

Perform this same movement pattern, but rather than using a straight arm for support with the weight on the wrist, place the forearm on the mat with the elbow under the shoulder and the fingers facing directly forward. In this version the legs will remain straight.

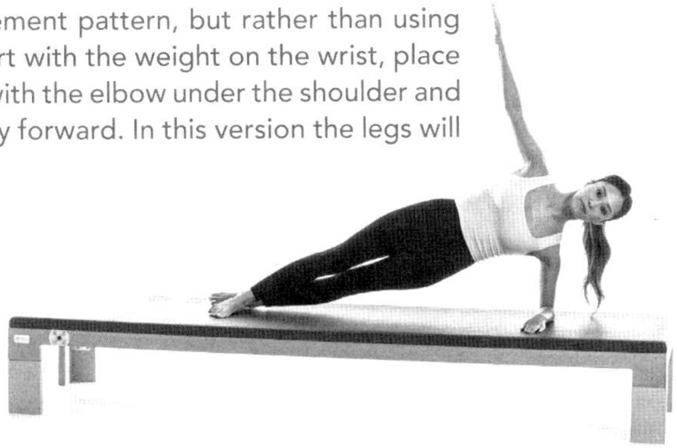

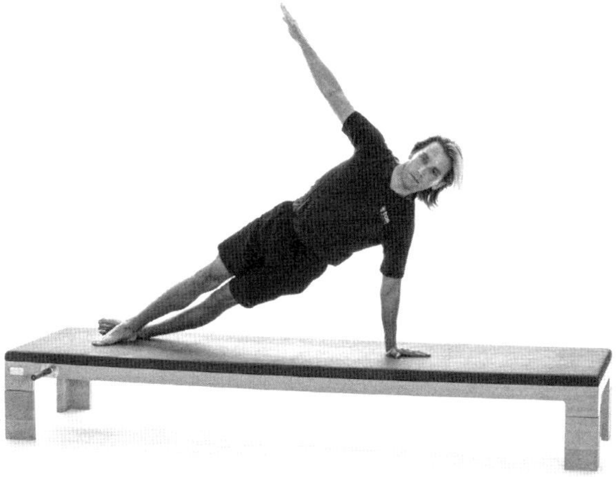

Inhale. Return to the previous position with the body in a straight diagonal line and the upper arm aligned with the shoulder.

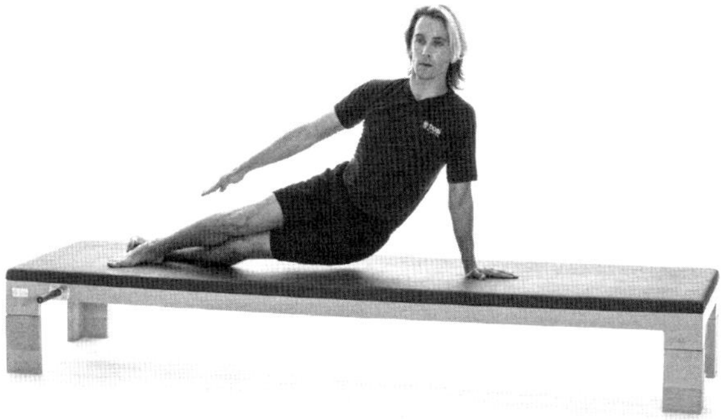

Exhale. Bend the knees and lower the body to the start position, keeping the pelvis slightly off the mat (if possible) or placing it lightly on the mat. Repeat 3-5 times before switching to the other side.

MAT

Rotation

INTERMEDIATE

Muscle Focus

- Abdominal obliques
- Back extensors

Objectives

- To improve abdominal oblique and back extensor strength
- To develop trunk stabilization and rotation

Spine Twist—Sitting

This exercise emphasizes organized rotation of the spine around the longitudinal axis. Proper engagement of the abdominal obliques, together with the support of the back extensors, allow correct rotation of the spine in the upright sitting position. Many movements in daily activities that demand rotation, such as cleaning and gardening, or recreational activities such as golf, volleyball, and tennis, can lead to backache or more severe injuries if not performed correctly. People tend to use the shoulders and arms excessively when doing rotational movements rather than using the powerful muscles of the trunk and focusing on spinal rotation. Typically this is to compensate for lack of mobility and strength in the trunk, or simply because of lack of awareness or skill. Tremendous improvement in performance can be gained when rotation of the trunk is maximized and the powerhouse is employed, rather than relying primarily on the arms and shoulders.

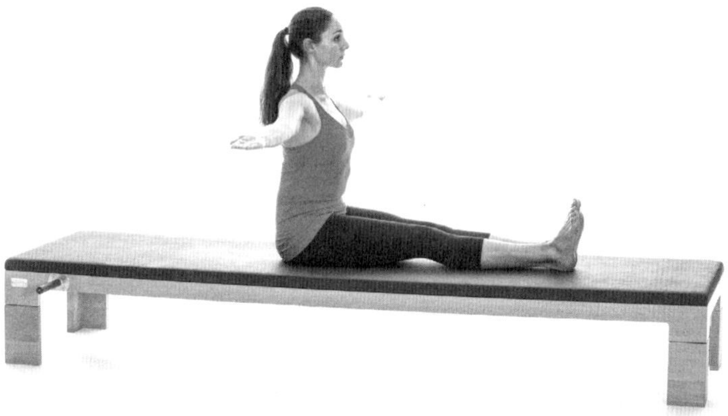

Setup. Sit upright with the legs straight and together, the feet dorsiflexed, heels on the mat. Hold the arms in a T position with the palms facing upward (shoulders in external rotation).

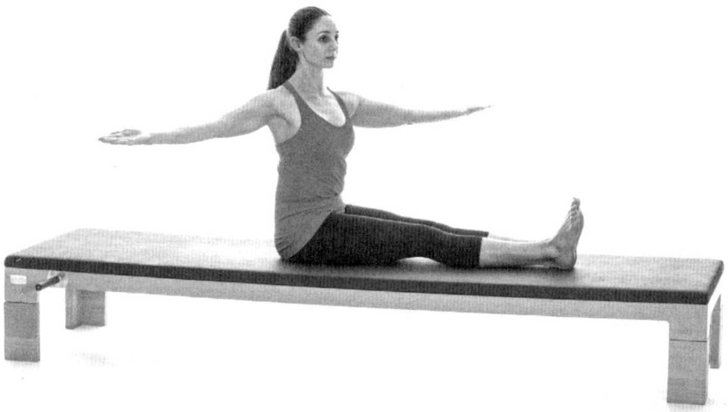

Exhale. Rotate the trunk to one side, pulsing twice when the trunk reaches maximum range (exhaling on each pulse).

Imagery

Imagine two poles or energy lines: one is vertical, running up and down the back, and the other is horizontal, running across the shoulders from the fingertips of one hand to the fingertips of the other. The horizontal pole rotates around the vertical one, while both poles remain in their respective planes of motion.

- Keep the pelvis and legs stable.
- Initiate the movement from the trunk, not from the shoulders or arms.
- Move the head, shoulders, and trunk as one unit.

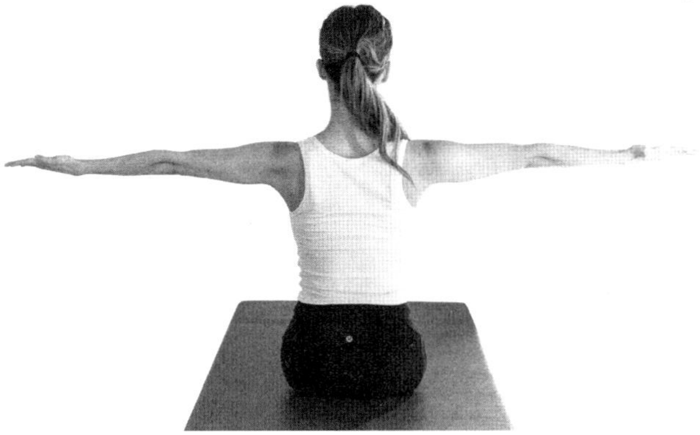

The arms should reach out in opposite directions, creating a straight line across the shoulders.

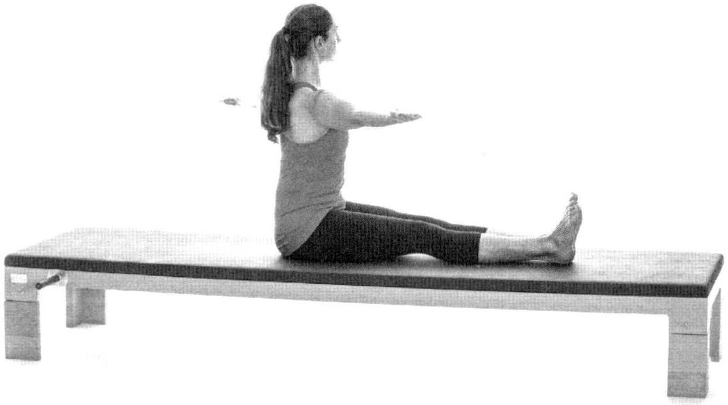

Inhale. Pass through the center and repeat the movement to the other side. Complete the exercise by returning to the start position. Repeat 5 times to each side.

Saw

Muscle Focus

- Hamstrings
- Adductors
- Abdominal obliques
- Back extensors

Objectives

- To improve hamstring and hip adductor flexibility
- To improve abdominal oblique and back extensor control

The Mat: Saw involves an intricate interplay of extending and rotating the trunk and stretching the hamstrings and adductors. Maintain an upright trunk as you rotate around the longitudinal axis in the initial phase prior to the stretch. Return to this exact upright position following the stretch. Only after sitting upright should you rotate back to face center. When sitting upright, whether facing front or rotating, keep the spine elongated over the stable base of the pelvis.

As the trunk and arm reach forward over the leg during the stretch phase, keep the back extensors engaged and the back as flat as possible. This maximizes the hamstring stretch and offers the added benefit of potentially strengthening the back extensors. This exercise is sometimes taught with flexion of the trunk in an endeavor to engage the abdominals more and stretch the back. However, this position is ineffective at doing either. It will not challenge the abdominals enough to achieve any significant strength gain and will not be a profound stretch for the back muscles. The only part of the back that might stretch is the mid- and upper back, a region that few people need to stretch.

When stretching over the leg, the trunk tips forward with the pelvis as one unit, hinging at the hip joint as opposed to segmental articulation of the spine. The tilt forward of the pelvis may be very slight, particularly if someone has tight hamstrings. Keep the spine aligned over the leg and the head aligned with the spine, looking down toward the leg. Some instructors recommend rotating the trunk in this position and looking toward the back arm. Adding rotation to this challenging position often results in severe compensations and bad alignment. Certainly, rotation can be added once proficiency in this version has been achieved.

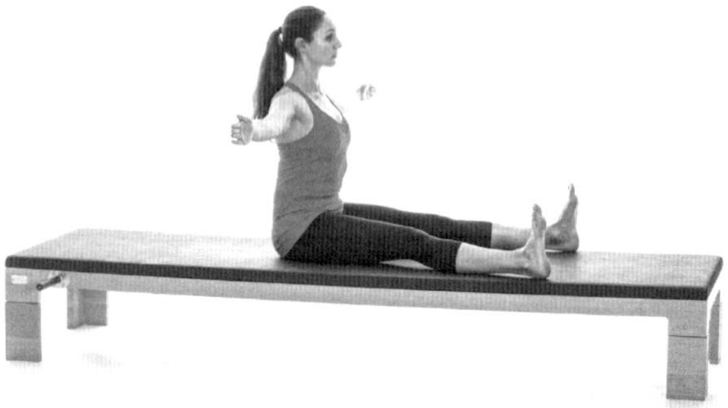

Setup. Sit upright, with the legs straight and open slightly beyond shoulder width, feet dorsiflexed. Hold the arms in a T position, reaching them as far out to the sides as possible, palms facing forward.

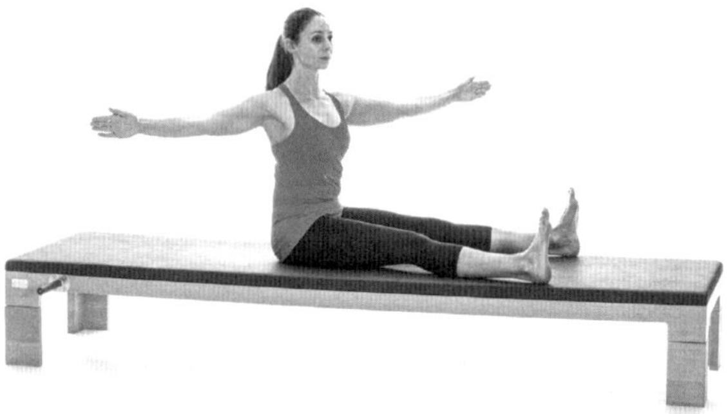

Inhale. Rotate the trunk around the longitudinal axis. Keep the pelvis anchored, and move the arms and head with the trunk.

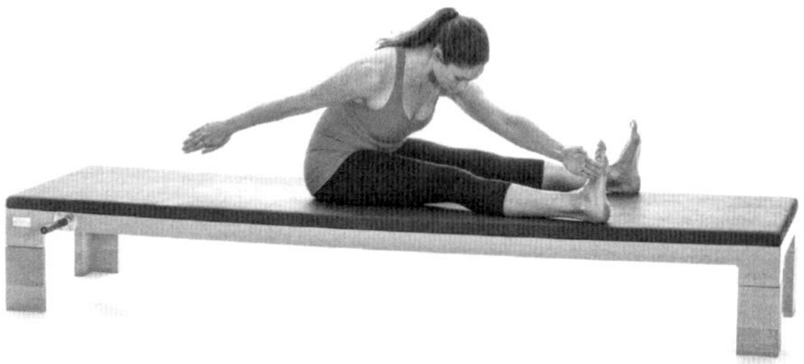

Exhale. Reach forward over the leg with the trunk. The front arm crosses the leg, and the hand extends past the small toe. The back arm reaches back with the palm of the hand facing the body. Feel the oppositional pull of the arms.

Imagery

Visualize a pole strapped to the back. Rotate around the pole when in the upright position. When folding the trunk over the leg for the stretch, hinging from the hip joint, maintain the feeling of the pole strapped to the back to accentuate spinal extension.

- Keep the back extensors engaged when reaching forward.
- Keep the feet dorsiflexed with the toes reaching toward the ceiling, heels on the mat.
- Anchor the pelvis and distribute your weight evenly on the sit bones.

VARIATION

In order to assist with the stretch phase, when the trunk is over the leg, place the back hand on the ground and push the trunk forward with the back arm. This offers support for the trunk and increases the stretch.

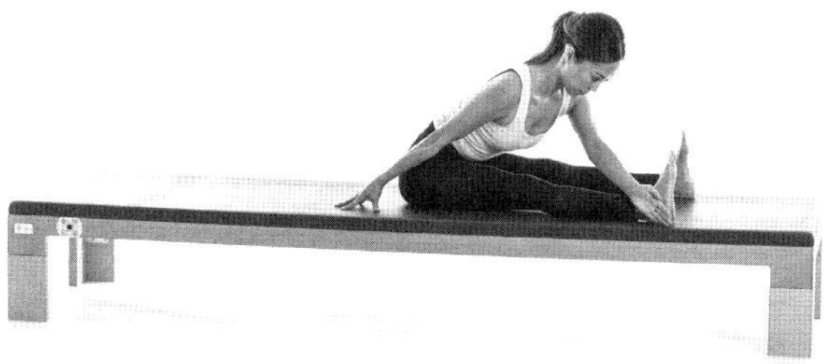

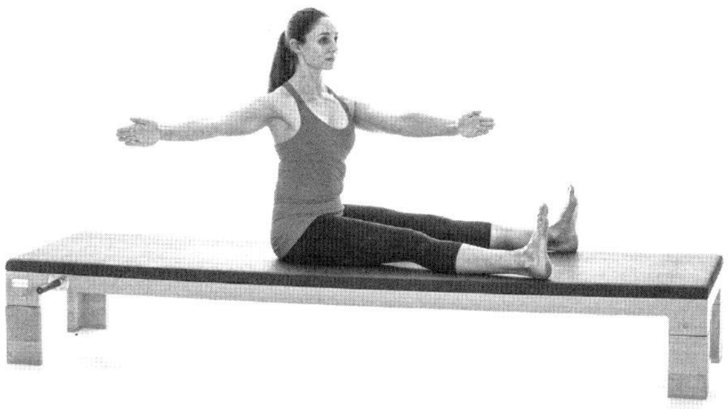

Inhale. Extend the spine further to accentuate the hamstring stretch as the body lifts to the vertical position while still rotated. The arms form an L shape momentarily before returning to the T position.

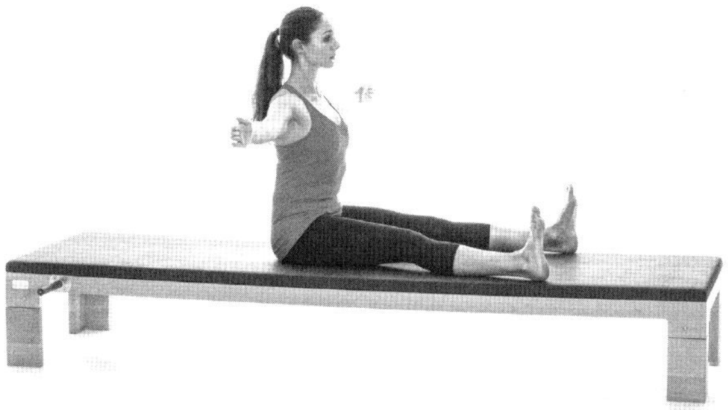

Exhale. Rotate back to the center start position before rotating to the other side. Repeat 3-5 times to each side.

MAT

Rotation

INTERMEDIATE

Muscle Focus

- Abdominals
- Hip flexors

Objectives

- To improve abdominal strength
- To improve hip flexor control
- To develop lumbopelvic stabilization

Corkscrew

This exercise builds on the principles of the Mat: Spine Twist—Supine but incorporates a longer lever (the legs), intensifying the work of the hip flexors and the abdominals, particularly that of the abdominal obliques. The pendulum motion and circling of the legs demand intricate control of the spine and coordination of the abdominals and hip flexors, which act alternately as movers and stabilizers at various points in the exercise. Note that the pelvis together with the legs rock from side to side, with one side of the pelvis briefly lifting off the mat as the legs move to the opposite side. However, the pelvis returns to center soon afterward, as the legs continue in an arc to the other side, at which point the opposite side of the pelvis lifts off the mat before anchoring itself in the center. The lower back should imprint into the mat as the legs pass through the center and should leave the mat only momentarily as the legs go out to the sides.

Imagery

Visualize drawing a big circle on the ceiling as the legs arc around in one direction and then in the reverse.

- ○ Keep the legs and feet together and aligned.
- ○ Keep the shoulder girdle, neck, and head as still and relaxed as possible.
- ○ Focus the movement in the waist area.
- ○ Keep the size of the circle moderate.

MODIFICATION

This modification mimics the Mat: Spine Twist—Supine but with the legs straight rather than in tabletop position. Move the legs from side to side rather than in a circle. This pendulum motion is less demanding on the hip flexors than the Mat: Corkscrew. The primary focus of the movement, which equates to rotation of the spine, is on the abdominal obliques. In both the Mat: Corkscrew and this modification the legs can be slightly bent if tight hamstrings are present to reduce load on the hip flexors and lower back.

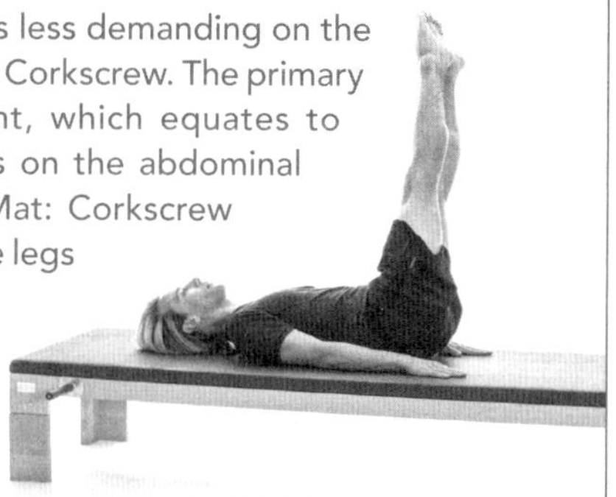

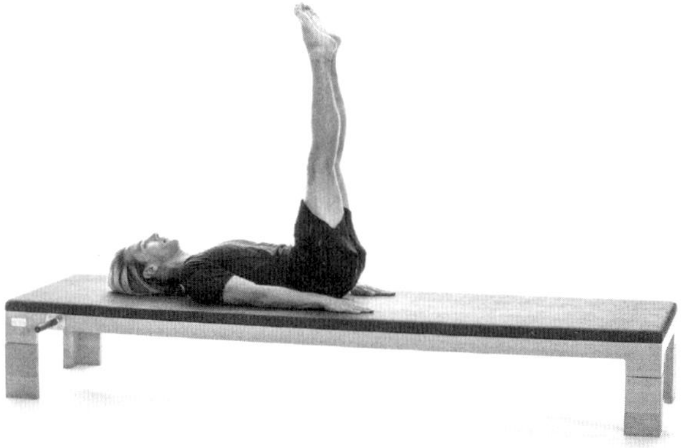

Setup. Lie supine, with the arms in a T position or at the sides of the body (which tends to be a more challenging position because it provides less stability) and the legs perpendicular to the floor. Imprint the lower back into the mat.

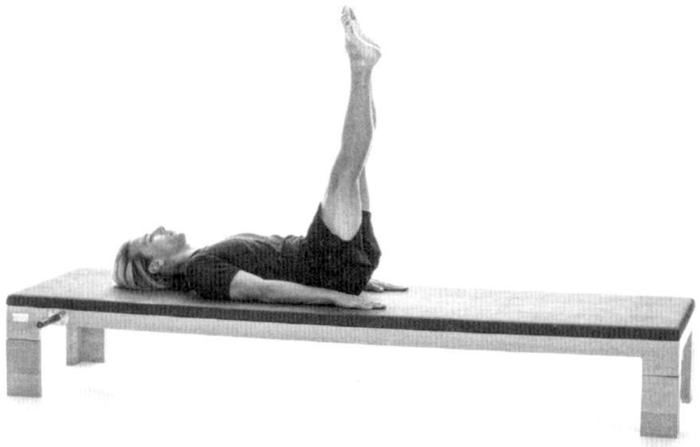

Inhale. Shift the pelvis and both legs to one side, keeping the shoulders stable and relaxed. Move the legs as one unit, which sometimes requires reaching out farther with the top leg in order to keep them together. However, this should be subtle; overcorrecting can result in overuse of the lower back extensors and hyperlordosis.

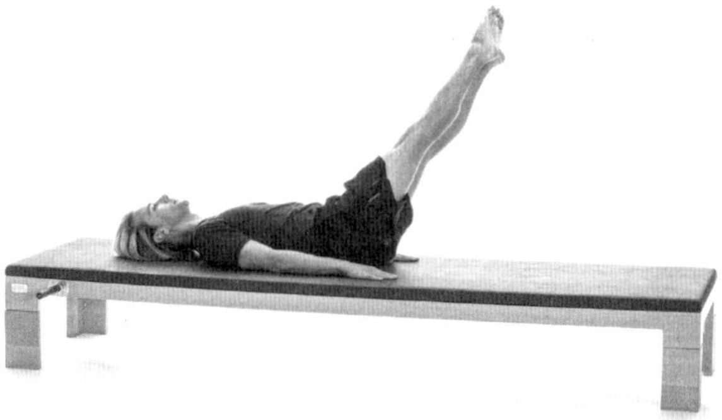

Exhale. Circle the legs downward in an arc through the center and around to the opposite side. As the legs pass through the center, imprint the lower back into the mat.

Once the legs reach the opposite side of the arc, bring them back to the start position and pause momentarily. Alternate the direction. Use the starting point (perpendicular) as the reference position. Repeat 5 times in each direction.

Hip Circle Prep

Certain elements of the Mat: Corkscrew apply to this exercise; however, the sitting V position of the body requires a higher level of stabilization, strength, and control. The shoulder girdle must remain stable, and abdominal support must be maintained in order to avoid stress on the lumbar spine as the legs reach out to one side, circle down and around to the other side, and return to center.

The spinal rotation, and the power it demands, can improve control of the powerhouse and enhance athletic performance.

Imagery

Imagine drawing a cone shape, with the pelvis at the apex and the feet tracing the large, round edge. The bigger the cone, the more support and stabilization you need.

- ○ Avoid hyperextending the lumbar spine as the legs circle.
- ○ Keep the shoulder girdle stable and the mid- and upper back extensors engaged.
- ○ Move the pelvis from side to side as the legs draw a large circle.
- ○ Keep the legs together as they move with the pelvis as one unit.

PROGRESSION

In the advanced version of this exercise, the arms and head move with the upper body as one unit in one direction, while the legs and pelvis move as one unit in the opposite direction. To start, the arms reach forward together with the legs. Move the trunk to one side and circle the arms up and around to the other side and back to center. Simultaneously the legs reach to the opposite side, and then circle down and around to the other side and meet the arms back in the center. The arms create one cone and the legs another: one clockwise and the other counterclockwise. Repeat 5 times in one direction, then repeat in the opposite direction.

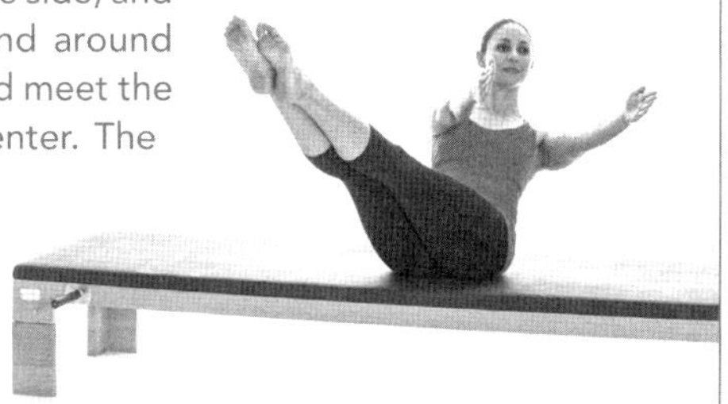

Muscle Focus

- Abdominals
- Hip flexors
- Back extensors

Objectives

- To improve abdominal oblique strength
- To improve hip flexor control
- To develop lumbopelvic and scapular stabilization
- To develop trunk rotation

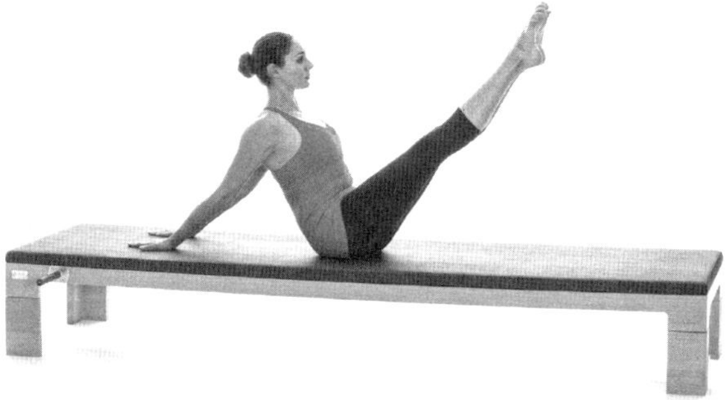

Setup. Sit with legs straight in front of you and the arms behind you, hands resting on the floor, fingers facing away from the body. The arms should lightly support the body, like training wheels on a bicycle. Bend the knees toward the chest and straighten the legs at approximately a 60-degree angle to the floor, keeping them together.

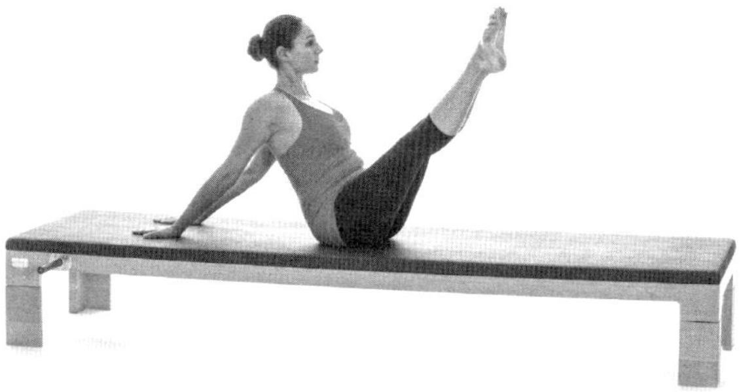

Inhale. Shift the pelvis and the legs as a unit to one side.

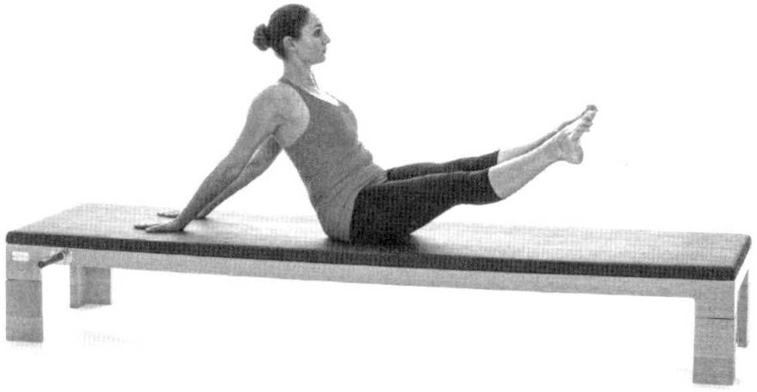

Exhale. Circle the legs down and around as the pelvis moves through the center to the opposite side and back to center. Return to the start position. Repeat 5 times in one direction to achieve a sense of flow, then repeat in the opposite direction.

Twist

Muscle Focus

- Abdominal obliques
- Scapular stabilizers
- Back extensors

Objectives

- To improve abdominal oblique strength
- To improve back extensor control
- To improve shoulder strength
- To develop scapular stabilization

This exercise adds the element of rotation to the Mat: Side Bend, making the movement three-dimensional. The rotation involves not only the trunk, but also, very significantly, the shoulder. A single shoulder supports the weight of the body in a suspended position and accommodates its rotation, with most of the movement occurring in the glenohumeral joint. This is a tall order for this small, relatively unstable, muscle-dependent joint. I like to teach the Mat: Side Bend before teaching the Mat: Twist. Once both have been learned I often combine them, doing 3 repetitions of one and then 3 of the other. This is a complex exercise that involves stabilization, movement in all planes of motion, and intricate coordination.

Imagery

I use several images in this exercise. The visual I give for the top position of the twist is a pyramid—the trunk and arm, as one unit, create one side of the pyramid and the legs, the other side. When the arm reaches under the body, the movement is like threading a needle, and the energy should be spiraling. The return to the diagonal position should create a well-defined line. In this position, feel the strong diagonal energy line running through the body and a second line running through the arms and shooting out of the top arm like a laser beam. Line is everything in this wonderful and

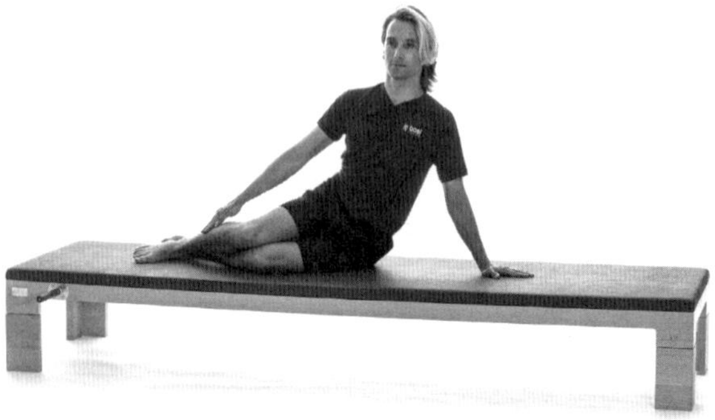

Setup. Sit sideways with the weight on one side of the pelvis. Bend the legs and place the top foot in front of the bottom one. Rest the upper body weight on the supporting arm while maintaining strong scapular stabilization and recruiting the abdominal obliques. Rest the other arm on the side of the legs.

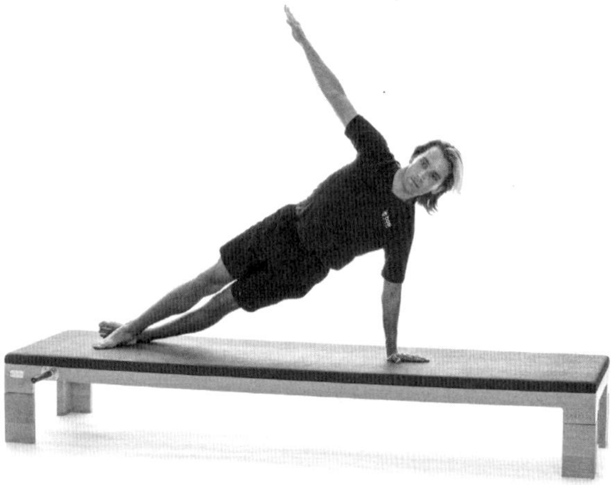

Inhale. Lift the pelvis away from the floor while straightening the legs, establishing a straight diagonal line with the body. Raise the upper arm to shoulder height, creating a 90-degree angle between the arm and the trunk, fingers directed diagonally toward the ceiling.

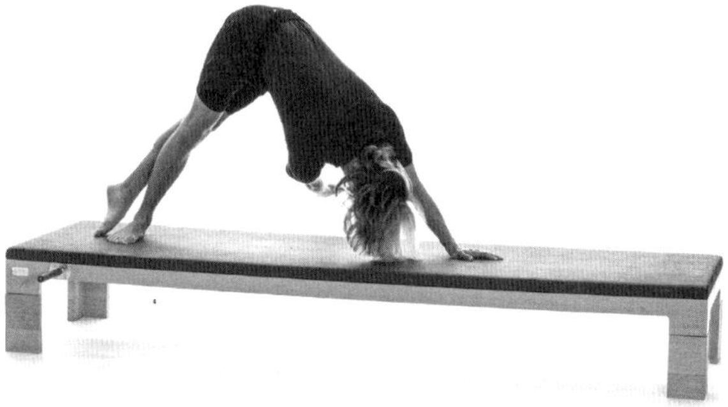

Exhale. Lift the pelvis as high as possible and rotate the trunk as the free arm reaches under the body. Distribute the weight between the hand on the floor and the front foot.

challenging exercise. It is a movement that is beautiful to watch and equally as enjoyable to do.

- Minimize the use of the legs and maximize the activation of the lateral flexors and rotators of the trunk.
- Keep the scapula stable, rotating around the glenohumeral joint.
- Allow the head to follow the line of the spine.

PROGRESSION

This is a very challenging exercise. When executed well, it creates beautiful shapes with spiraling movement. To make it even more challenging in terms of both strength and flexibility, lower the pelvis toward the mat (not quite touching) as described in the final phase of the exercise, but keep the legs straight. This provides a tremendous stretch for the lateral flexors of the trunk on the lower side and demands exceptional stability and control of the scapula and shoulder joint of the working arm. The free arm is lowered to shoulder height, parallel to the floor, and the gaze is directed beyond the hand of this arm. Lifting the pelvis again to form the straight diagonal line with the body demands great focus on the lateral flexors of the lower side. Repeat 3-5 times before switching to the other side.

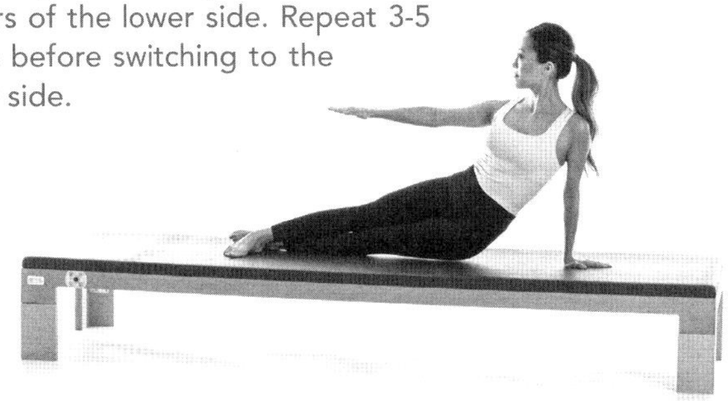

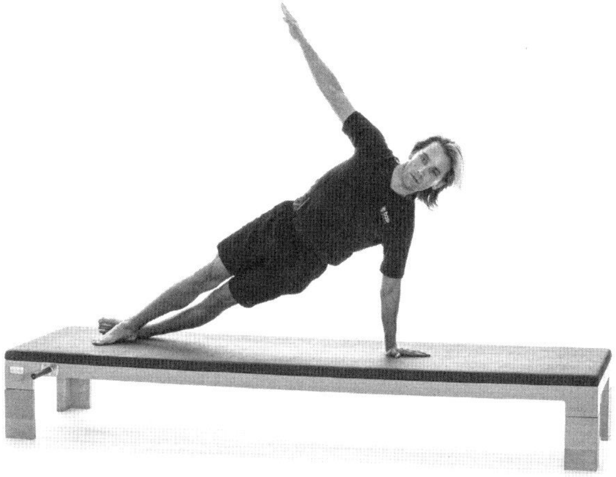

Inhale. Return to the previous position with the body on a straight diagonal line and the free arm reaching up, creating a 90-degree angle at the shoulder joint.

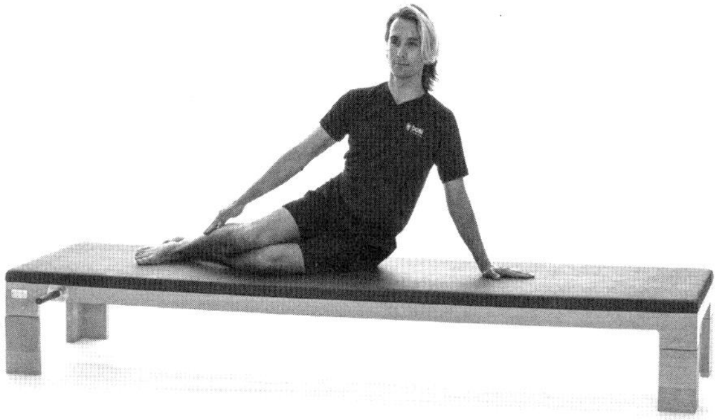

Exhale. Bend the knees and lower the body to the start position, keeping the pelvis slightly off the mat (if possible) or placing it lightly on the mat. Repeat 3-5 times before switching to the other side.

Back Extension

The importance of this block cannot be overemphasized. The following exercises focus on improving all aspects of function of the back extensors: strength, muscular endurance, and controlled activation. The spinal extensors are used to produce or maintain spinal extension, while the abdominals function as stabilizers to distribute the work through the entire back and reduce the potentially harmful forces on the spine. Integrating spinal extension into your Pilates program is vital for maintaining muscle balance, particularly because so many Pilates exercises emphasize spinal flexion. In addition, many everyday activities of modern day living such as working at a desk, typing on a keyboard, using a smartphone and tablet, and driving tend to draw the spine forward into flexion, as do many recreational activities. Additionally, the nature of aging and the effect of gravity on the human body further underscores the need to build strength and endurance of the spinal extensors. Conditioning these muscles properly may also reduce the risk of osteoporosis and lower back injury.

However, it is also important to note that spinal extension is a common mechanism for producing injury to the back, particularly the lower back. Optimal technique and a safe and well-planned progression to the more demanding exercises must be implemented to reap the benefits and reduce the risks of these exercises. The back muscles cannot be viewed simply as one group. In fact, it is possible (and advisable) to work the different regions of the back while minimally involving the other regions. It is preferable to initially focus on the mid- and upper back while keeping the lower back stable before forging ahead into more extreme ranges that involve the lower back extensors. The advanced exercises presented in this block should be attempted only after you have achieved proficiency with the more fundamental exercises. If you experience discomfort or have a condition for which back extension would be contraindicated, proceed with caution and seek advice from a medical professional.

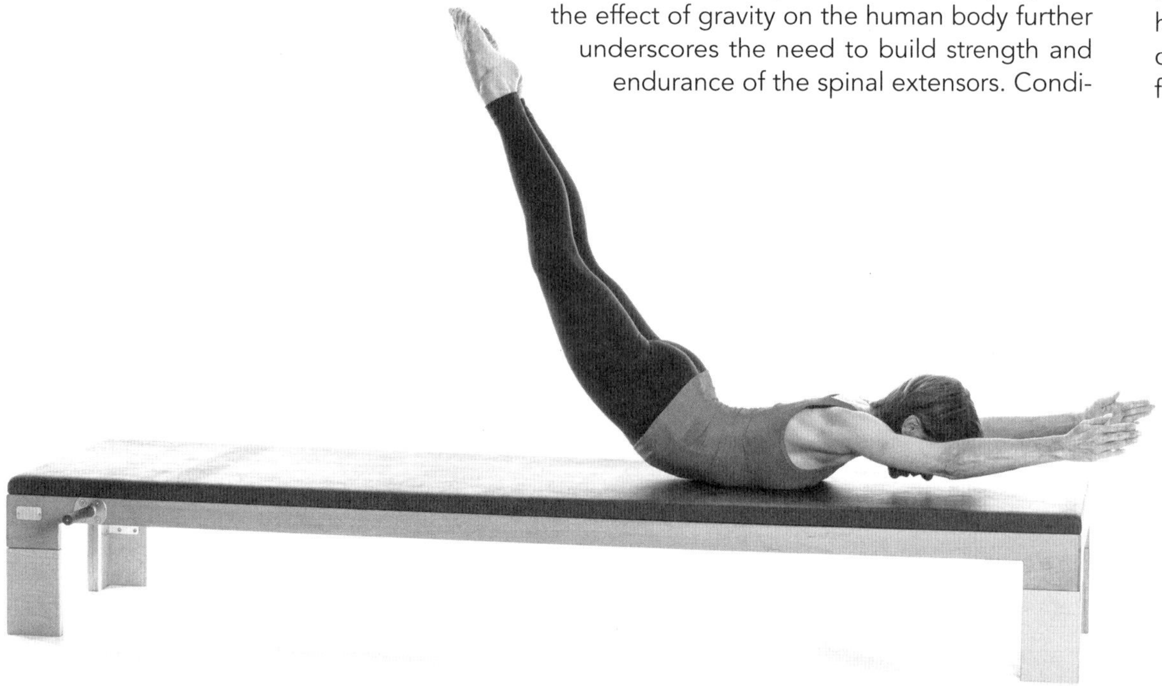

Back Extension

Muscle Focus

- Back extensors
- Abdominals

Objectives

- To improve back extensor strength
- To improve abdominal control
- To develop scapular stabilization

This exercise provides a good foundation for the subsequent mat work back extension exercises. Proper abdominal recruitment plays a crucial role in supporting the back and achieving correct alignment during this exercise. Distributing the load through the entire vertebral column and mobilizing each intravertebral joint helps to prevent the shearing forces on the spine that commonly occur when extension is concentrated in the lower back.

Just as the abdominals help stabilize the lumbar spine, so the scapular stabilizers help stabilize the thoracic spine. These muscles, particularly the lower trapezius, also serve as mid-back extensors. Take advantage of this muscular interplay at work in back extension exercises. Practice establishing good alignment, movement mechanics, and function of the back and shoulders. Allow the pelvis to serve as an anchor for the movement as the spine is allowed to move freely.

Imagery

Use the image of an airplane hovering just above the ground to help achieve an elongated (as opposed to an excessively arched) position and a feeling of flight; light and unencumbered.

- ○ Maintain abdominal support.
- ○ Maintain scapular stabilization.
- ○ Keep the head aligned with the spine.
- ○ Press the arms against the sides of the body and reach the fingers toward the feet.

PROGRESSION

Adding challenge to this exercise when the back is in extension and the arms are out to the sides in the T position will prove extremely rewarding. At this point in the exercise, externally rotate the shoulders further so the thumbs face the ceiling. Lift the arms toward the ceiling, adducting the scapulae. Lower the arms slightly, abducting the scapulae while maintaining back extension. The movement of the arms and that of the scapulae should be separate movements. Repeat the arm and scapula movement 5 times before rotating the shoulders so the palms face the floor. Internally rotate the shoulders and return arms to the sides of the body. Lower the trunk. Repeat the entire sequence 3-5 times.

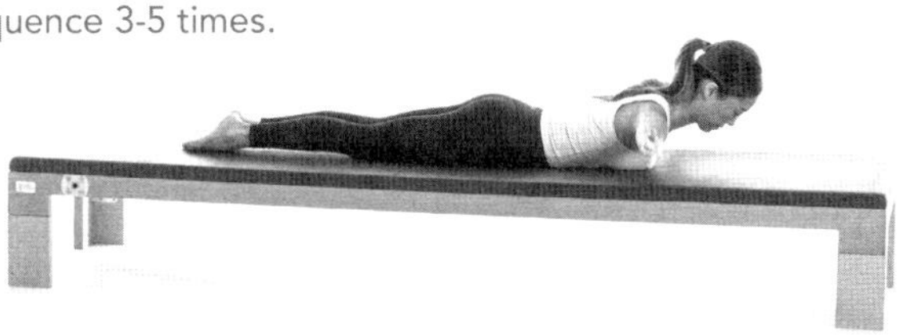

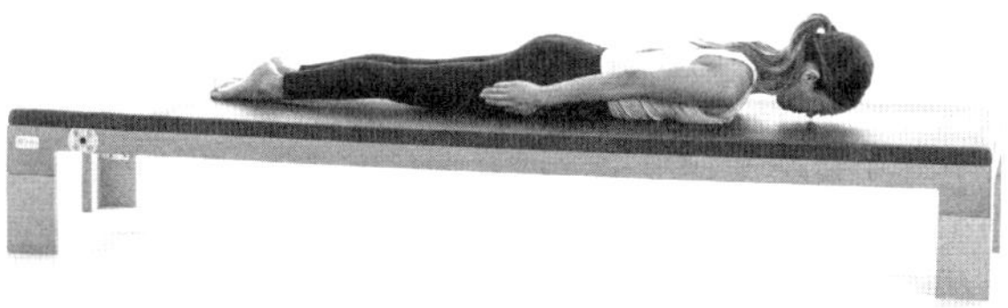

Setup. Lie prone with the forehead hovering slightly above the floor (place a rolled towel under the forehead if necessary to maintain good alignment of the head and spine). Keep the arms by the sides, pressing the palms against the legs. Keep the legs together and the feet plantarflexed.

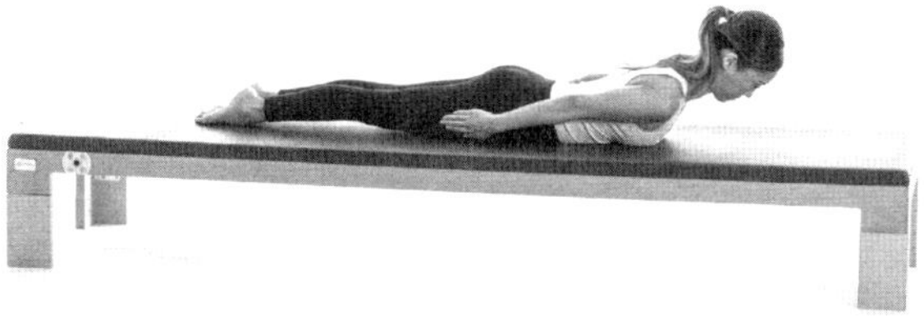

Inhale. Lift the head, shoulder girdle, and chest off the mat. Keep the legs stable and together. Press the pubic symphysis gently into the mat, engaging the abdominals and the gluteals.

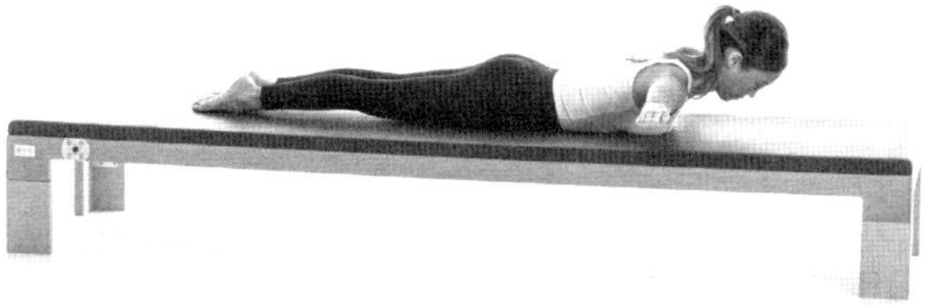

Exhale. Reach the arms out to the sides into a T position, externally rotating the shoulders, palms facing the floor.

Inhale. Move the arms back to the sides of the body, internally rotating the shoulders, palms facing the body, and keeping the trunk stable.

Exhale. Lower the upper body (not completely), keeping the back extensors, abdominals, and gluteals activated. After the final repetition, lower the body to the start position. Repeat 5-10 times.

Single-Leg Kick

Muscle Focus

- Back extensors
- Abdominals
- Hamstrings
- Scapular stabilizers

Objectives

- To improve mid- and upper back extensor strength
- To improve hip extensor and knee flexor control
- To develop trunk and scapular stabilization

The setup in this exercise is very important. Incorrect positioning of the body and inadequate support for the spine can place excessive pressure on the lower back. The back extensor work should be focused on the mid- and upper back, while the abdominals support the lower back. The arms, of course, also add support, and good scapular stabilization is imperative. The elbows should be directly under the shoulders and forearms placed either in a triangular shape with the fingers interlaced or parallel to each other, palms down. In either case, the scapulae should sit in a stable, neutral position.

Imagery

The body shape should be like a sphinx. The leg movement is disassociated from the rest of the body's stable position, with the lower legs bending and straightening like the opening and closing of a handheld fan (when viewed from the side).

- ○ Develop scapular stabilization.
- ○ Keep the pubic symphysis lifting up toward the sternum.
- ○ Keep the lower legs lifted off the mat.
- ○ Maintain hip extension.

VARIATION

In the case of discomfort or excessive pressure in the lower back, this exercise can be performed in a prone position with the hands one on top of the other and the forehead resting on the hands. This will immediately decrease the pressure on the lower back but be equally as demanding on the upper back extensors and hamstrings.

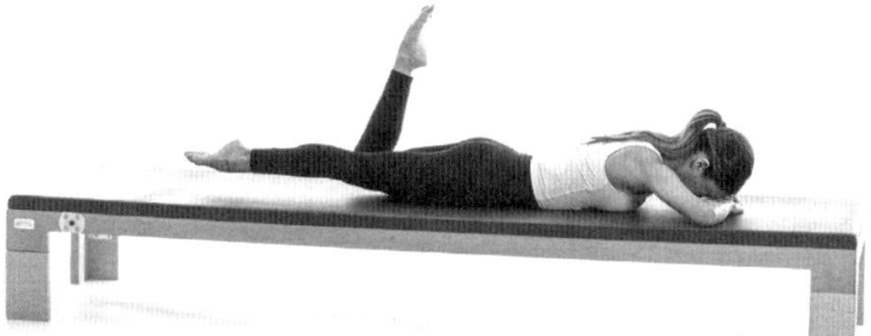

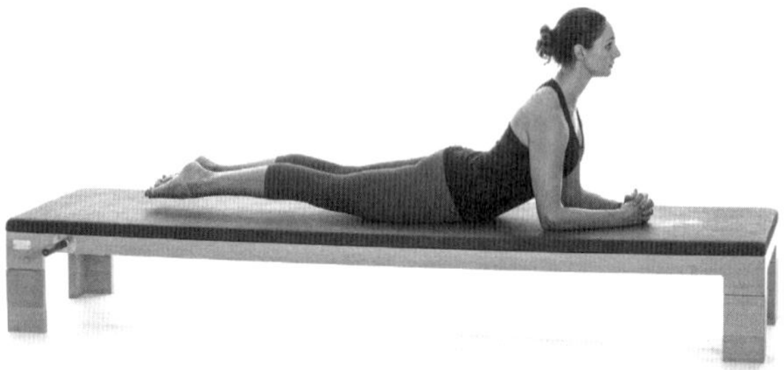

Setup. Lie prone, place the elbows under the shoulders and engage the abdominals, and lift the chest and extend the back. Position the forearms in a triangular shape with the fingers interlaced or parallel to each other. Keep the legs straight and lift them slightly off the mat.

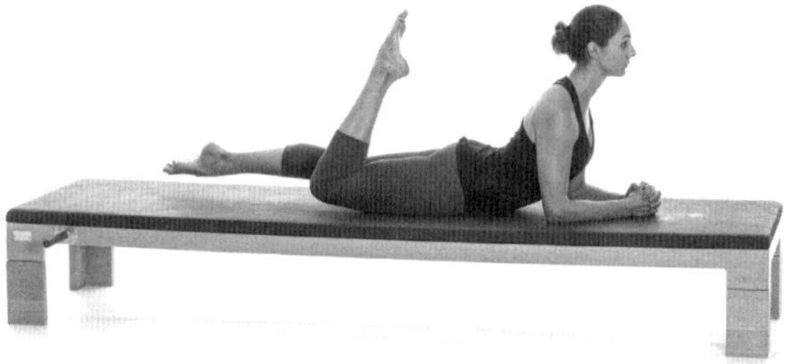

Exhale. Bend the leg, pulsing twice when in maximum knee flexion, then straighten it while simultaneously bending the other leg and pulsing it twice.

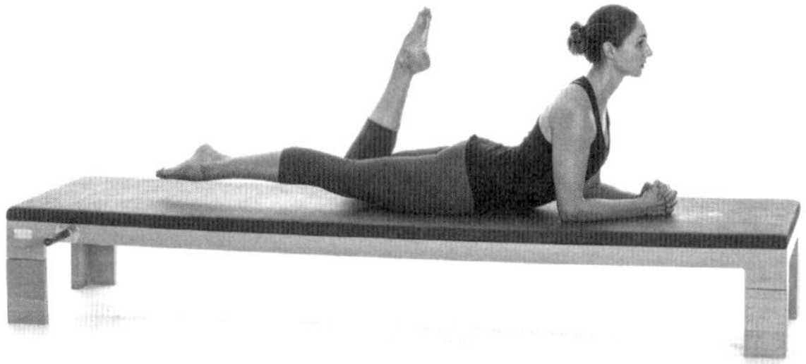

Inhale. Bend the leg, pulsing twice when in maximum knee flexion, then straighten it while simultaneously bending the other leg and pulsing it twice.

Repeat the same pattern of alternately bending and pulsing one leg as the other straightens, performing one cycle (both legs) on an exhale and one cycle (both legs) on an inhale. There is no change in the body position. Repeat the breath cycle (inhale and exhale) 10 times.

MAT

Back Extension

INTERMEDIATE

Double-Leg Kick

This is an exceptional back extension exercise with several important benefits in addition to strengthening the back extensors. First, the arms add support to the back extension, helping monitor the load on the back. Second, holding the arms together provides an excellent stretch for the chest and shoulders. This exercise also provides good hamstring work and prepares you for the Mat: Rocking. An elongated body position emphasizes the activation of the mid- and upper back (as opposed to a high arched position, which would focus the work on the lower back).

Imagery

Visualize the body as an archer's bow, with the arms forming the twine. This powerful image also reinforces the elongation desired in this exercise.

- Keep the hip extensors and the hip adductors engaged.
- Relax the elbows to the floor during the down phase, placing the hands high up on the back.
- Keep the head aligned with the spine when lifting into back extension.
- Keep the scapulae apart and straighten the arms completely during the back extension.

VARIATION

Those with tight chest muscles and tight shoulders may lack the mobility to interlace the hands behind the back. Holding a small towel will enable them to reap the benefits of this exercise without placing excessive strain on the shoulders.

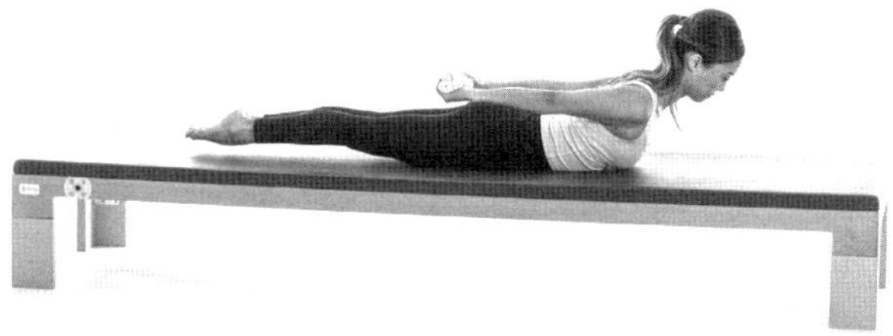

Muscle Focus

- Back extensors
- Abdominals
- Hip extensors
- Triceps
- Scapular stabilizers

Objectives

- To improve back extensor strength
- To improve hip extensor, elbow extensor, and knee flexor control
- To improve thoracic flexibility

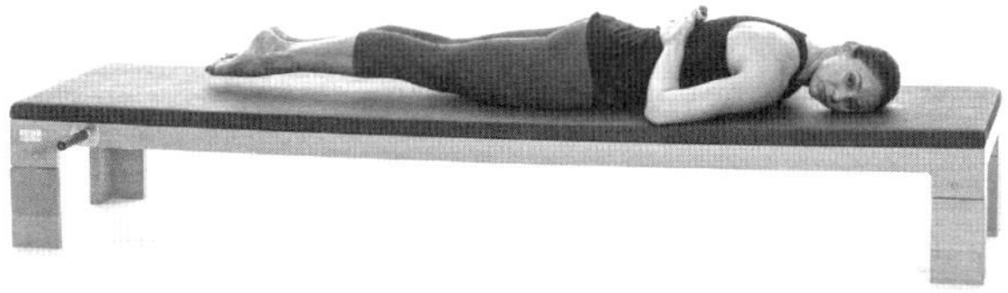

Setup. Lie prone with the fingers interlaced behind the back, and allow the elbows to fall to the floor. Turn the head to one side, resting the cheek on the floor. Lift the legs slightly off the mat, keeping them straight and together.

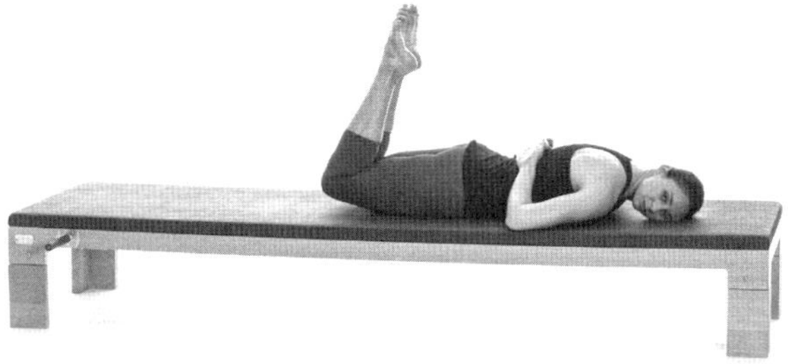

Exhale. Bend both legs together, pulsing 3 times when in maximum knee flexion, keeping the lower thighs lifted.

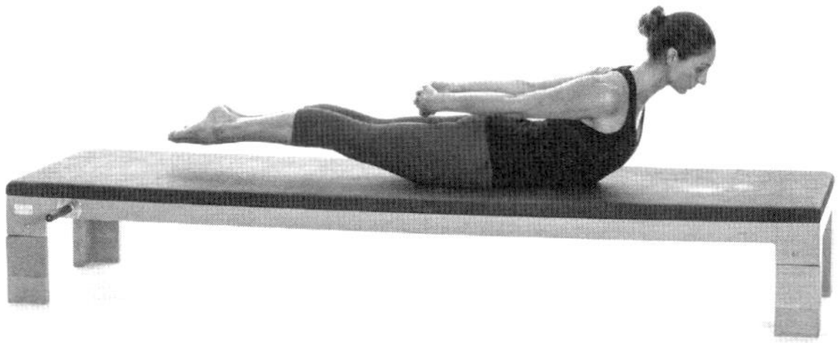

Inhale. Extend the back, lifting the chest off the mat. Simultaneously straighten the arms and the legs, and bring the head to the center.

Exhale. Lower the body to the start position, placing the back of the hands high on the back, elbows falling toward the mat, and resting the opposite cheek on the floor. Alternate the cheek each repetition. Repeat 10 times.

Swimming

Muscle Focus

- Back extensors
- Hip extensors
- Shoulder flexors

Objectives

- To improve back extensor strength
- To improve shoulder flexor and hip extensor control
- To develop trunk stabilization
- To develop coordination and cross-patterning

This exercise is invaluable in terms of developing strength and cross-pattern coordination of the back extensors, shoulder flexors, and hip extensors. When the right side of the back and right shoulder are working, the left hip extensors are activated, and vice versa. This pattern is used frequently in everyday movements and recreational activities, most commonly in the normal gait cycle (walking). As we stride forward with the right leg, the left leg goes backward while the trunk rotates slightly to the right, resulting in the exact pattern of this exercise.

I use the same breath pattern for this exercise as the Mat: Hundred: 5 counts to inhale and 5 counts to exhale, moving the limbs in a small, brisk flutter motion without pausing. (I refer to the Mat: Swimming as the Mat: Hundred for the back.)

Imagery

Imagine doing little flutter kicks with the arms and legs, as if both are doing the leg movement of the crawl stroke, swimming in opposite directions. The trunk, from head to pelvis, is like a solid plank, remaining stable while the arms and legs hinge around small, independent axes and have no effect on the stability of the plank.

- Maintain trunk and pelvic stabilization.
- Avoid elevating the shoulders.
- Keep the movements of the arms and legs small.

MODIFICATION

Beginners can make this exercise easier by pausing in the neutral position before switching to the opposite side. In order to modify it further, allow the arm and leg that are not being lifted to remain on the mat. This provides some support and recuperation time for the limbs not being lifted.

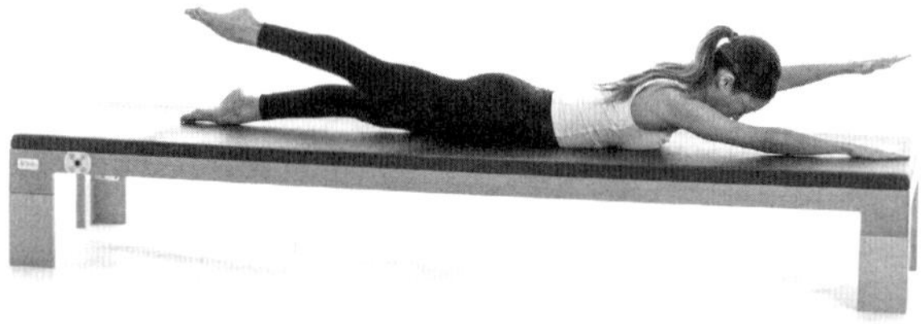

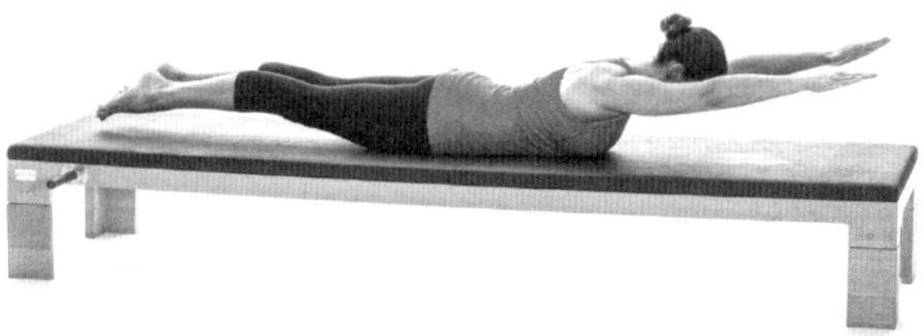

Setup. Lie prone with the arms reaching forward and the legs together. Lift the chest, arms, and legs slightly off the mat.

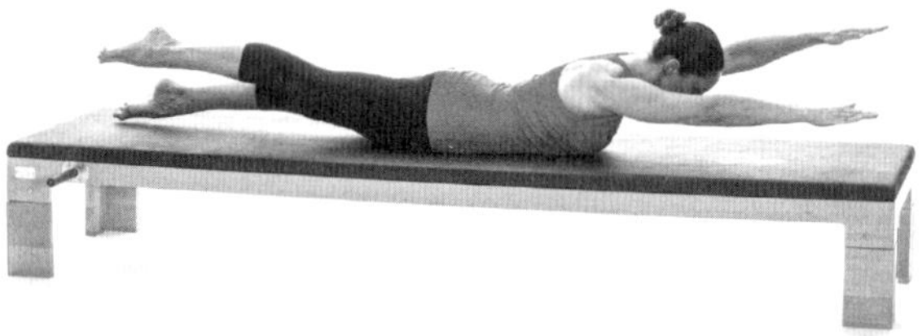

Inhale. Lift the left arm and right leg simultaneously. Switch to lifting the right arm and left leg simultaneously. Start slowly and then speed up the movement, alternating arms and legs, until the movement flows. Continue this movement cycle while inhaling for 5 counts.

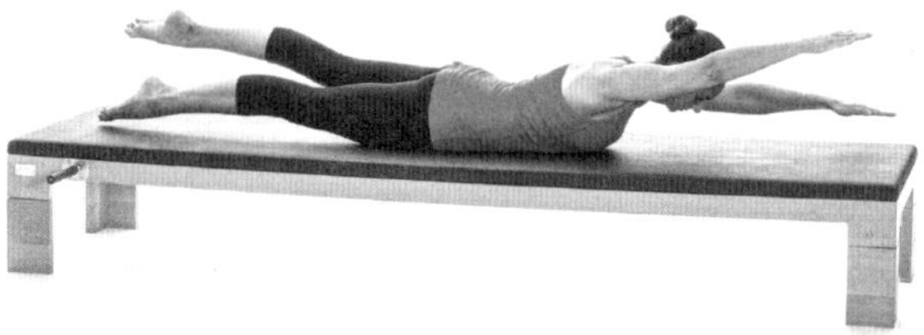

Exhale. Repeat the arm and leg movement cycle while exhaling for 5 counts. Continue this pattern for 5-10 breath cycles (inhale and exhale).

Complete the exercise by suspending the body in space for a moment before lowering the legs and upper body to the mat.

Rocking

Mat: Rocking relies on the stable shape of the body and intricate shifts of weight to "get the ball rolling." It is difficult to articulate how this happens because the process is internal and not visually apparent; once you establish the shape, you shift the center of gravity slightly forward and away you rock—back and forth! Once in motion, it is about maintaining a solid position and utilizing momentum. I cannot overemphasize the importance of the hip extension. Reach the feet to the ceiling at the same time as you extend the back. I recommend actually engaging the knee extensors as if straightening the legs; however, with the hands holding on to the ankles, it forces the legs higher toward the ceiling and lifts the trunk higher into an arc shape. To start the rocking, use the hip extensors to lift the legs even higher and reach the feet to the ceiling. This will cause the body to tip forward. Once it has tipped forward, use the back extensors to lift back up. Alternate between lifting the legs higher and the trunk higher to keep the momentum going. Like the Mat: Swan Dive, this exercise relies more on stability and intricate muscle coordination than on pure flexibility or strength.

Imagery

As in the Mat: Double-Leg Kick, the body is the shape of an archer's bow; the arms are the twine. However, in this case, the position is far more arched: The bow is taut in preparation for shooting the arrow. Another good image is that of a boat rocking back and forth as it sails over waves.

- Keep the head stable and aligned with the spine.
- Maintain scapular stabilization with the arms straight.
- Keep the legs adducting, only opening as much as is needed to avoid pressure on the pelvis and the lower back.

MODIFICATION

A good preparation for this exercise is to lift into the rocking position and then lower down to the floor. Repeat this action several times without the rocking to develop flexibility, strength, and coordination.

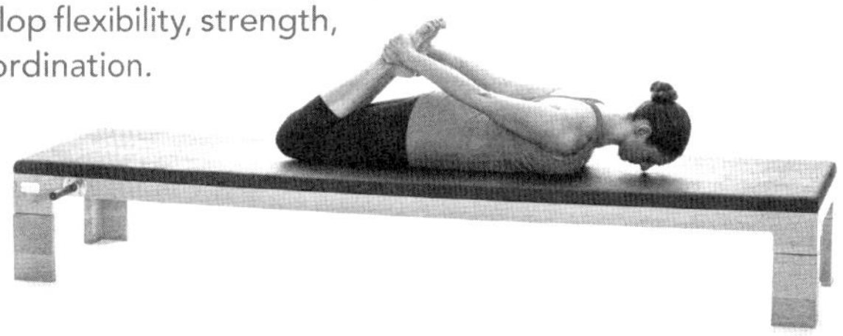

Muscle Focus

- Back extensors
- Abdominals
- Hip extensors
- Knee extensors

Objectives

- To improve back extensor and hip extensor strength
- To improve knee extensor control
- To improve hip flexor and thoracic flexibility
- To develop trunk stabilization

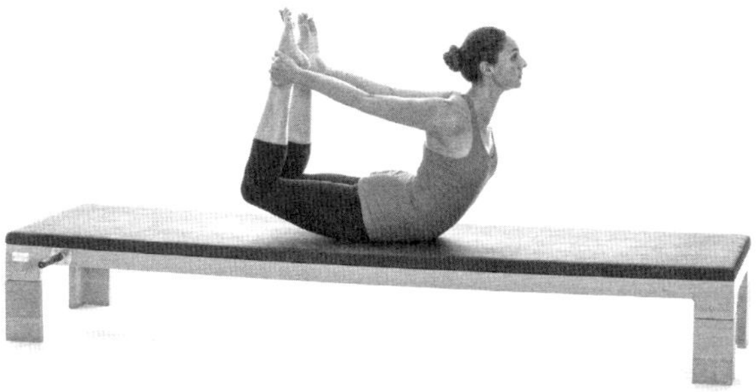

Setup. Lie prone. Bend the knees and reach back with the arms, taking hold of the legs just above the ankles. Lift the trunk and legs into an arch.

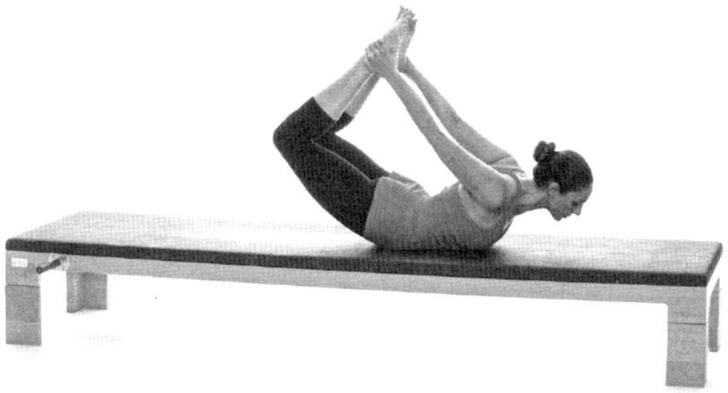

Exhale. Rock forward.

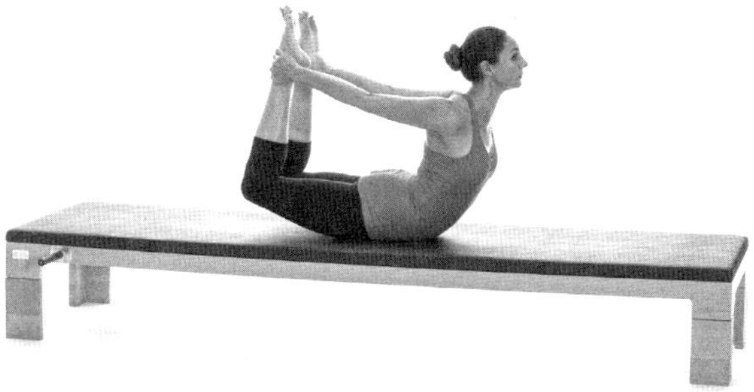

Inhale. Rock backward. Repeat 5 times.

Swan Dive

Muscle Focus

- Back extensors
- Hip extensors
- Abdominals
- Shoulder flexors

Objectives

- To improve back extensor and hip extensor strength
- To improve trunk stabilization
- To develop coordinated interplay of the back extensors and hip extensors

The Mat: Swan Dive is a beautiful exercise to watch and a very difficult one to execute well. It embodies many of the movement principles of Pilates, particularly flow. This exercise is all about harnessing energy and keeping it moving. Although it appears to rely primarily on flexibility of the spine in extension, the essence of performing the exercise well lies in trunk stabilization and activating the correct muscles in the correct sequence with immaculate timing.

You must hold the trunk in a firm position, created by the back extensors and hip extensors and supported by the abdominals. The abdominals assist in achieving the desired shape of the body and in distributing the extension through the entire back, working each vertebral joint rather than concentrating the forces in the lumbar region.

I have seen many a young dancer with a spine like rubber struggle to do this exercise well. I am not blessed with a spine like rubber, particularly now as my body gallops toward 70 years of age. Yet I can still manage to achieve good height and flow in this exercise, sometimes even better than the young, and far more flexible movers, who tend to rely primarily on the hypermobility of their spines. Success comes from the organization of the joints up and down the kinetic chain (hips, spine, shoulders)—and most importantly, years of practice in harnessing the enormous energy that becomes available when the body is unleashed into the forward dive. From that point it is all about maintaining that momentum. Hold the body stable and keep all the necessary muscles activated. Focus on the back extensors and shoulder flexors to lift the trunk high, and on the hip extensors to lift the legs high.

Imagery

Visualize a big, well-inflated tire rolling back and forth. If it is not fully inflated, it will make jarring movements, getting stuck at certain points. So it is with the body: It will stop and start, even with the back extensors and hip extensors engaged, if the trunk is not held firmly in an arc shape.

- Engage the abdominals.
- Maximize momentum and fluidity of movement.
- Maintain the arc shape of the body.

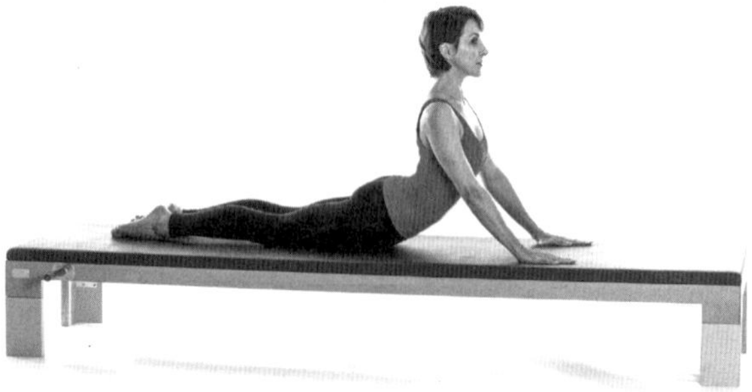

Setup. Lie prone with the hands under the shoulders and the forearms on the mat. Contract the abdominals and sequentially extend the back, starting from the crown of the head and moving down through the neck, chest, and lower back. Keep the elbows by the sides and maintain contact between the forearms and the mat as long as possible. Straighten the arms (without elevating the scapulae) and lift high into the arc position. (It is not imperative to straighten the arms completely, only as far as possible without the scapulae elevating.)

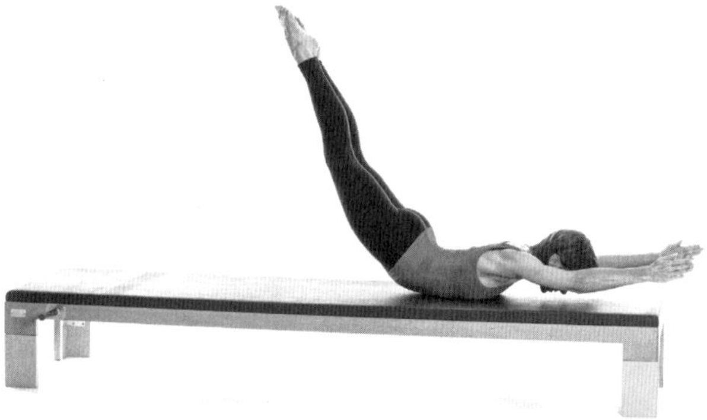

Exhale. Release the arms, dropping the body forward toward the mat. Reach the arms overhead, in line with the ears, and extend the legs up toward the ceiling.

It is helpful on the first drop forward to place the hands on the forehead with the arms bent and to straighten them toward the ceiling as you rock back in the next step. From this point on, they remain straight overhead.

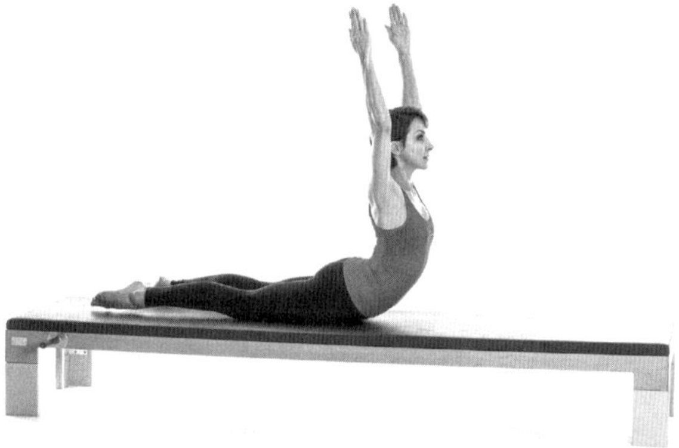

Inhale. Rock backward in an arc shape with the trunk upright, reaching the arms toward the ceiling and lowering the legs to the mat. Maintain the momentum and continue rocking, increasing the height of the legs and arms on each repetition. Repeat 5 times.

On the final repetition, place the hands down to catch the body in the supported arc position. Bend the arms and lower the body to the prone position.

Rest Position

Although I categorize this exercise as part of the foundation block, it is typically offered after back extension work. For this reason, I have placed it at this point in the book. The Mat: Rest Position can serve many purposes and appear at different points in a mat work routine. It may be a momentary rest, it could be a transition into other exercises, and as stated, it could be a stretch and relaxation following back extension exercises. In the kneeling position, rest the trunk on the thighs and reach the arms forward. Allow the pelvis to sink toward the heels, releasing the neck, shoulders, and lower back muscles.

Imagery

Imagine the back, pelvis, and shoulders are draped over the thighs. With each breath the back expands laterally and the relaxation deepens, allowing a sensation of the body melting over the legs.

- ○ Breathe naturally and deeply.
- ○ Allow the pelvis to sink toward the heels and the shoulders to relax.
- ○ Close the eyes if it feels more comfortable.

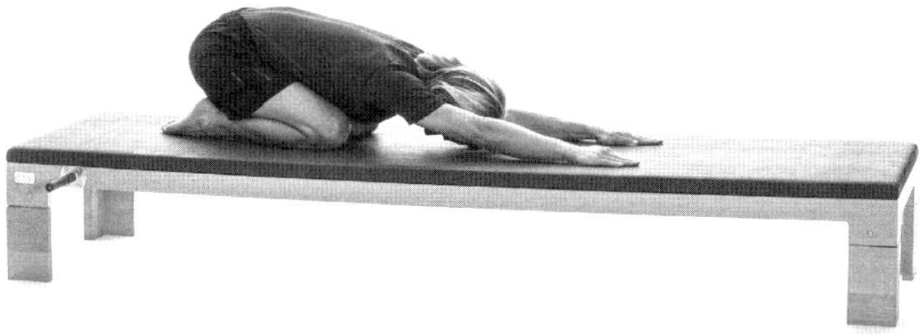

Kneel with the chest on the thighs and the pelvis resting on the heels. Place your forehead on the ground (on a rolled towel if necessary) with the arms reaching forward or at the sides of the body, whichever feels more comfortable. Comfort is key.

VARIATION

If you have a preexisting knee condition, place a cushion between the pelvis and the legs so that the flexion of the knees is not as extreme and pressure on the knees is diminished. If you have back problems or other restrictions, you can drape yourself, prone, over a large ball. This will offer support to the trunk and reduce the stress on the knees, hips, and back.

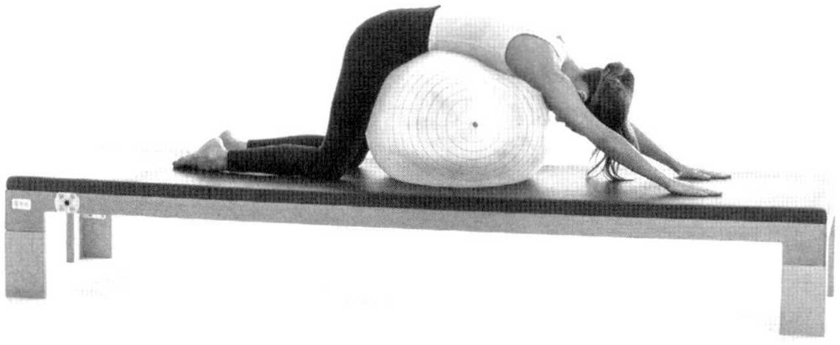

Muscle Focus

- Lower back extensors
- Shoulder extensors

Objectives

- To relax the back and shoulders
- To rest the body, particularly after back extension exercises
- To improve back extensor flexibility, particularly the lower back

5

Reformer

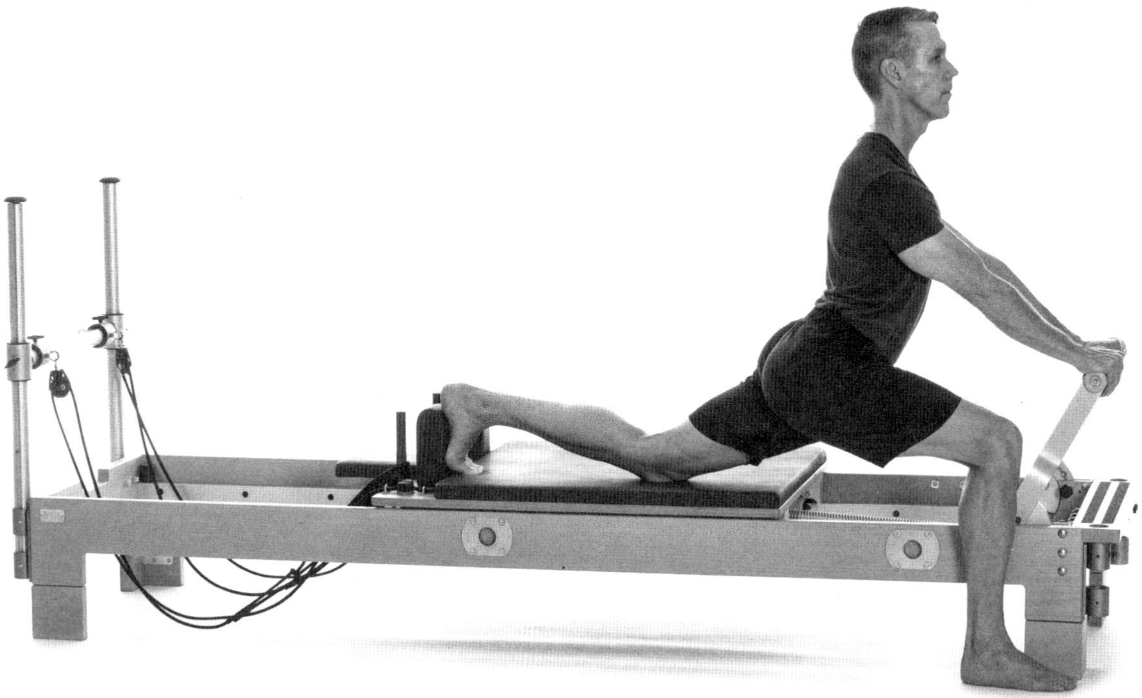

The universal reformer, commonly known simply as the reformer, is undoubtedly the most recognizable and popular piece of equipment in the Pilates menagerie. The scope of this piece of equipment is vast, limited only by our own imagination and the constraints of the human body. It is the creation of a man referred to as a genius of the body, certainly a man way ahead of his time. The movements performed on the reformer range from fundamental to extremely advanced; they are performed in every conceivable position and for every possible purpose. This versatility exemplifies the method itself.

Each piece of Pilates apparatus has specific advantages and unique features. Just as a good carpenter chooses the correct tool for the job, so it is with the choice of Pilates apparatus—the device should be well suited to the task at hand. For instance, the reformer is probably the most user-friendly apparatus on which to perform the foot work; it places the body in a comfortable, non-weight-bearing, supine position, facilitating balanced muscle recruitment. Performing foot work on the reformer is less demanding than doing the same exercises on the cadillac or wunda chair, and the stabilization of the pelvis and trunk, although emphasized on all the apparatus, is most easily achieved on the reformer. The reformer also provides the teacher with a good vantage point to observe and correct alignment and muscle action.

The upper body exercises that can be done on the reformer are unsurpassed in their diversity and comprehensiveness. The stretches performed on the reformer for the hip flexors, hamstrings, and hip adductors cannot be duplicated as effectively on the other apparatus. The reformer readily accommodates full ranges of motion, with a wide array of body position and resistance options.

The reformer also uniquely facilitates jumping, as one would on a trampoline, while lying supine using the jumpboard (also called the foot platform). The jumpboard offers exercises for athletes, dancers, and fitness enthusiasts to practice and improve jumping technique. It also facilitates elevated challenge by adding resistance and complex movement combinations to jumping. Conversely, it can also be used by those with physical restrictions who have difficulty placing their feet on the footbar.

Foot Work

Foot work is a fundamental part of the Pilates workout. It is commonly done on the reformer, cadillac, and wunda chair. Yet it can also be done on other pieces of apparatus, although not as mainstream, such as the F2 spine corrector and F2 chair, which both have integrated resistance mechanisms. In order to be consistent, I teach

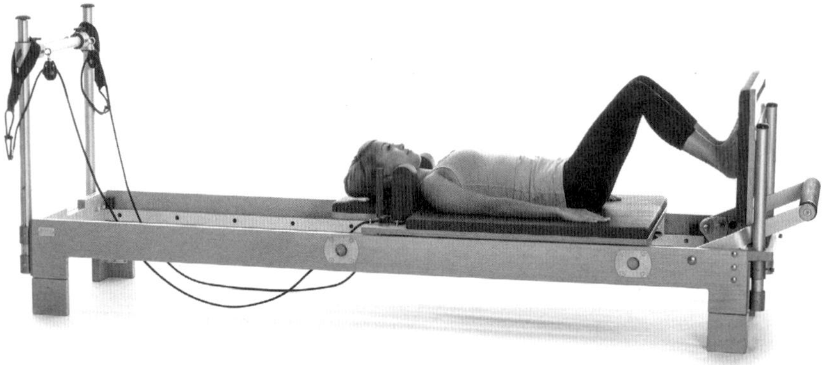

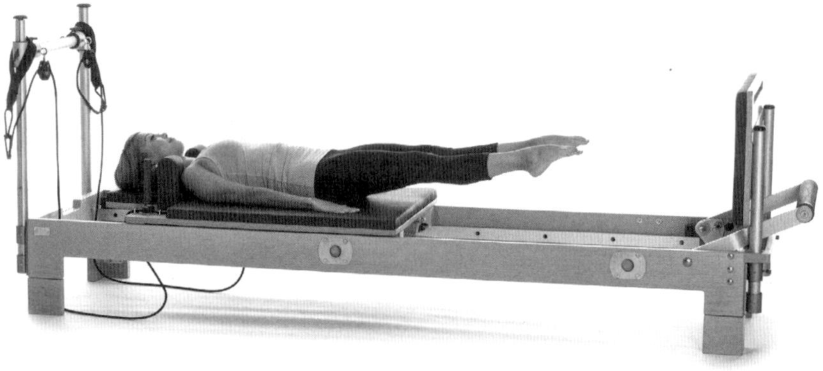

the same comprehensive foot work routine on each apparatus. In the comprehensive block system, the foot work typically follows the warm-up (described on page 31). I view the foot work as an extension of the warm-up, providing a transition into the main body of the session. Although labeled *foot work*, it clearly involves the entire leg. In fact, it involves the entire body.

Focus initially on the positioning of the pelvis and the spine, because this forms the foundation of the work. I recommend maintaining a neutral pelvis and neutral spine position throughout the foot work. However, this ideal cannot always be achieved. In specific cases—for example, if hyperlordosis is present and the lower back muscles are hypertonic—it may be best to deviate from a neutral pelvis and spine. In this case we would possibly work with a slight posterior tilt of the pelvis and the corresponding spinal position to achieve correct muscle activation, void of excessive tension, particularly in the lower back. Once normal movement patterns have been achieved, then a neutral position of the pelvis and spine should be implemented.

The position of the pelvis and trunk is essentially the same throughout the foot work. The musculature of the lower body is challenged in subtly different ways through different positions of the feet and legs while the core remains constant. The focus of the muscle activation in this block is the hip extensors and knee extensors, with particular attention to the hamstrings. It is important to ensure that the hamstrings engage because they tend to be overpowered by their antagonist, the larger and typically stronger quadriceps. This is more apparent when working with higher resistance. I prefer that the gluteals, which are also hip extensors, be relaxed during these exercises. This allows smooth, unrestricted hip movement and increases the probability of maintaining a neutral pelvic position.

Be sure to focus on both the concentric and eccentric contractions as the legs straighten and bend. The eccentric phase (as the legs bend) is often overlooked. This dual focus is among the factors that make Pilates such an excellent regimen for functional training, because both concentric and eccentric contractions are employed continually throughout our daily activities and athletic pursuits.

When doing the foot work, I encourage straightening the legs completely. There is a tendency to stop short of fully straightening the legs out of fear of locking the knees. However, failing to fully straighten the legs can lead to both muscular and neuromuscular problems. Not only are the muscles not strengthened in the last few degrees of their range, but the sensation of completely straightening the legs fades from memory, and *almost* straight begins to feel like *completely* straight. The knee joint was built to reach full extension and it should be used to its maximum potential.

Teachers sometimes speak of straightening the legs, or conversely, bending the legs (drawing them in), from the abdominals. Anatomically, this is clearly not accurate—there is no muscular connection between the abdominals and the legs. Conceptually, however, the movement of the legs emanates from the powerhouse. Visualizing pushing the legs out or drawing the legs in from deep within the pelvic bowl—essentially recruiting the muscles of the internal support system (ISS)—encourages a stable foundation and smooth, flowing movement. I like to visualize the ISS as a steam

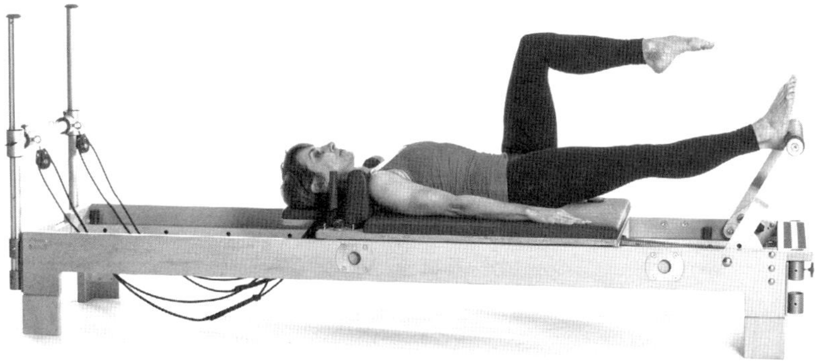

engine, and the legs as cranks that are driven by that engine. This image helps create the desired movement pattern as well as a sensation of warming up.

The foot work offers the teacher and the student a great deal of information regarding strength, flexibility, stabilization, alignment, asymmetries, and movement habits. In many ways the foot work resembles the gait cycle and, as such, gives insight into the way a person walks and runs. It is a fascinating area of study and should be observed from various angles.

Parallel Heels

The heel position has two major benefits. The first is that it allows you to align and use the legs while initially taking the complex mechanism of the foot partially out of the equation. Although the foot is the foundation, it remains still; the movement occurs primarily in the ankle, knee, and hip joints. The second benefit of bearing weight on the heel is that you can more readily connect with the hamstrings when straightening the leg.

In the various heel positions, the feet should remain still, as if there were a floor beneath them. The position of the feet in this scenario is determined by placing them in maximum dorsiflexion when the knees are bent and then keeping them still as the legs straighten and bend. The pivot point is the ankle joint; in contrast, if the feet were in full dorsiflexion throughout, the ankle and foot would remain at the same angle and the feet would rock back and forth on the heel.

Imagery

Visualize a rubber band connecting the heels to the sit bones. As the legs straighten, the band stretches, creating a strong pull between the heels and the sit bones. Once the legs are straight, imagine the band overpowering your musculature and pulling the heels backward, despite your attempts to keep the legs straight. This process of creating internal resistance amplifies the eccentric contraction.

- Initiate the movement with the hamstrings.
- Keep the feet still, as if standing on the floor.
- Use the ankles as the pivot point of the movement.
- Maintain lumbopelvic stabilization.

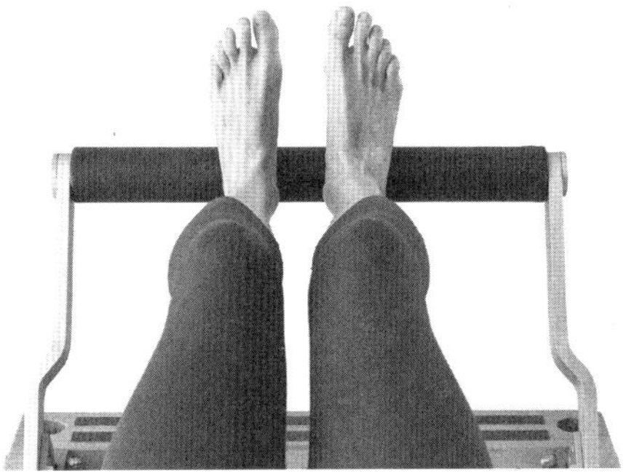

The parallel heels position allows full use of the ankle, knee, and hip joints.

Muscle Focus

- Hamstrings
- Quadriceps

Objectives

- To improve hip extensor and knee extensor strength
- To develop lumbopelvic stabilization

RESISTANCE

Light Medium Heavy

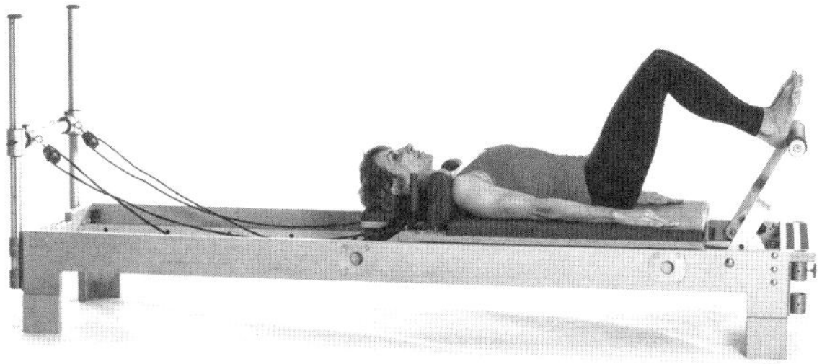

Setup. Lie supine in a neutral spine position. Place the heels on the footbar with the feet 2-4 inches (5-10 centimeters) apart and the legs parallel. We commonly call this position *hip width*. This should not be misunderstood as the width of the pelvis, but rather the distance between the insides of the acetabula, the sockets of the hip joint. A good gauge is placing the feet in line with the ischial tuberosities, or the sit bones. Relax the arms by the sides of the body, shoulders positioned firmly against the shoulder rests. Place the head on the headrest (adjusted to provide optimal spinal alignment, free of tension).

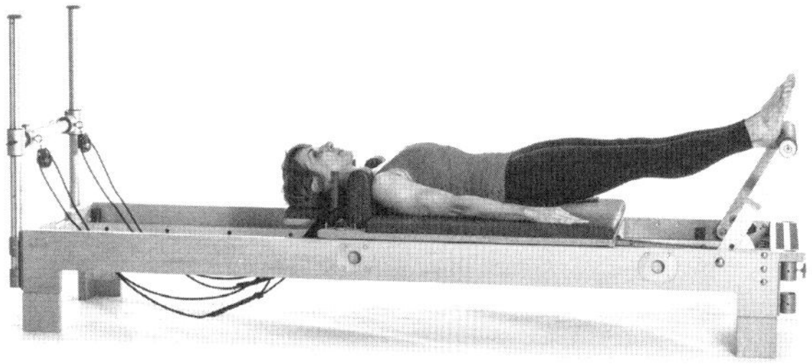

Exhale. Straighten the legs completely, extending the hips and knees while maintaining stability in the pelvis and trunk.

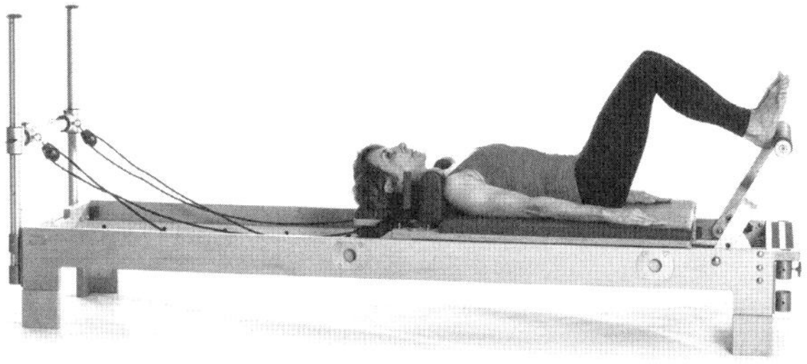

Inhale. Bend the knees and flex the hips, returning toward the stopper without necessarily touching it or halting the movement. Maintain a consistent angle between the feet and the footbar. Repeat 10 times.

Parallel Toes

Muscle Focus

- Hamstrings
- Quadriceps
- Ankle–foot plantarflexors

Objectives

- To improve hip extensor and knee extensor strength
- To improve ankle–foot plantarflexor control
- To develop lumbopelvic stabilization

RESISTANCE

Light Medium Heavy

During foot work exercises in the toe position on the reformer, cadillac, and wunda chair, the foot should remain active, maintaining a consistent angle between the foot and the footbar (as determined by the maximum plantarflexion that can be achieved when the knees are fully extended). As the knees bend, maintain this angle, keeping the heels still and pivoting at the ankle joint (not the metatarsal–phalange joint). There is a tendency, particularly among dancers, to maintain maximum plantarflexion throughout the movement. This results in rocking back and forth on the balls of the feet, eliminating the ankle as the pivot point.

Pressure should be evenly distributed throughout the front of the feet when pushing through the balls of the feet and the toes. The toes wrap gently around the footbar.

The toe position is more challenging than the heel position. Not only is it more complex, with more joints involved, but it also generates greater resistance due to the added height of the feet. There is a tendency to drop the heels as the legs straighten, releasing the resistance, and then to lift the heels as the legs bend, placing the feet in full plantarflexion. This typically occurs when there is a lack of strength and the resistance is too high. Lower the resistance and focus on keeping the heels still and achieving good alignment of the feet. Working with less resistance in order to maintain the correct position of the feet is preferable to loading on the weight and compromising the form.

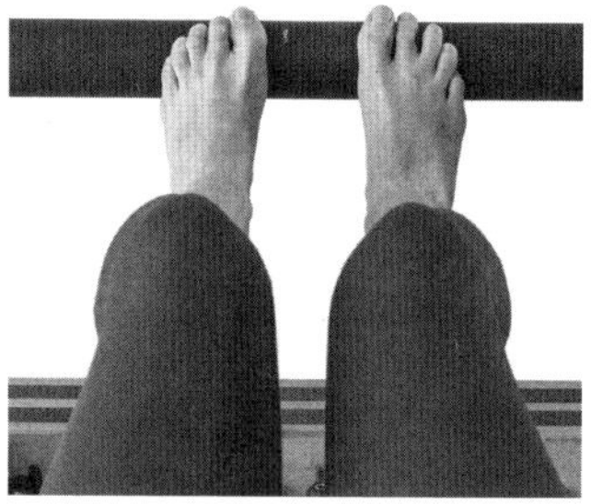

Sometimes the feet roll out (supinate); if this happens, adjust the subtalar joint such that slightly more weight is placed on the inner aspect of the feet and increase engagement of the peroneal muscles. Less commonly, in my experience, the feet roll in (pronate); to correct this, place more weight on the outer aspect of the feet and increase engagement of the tibialis posterior.

Imagery

Visualizing a rubber band connecting the heels to the sit bones works for all the foot work positions. When pushing off the toes, you should feel a lifted sensation, as if you are pushing off a springboard.

- Initiate the movement from the hamstrings.
- Keep the heels still and the angle of the feet relative to the footbar consistent.
- Maintain lumbopelvic stabilization.

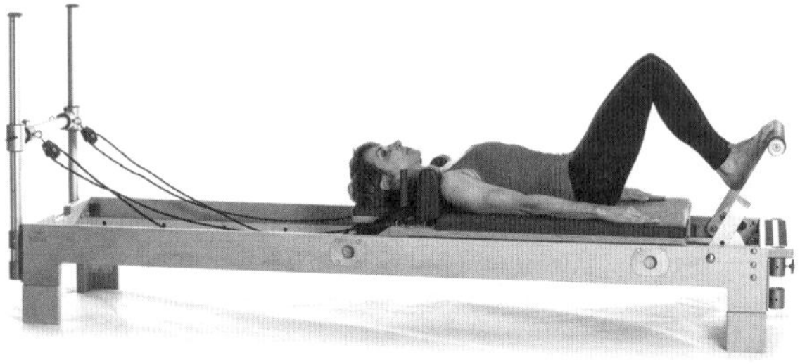

Setup. Lie supine in a neutral spine position, with the weight evenly distributed through the balls of the feet and the toes gently wrapped around the footbar. Position the feet 2-4 inches (5-10 centimeters) apart, with the legs parallel. Relax the arms by the sides of the body, shoulders positioned firmly against the shoulder rests. Place the head on the headrest (adjusted to provide optimal spinal alignment, free of tension).

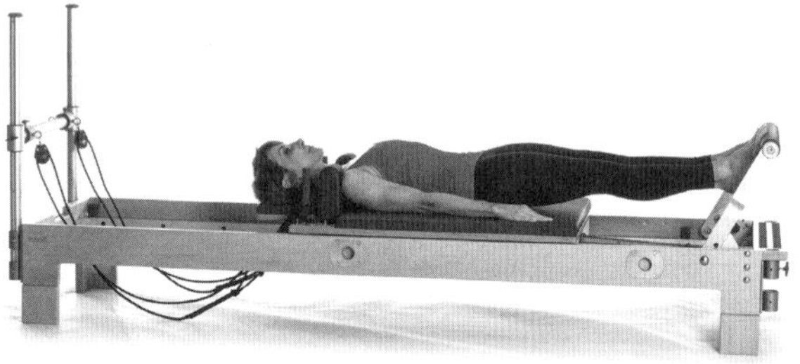

Exhale. Straighten the legs completely, extending the hips and knees while keeping the pelvis and trunk stable.

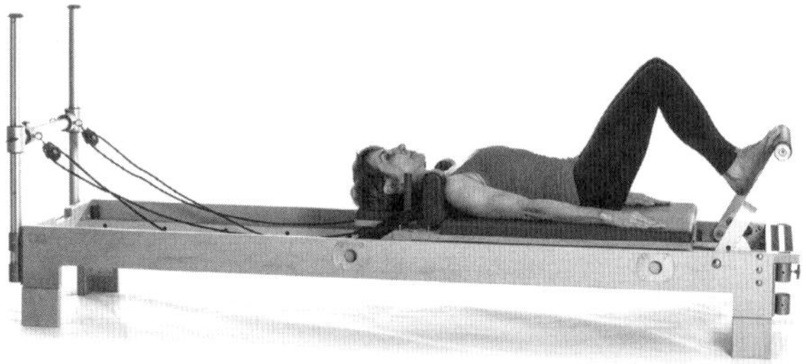

Inhale. Bend the knees and flex the hips, returning toward the stopper without necessarily touching it or halting the movement. Repeat 10 times.

V Position Toes

The extent of external rotation of the hip joints in this exercise is approximately 30 degrees between the two hip joints, although this will vary somewhat by individual. Dancers who are accustomed to working with much greater hip external rotation (turnout) should not compare this position to a first position in ballet—it is not. It is a classic Pilates position that can be more accurately compared to a military stance. (Dancers can add exercises that are specifically adapted to incorporate turnout, but it is not the norm.)

The exact position can be achieved when transitioning from the Reformer: Parallel Toes by simply bringing the heels together without adjusting the distance between the feet. Note that the V position is typically done on the toes only, making the transition seamless.

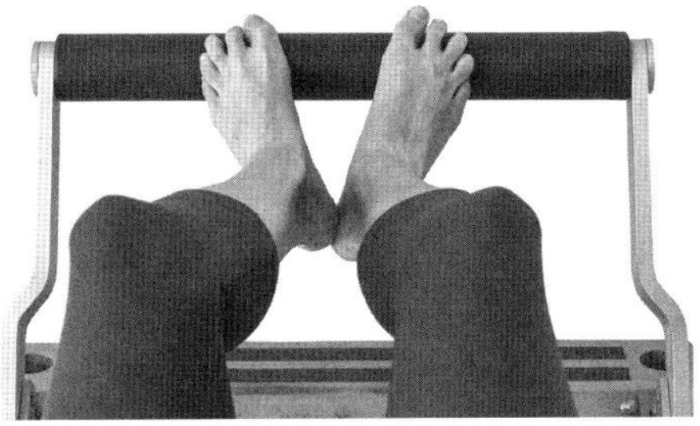

The V position offers moderate, rather than maximal, hip external rotation.

Imagery

Imagine straightening the legs and squeezing them together at the same time, as if holding a big ball or balloon between the legs.

- Initiate the movement from the hamstrings.
- Keep the heels still while squeezing them together.
- Straighten the legs completely.
- Maintain lumbopelvic stabilization.

Muscle Focus

- Hamstrings
- Quadriceps
- Hip adductors
- Ankle–foot plantarflexors

Objectives

- To improve hip extensor and knee extensor strength
- To improve hip adductor control
- To improve ankle–foot plantarflexor control

RESISTANCE

Light Medium Heavy

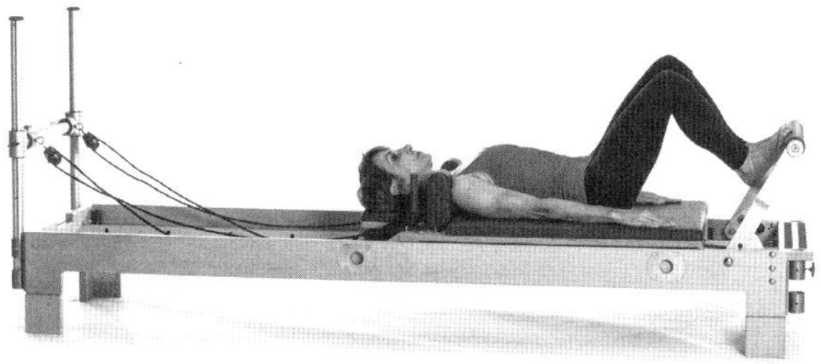

Setup. Lie supine in a neutral spine position. Position the toes on the footbar 2-4 inches (5-10 centimeters) apart with the heels together, creating a V position with the feet. Relax the arms by the sides of the body, shoulders positioned firmly against the shoulder rests. Place the head on the headrest (adjusted to provide optimal spinal alignment, free of tension).

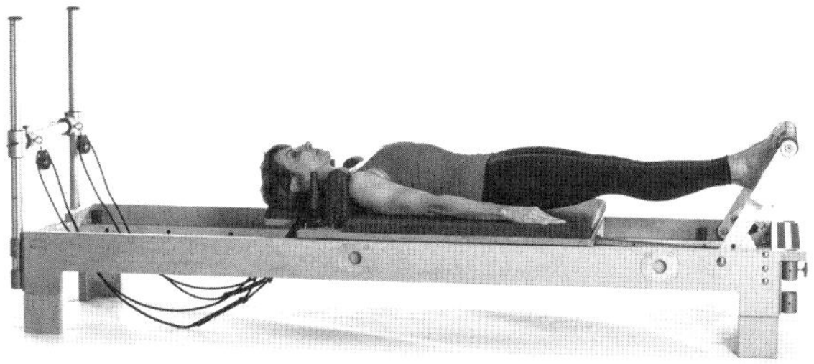

Exhale. Straighten the legs completely, extending the hips and knees while maintaining stability in the remainder of the body.

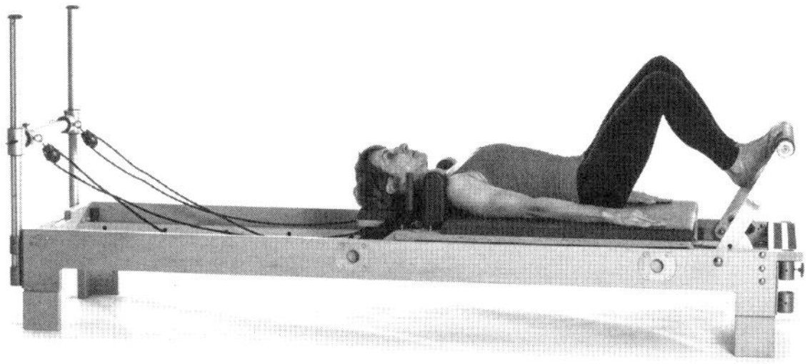

Inhale. Bend the knees and flex the hips, returning toward the stopper without necessarily touching it or halting the movement. Maintain the same degree of hip external rotation and a consistent angle between the feet and the footbar. Repeat 10 times.

Open V Position Heels

Muscle Focus

- Hamstrings
- Quadriceps
- Hip adductors

Objectives

- To improve hip extensor and knee extensor strength
- To improve hip adductor control
- To improve hip flexibility

RESISTANCE

Light — Medium — Heavy

The open V positions of both the heels and toes are not from the classic Pilates repertoire but offer valuable benefits. They take the hip joint into a wider, more challenging range of motion than most people are used to, in terms of both hip abduction and external rotation. I encourage you to explore this range as a means of achieving and maintaining optimal function of the hip joint. These open V positions also allow dancers (and other athletes who use similar movements) to correct their technique and develop strength in this range.

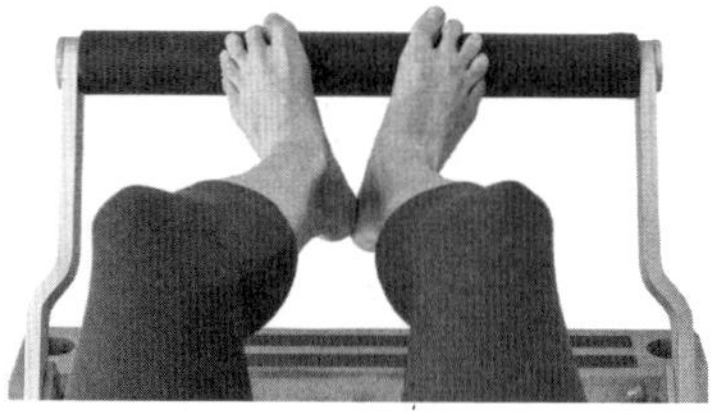

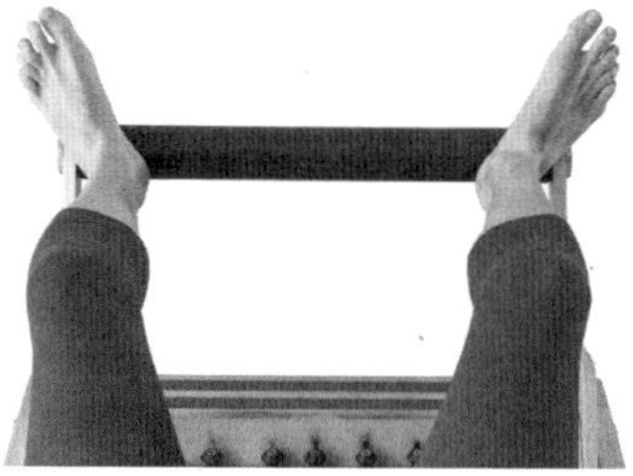

I suggest finding the position by keeping the shape of the Reformer: V Position Toes (consistent hip external rotation), then opening the legs wider and placing the feet toward the outside of the footbar.

Imagery

As with the Reformer: V Position Toes, imagine straightening the legs and simultaneously squeezing them together, emphasizing the involvement of the hip adductors as the legs straighten and bend. When the knees bend, visualize them reaching out to the sides of the body along a diagonal energy line.

- ○ Focus on engaging the hip adductors.
- ○ Keep the feet still, as if standing on the floor.
- ○ Maintain correct tracking of the leg, aligning the hip, knee, and foot.
- ○ Maintain lumbopelvic stabilization.

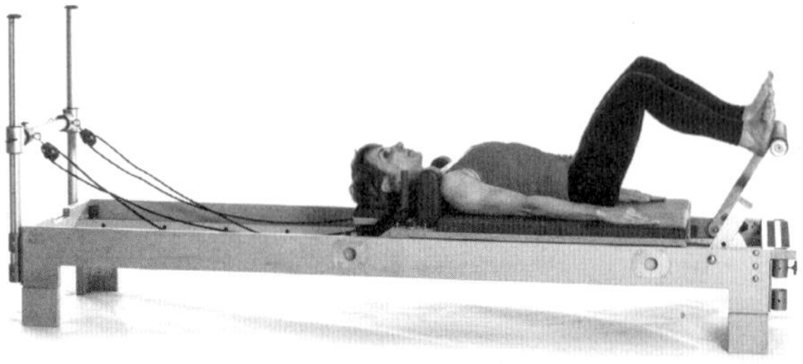

Setup. Lie supine in a neutral spine position, with the heels toward the ends of the footbar and the hips externally rotated, creating an open V position with the legs. Relax the arms by the sides of the body, with the shoulders positioned firmly against the shoulder rests. Place the head on the headrest (adjusted to provide optimal spinal alignment, free of tension).

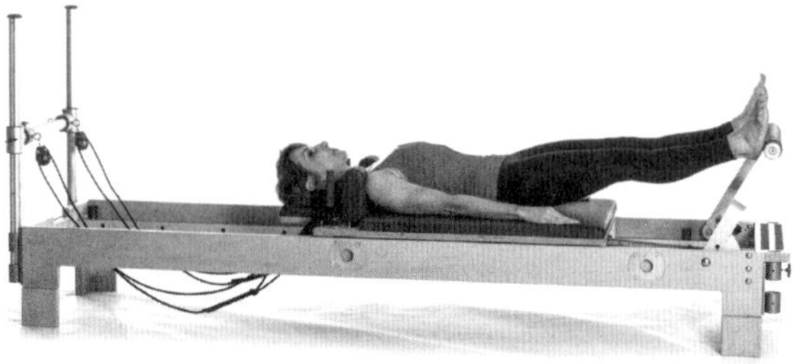

Exhale. Straighten the legs completely, extending the hips and knees while maintaining stability in the pelvis and trunk.

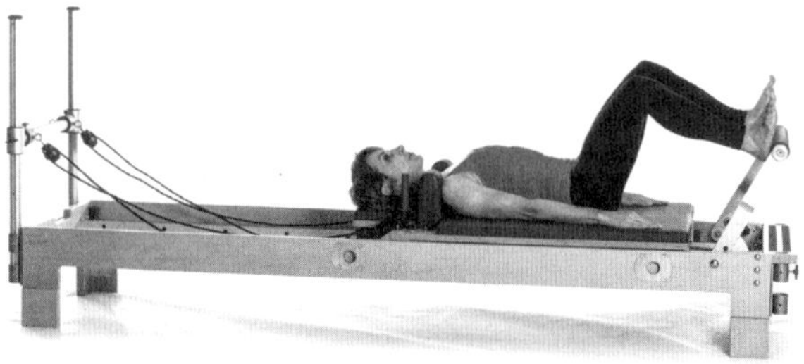

Inhale. Return toward the stopper without necessarily touching it or halting the movement. Maintain the same degree of hip external rotation and a consistent angle between the feet and the footbar. Repeat 10 times.

Open V Position Toes

This open V position on the toes is possibly the most complex position in the foot work block, because it requires tremendous control of the hip and knee joints and the feet. In addition, it offers the most stretch in the hip joint and a unique angle of challenge for the hamstrings and quadriceps. Although dancers will find this position particularly familiar and beneficial, many people can benefit from this opening of the hip joint.

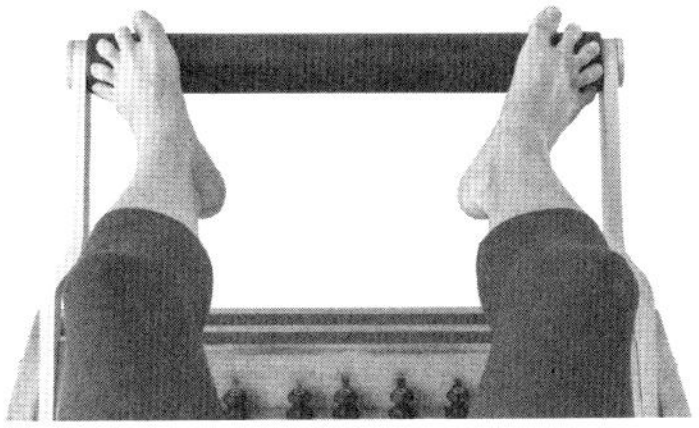

The vastus medialis oblique muscle can be distinctly felt and strengthened (often a goal in corrective work of the knee) during this exercise.

Imagery

Employ the rubber band, springboard, and straightening-while-squeezing concepts used in the previous foot positions. In addition, the image of an open-leg squat may help you release tension in the hip joint and create a sensation of the pelvis opening and relaxing.

- ○ Straighten the legs completely.
- ○ Keep the heels still.
- ○ Maintain correct tracking of the leg, aligning the hip, knee, and foot.
- ○ Maintain lumbopelvic stabilization.

Muscle Focus

- Hamstrings
- Quadriceps
- Hip adductors
- Ankle–foot plantarflexors

Objectives

- To improve hip extensor and knee extensor strength
- To improve hip adductor control
- To improve ankle–foot plantarflexor control
- To improve hip flexibility

RESISTANCE

Light Medium Heavy

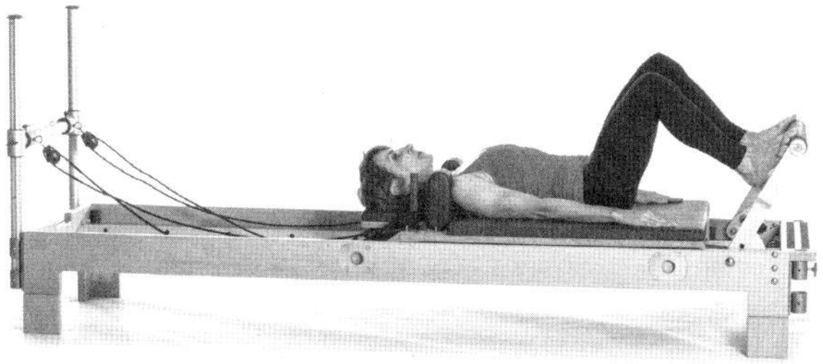

Setup. Lie supine in a neutral spine position, with the toes toward the ends of the footbar and the hips externally rotated, creating an open V position with the legs. Relax the arms by the sides of the body, with the shoulders positioned firmly against the shoulder rests. Place the head on the headrest (adjusted to provide optimal spinal alignment, free of tension).

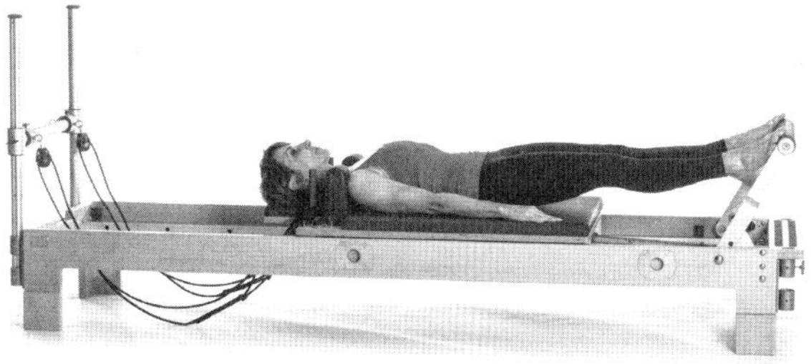

Exhale. Straighten the legs completely, extending the hips and knees while maintaining stability in the pelvis and trunk.

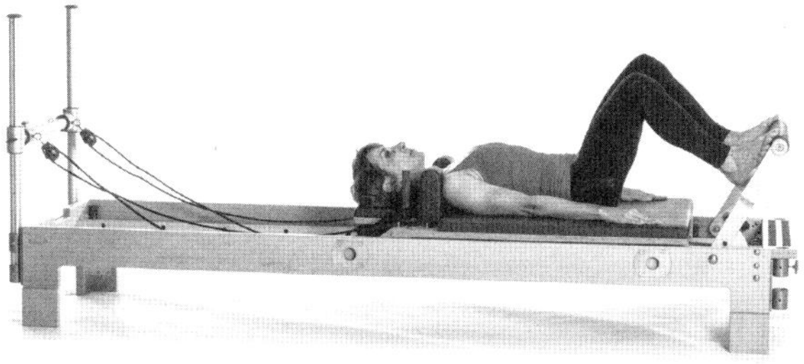

Inhale. Return toward the stopper without necessarily touching it or halting the movement, keeping the heels still. Maintain the same degree of hip external rotation and a consistent angle between the feet and the footbar. Repeat 10 times.

Calf Raises

Muscle Focus

- Ankle–foot plantarflexors

Objectives

- To improve ankle–foot plantarflexor strength and flexibility
- To develop foot control and alignment

RESISTANCE

Light Medium Heavy

This is an exceptional exercise for developing range of motion and strength of the foot and ankle complex, including the many muscles and joints that contribute to its movement. It also allows you to focus on correcting alignment of the foot, which is so important in walking, running, and other everyday movements, as well as many athletic pursuits. Imagine the importance of exact and efficient foot alignment for a marathon runner, who repeats the same movement pattern thousands of times in one event, not to mention the countless repetitions during training.

Pay particular attention to the eccentric contraction as you lower the heels. Do not succumb to the pull of the springs by dropping the heels; instead, resist the pull and actively dorsiflex the feet at the end range. Avoid the tendency to roll onto the outside or inside of the feet as you reach maximum plantarflexion. Limiting the range of the ankle joint and maintaining correct alignment, with weight proportionately distributed through the toes, is preferable to going higher and deviating from the centerline.

Imagery

The image of pushing the footbar away from the body helps to achieve the desired amount of plantarflexion. The more stable the body is, particularly the pelvis, the more powerful each thrust will be. Think of 50 percent of the weight being concentrated around the big toe and the remaining 50 percent distributed through the remaining toes proportionately, according to size of the toe. This is an approximation but provides a good image.

- ○ Use the full range of motion of the ankle.
- ○ Align the feet correctly, focusing on the subtalar joint.
- ○ Actively dorsiflex the feet when lowering.
- ○ Maintain lumbopelvic stabilization.

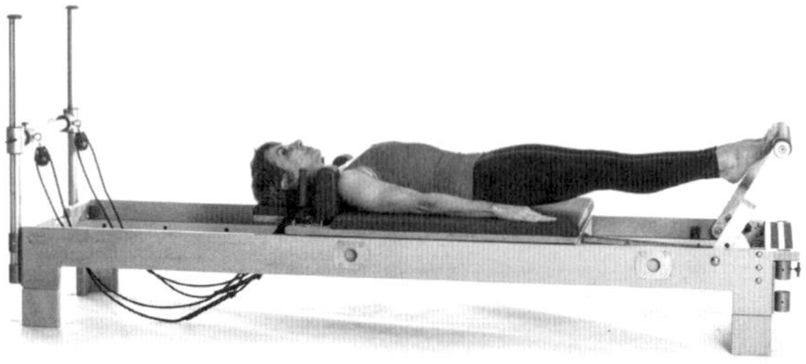

Setup. Lie supine in a neutral spine position with the feet plantarflexed and the weight evenly distributed through the balls of the feet, toes gently wrapped around the footbar. Position the feet 2-4 inches (5-10 centimeters) apart with the legs straight and parallel. Relax the arms by the sides of the body, with the shoulders positioned firmly against the shoulder rests. Place the head on the headrest (adjusted to provide optimal spinal alignment, free of tension).

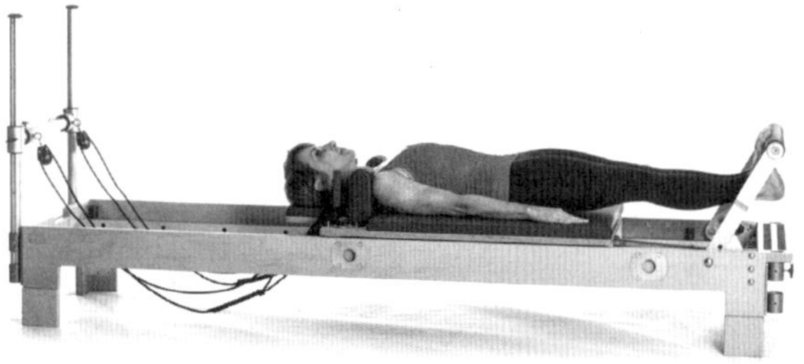

Exhale. Dorsiflex the feet, pressing the heels under the footbar.

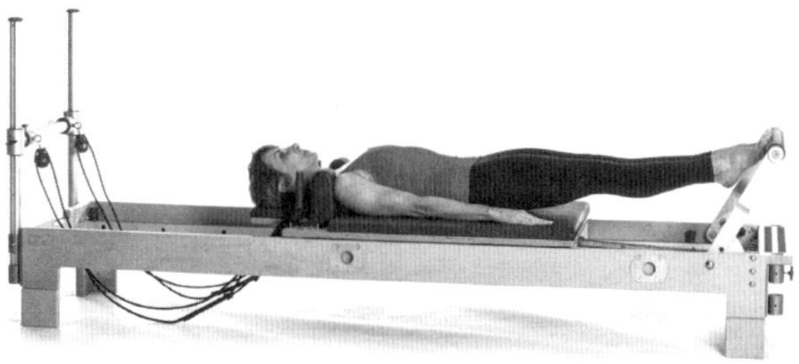

Inhale. Plantarflex the feet. Repeat 10-20 times.

Prances

Like the Reformer: Calf Raises, this exercise begins with the legs straight and the feet in maximum plantarflexion. One foot dorsiflexes while the other plantarflexes, both return to the start position, then the feet switch roles. It is important to go through the start position, with legs completely straight and both feet in maximal plantarflexion, to achieve a sense of height and elongation through each cycle. The stability of the pelvis and the profound work of the feet give this exercise the desired sense of flow, elevation, and lightness. The breath pattern also helps greatly in creating the desired flow.

Imagery

The image of a horse prancing is commonly used for this movement in dance training. Aim to achieve the grace, flow, and proud, upright feeling of a beautiful dancer or a horse, barely touching the ground. Another image is to think of the footbar as a trampoline, adding lift and buoyancy to the movement and emphasizing the upward thrust.

- Work both feet equally in their respective full ranges of motion; as one lifts into plantarflexion, the other presses down into dorsiflexion.
- Maintain lumbopelvic stabilization.

PROGRESSION

This exercise has a distinct rhythm. To add complexity to the rhythm and extra challenge for the calf muscles, perform a double pulse with each foot. This can be felt particularly in the foot that is dorsiflexing (but do not ignore the foot that is plantarflexing). This will give the exercise even more of a springy, bouncy feel. Keep the breath pattern the same as before. This will necessitate extending the breath, which is an excellent breathing exercise in itself.

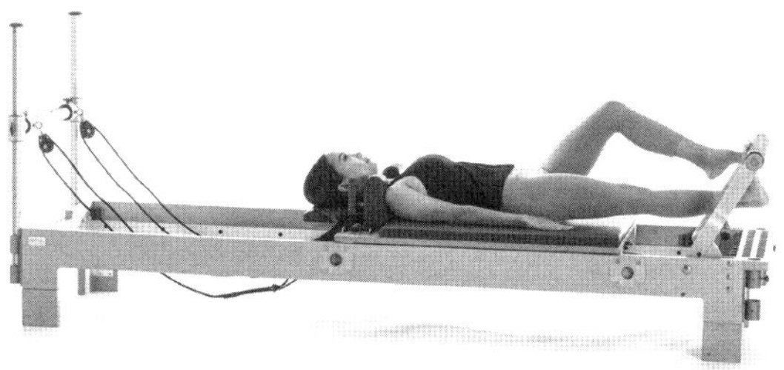

Muscle Focus

- Ankle–foot plantarflexors

Objectives

- To improve ankle–foot plantarflexor strength and flexibility
- To develop foot control and alignment
- To develop lumbopelvic stabilization

RESISTANCE

Light — Medium — Heavy

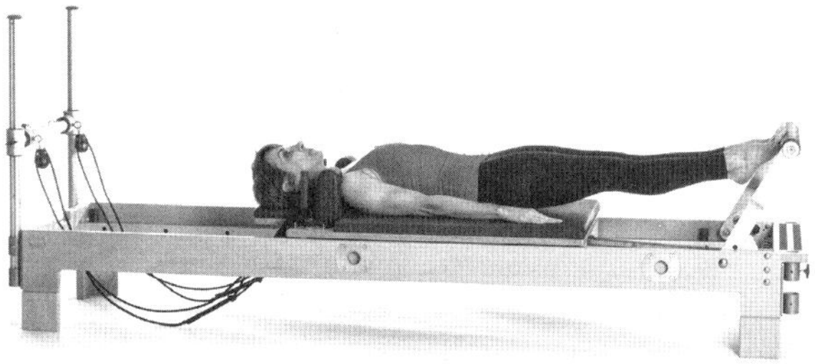

Setup. Lie supine in a neutral spine position with the feet plantarflexed and the weight evenly distributed through the balls of the feet, toes gently wrapped around the footbar. Position the feet 2-4 inches (5-10 centimeters) apart with the legs straight and parallel. Relax the arms by the sides of the body, with the shoulders positioned firmly against the shoulder rests. Place the head on the headrest (adjusted to provide optimal spinal alignment, free of tension).

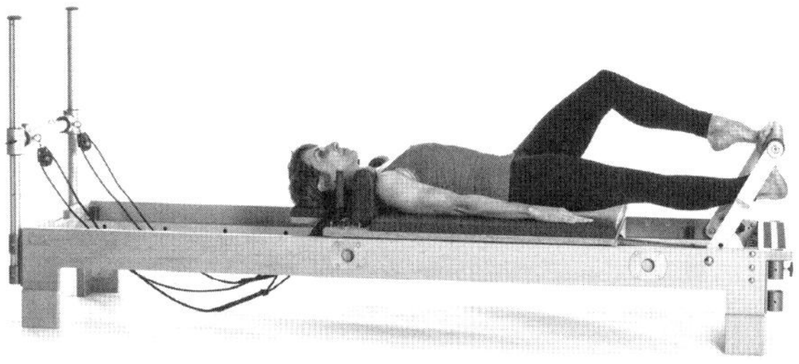

Exhale. Dorsiflex one foot and plantarflex the other. Switch the feet after transitioning through the start position.

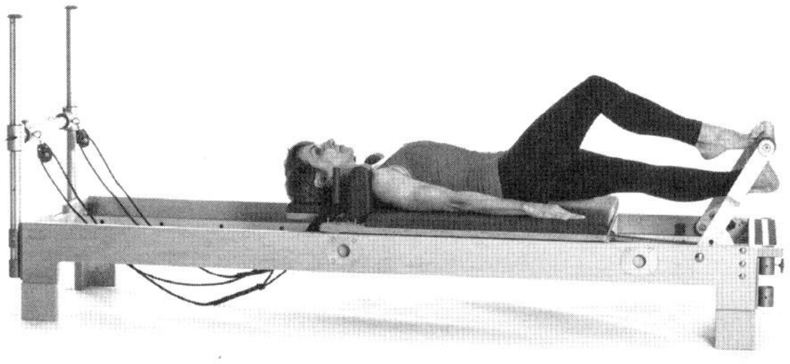

Inhale. Repeat the cycle with each foot plantarflexing and dorsiflexing once. Continue for 10 complete cycles (10 plantarflexions and dorsiflexions on each foot).

Prehensile

Muscle Focus

- Hamstrings
- Quadriceps

Objectives

- To improve foot and ankle–foot plantarflexor flexibility
- To improve hip extensor and knee extensor strength
- To develop lumbopelvic stabilization

RESISTANCE

Light Medium Heavy

Although this is one of the classic Pilates positions, the unusual position of the feet and relatively complex movement pattern makes the Reformer: Prehensile difficult to execute well, and therefore I don't necessarily offer it to students early in their training. When done well and used appropriately, it is a very valuable position that provides an effective stretch for the fasciae and intrinsic muscles of the feet as well as the ankle–foot plantarflexors. For this reason, I recommend this exercise follow Reformer: Calf Raises and Reformer: Prances, providing a welcome stretch for the calves.

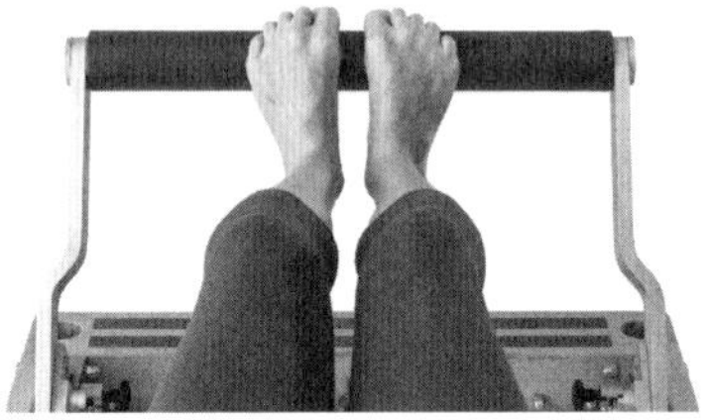

Interestingly, the prehensile position places pressure on areas of the feet that correlate with reflexology pressure points. An excellent stretch can be felt in the feet and calf muscles.

Imagery

The most effective image is a bird wrapping its talons around a branch and holding it firmly.

- Keep reaching the heels under the footbar to maximize the calf stretch.
- Wrap the forefeet around the footbar stretching the tops of the feet.
- Keep the toes spread out rather than clenched.
- Maintain lumbopelvic stabilization.

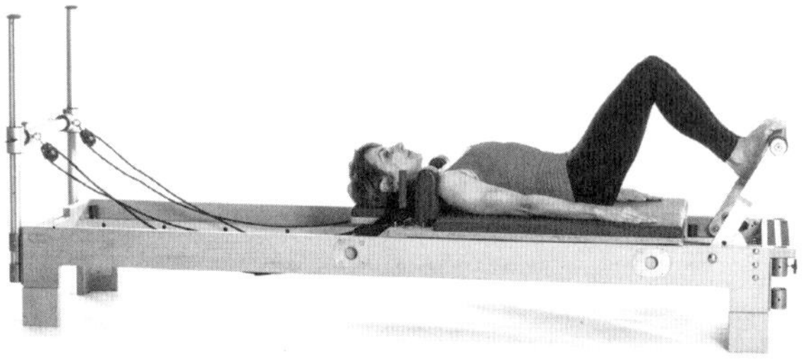

Setup. Lie supine in a neutral spine position, with the forefeet wrapped around the footbar. Position the feet 2-4 inches (5-10 centimeters) apart with the legs parallel. Relax the arms by the sides of the body, with the shoulders positioned firmly against the shoulder rests. Place the head on the headrest (adjusted to provide optimal spinal alignment, free of tension).

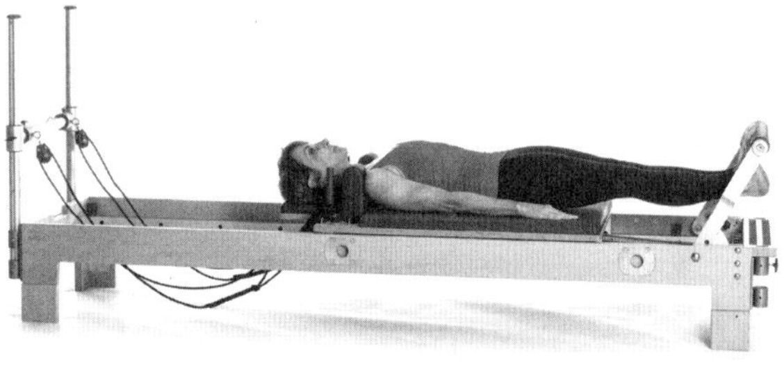

Exhale. Straighten the legs, extending the hips and knees while pushing the heels under the footbar. Keep the pelvis and trunk stable.

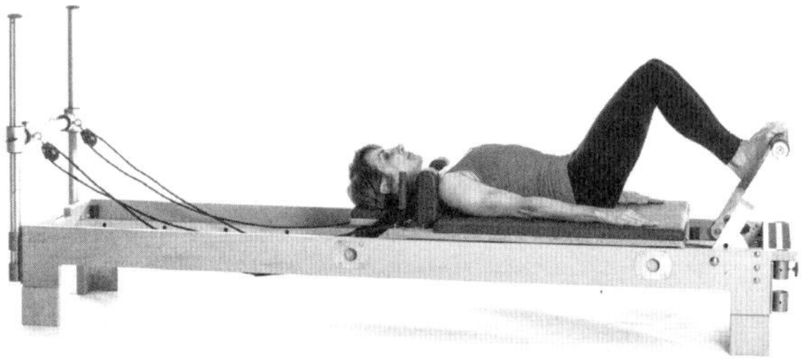

Inhale. Bend the knees, returning toward the stopper without necessarily touching it or halting the movement. Continue pushing the heels under the footbar. Repeat 10 times.

Single-Leg Heel

Working a single leg is invaluable for several reasons. First, it allows each leg to work independently without relying on the other. Often one leg is dominant, whether noticeably or not, and will tend to get stronger while the less dominant side becomes weaker. This is particularly common following an injury or surgery. Working unilaterally (typically starting with the weaker side) will strengthen the weaker leg in an endeavor to create balance. It will also magnify compensations and misalignments, making it easier to detect them. Finally, exercising a single leg increases the challenge of keeping the pelvis stable. The single-leg series should be included in your program, if at all possible. I recommend preparing by placing both feet on the footbar, then once good alignment has been achieved, lifting one foot off without readjusting the other foot, the pelvis, or the trunk.

Imagery

Imagine that both legs are on the footbar and that you are pushing off both legs. Visualizing the invisible leg helps keep the structure stable and balanced.

- ○ Keep the working foot dorsiflexed as if standing on the floor.
- ○ Keep the supporting leg stable in a tabletop position.
- ○ Maintain lumbopelvic stabilization.

VARIATION

There are many single-leg footwork variations that are very beneficial. A good option for the Reformer: Single-Leg Heel is to straighten the supporting leg toward the ceiling, as close to perpendicular as possible, as you straighten the working leg. The legs straighten and bend simultaneously. Keep both feet dorsiflexed.

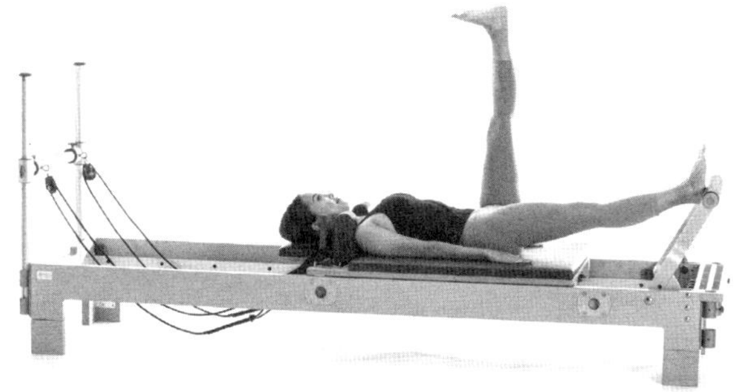

Muscle Focus

- Hamstrings
- Quadriceps

Objectives

- To improve hip extensor and knee extensor strength
- To develop lumbopelvic stabilization

RESISTANCE

Light — Medium — Heavy

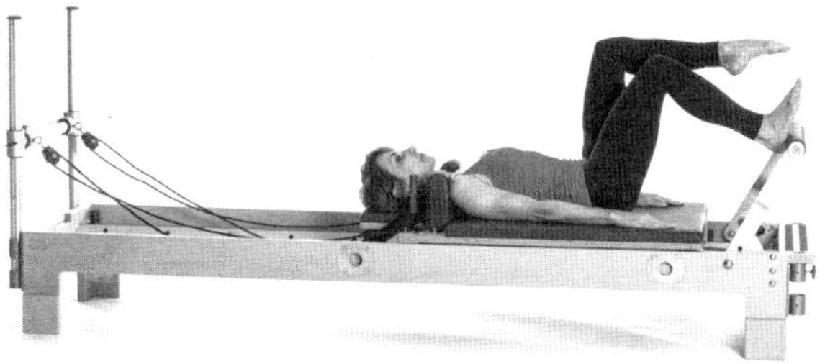

Setup. Lie supine in a neutral spine position, with the heels on the footbar. Position the feet 2-4 inches (5-10 centimeters) apart with the legs parallel. Relax the arms by the sides of the body, with the shoulders positioned firmly against the shoulder rests. Place the head on the headrest (adjusted to provide optimal spinal alignment, free of tension). Lift one leg and hold it in a tabletop position.

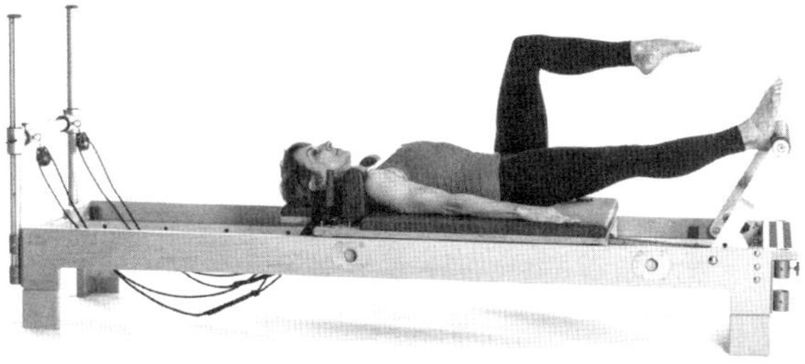

Exhale. Straighten the leg that is on the footbar completely, extending the hip and knee. Keep the pelvis and trunk stable.

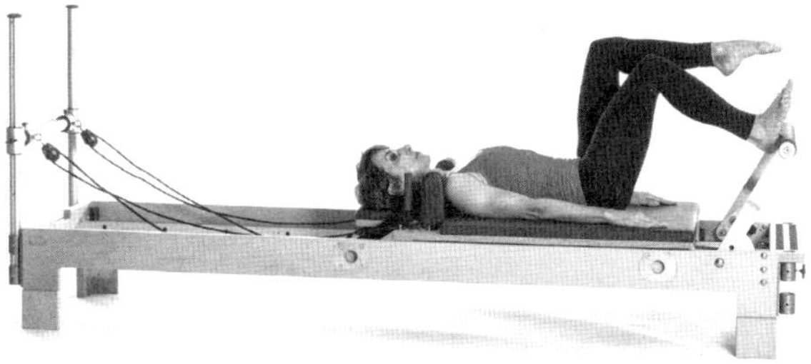

Inhale. Bend the leg, returning toward the stopper without necessarily touching it or halting the movement. Repeat 10 times before switching to the other side.

REFORMER
Foot Work
FUNDAMENTAL

Single-Leg Toes

Muscle Focus

- Hamstrings
- Quadriceps
- Ankle–foot plantarflexors

Objectives

- To improve hip extensor and knee extensor strength
- To improve ankle–foot plantarflexor control
- To develop lumbopelvic stabilization

RESISTANCE

Light — Medium — Heavy

In this exercise, the feet and legs begin in a parallel position, with the toes gently wrapped around the footbar. This is the most challenging position in the foot work in terms of load. Remember, working with a lighter load and correct alignment is always preferable to compromising good form for the sake of load. However, once you have achieved good form and control, increasing the load to challenge the musculature of the foot and improve strength can prove valuable.

Imagery

The desired sense of elongation of the movement is easier to feel in the toe position than in the heel position (see also Reformer: Single-Leg Heel).

- Keep the heel of the working foot still.
- Straighten the working leg completely with each repetition.
- Keep the supporting leg stable in a tabletop position.
- Maintain lumbopelvic stabilization.

VARIATION

A good variation for Reformer: Single-Leg Toes is to straighten the supporting leg just above the footbar. As the working leg straightens, lift the other leg up so that it is perpendicular to the floor. In this position, dorsiflex both feet, plantarflex both feet, then bend the working leg and lower the supporting leg.

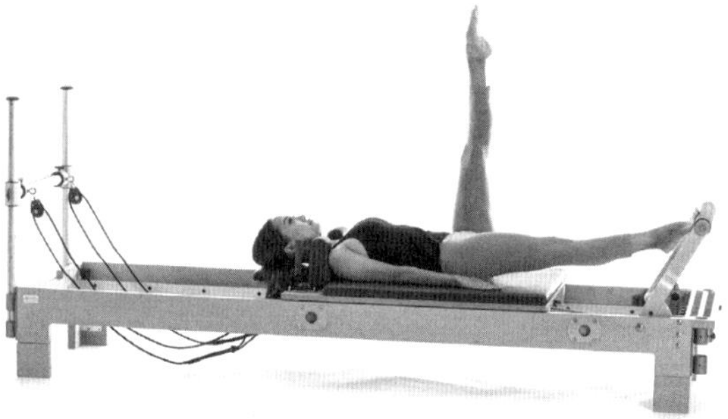

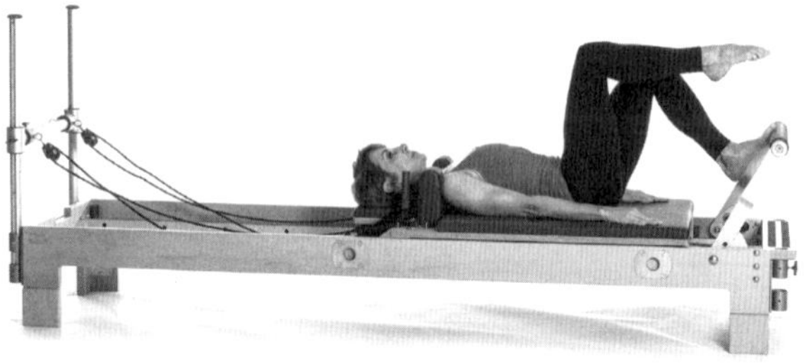

Setup. Lie supine in a neutral spine position, with the weight evenly distributed through the balls of the feet and the toes gently wrapped around the footbar. Position the feet 2-4 inches (5-10 centimeters) apart with the legs parallel. Relax the arms by the sides of the body, with the shoulders positioned firmly against the shoulder rests. Place the head on the headrest (adjusted to provide optimal spinal alignment, free of tension). Lift one leg and hold it in a tabletop position.

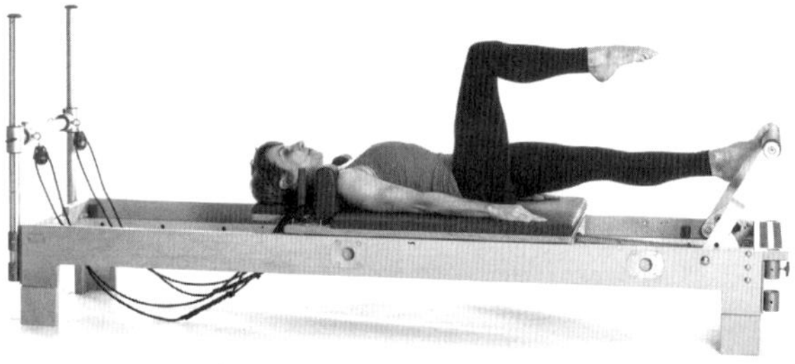

Exhale. Straighten the leg that is on the footbar completely, extending the hip and knee while maintaining stability of the pelvis and trunk.

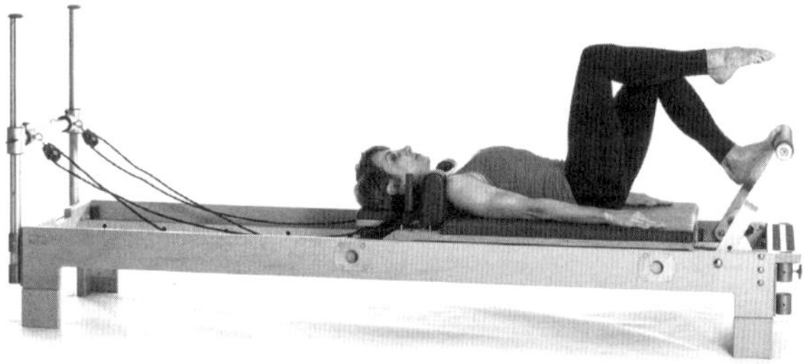

Inhale. Bend the leg, returning toward the stopper without necessarily touching it or halting the movement. Maintain a consistent angle of the foot to the footbar as the knee bends. Repeat 10 times and switch to the other side.

Abdominal Work

The abdominal work in Pilates cannot be overemphasized. As part of the powerhouse, the abdominals play a prominent role in a healthy functioning ISS. Even so, the abdominals are only part of the whole and not the entire picture. People tend to view abdominal strength and abdominal exercises as the be-all and end-all of a strong core and of the practice of Pilates. They are not! Unfortunately, this distorted view has only increased with the popularity of core training. Abdominals that are overdeveloped and possibly tight relative to the other muscles of the ISS can lead to multiple problems, including malalignment. A healthy balance of the musculature of the body, in particular the muscles of the ISS, is the goal, and therefore it is important to create some guidelines from the outset.

There are four layers of abdominal muscle: rectus abdominis, external oblique, internal oblique, and the deepest layer, transversus abdominis (TA). The TA is a fundamental ingredient in the powerhouse concept, which is part of every movement in Pilates. The TA plays a key role in the stabilization and protection of the spine and should be engaged throughout the Pilates session. Engaging the TA is a prerequisite to achieving the desired effect from abdominal work and the correct quality of movement.

It is interesting to compare, for instance, the typical abdominal crunch, a part of many fitness regimens, to the Mat: Chest Lift. They are seemingly similar, yet the focus, the quality, and arguably the outcome of each is entirely different, in large part because of the emphasis on TA engagement in the chest lift position. This emphasis should not overshadow the importance of the other abdominal muscles, which, when working together as an integrated complex, serve as both a brace for the trunk and a powerful initiator for any trunk movement. Working the abdominals all together, precisely and in a coordinated manner, is challenging to say the least. I have witnessed many tough and seasoned athletes—who were accustomed to performing hundreds of repetitions of abdominal crunches—crumble after attempting 10 well-executed Mat: Chest Lifts.

When compiling the abdominal work section of the Pilates session, take care to make it balanced. Use both isometric and isotonic (dynamic) exercises, because each type of muscle contraction develops the muscles differently and plays a part in optimal function. In addition, integrate sequences that are biased toward developing muscle strength and those that are biased toward muscle endurance. Remember also that the recruitment of the abdominals is important not only during forward flexion but during all ranges of motion, including spinal extension.

An image commonly used in Pilates to achieve the correct recruitment of the abdominals is that of "hollowing" the midsection of the body, specifically the abdominal cavity. It is this drawing in of the navel to the spine that encourages the recruitment of the TA. I like to visualize a hollow, deep, carved-out wooden bowl. The bowl is solid and stable, able to hold large amounts of energy and life force within it. At the same time, it is important to mention the concept of bracing, similar to the effect of a corset. An excellent visual is that of a tree trunk. If the trunk were hollowed or thinned in one section, it would be weaker at this point, whereas if the trunk is wide and round, it is strong and stable. I believe that both approaches have their place in our movement vocabulary and are equally valid. The common goal is a stable and supportive trunk, which is at the same time mobile and functional, forming the foundation of our movement.

Finally, although we speak a great deal about the importance of spinal stabilization and of the vital role the abdominals play in this process, it is important to keep in mind that stabilization is dynamic and ever-adapting. It is not static. The work of the abdominals, although powerful, is pliable. Dynamic stabilization also facilitates efficient, natural breathing during physical activity, providing support for the spine.

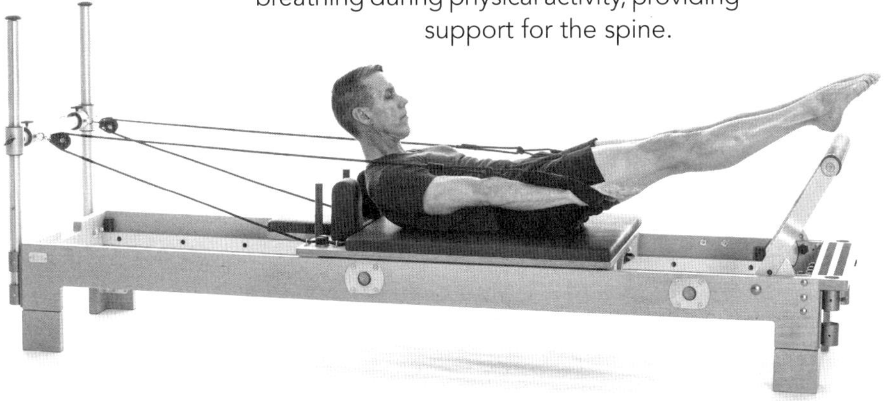

Hundred Prep

Muscle Focus

- Abdominals
- Shoulder extensors
- Hip flexors

Objectives

- To improve abdominal strength
- To improve shoulder extensor and hip flexor control
- To develop lumbopelvic stabilization

RESISTANCE

Light Medium Heavy

The Reformer: Hundred Prep is simple and very effective. You can immediately feel the abdominals working and sense the synergy between the trunk flexors and the shoulder extensors. This exercise is a challenge for people of every fitness level, and it can be adapted to meet different goals. It serves as an excellent preparation for the more advanced Reformer: Hundred and Coordination because it includes elements of both. The Reformer: Hundred Prep is a dynamic (isotonic) exercise, which complements the many isometric abdominal exercises.

Imagery

The movement of the upper body and the arms during this exercise can be likened to a seesaw, alternately lifting and lowering as one unit. Achieving the feeling of synergy between the abdominals and arms early in the process of the abdominal work is important because it is a recurring theme in many of the abdominal exercises that follow.

- ○ Maintain lumbopelvic stabilization.
- ○ Contract the abdominals prior to the movement and keep them engaged.
- ○ Avoid hyperlordosis and bulging of the abdominal region.
- ○ Keep the head aligned with the spine.

PROGRESSION

The first part of the exercise remains the same. However, in the second part (inhale), rather than lowering the body as the arms lift, keep the trunk as lifted and stable as possible as you lift the arms to a 90-degree angle in the shoulder joint (approximately 10 degrees shy of perpendicular to the floor depending on the height of the trunk in flexion) before lowering the upper body and arms as one unit. Continue maintaining muscle engagement and slight tension in the straps. Repeat 5-10 times.

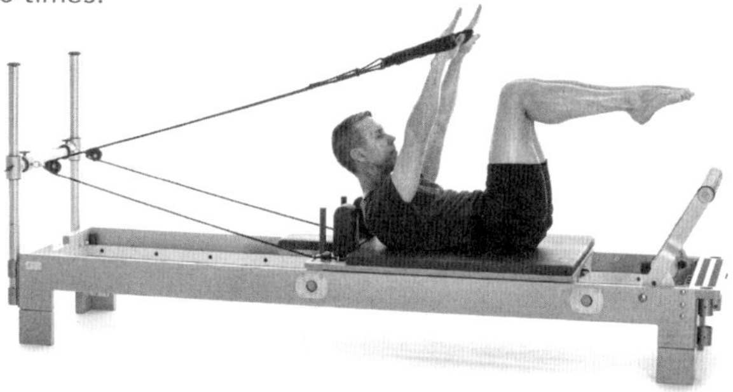

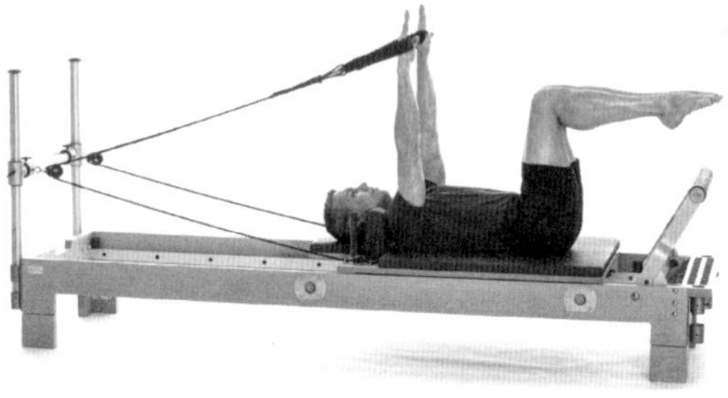

Setup. Lie supine in a neutral spine position with the legs in a tabletop position (hips and knees at a 90-degree angle). Place the hands in the straps with the arms perpendicular to the body, maintaining slight tension in the straps.

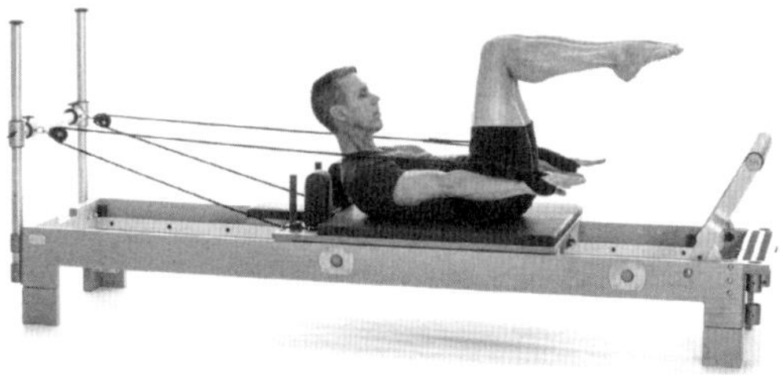

Exhale. Lift the head and chest while pressing the arms down to the sides of the body and keeping the legs in the tabletop position.

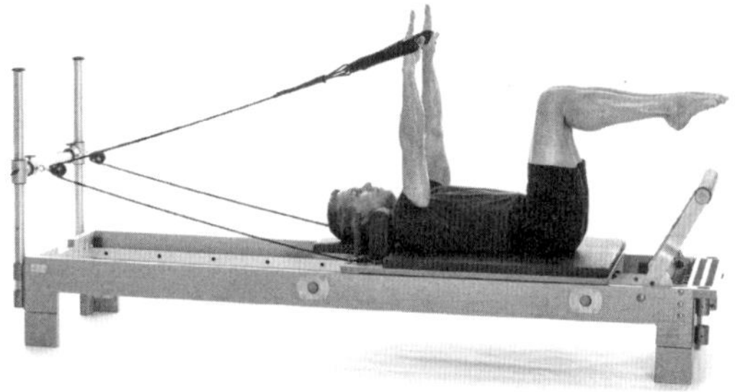

Inhale. Lift the arms and lower the upper body as one unit. Continue maintaining muscle engagement and slight tension in the straps. Return to the start position. Repeat 5-10 times.

Hundred

This exercise is a signature exercise of the classic Pilates repertoire. Like the Reformer: Hundred Prep, it emphasizes integration of the abdominals and shoulder extensors. The slight up-and-down beating motion of the arms adds movement to the isometric activity of the abdominals and stimulates circulation and deep breathing.

This challenging exercise demands a high level of awareness, control, abdominal strength, and understanding of the concept of the ISS. The Reformer: Hundred and several other similar exercises involve isometrically contracting the abdominals and holding the trunk stable in the same position. Therefore supplementing them with dynamic (isotonic) exercises is important in creating a balanced abdominal conditioning program.

Imagery

Visualize the pumping action of the arms as a generator creating energy that gushes through the body, with the epicenter in the abdominal region. The hollow bowl image mentioned previously also helps to fortify the position of the trunk.

- Imprint the lower back into the mat.
- Keep the head aligned with the spine and the eyes focused forward.
- Keep the carriage as still as possible as the arms pump up and down with small, calm movements.

MODIFICATION

To make the Reformer: Hundred easier on the abdominals and alleviate potential strain on the lower back, keep the legs in a tabletop position.

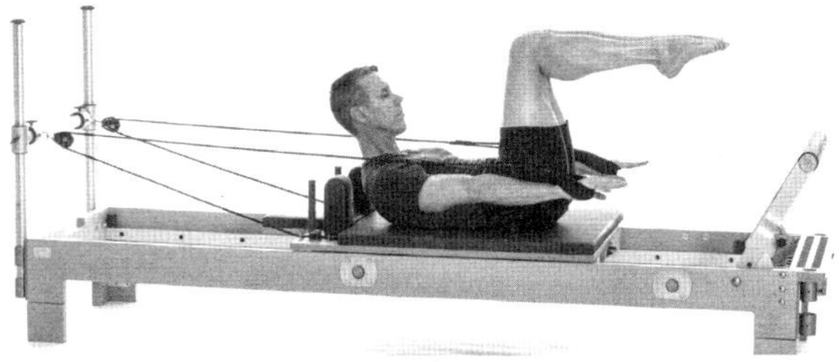

Muscle Focus

- Abdominals
- Shoulder extensors
- Hip flexors

Objectives

- To improve abdominal strength
- To improve shoulder extensor and hip flexor control
- To develop lumbopelvic stabilization

RESISTANCE

Light — Medium — Heavy

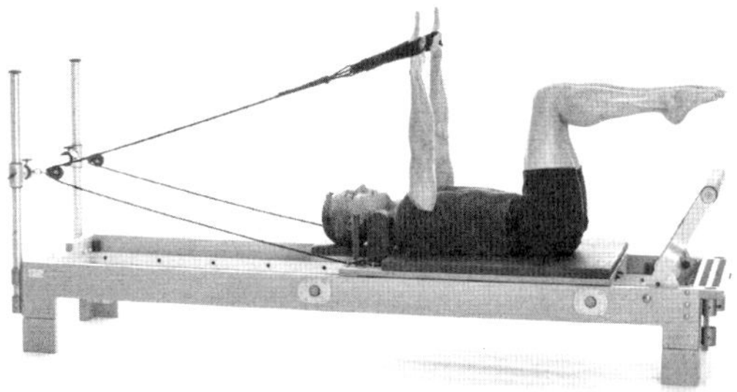

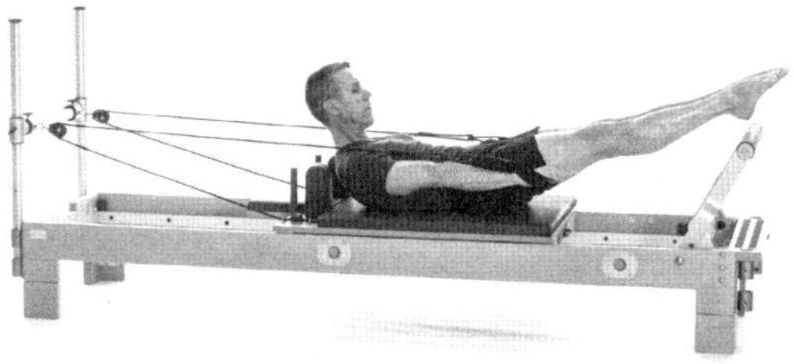

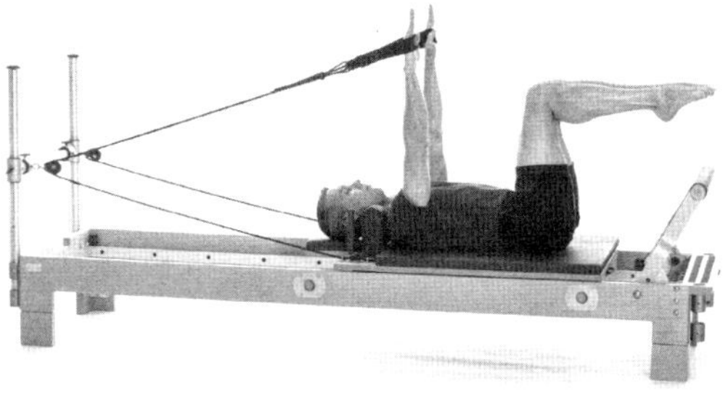

Setup. Lie supine in a neutral spine position with the legs in a tabletop position. Place the hands in the straps with the arms perpendicular to the body, maintaining slight tension in the straps.

Exhale. Lift the head and chest while pressing the arms down to the sides of the body and straightening the legs. The height of the legs and angle of the hip joints will be dictated by your abdominal strength and control. The classic position is performed with the feet opposite the eyes—however, if you are unable to maintain this difficult position, it is quite legitimate to lift the legs higher (toward perpendicular) to make the exercise more accessible.

Inhale. Pause, deepening the abdominal contraction.

Exhale. Pump the arms up and down in a small, rhythmic motion for 5 counts.

Inhale. Continue pumping the arms up and down for 5 counts. Repeat for 10 breath cycles, a total of 100 counts (hence the name). Focus on the stabilization of the trunk and pelvis, maintaining forward flexion.

After the final inhale, bend the legs to tabletop position. Lift the arms to a 90-degree angle in the shoulder joint (approximately 10 degrees shy of perpendicular to the floor depending on the height of the trunk in flexion) before lowering the upper body and arms as one unit. Continue maintaining abdominal engagement and slight tension in the straps. Return to the start position.

Coordination

Muscle Focus

- Abdominals
- Shoulder extensors
- Hip flexors

Objectives

- To improve abdominal strength
- To improve hip flexor and shoulder extensor control
- To develop lumbopelvic stabilization
- To develop coordination

RESISTANCE

Light Medium Heavy

The name of this exercise hints at its complexity, particularly the coordination of breath with the movement, which is especially challenging. Although coordinating four distinct breaths with four movements might seem to be simpler and make more intuitive sense, I prefer to use two breaths for the four movements. Doing so creates better flow and encourages deeper breathing, with more active use of the respiratory muscles. It also makes coordinating the movements more challenging.

Note the coordinated movement pattern of the shoulder extensors working in concert with the trunk flexors is similar to Reformer: Hundred Prep and Hundred. This powerful synergy forms the foundation of this exercise. The sequencing of the movements and muscle recruitment is of utmost importance.

Imagery

This exercise requires a rub-your-stomach-while-patting-your-head type of action. Picture a closed-loop mechanical toy that repeatedly goes through an identical sequence of movements. However, making your actions too mechanical will sacrifice the dynamic of the exercise and flow of the movement. The motion should be smooth, with the opening and closing of the legs a little sharper in dynamic than the lifting and lowering of the body as the legs straighten and bend.

- Keep the feet opposite the eyes when the legs are straight.
- Imprint the lower back into the mat when the trunk is lifted into flexion.
- Draw the knees in toward the chest before lifting the arms and then lowering the trunk and head.

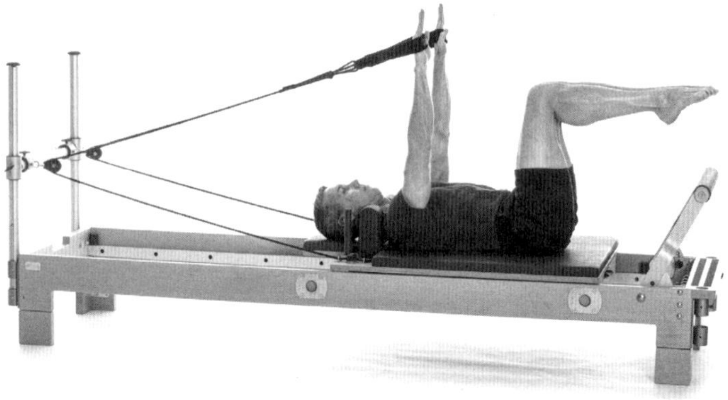

Setup. Lie supine in a neutral spine position with the legs in a tabletop position. Place the hands in the straps with the arms perpendicular to the body, maintaining slight tension in the straps.

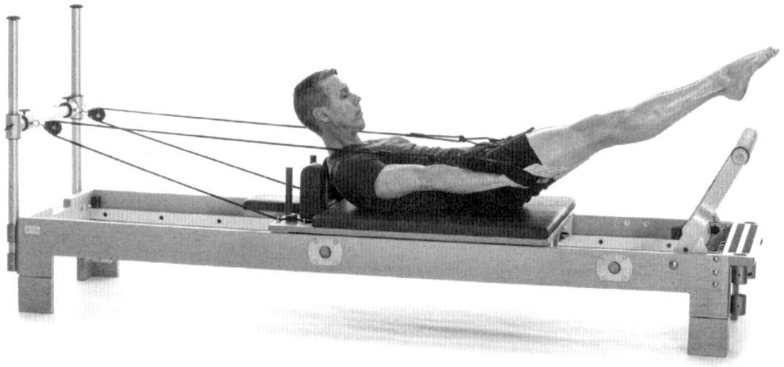

Exhale. Lift the head and chest while pressing the arms down to the sides of the body, straightening the legs and keeping the feet at eye level.

VARIATION

The trunk is lowered after each repetition (isotonic contraction). If coupled with the Reformer: Hundred (the trunk remains lifted and stable throughout), it provides a good balance. However, Reformer: Coordination can also be performed as an isometric exercise (the same trunk position as the Reformer: Hundred) by drawing the legs in and lifting the arms between each repetition, but not lowering the trunk. Each version has benefits. However, whichever version you choose, the head must move together with the trunk—go all the way down and all the way up between each repetition (isotonic) or stay raised up with the trunk (isometric). It should never go halfway up and down (an area I call the *danger zone*) because this position will inevitably result in excessive tension and discomfort in the neck.

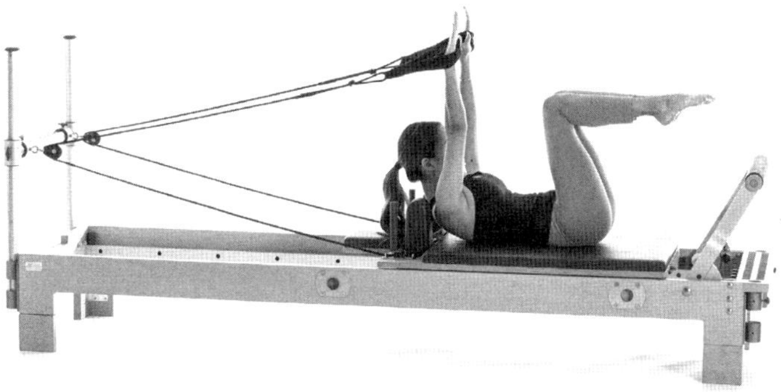

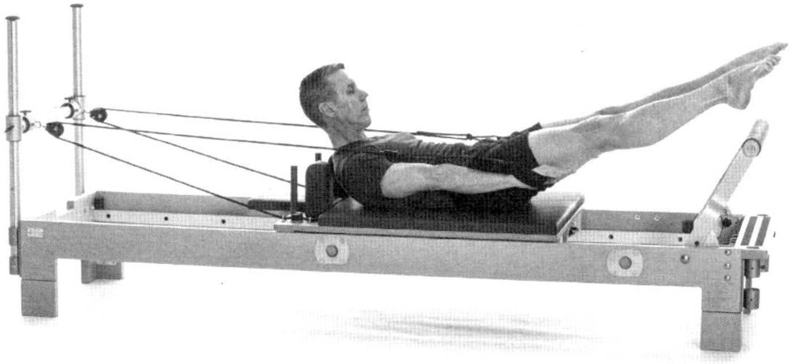

Continuing to exhale, open and close the legs (no wider than the footbar) in a brisk motion.

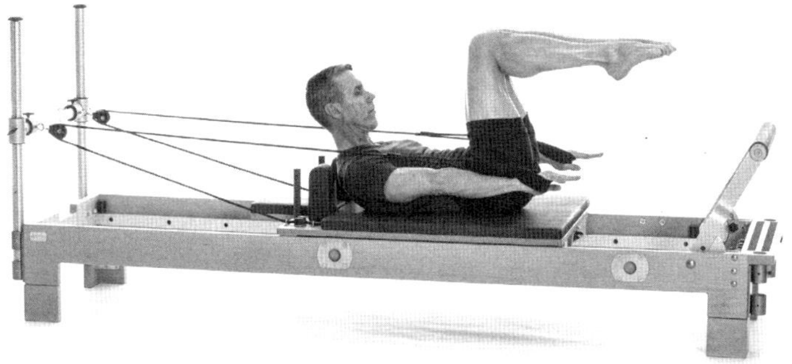

Inhale. Bend the legs beyond the tabletop position, drawing the knees toward the chest, and lift the arms to a 90-degree angle in the shoulder joint (approximately 10 degrees shy of perpendicular to the floor depending on the height of the trunk in flexion) before lowering the upper body and arms as one unit. Maintain abdominal engagement and slight tension in the straps. Return to the start position. Repeat 5-10 times.

REFORMER
Abdominal Work
FUNDAMENTAL

Muscle Focus

- Abdominals
- Hip flexors
- Back extensors

Objectives

- To improve abdominal strength
- To improve back extensor and hip flexor control
- To develop trunk stabilization

RESISTANCE
Light — Medium — Heavy

Short Box—Round Back

The Reformer: Short Box—Round Back exercise introduces the short box series, a progression of six exercises in which the Pilates box is placed on the reformer sideways to the carriage. Although the entire series focuses on the muscles of the trunk, particularly the abdominals, each exercise uses the muscles of the trunk in a slightly different way. Certain exercises in the series fit comfortably into more than one block. Due to this overlap, they can be used in different blocks depending on the structure of the session. For instance, the Reformer: Short Box—Tilt, Short Box—Twist, and Short Box—Round-About (not included in this book) exercises, although they work the abdominals, appear in the lateral flexion and rotation block due to their emphasis on the abdominal obliques.

The round back comprises two distinct positions: the initial upright position and the round back C curve position. To create the C curve, engage the abdominals, focusing the flexion of the spine in the lumbar region. Allow the thoracic spine and the pelvis to respond to the action in the lower back while keeping the shoulders above the hips. The back extensors contract eccentrically, working in concert with the abdominals to create the elongated C curve (think uppercase C). Once you have established the shape (and only then), take the trunk back, pivoting at the hip joint, ideally to the point where the lower back rests on the box. Then lift the trunk again, maintaining the C curve and returning to the position in which the shoulders are above the hips. At this point, extend the trunk into the upright start position. Imprinting these two positions of the trunk, upright and round back, into the muscle memory is important, because they form the basis of many of the abdominal exercises in Pilates.

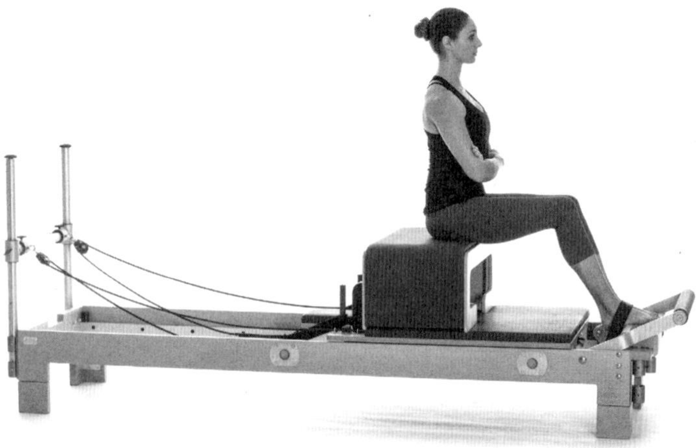

Setup. Place the footbar in the down position. Sit upright on the box close to the front. Place the feet under the foot strap, hip width apart. Cross the arms in front of the body. Bend the legs and anchor the feet so that the movement occurs in the hip joint, with only the pelvis and trunk changing position. Make sure all the springs are attached during the entire series to prevent the carriage from moving.

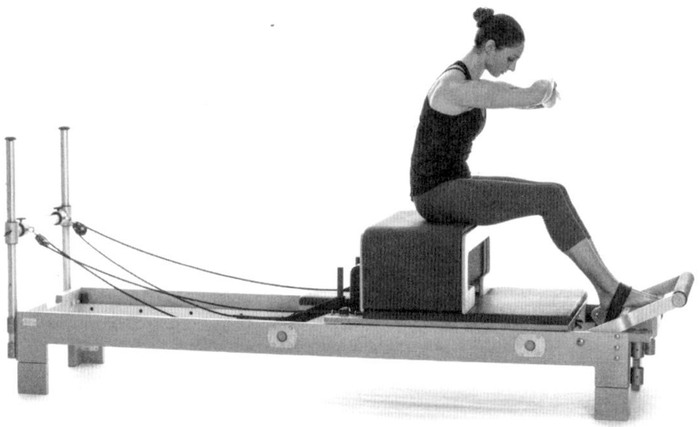

Exhale. Round the trunk into a C curve position, shoulders above the hip joints. Simultaneously lift the arms to shoulder height (parallel to the floor).

Continuing to exhale, lower the body backward with the trunk in the rounded position until the lower back rests on the box (or as close to it as possible), keeping the arms floating parallel to the floor.

Imagery

In the sitting position, the placement of the shoulders is above the hips. As the trunk is rounded, you should feel that the spine is being stretched from the back like a rubber band, creating the C curve. However, it is important to keep the shoulders above the hips. This alignment does not change as the spine is rounded. The spine continues being pulled back until the lumbar spine rests on the box, and then rises again so the shoulders are above the hips. Only at this point is the rubber band released, and the trunk returns to the upright position. Visualizing the opening of the vertebrae in the round position will make the spine feel longer and will help prevent it from collapsing. You should feel even more lifted and taller in the round back position than in the upright position. When tipping back in the round back position, the action resembles pouring tea from a teapot.

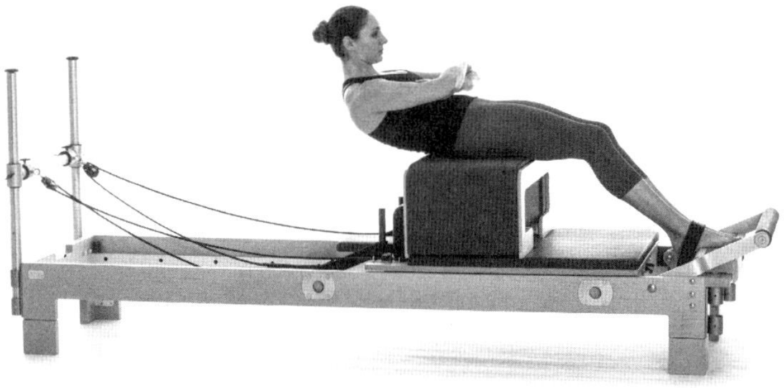

Inhale. Pause in this position.

Exhale. Raise the body, maintaining the C curve of the trunk, until the shoulders are above the hips. Move the arms with the trunk, parallel to the floor.

Inhale. Extend the trunk, sitting upright and lowering the arms. Return to the start position. Repeat 5 times.

- Establish the round back position prior to tipping back.
- Maintain the stable, round position of the trunk as it tips back and then lifts up again.
- Straighten into the upright position once the shoulders are above the hips to conclude the exercise.

PROGRESSION

After the trunk has been lowered to the box, maintain a stable trunk with no changes in the position. Lift the arms overhead (arms folded) and return them to the chest, keeping them folded. Maintaining the C curve, return to the sitting position. Complete the movement by sitting upright as in the original exercise. This is an excellent progression that challenges abdominal strength and trunk stabilization.

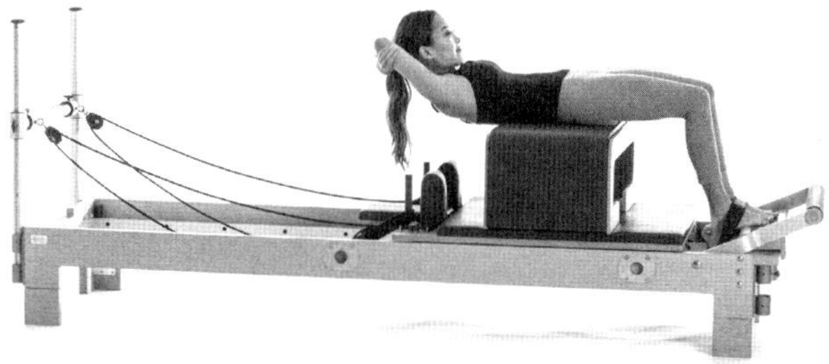

Short Box—Flat Back

Muscle Focus

- Abdominals
- Back extensors
- Hip flexors

Objectives

- To improve abdominal and hip flexor strength
- To improve back extensor control
- To develop trunk stabilization

RESISTANCE

Light Medium Heavy

This exercise has similarities to the Reformer: Short Box—Round Back in terms of the action of the abdominals and the hip joint being the pivot point of the movement. Both exercises work the abdominals, maintain a stable trunk as the body is lowered and lifted, and feature movement in the sagittal plane. In the Reformer: Short Box—Round Back, the abdominals do the bulk of the work to maintain the C curve position as the body is lowered and lifted and are supported by the back extensors only insofar as creating and maintaining the C curve shape. However, in the Reformer: Short Box—Flat Back, the abdominals and the back extensors co-contract to hold the trunk in a neutral spine position (not actually a flat back, as the name implies) as it is lowered and lifted. The hip flexors play an important role in both exercises, contracting eccentrically as the body is lowered and concentrically as it returns to the upright position, but they bear a greater load in this exercise because of the longer lever arm.

The back-and-forth movement of the trunk is relatively contained and should not exceed 45 degrees when hinging back. Beyond this angle, there is a high risk of hyperextending the back; to avoid this, the pelvis and the trunk must move as one unit, hinging at the hip joint. If the pelvis stops and the upper body continues to tilt back, the result is hyperlordosis and excessive pressure on the lower back.

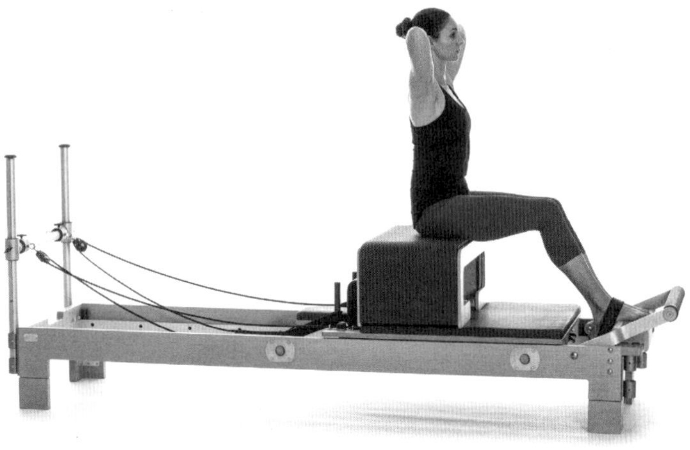

Setup. Place the footbar in the down position. Sit upright on the box close to the front. Place the feet under the foot strap, hip width apart, hands behind the head. Keep the legs bent and stable. Every effort should be made to keep the lower body uninvolved in the exercise.

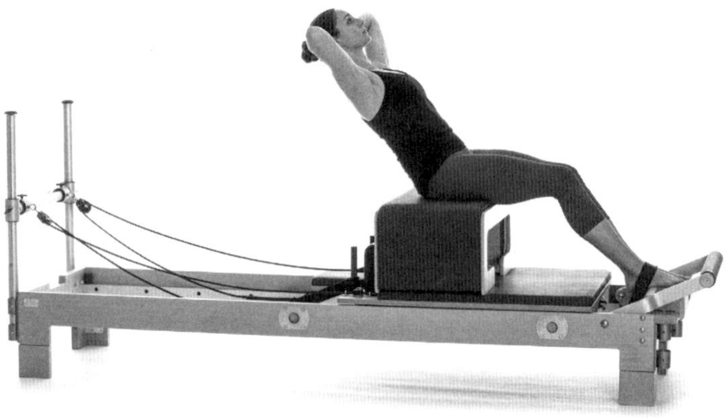

Inhale. Hinge back, moving the trunk and pelvis as one unit.

Imagery

The image of a closed door lying on its side, opening slightly on its hinge and then closing again, helps achieve the correct movement and form.

- Co-contract the abdominals and back extensors.
- Move the pelvis and trunk as one unit, hinging at the hip joint.
- Keep the head aligned with the spine.

PROGRESSION

The Reformer: Short Box—Flat Back can be performed with the arms overhead holding a pole. This lengthens the lever arm greatly and, as a result, increases the challenge exponentially.

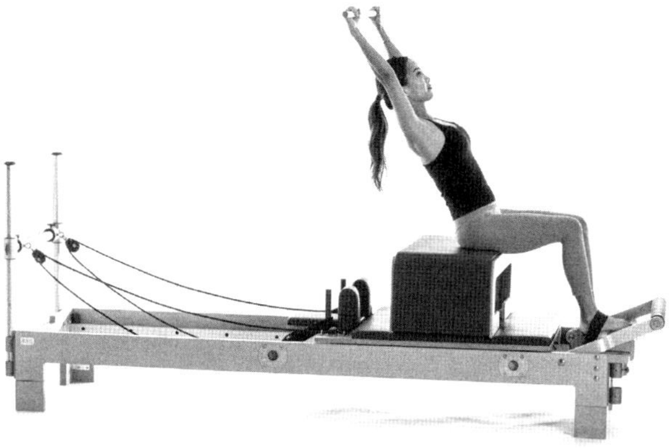

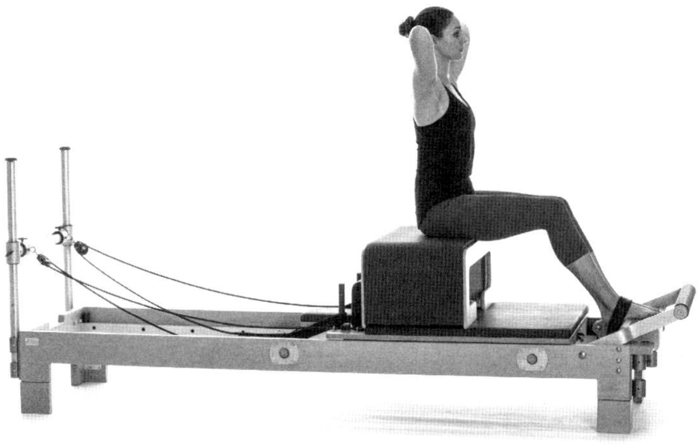

Exhale. Lift the trunk. Return to the start position. Repeat 5 times.

Long Box—Climb-a-Tree

Muscle Focus

- Abdominals
- Back extensors
- Hip flexors

Objectives

- To improve abdominal strength
- To improve hip flexor and back extensor control
- To improve hamstring and thoracic flexibility

RESISTANCE

Light — Medium — Heavy

Although this exercise in its classic form is performed on the short box and is regarded as part of the short box series, I recommend learning it on the long box (box longways on the carriage). The long box offers far more support for the lower back and facilitates a better stretch for the thoracic region. This makes it accessible to many more people and increases the potential benefits without the potential danger of excessive pressure on the lower back. When performing this movement on the short box, the hinge point (the point of movement between the spine and the box) is centered on the lumbar spine, potentially creating a shearing force on the vertebrae of the lower back. Therefore, I recommend mastering this exercise on the long box before attempting it on the short box.

I encourage you to maximize the stretch of the hamstrings in the sitting position when the leg is straight by keeping the back extensors engaged and the trunk as upright as possible. It is important to maintain abdominal contraction throughout the exercise, particularly during the arm circling phase, to avoid excessive pressure on the lower back. Strive for deep flexion of the trunk as you climb down and then up the "tree" (leg), highlighting abdominal activation. It is important for the upright leg to be perpendicular to the box during the climbing phases. When the leg is not high enough there will potentially be excessive load on the lower back and the probability of hyperlordosis. This typically occurs when the hamstrings are tight, possibly coupled with weak hip flexors and lack of abdominal support. Conversely, when the leg is taken beyond perpendicular, there is a tendency to hang on the leg. This scenario occurs when the hamstrings are extremely flexible.

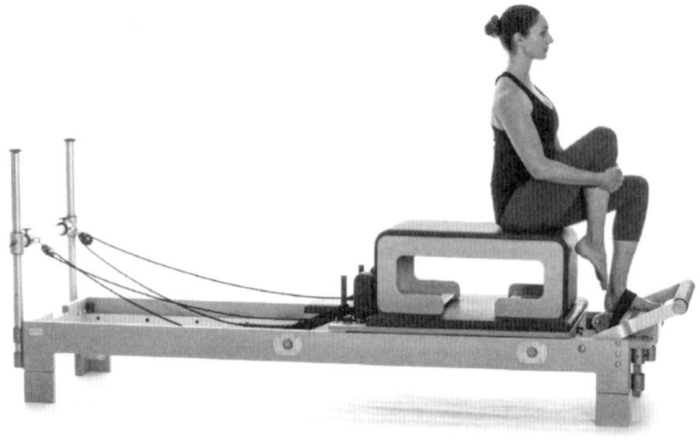

Setup. Place the footbar in the down position. Sit upright on the box (long box) close to the front. Place the feet under the foot strap, hip width apart. Remove one foot from the foot strap, bend the leg, hold below the knee, and draw the thigh to the chest.

Exhale. Pull the thigh to the chest and do 3 pulses, elongating the back and sitting more upright with each pulse.

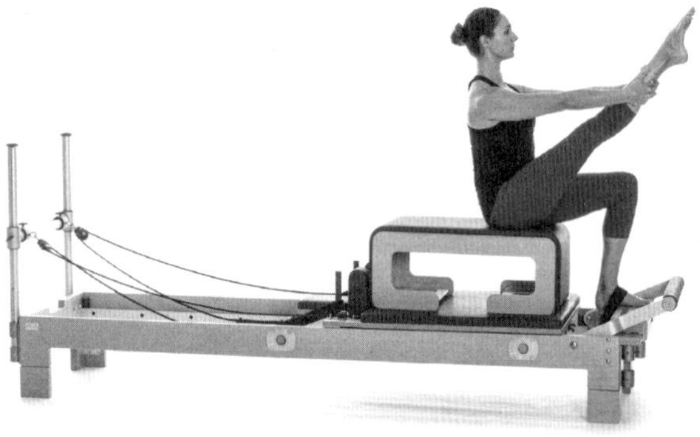

Inhale. Hold the ankle and straighten the leg while keeping the back as straight as possible.

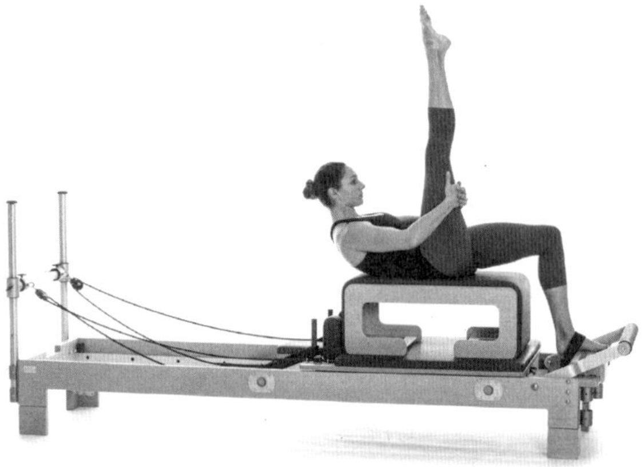

Exhale. Walk the hands down the leg (3 hand changes), lowering the trunk to the box in flexion. The upright leg moves to a perpendicular position to the box and remains stable.

Imagery

Imagine climbing down and then up a tree, keeping the body as close to the trunk of the tree as possible by maximizing spinal flexion. The tree (leg) must be firm and stable in an upright position, reaching toward the ceiling.

- Begin the movement by sitting upright with the back extensors engaged.
- Emphasize trunk flexion when "climbing" down and up the leg.
- Keep the abdominals engaged, particularly during the arm circling phase to avoid the ribs thrusting forward.

MODIFICATION

The first part of the exercise remains exactly the same as described. After lowering the trunk to the box, rather than arching the back over the box and circling the arms around during the inhale, hold the trunk stable with the lower back imprinted into the box and reach the arms forward, parallel to the floor. Place the hands back behind the leg before continuing to walk up the leg, and complete the exercise exactly as described.

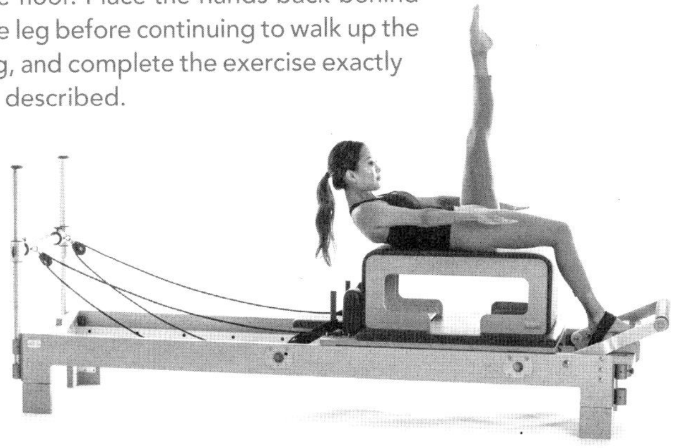

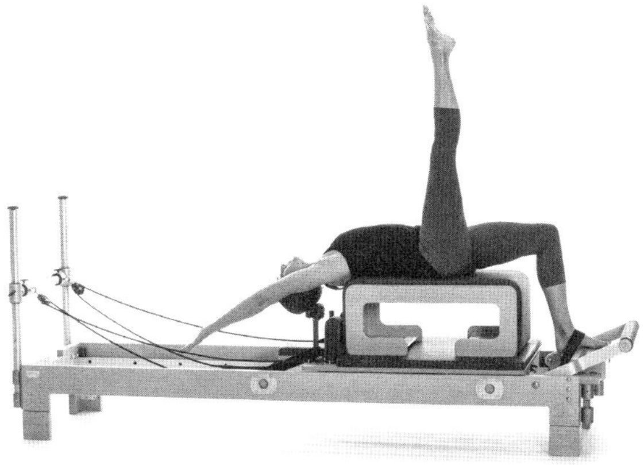

Inhale. Arch the mid- and upper back over the box while reaching the arms overhead, then circle them around to the sides of the body.

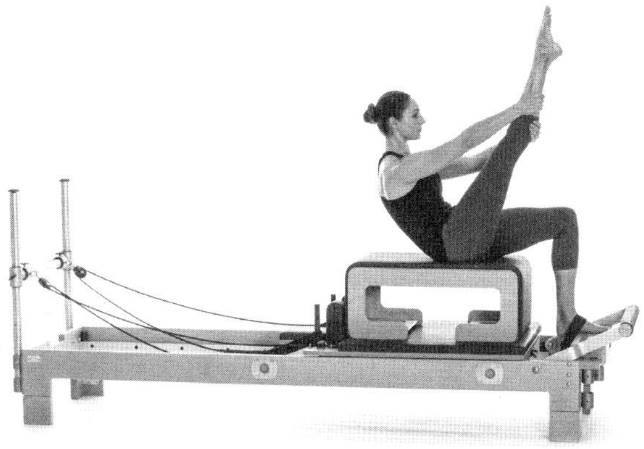

Exhale. Return to trunk flexion and place the hands on the back of the leg. Climb up the leg (3 hand changes), maintaining flexion of the trunk.

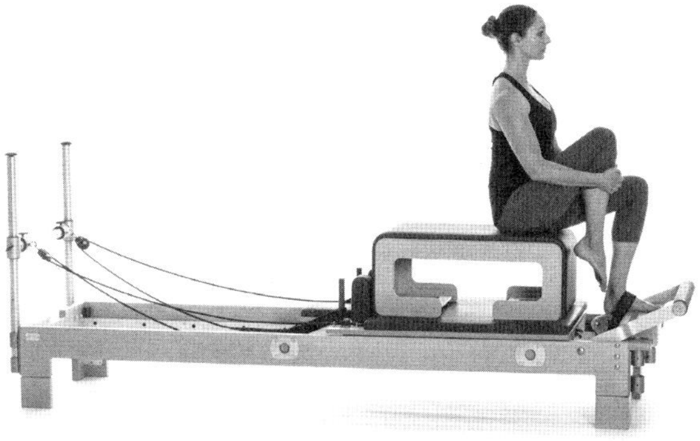

Inhale. Extend the spine while keeping the leg straight. Continuing to inhale, bend the leg, and sit upright. Return to the start position. Repeat 3-5 times before switching to the other side.

Backstroke

Muscle Focus

- Abdominals

Objectives

- To improve abdominal strength
- To develop lumbopelvic stabilization
- To develop shoulder and hip joint mobility

RESISTANCE

Light — Medium — Heavy

The Reformer: Backstroke is a complex, high-level exercise that demands coordination and strength. The position on the box and the resistance from the straps result in an enormous demand on the abdominals. Lack of abdominal strength will potentially lead to stress on the lower back and compromised head alignment resulting in neck strain. Keeping the trunk stable and the head in an optimum position as the arms and legs move independently is the key to the success of this exercise. It is helpful to introduce this exercise on the mat or on the box without the straps, adding resistance only once good coordination, muscle recruitment, and strength have been achieved. The eyes must focus forward throughout the exercise and must not follow the arms as they straighten toward the ceiling and then circle around, which is a very common mistake.

Imagery

Imagine the trunk is a rowing boat, sturdy and stable. Think of the legs and arms as oars moving in a circular motion independently of the trunk. The pause following the circling motion, with the arms pressing against the legs, places the body in a streamlined position. This is the point you should feel as if you are a boat gliding through the water after a powerful stroke of the oars.

- ○ Keep the eyes focused directly forward.
- ○ Maintain maximum trunk flexion, keeping the head aligned with the spine.
- ○ Synchronize the movement of the arms and legs.

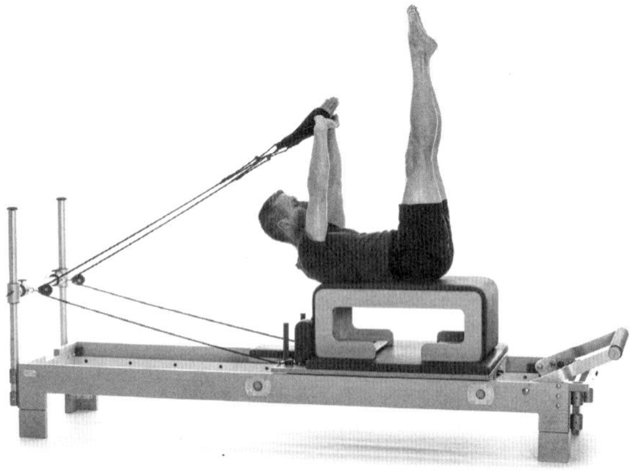

Setup. Lie supine on the long box, facing the footbar, with the base of the scapulae placed at the back edge of the box. Lift the trunk into maximal spinal flexion and the legs into a tabletop position. Hold the straps with the hands in a fist or open-hand position, palms facing up and elbows pointing outward. Hold the hands directly above the sternum. Keep the eyes focused forward.

Inhale. Straighten the arms and legs directly up toward the ceiling (perpendicular to the box).

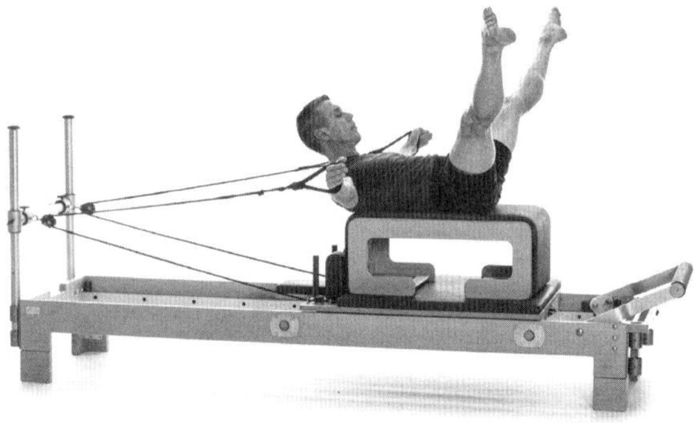

Continuing to inhale, take the arms and legs out to the sides.

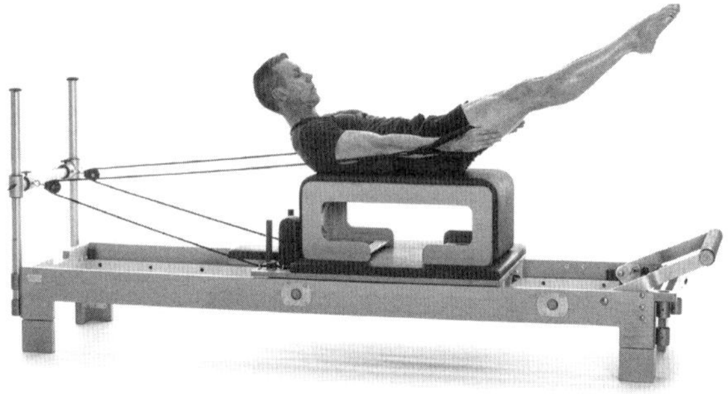

Exhale. Bring the legs together and the arms to the sides of the body. Pause momentarily in this position before rotating the legs back to parallel and bending the arms and legs simultaneously. Return to the start position. Repeat 5 times.

Abdominals With Legs in Straps

An understanding of the concepts of trunk stabilization and hip disassociation are prerequisites to proper execution of this exercise. If you have not already learned the Reformer: Scooter and Knee Stretch—Round Back exercises described later in this chapter, I highly recommend that you do so. You can apply these learned movement patterns to this exercise, which is essentially the Reformer: Knee Stretch—Round Back in a supine position.

Because of the significant load on the hip flexors, this exercise can potentially create hazardous stresses on the spine, particularly if the lumbopelvic stabilization (provided largely by the abdominals) is insufficient. This makes the exercise very challenging. Developing a good strength ratio between the hip flexors and the abdominals is critical. Problems arise when the hip flexors overpower the abdominals, likely resulting in excessive load on the lower back.

A distinction must be made between the rectus femoris, a two-joint hip flexor, and the psoas and iliopsoas, which are single-joint hip flexors. The objective should be to focus on the latter, which are often overshadowed by the former. To encourage use of the psoas and iliopsoas, the feeling should be that the movement is emanating from deep in the pelvic bowl, rather than from the legs. It sometimes helps to imagine the legs being almost weightless and the abdominals pulling the legs in (in reality, the abdominals only stabilize and it is the hip flexors creating the movement).

Imagery

Combine two images: the abdominals creating a hollow bowl, anchored into the carriage, and the legs moving like pistons pumping in and out (with the emphasis on the "in" phase toward the body). The feet remain at eye level, moving along a horizontal plane.

- ○ Draw the knees in toward the forehead.
- ○ Move the feet along a horizontal plane, avoiding dropping them down or bending the knees excessively.
- ○ Maintain lumbopelvic stabilization, imprinting the lower back into the carriage.

Muscle Focus

- Abdominals
- Hip flexors

Objectives

- To improve abdominal and hip flexor strength
- To develop lumbopelvic stabilization

RESISTANCE

Light | Medium | Heavy

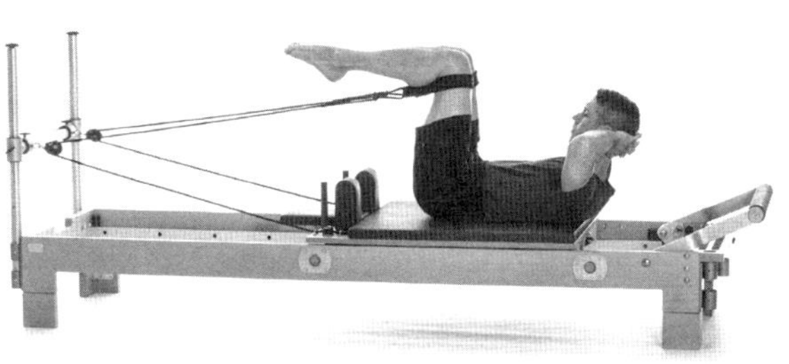

Setup. Place the footbar in the down position. Lie supine in the Mat: Chest Lift position, with the back of the head toward the footbar. To determine how far from the shoulder rests the pelvis should be, reach straight arms toward the shoulder rests and touch them with the fingertips. Thread the legs through the straps, placing them just above the knees, and bring the legs into a tabletop position. Hold the trunk in forward flexion and place the hands behind the head.

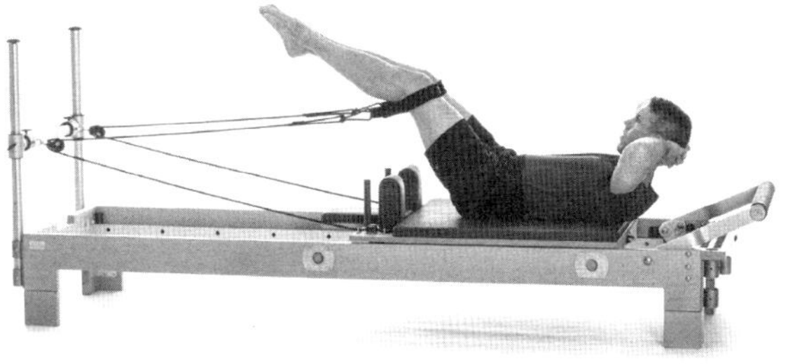

Inhale. Straighten the legs most of the way, keeping some tension in the straps, maintaining lumbopelvic stabilization, and gliding the feet along a horizontal line.

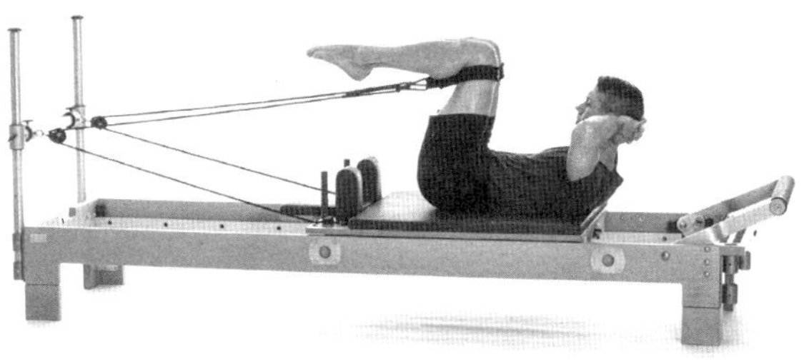

Exhale. Draw the thighs toward the chest, going beyond the tabletop position (approximately a 100-degree angle in the hip joint). Repeat 5-10 times.

Muscle Focus

- Abdominal obliques
- Hip flexors

Objectives

- To improve abdominal oblique and hip flexor strength
- To develop lumbopelvic stabilization

RESISTANCE

Light Medium Heavy

Abdominals With Legs in Straps With Rotation

This exercise is very similar to the Reformer: Abdominals With Legs in Straps, but incorporates trunk rotation. The element of rotation increases the challenge of maintaining pelvic stabilization and works the abdominal obliques more intensely. The upper body should move as one unit, with the elbows absolutely stable and pointing outward. Although the rotation of the vertebrae occurs largely in the thoracic spine, the sense should be that the upper body moves as a unit while the lower body is stable, with the movement occurring in the area of the waist. Think of the body as a series of discs; the lower disc (the pelvis) is stable while the upper disc (the trunk) rotates around the center. Mastery of the Mat: Chest Lift With Rotation and Criss-Cross are recommended prerequisites for this exercise.

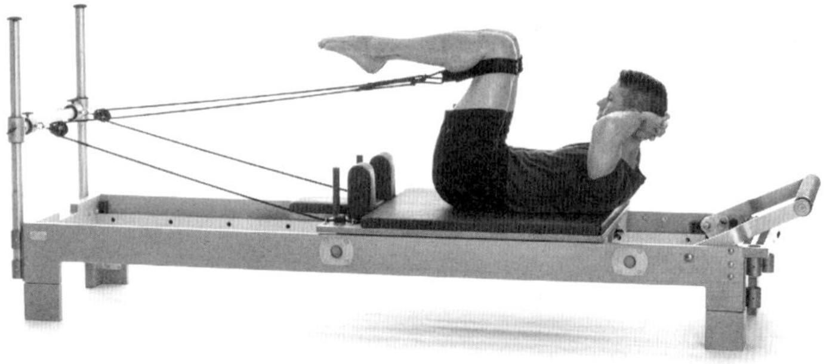

Setup. Place the footbar in the down position. Lie supine in the Mat: Chest Lift position, with the back of the head toward the footbar. To determine how far from the shoulder rests the pelvis should be, reach straight arms toward the shoulder rests and touch them with the fingertips. Thread the legs through the straps, placing them just above the knees, and bring the legs into a tabletop position. Hold the trunk in forward flexion and place the hands behind the head.

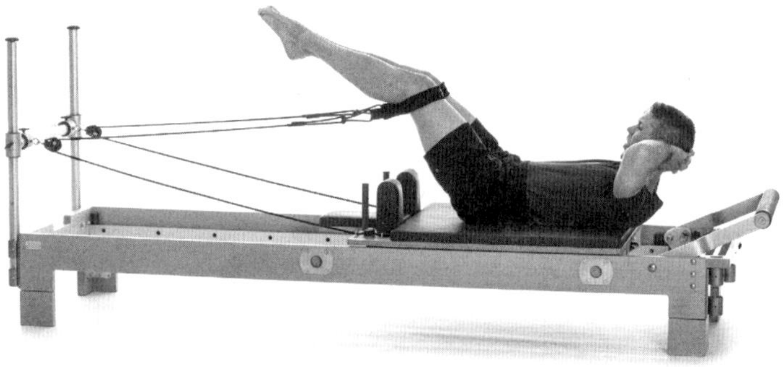

Inhale. Straighten the legs most of the way, keeping some tension in the straps, maintaining lumbopelvic stabilization, and gliding the feet along a horizontal line.

Imagery

As with the Reformer: Abdominals With Legs in Straps, think of the abdominal region as a hollow bowl and the legs as moving pistons of an engine. Emphasize the inward movement of the legs toward the body.

- Rotate the trunk, as opposed to swiveling it (lateral flexion).
- Maintain maximum flexion of the trunk as it rotates from side to side.
- Keep the lower scapula off the carriage during the rotation.
- Keep the elbows wide and stable and the shoulders relaxed.
- Maintain lumbopelvic stabilization.

MODIFICATION

There is a strong tendency in this exercise to over-rotate, resulting in more lateral flexion than rotation (swiveling). The lower back then starts to lift off the carriage and the back muscles become overactive while the abdominals are underactive. I encourage using the arms to assist in achieving an optimum position. Place the hands behind the thighs. As you draw the legs in and rotate the trunk, bend the arms and pull the trunk toward the knees. Note that the hands are aligned with the shoulders, therefore one hand will be higher than the other during the rotation. As the legs straighten and the trunk returns to the center, keep the hands behind the thighs (even if the legs do not straighten as much) and use the assistance of the arms to keep the trunk at a consistent height. Alternate sides.

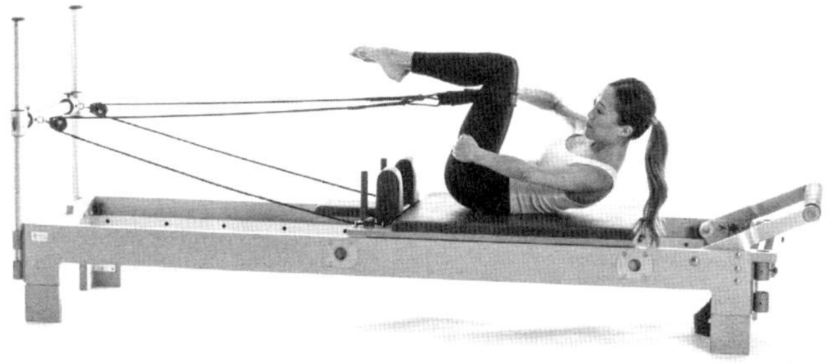

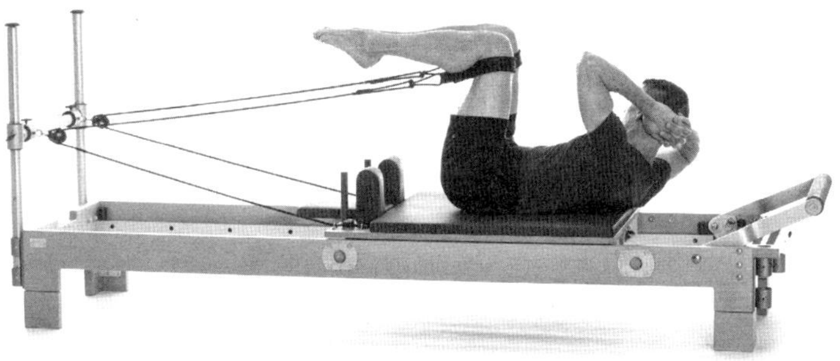

Exhale. Draw the thighs toward the chest, going beyond tabletop position (approximately a 100-degree angle in the hip joint), and simultaneously rotate the trunk to one side, bringing the upper shoulder toward the knees.

Inhale. Straighten the legs, gliding the feet along a horizontal line as the trunk returns to center, preparing to rotate to the opposite side.

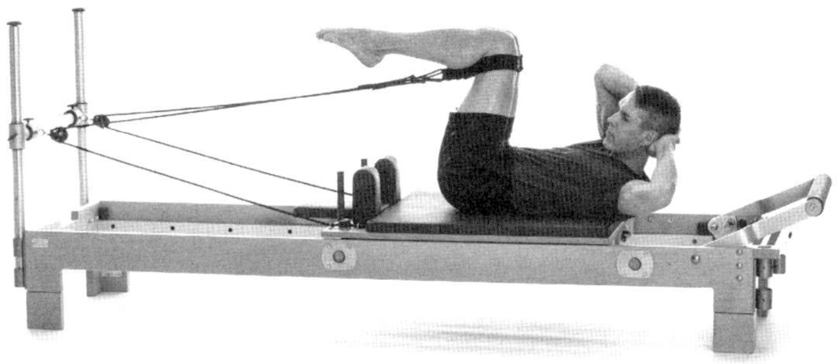

Exhale. Draw the thighs toward the chest and simultaneously rotate the trunk to the other side, bringing the upper shoulder toward the knees. Continue alternating sides, straightening the legs and bringing the upper body to center prior to each rotation. Repeat 5-10 times.

Hip Work

The hip joint deserves special consideration and has earned a block unto itself. Its close proximity to—and profound influence on—the pelvis affects the whole body, up and down the kinetic chain. The hips play a key role in the gait cycle and many other daily activities, from climbing stairs to sitting down and rising up from a chair. Many muscle groups act on the hip joint, and they are prone to imbalance. For instance, the gluteus medius, so vital in hip support and pelvic alignment, tends to be weak in relation to the other gluteal muscles. The hip flexors often become tight while the hip extensors become relatively weak, due in part to a modern lifestyle that has many of us spending hours a day sitting. Imbalances of the musculature in this region are further compounded by activities with highly repetitive motions, such as cycling and running, as well as dance (particularly classical ballet), in which the hip joint is in external rotation (turnout) much of the time.

A concept that is emphasized in the hip work block is *hip disassociation*—the performance of a smooth, uninterrupted movement of the hip joint while the adjacent pelvis is kept absolutely stable. Mastering the concept of disassociation is important, not only in relation to the hip joint but also to other parts of the body, such as the shoulder joint.

The hip joint can be viewed as a big spoon in a pot. The circular action used when stirring a pot is similar to the smooth movement desired when mobilizing the hip joint. The balance of the musculature is critical, and a good choice of imagery can assist in mastering the often-intricate process of moving and stabilizing different muscle groups.

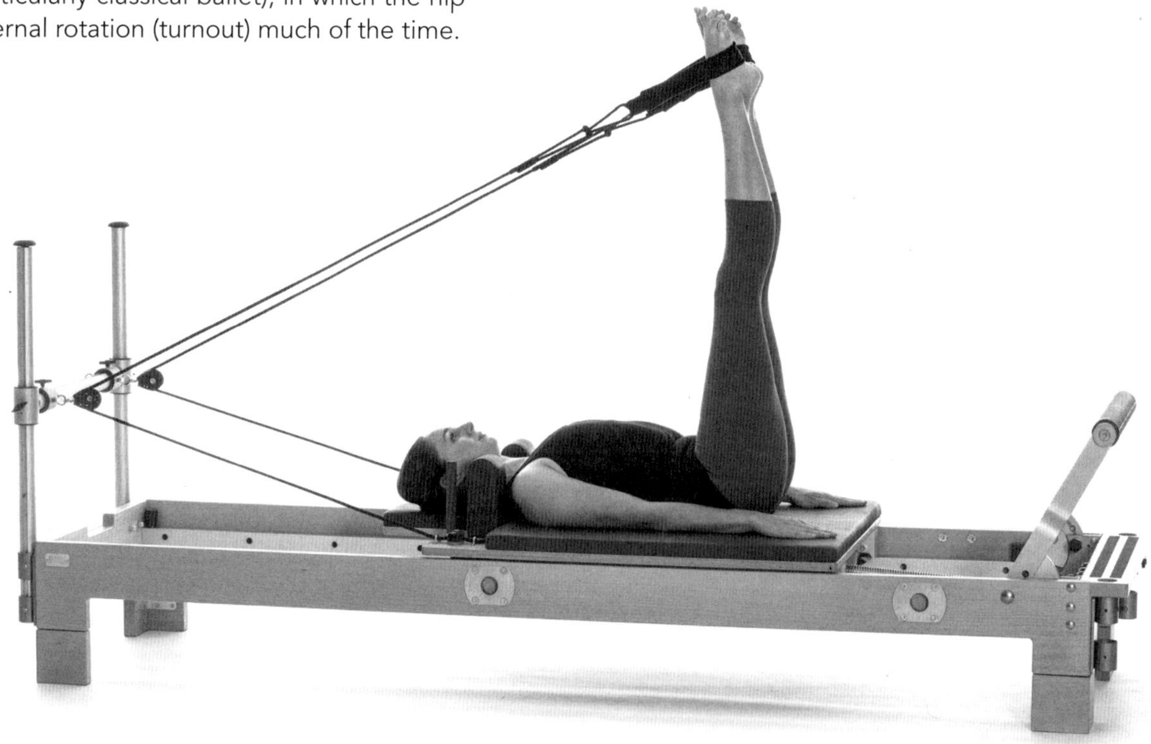

Frog

REFORMER
Hip Work
FUNDAMENTAL

This exercise resembles the Reformer: V Position Toes. Stability and alignment of the trunk and pelvis are the same, as is the basic action of the legs. However, here the focus is on the hip adductors in addition to the knee extensors and hip extensors. As with all the exercises in the hip work block, the Reformer: Frog demands a high degree of pelvic stabilization because the feet are in the straps instead of on the stable footbar. Note that the resistance is light, orienting the work toward stabilization as opposed to strength. The lighter resistance also facilitates the weaker muscle groups of the hip joint, such as the hip adductors and hip extensors, doing more of the work. When the resistance is higher, the larger and stronger quadriceps tend to be dominant and the lumbopelvic stabilizers are not required to work quite as hard.

Imagery

The image of a frog jumping works well, although the dynamic of the exercise is relatively slow. Focus on squeezing the legs together as you straighten the knees, as if you were holding a big balloon between the legs. This squeezing encourages activation of the hip adductors and prevents overactivation of the knee extensors.

- Maintain lumbopelvic stabilization.
- Bend the knees only to 90 degrees to avoid posterior pelvic tilt and the tailbone lifting.
- Squeeze the heels together continuously (even at the expense of straightening the legs completely).
- Travel along a horizontal line with the heels.

Muscle Focus

- Hip adductors
- Hamstrings
- Quadriceps

Objectives

- To improve hip adductor, hip extensor, and knee extensor control
- To develop lumbopelvic stabilization

RESISTANCE
Light Medium Heavy

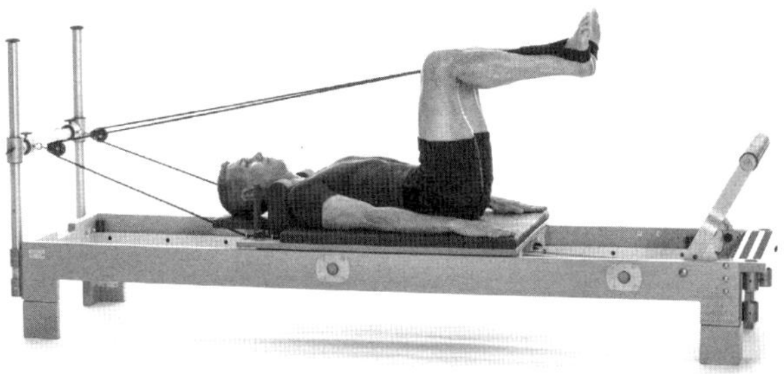

Setup. Lie supine in a neutral spine position. Place the feet in the straps and bend the knees to a 90-degree angle, with the hips externally rotated. Dorsiflex the feet and press the heels together.

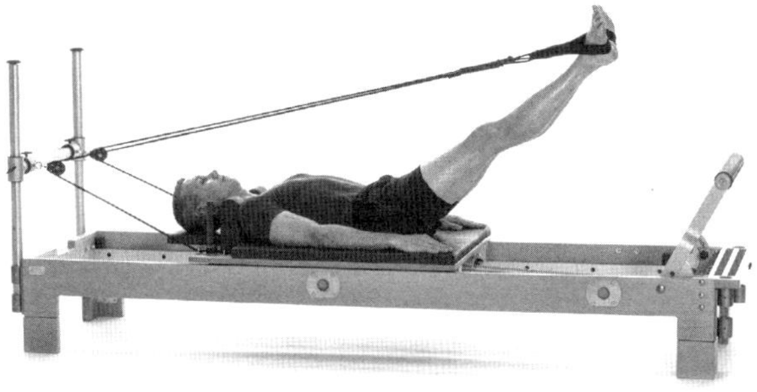

Exhale. Straighten the legs with the heels traveling along a horizontal line, parallel to the floor. Finish with the legs in a diagonal line, approximately 45 degrees to the carriage.

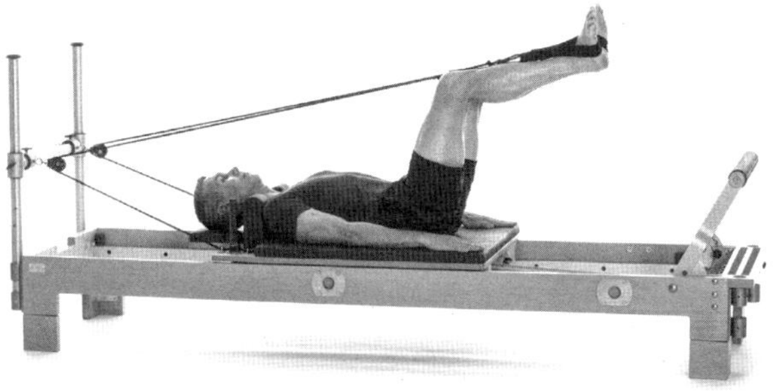

Inhale. Bend the knees. Return to the start position. Repeat 10 times.

Hip Circle Down

Muscle Focus

- Hip adductors
- Hamstrings

Objectives

- To improve hip adductor and hip extensor control
- To develop hip joint mobility
- To develop lumbopelvic stabilization

RESISTANCE

Light — Medium — Heavy

The Reformer: Hip Circle Down highlights the concept of hip disassociation and demands a great deal of skill. It also activates the hip adductors prominently, emphasizing control and precision. A micro-bend (slight bend) in the knees can be beneficial in order to de-emphasize the quadriceps and emphasize the hip adductors and hamstrings. The hamstrings tend to overpower the hip adductors at certain points in the exercise, both because of the nature of the movement and also because most people are more familiar with using them and they are generally better conditioned. Keeping the pelvis stable and in a neutral position encourages correct muscle activation, with a good balance between the hip adductors and the hamstrings. I recommend using a light weight (1-1.5 springs), which will amplify lumbopelvic stabilization and hip disassociation. However, after good control has been achieved, resistance can be increased to shift the focus from muscular control to muscular strength. In addition, range of motion can be increased, which will typically make the exercise more challenging. That said, people who are very flexible will benefit from restricting the range of motion. This same concept can be applied to the Reformer: Hip Circle Up and Opening.

Imagery

Imagine drawing the desired circular shape (two back-to-back semi-circles as opposed to two true circles) in space with the feet. The legs squeeze together as they draw a line down the center and then part as they trace the semi-circles, meeting again at the top. The size of the circle can be increased as more control is achieved. The movement should be fluid, and the lines of the drawing should be smooth and continuous.

- ○ Maximize the hip adductor work.
- ○ Keep the pace of the exercise consistent and the movement smooth and unrestricted.
- ○ Maintain lumbopelvic stabilization.

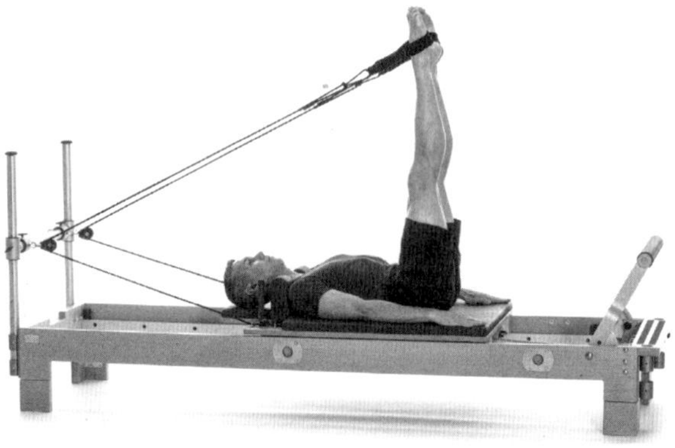

Setup. Lie supine in a neutral spine position. Place the feet in the straps and straighten the legs toward the ceiling in a perpendicular position (or as close as possible) without tilting the pelvis. Externally rotate the hips and plantarflex the feet.

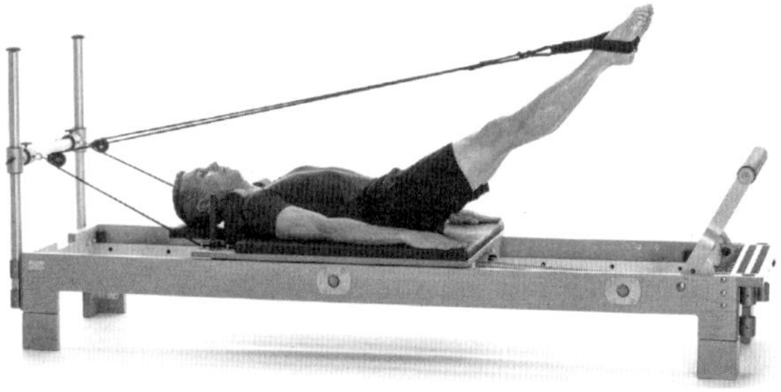

Exhale. Lower the legs straight down the center.

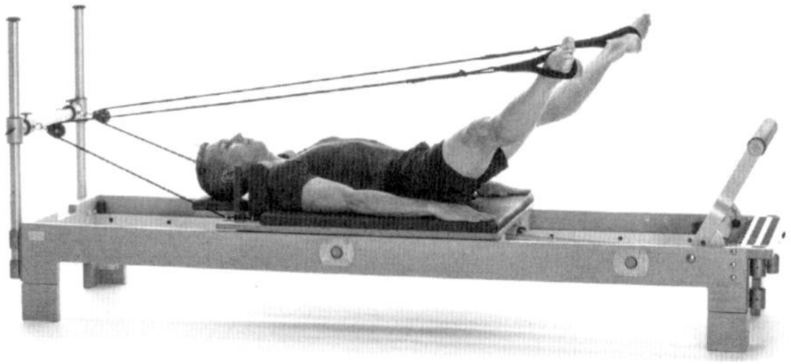

Inhale. Open the legs and circle them around and up to the perpendicular position. Return to the start position. Repeat 10 times.

Hip Circle Up

REFORMER
Hip Work
FUNDAMENTAL

Muscle Focus
- Hip adductors
- Hamstrings

Objectives
- To improve hip adductor and hip extensor control
- To develop lumbopelvic stabilization

RESISTANCE
Light Medium Heavy

It is often easier to feel the adductors working in the Reformer: Hip Circle Up than in the Reformer: Hip Circle Down. The load on the adductors is clearly felt as the legs are brought together following the circle during the concentric phase of the exercise. In the Reformer: Hip Circle Down, the adductors work eccentrically during this phase, resisting the pull of the springs as they open. In both versions, the adductors should work isometrically as the legs press against each other when moving up and down the centerline.

Imagery

Imagine drawing the desired circular shape (two back-to-back semi-circles as opposed to two true circles) with the feet. In addition, the feeling of the hip being a big spoon stirring thick syrup or porridge, the spoon being the femur and head of the femur, may be helpful. This encourages a smooth, fluid motion, free of tension, which often restricts the movement of the hip. Note that if the movement of the hip joint is restricted, the pelvis will tend to move around to compensate for the restriction. Increase resistance and range of motion for potential strength gains.

- ○ Maximize the hip adductor work.
- ○ Keep the pace of the exercise consistent and the movement smooth and unrestricted.
- ○ Maintain lumbopelvic stabilization.

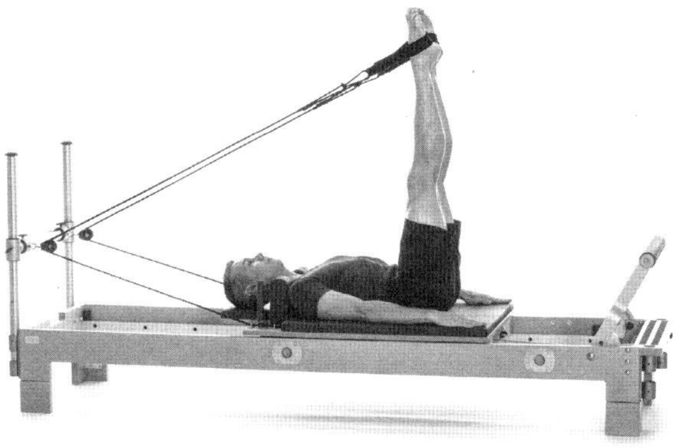

Setup. Lie supine in a neutral spine position. Place the feet in the straps and straighten the legs toward the ceiling in a perpendicular position (or as close as possible) without tilting the pelvis. Externally rotate the hips and plantarflex the feet.

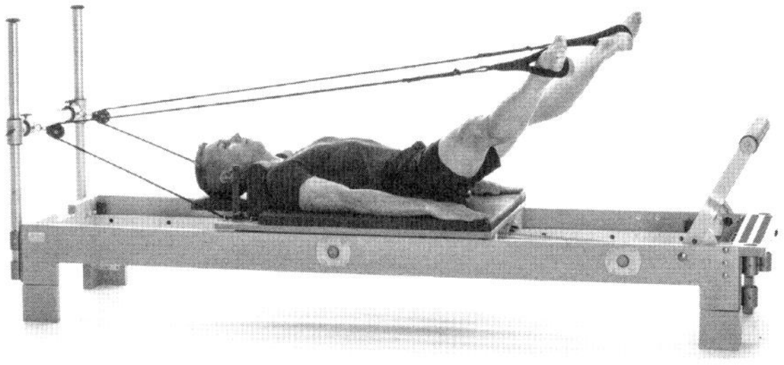

Exhale. Circle the legs out to the sides, around, and together to connect with each other at the bottom of the centerline.

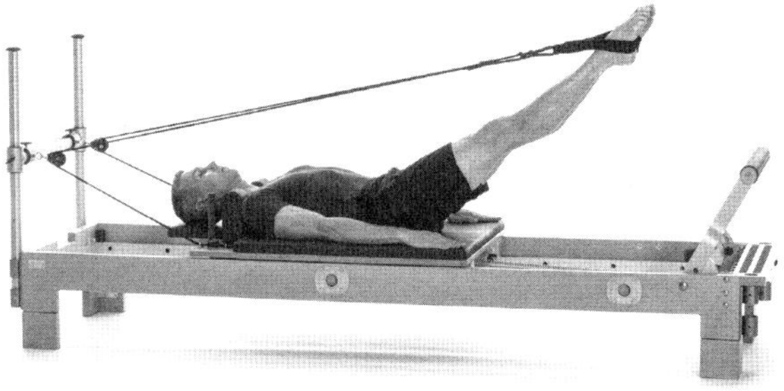

Inhale. Keeping the legs pressed together, lift them straight up the centerline to the perpendicular position (or as close as possible). Return to the start position. Repeat 10 times.

REFORMER

Hip Work

INTERMEDIATE

Muscle Focus

- Hip adductors

Objectives

- To improve hip adductor strength and flexibility
- To develop lumbopelvic stabilization

RESISTANCE

Light Medium Heavy

Opening

This exercise is a particularly valuable part of the hip work supine series because it places the body in an optimal position to explore the hip joint's functional range of motion—the maximum range of motion that can be achieved while maintaining the integrity of pelvic and spinal stability and alignment. This exercise has the potential to develop control and strength in these extreme ranges, which is particularly important for activities like dance, figure skating, and gymnastics. Athletes involved in these endeavors typically have exceptional flexibility, but they sometimes lack the muscular strength to support their expansive ranges of motion, which can result in injury. It is important that the feet travel along a horizontal path, drawing a semi-circle parallel to the floor, and do not drop as the legs are opened. Once good control has been achieved, resistance and range of motion can be progressively increased to add load to the musculature with the goal of gains in strength.

Imagery

Imagine squeezing the legs against a large balloon. Another image that works well to help keep the feet at a consistent height is to imagine lying underwater at the bottom of a swimming pool and opening and closing the legs while keeping the feet touching the surface of the water.

- ○ Keep the feet at a consistent distance from the floor.
- ○ Maximize hip adductor range of motion and activation.
- ○ Maintain lumbopelvic stabilization.

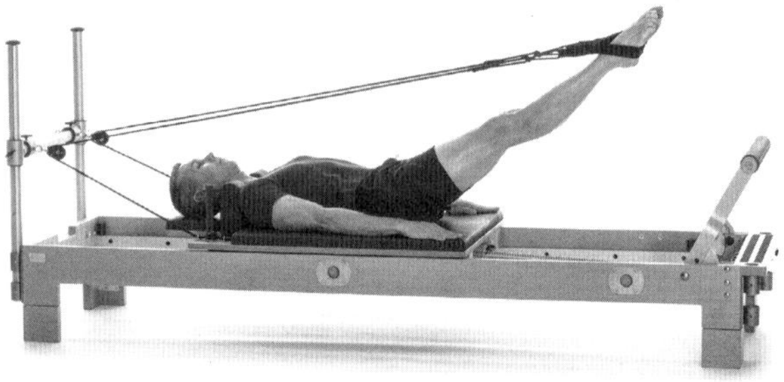

Setup. Lie supine in a neutral spine position. Place the feet in the straps and straighten the legs on a 45-degree angle without tilting the pelvis. Externally rotate the hips and plantarflex the feet.

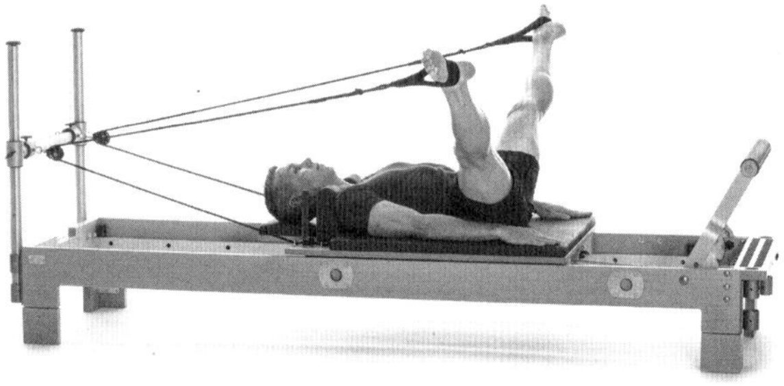

Inhale. Open the legs wide.

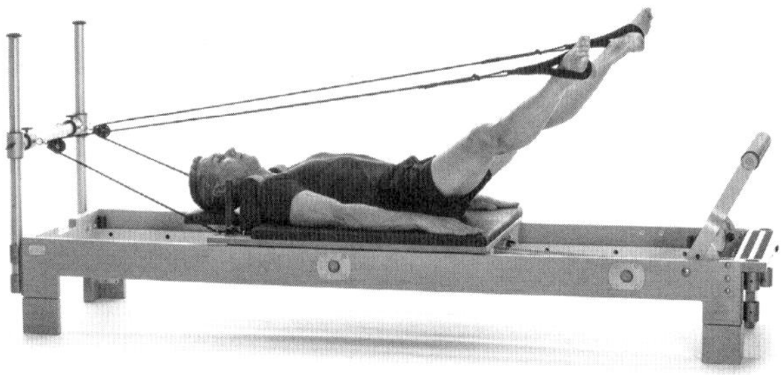

Exhale. Close the legs, maintaining a micro-bend in the knees. Return to the start position. Repeat 10 times.

Frog—Extended

The Reformer: Frog—Extended combines the Reformer: Frog with the Reformer: Opening, but it requires more control and coordination than either of those exercises. Maintain tension in the straps as the legs bend from the open-leg position into the frog position in the final phase by keeping the hamstrings engaged and the carriage still. I like to think of the movement as circular rather than linear, originating in the hip joints. The positioning and stability of the pelvis is critical; it provides a foundation for the exercise and accommodates the stretch by serving as an anchor for the movement.

Imagery

Imagine you are stirring an enormous pot of porridge, performing large circular movements with the feet and legs.

- Keep the carriage still as the legs bend from the open position to the frog position.
- Maintain hip extensor engagement as the legs bend to prevent the legs from coming too close to the chest, causing the pelvis to tuck.
- Maintain lumbopelvic stabilization.

Muscle Focus

- Hip adductors
- Quadriceps

Objectives

- To improve hip adductor strength and flexibility
- To improve knee extensor control
- To develop lumbopelvic stabilization

RESISTANCE

Light (selected) — Medium — Heavy

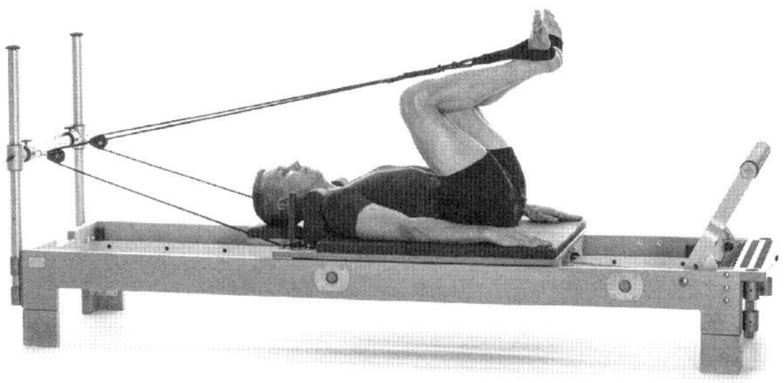

Setup. Lie supine in a neutral spine position. Place the feet in the straps and bend the knees (beyond a 90-degree angle), with the hips externally rotated. Dorsiflex the feet and press the heels together.

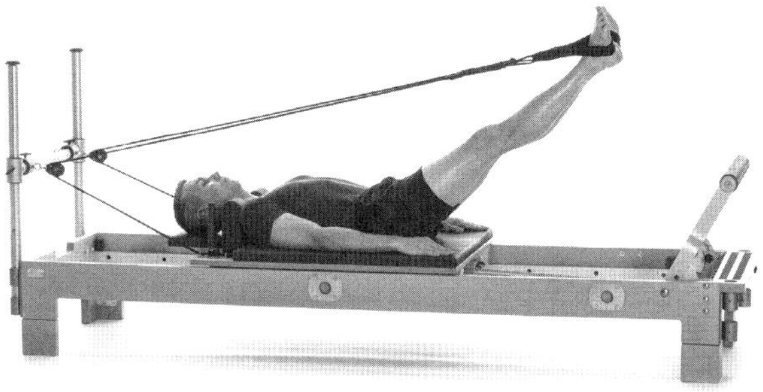

Exhale. Straighten the legs with the heels traveling along a horizontal plane, parallel to the floor. Finish with the legs in a diagonal line, approximately 45 degrees to the carriage.

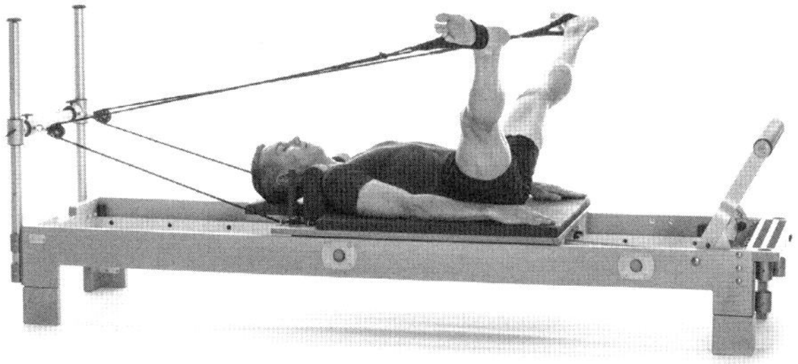

Inhale. Open the legs wide, as in the Reformer: Opening.

Exhale. Bend the knees, bringing the heels together to the frog position, maintaining tension in the straps.

Inhale. Pause in the frog position, preparing to straighten the legs. Repeat 5 times.

Frog—Extended Reverse

Muscle Focus

- Hip adductors
- Quadriceps

Objectives

- To improve hip adductor strength and flexibility
- To improve knee extensor control
- To develop lumbopelvic stabilization

RESISTANCE

Light — Medium — Heavy

Although very similar to its sibling the Reformer: Frog—Extended, the Reformer: Frog—Extended Reverse feels quite different. The stretch in the adductors is more intense as the legs are straightened out to the sides, and the work of the adductors is more challenging as the legs are brought together. Keeping tension in the straps and the carriage still as the legs straighten out to the sides from the frog position to the open position is important. Maintaining hamstring engagement helps keep tension in the straps. Emphasize the circular action that occurs in the hip joints. The position and stability of the pelvis should not be compromised—if it tilts, the full potential of the adductor stretch will be lost.

Imagery

The movement should feel as if you had been stirring an enormous pot of porridge in one direction and have just reversed the direction of the stirring, using large circular movements with the feet and legs.

- Keep the carriage still as the legs straighten out to the sides.
- Keep a micro-bend in the knees as the legs close, focusing the work on the hip adductors.
- Maintain lumbopelvic stabilization.

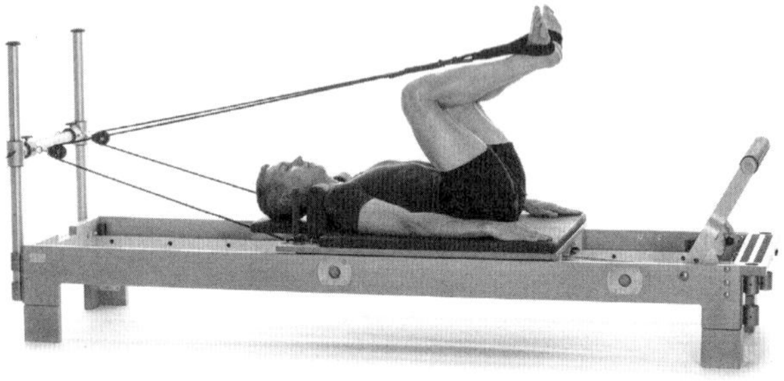

Setup. Lie supine in a neutral spine position. Place the feet in the straps and bend the knees (beyond a 90-degree angle), with the hips externally rotated. Dorsiflex the feet and press the heels together.

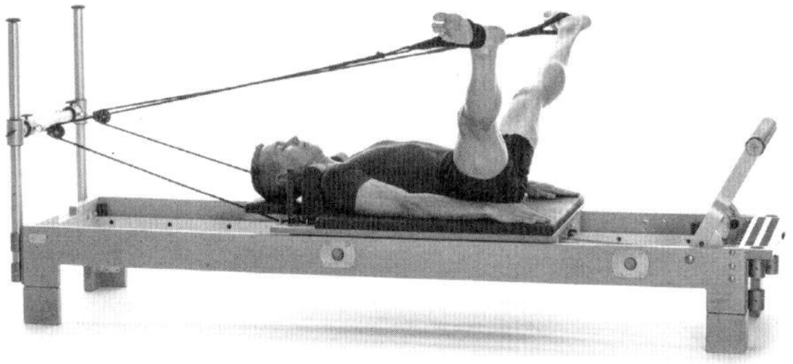

Exhale. Straighten the legs out to the sides into an open position without moving the carriage.

Inhale. Pause in the open position, preparing to close the legs.

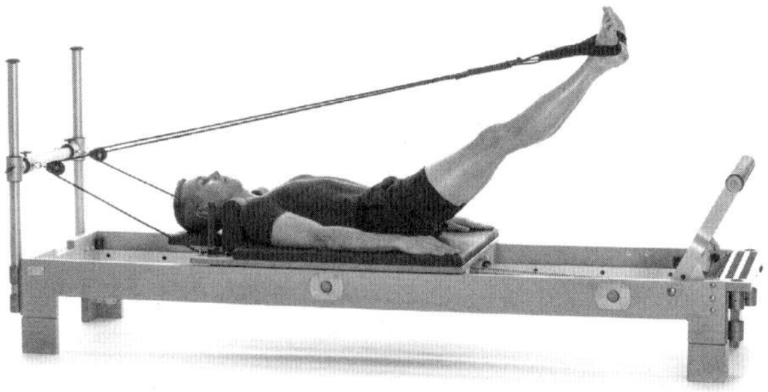

Exhale. Close the legs, maintaining a micro-bend in the knees, and bring the heels together.

Inhale. Bend the knees. Return to the start position. Repeat 5 times.

Spinal Articulation

The spinal articulation block incorporates principles and targets muscle groups that are fundamental to Pilates. The spine is the central pillar of the body, not only in terms of bone structure but also in terms of muscular support and neurological well-being. As Joseph Pilates wrote in *Return to Life Through Contrology,* "If your spine is inflexibly stiff at 30, you are old; if it is completely flexible at 60, you are young." Cultivating awareness and control of the intricate intersegmental movements of the spine is a lifelong process. Joseph Pilates specifically addresses the vertebra-by-vertebra movement of the spine in *Return to Life Through Contrology* and claims that this "rolling" and "unrolling" movement "gradually but surely restores the spine."

In order to achieve the desired flowing movement, you must be acutely aware of the small intervertebral muscles and be able to control them. Breath is also an important component in spinal articulation; not only does it provide a rhythm to the movement, but it also encourages the recruitment of key muscles. In addition, spinal articulation can enhance the breathing process by "wringing" the lungs out as you would a sponge, which in turn allows them to be filled to their full capacity.

The majority of the spinal articulation exercises move through spinal flexion, and it is typically this range of motion that we associate with the term *spinal articulation*. However, at times you may reap great benefits by visualizing spinal articulation as the spine extends as well. This is a difficult concept to grasp initially and even more difficult to achieve. It is not recommended in all back extension exercises, but when used appropriately, it can serve as an excellent cue with invaluable results.

The abdominals play a prominent role in spinal articulation, whether through spinal flexion or spinal extension. Good abdominal control is a required ingredient for successful spinal articulation. Furthermore, the TA has a particularly profound role in facilitating efficient spinal articulation. Thus, spinal articulation should be practiced and mastered at all levels of Pilates work.

The image of a rolling wave describes spinal articulation exceptionally well. It conjures up not only the progressive curling action but also the feeling of the continuous flow of the waves. Being a person who loves the ocean, any image relating to water inspires me. But even those who have only seen the ocean and not felt it can appreciate the smooth, natural, rhythmic power of a rolling wave!

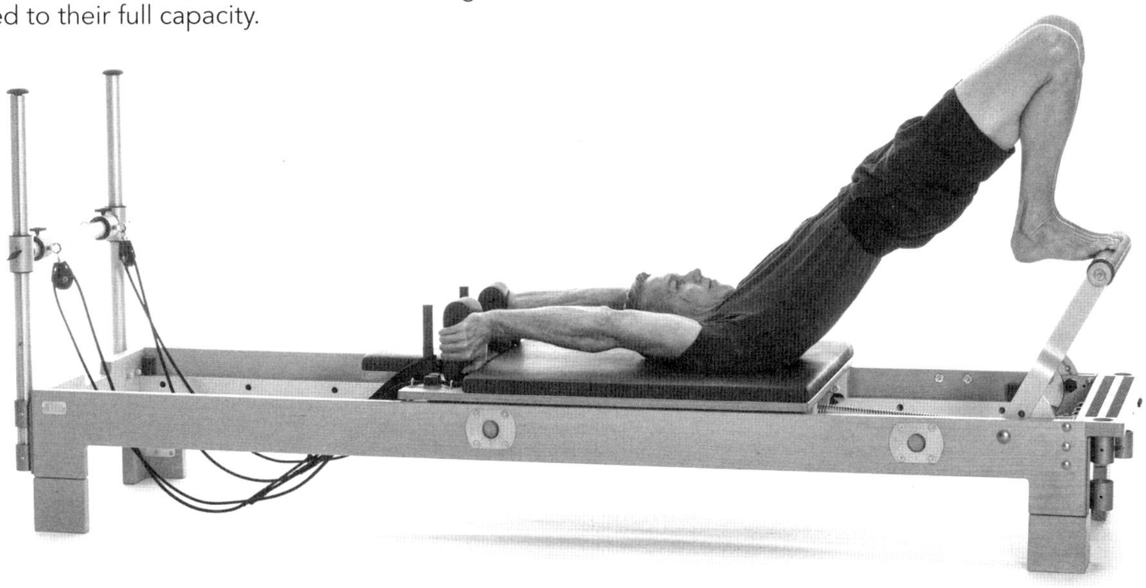

REFORMER

Spinal Articulation

FUNDAMENTAL

Bottom Lift

Muscle Focus

- Abdominals
- Hamstrings

Objectives

- To develop spinal articulation
- To improve abdominal and hip extensor control

RESISTANCE

Light Medium Heavy

This introductory exercise in the spinal articulation block is essentially a Mat: Pelvic Curl, which is typically the first exercise in the mat work, performed on the reformer. However, the element of instability due to the mobile carriage makes this exercise far more challenging. In addition, the range of motion is greater because the feet are placed much higher—on the footbar rather than on the floor. Pelvic stabilization and spinal articulation should be mastered on the mat before proceeding to the Reformer: Bottom Lift. The hamstrings, which are crucial to the lifting and lowering of the pelvis, play an even greater role in this version; they act not only as hip extensors but also as knee flexors in order to keep the carriage in place. The movement of the carriage should be minimal; strive to keep it stable and as close to the stopper as possible. The lower the spring tension is set, the more challenging it is to prevent the carriage from moving and to keep it close to the stopper. The demand on the hamstrings increases exponentially as the spring tension is decreased. Start with a comfortable spring setting, and as you become progressively proficient at this exercise, lower the tension. Note that the weight is on the balls of the feet, which demands foot stability and exceptional control of the ankle and subtalar joint to maintain good alignment. There is a strong tendency to lift the heels high and rely on plantarflexion to raise the body. Avoid this tendency by establishing the correct position of the heels and then not moving them as you articulate the spine up and down. The feeling should be as if there is a floor beneath the feet.

Imagery

Use the image of a banana peel being peeled off the fruit, just as the spine is peeled off the reformer, and then the image of the peel being returned to the fruit as the spine is lowered.

- ○ Minimize movement of the carriage.
- ○ Align the feet as in Reformer: Parallel Toes and keep the heels stable. Keep the legs parallel and the hip adductors engaged.

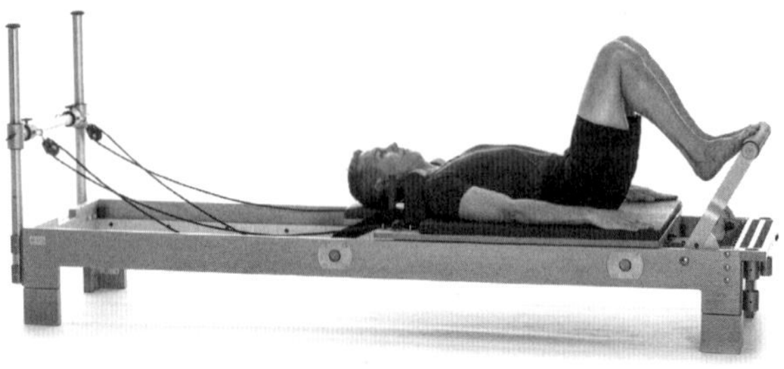

Setup. Lie supine in a neutral spine position, with the headrest down (flat). Place the toes on the footbar, with the legs parallel and the knees bent.

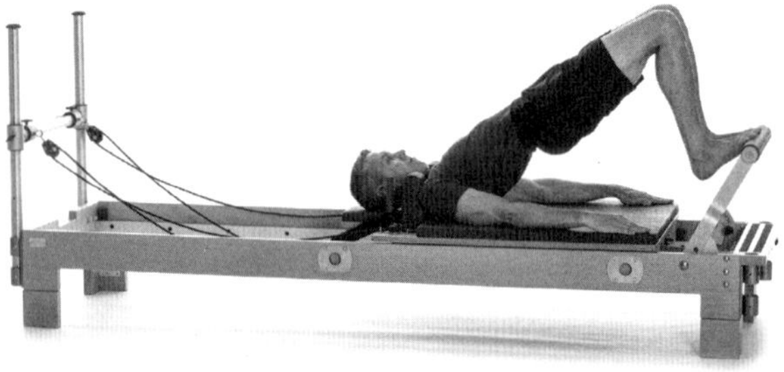

Exhale. Draw in the abdominals and tilt the pelvis in a posterior direction. Articulate the spine upward, one vertebra at a time, extending the hips (but not the knees) and lifting onto the shoulder girdle. Establish a straight line from the shoulders through the front of the hips to the knees, avoiding hyperlordosis.

Inhale. Pause, holding this position.

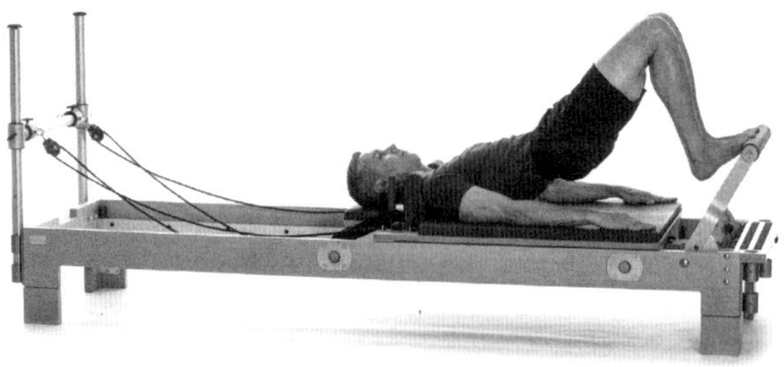

Exhale. Articulate the spine down. Return to the start position. Repeat 5-10 times.

Bottom Lift With Extension

Adding knee extension when in the lifted position accentuates the hip extensor component of the exercise and requires excellent lumbopelvic stabilization. Activating the hip extensors and the knee extensors facilitates the straightening of the legs, creating a suspended bridge position. Although the gluteals may be recruited to help support the position, they are not the prime focus. There is a tendency for the gluteals to overshadow the hamstrings and to disrupt pelvic alignment; therefore, an effort should be made to engage the hamstrings prior to the gluteals during hip extension.

Avoid straightening the legs completely, which can place undue strain on the lower back. When returning to the stopper, maintain the strong energy line from shoulders through the front of the hips to the knees; this helps offset the natural tendency to drop the pelvis and flex at the hip joint.

Imagery

The extended position resembles a suspension bridge—well supported and stable, with no breaks in the line of the body from feet to shoulders.

- ○ Keep the heels stable.
- ○ Keep the knees slightly bent when straightening the legs, do not extend them completely.
- ○ Lift the pelvis and keep the hips extended as you bring the carriage toward the stopper.

VARIATION

This exercise can be performed with the feet in the small V position and the hips externally rotated as in the Reformer: V Position Toes. This serves as a good preparation for the Reformer: Semi-Circle.

Muscle Focus

- Abdominals
- Hamstrings
- Quadriceps

Objectives

- To develop spinal articulation
- To improve abdominal, hip extensor, and knee extensor control

RESISTANCE

Light Medium Heavy

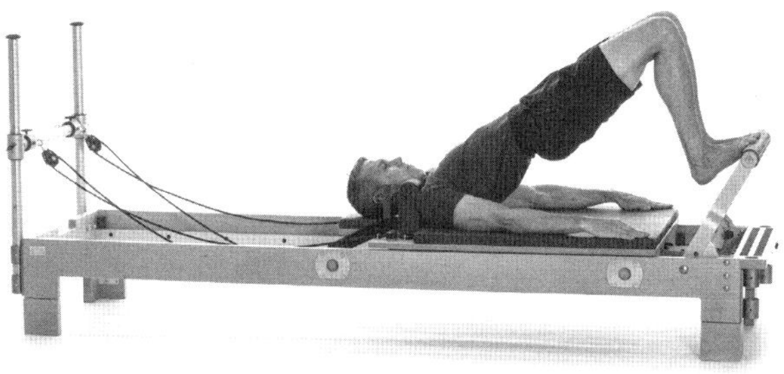

Setup. Lie supine, with the spine in a neutral position and the headrest down (flat). Place the toes on the footbar, with the legs parallel and the knees bent.

Exhale. Draw in the abdominals and tilt the pelvis in a posterior direction. Articulate the spine upward, one vertebra at a time, extending the hips and lifting onto the shoulder girdle. Form a straight line from the shoulders to the knees, avoiding hyperlordosis.

Inhale. Pause in this position.

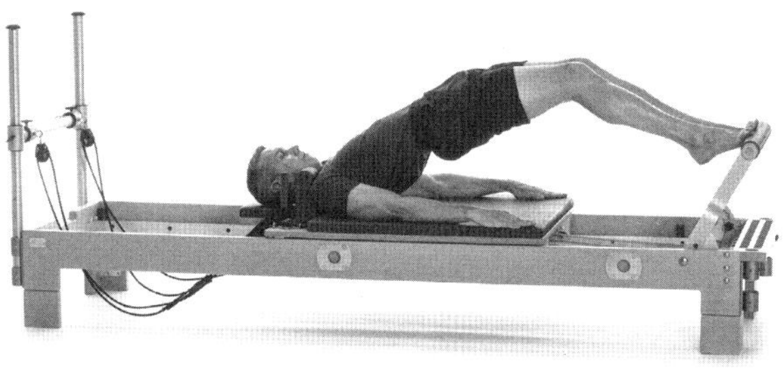

Exhale. Extend the knees (not completely) and the hips, without lowering the pelvis.

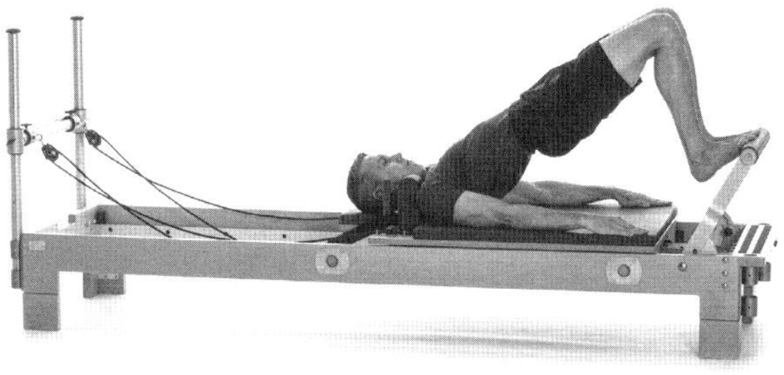

Inhale. Bend the knees, keeping the pelvis high, the legs parallel, and the heels stable. Repeat 5-10 times.

Exhale. Articulate the spine down. Return to the start position.

REFORMER

Spinal Articulation

INTERMEDIATE

Semi-Circle

Muscle Focus

- Abdominals
- Hamstrings
- Triceps

Objectives

- To develop spinal articulation
- To develop scapular stabilization
- To improve hip extensor and elbow extensor control

RESISTANCE

Light Medium Heavy

The Reformer: Semi-Circle is a progression of the Reformer: Bottom Lift With Extension; the position is more challenging and the ranges of motion are more demanding. Greater control and the recruitment of several additional muscle groups are required. The raised position of the pelvis and the V position of the feet demand increased abdominal and hip adductor and extensor control to keep the pelvis in a neutral position (or as close as possible), the hip flexors stretched, and the legs well aligned. (The legs tend to splay due to tight hip flexors and overuse of the gluteals.) Keeping the pelvis lifted and the feet in a moderate V position as the carriage returns toward the stopper ensures an effective stretch of the hip flexors. It is important to keep the heels stable, as in the Reformer: V Position Toes. There is a tendency to raise the heels high in order to lift the pelvis when the carriage is close to the stopper. The hip extensors, not the ankle–foot plantarflexors, should be used to maintain the height of the pelvis.

This exercise offers an opportunity to take advantage of the mobility of the spine by not stopping in a neutral position of the spine and pelvis, but continuing into hyperextension. The increased range benefits not only the lower spine but also the upper body. It emphasizes scapular stability and flexibility, as well as extension of the thoracic spine. This stretch of the thoracic region is particularly beneficial for people who have tight shoulder and chest muscles as well as round-shoulder posture.

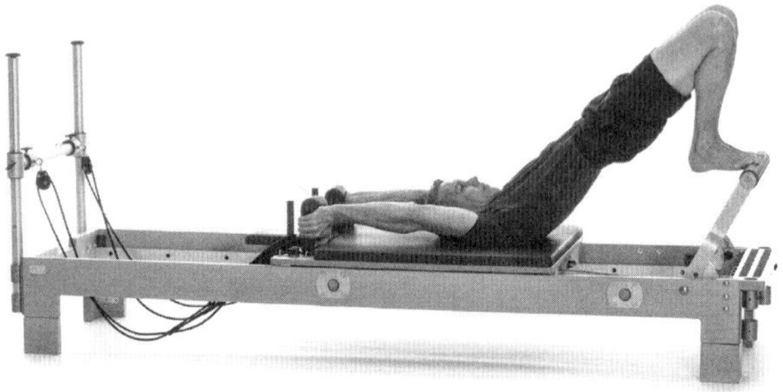

Setup. Lie on the carriage with the feet in a V position, toes on the footbar and heels together. Lift the pelvis and fully extend the hips, resting on the shoulder girdle. Press the hands against the shoulder rests and straighten the arms, keeping the pelvis elevated.

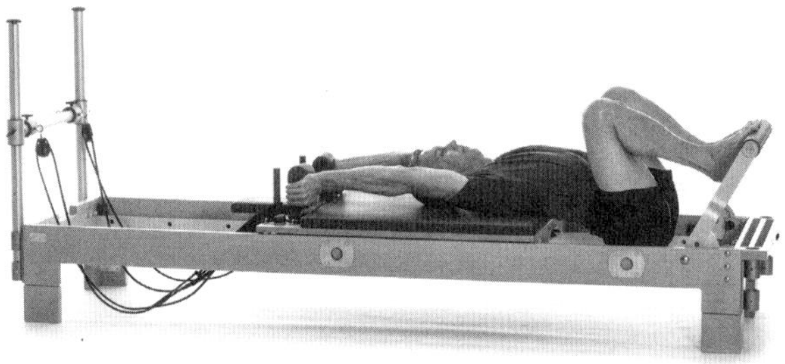

Exhale. Articulate the spine downward, one vertebra at a time, beginning the movement from the top of the thoracic spine and continuing until the pelvis is touching the springs. The spine will be hyperextended. Keep the carriage as still as possible during this phase.

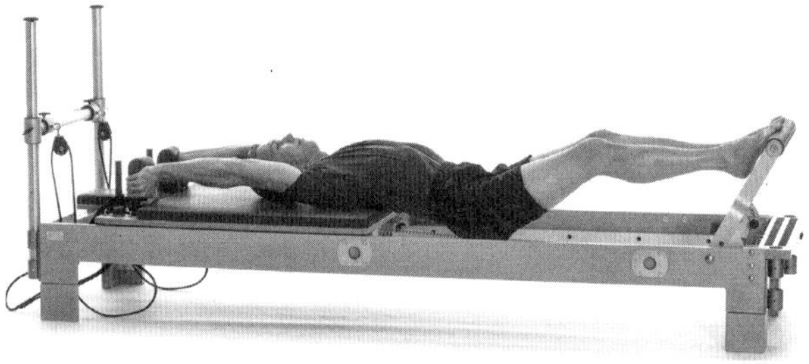

Inhale. Extend the knees without straightening the legs completely (5-10 degrees shy of straight), keeping the pelvis just above the springs and the spine hyperextended.

Imagery

The movement of the Reformer: Semi-Circle should feel like a rolling wave with no beginning and no end. The sensation of flow is extremely profound. It is a beautiful exercise to do and watch.

- Minimize the movement of the carriage when articulating the spine up and down.
- Squeeze the heels together, keeping them stable in a V position.
- Keep the arms straight.

VARIATION

The direction of this sequence can be reversed. From the start position, extend the knees without straightening the legs completely. Roll the spine down and place the pelvis close to the springs. Keep the carriage as still as possible during this phase. Bend the knees, bringing the carriage in toward the stopper. When it will not move any further, roll up, articulating the spine to the start position. Continue to keep the carriage as still as possible.

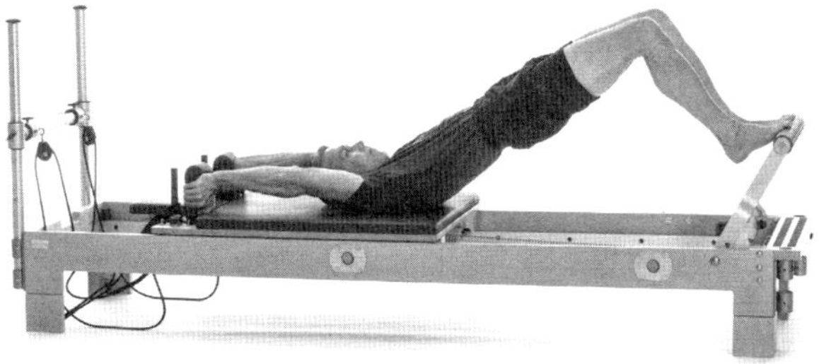

Exhale. Draw in the abdominals, tilt the pelvis in a posterior direction, and articulate the spine upward, one vertebra at a time, lifting onto the shoulder girdle and reaching full hip extension. Keep the carriage as still as possible during this phase.

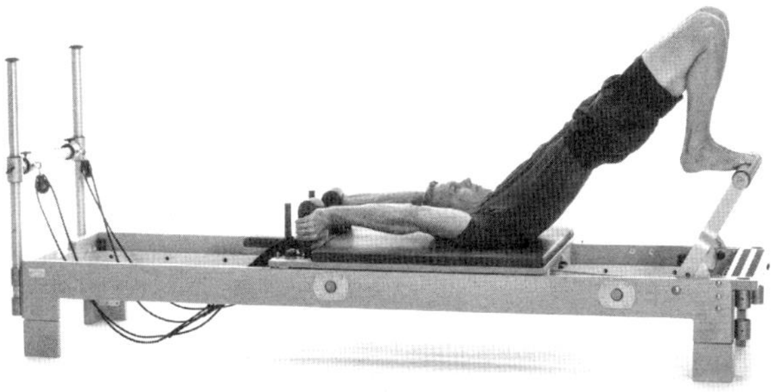

Inhale. Bend the knees, keeping the heels stable, the hips extended, and the pelvis lifted. Return to the start position. Repeat 5 times.

REFORMER
Spinal Articulation
INTERMEDIATE

Muscle Focus

- Abdominals
- Back extensors
- Hamstrings

Objectives

- To develop spinal articulation
- To improve lower back and hamstring flexibility

RESISTANCE
Light Medium Heavy

Short Spine

The Reformer: Short Spine, as presented here, is slightly different from the version originally created by Joseph Pilates. In the classic version, the roll-up onto the shoulders is performed as the carriage moves toward the stopper. In this version, the roll-up is performed with the carriage stationary and positioned firmly against the stopper. Not relying on the springs or straps during the roll-up requires greater abdominal control and back extensor flexibility. In addition, by taking the carriage all the way to the stopper first, you will achieve a more effective hamstring stretch as you bring the legs over the face. During this phase, keep the pelvis as stable as possible and the sacrum as close to the carriage as possible. Most people find it impossible to keep the pelvis in a neutral position, or even close to neutral, as the legs go over. However, the action of anchoring the sacrum and actively drawing it toward the carriage helps stabilize the pelvis and ensure a significant hamstring stretch.

When the legs are overhead and the trunk is stable and resting on the shoulder girdle, bend the knees, maintaining tension in the straps and preventing the trunk from collapsing. Keep the feet positioned above the face and the legs in a diamond shape as the spine rolls down, vertebra by vertebra, onto the carriage. Allow the knees to straighten slightly during the roll-down, facilitating the "melting" of the spine into the carriage. This provides a wonderful stretch for the lower back. Once the pelvis can move no further, dorsiflex the feet and take the legs across the body, extending the hips without bending the knees further, maintaining the diamond shape. Finally, place the pelvis in a neutral position on the carriage, returning to the start position.

Note that the extreme flexion of the spine, plus the potential weight placed on the cervical spine, precludes those with back and neck problems—particularly if discs are involved—from performing this exercise.

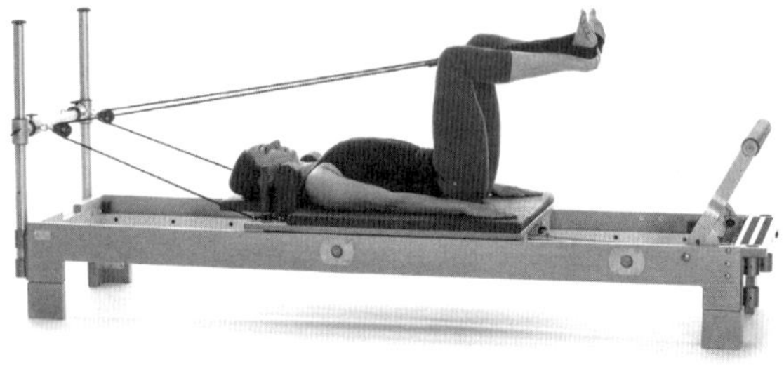

Setup. Lie supine, with the feet in the straps in the Reformer: Frog—Extended start position, hips in external rotation, knees bent, heels together, and feet dorsiflexed. Note that the headrest must be down (flat).

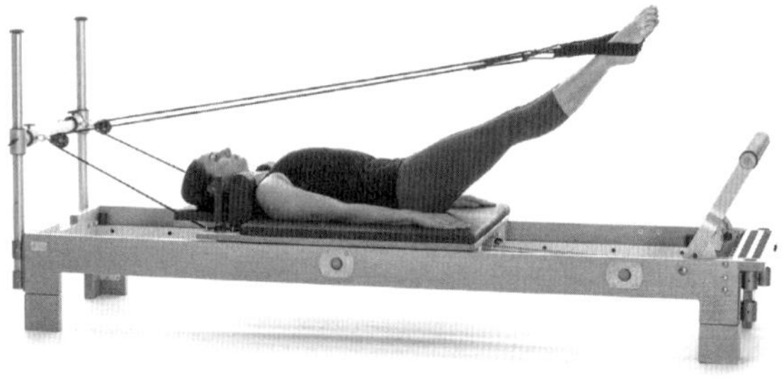

Exhale. Straighten the legs and plantarflex the feet.

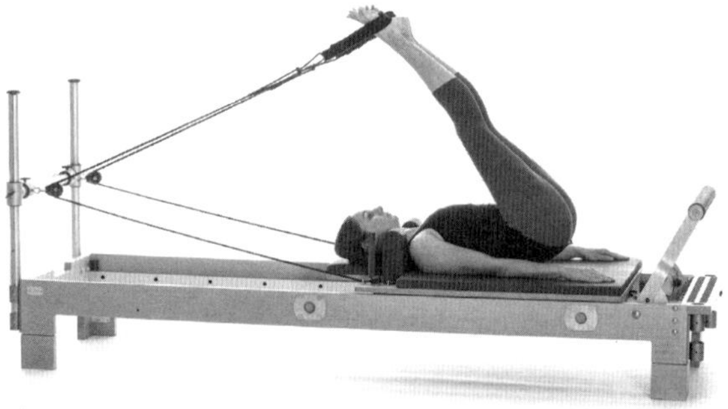

Inhale. Bring the legs overhead, moving the carriage to the stopper.

Imagery

Enjoy the flowing wave-like motion of this exercise. The energy should feel circular and endless. The sensation is similar to the Reformer: Semi-Circle.

- Bring the carriage all the way to the stopper before rolling up.
- Keep tension in the straps when rolling up onto the shoulders and bending the legs into the diamond shape.
- Maintain back extensor engagement when on the shoulders and bending the knees to help protect the spine.
- Keep the feet opposite the eyes when rolling down in the diamond shape, allowing the knees to hug the sides of the chest and to straighten slightly.
- Maintain the diamond shape of the legs during the final phase, emphasizing hip extension and not bending the knees further.

VARIATION

This variation is closer to the classical version. When the legs are brought over the body, rather than trying to keep the sacrum anchored, allow the pelvis to lift. Roll up onto the shoulders as the carriage moves all the way to the stopper. Once the carriage reaches the stopper, extend the hips, and lift as high as possible onto the shoulders. The second part of the exercise is as described in the Reformer: Short Spine.

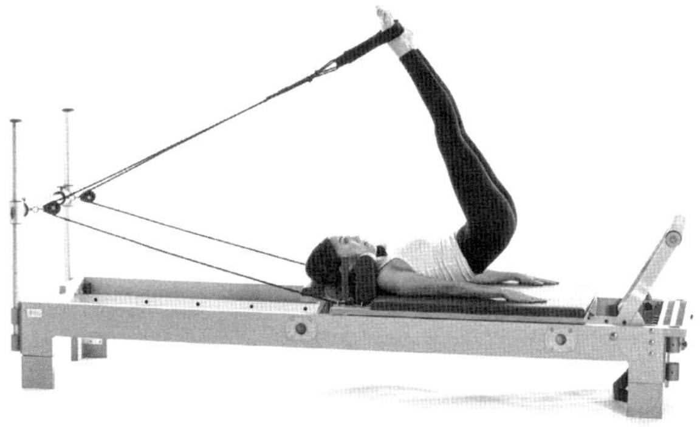

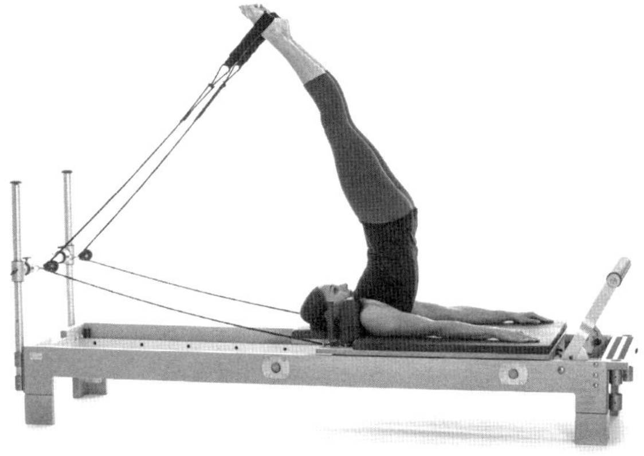

Exhale. Articulate the spine, rolling up onto the shoulders.

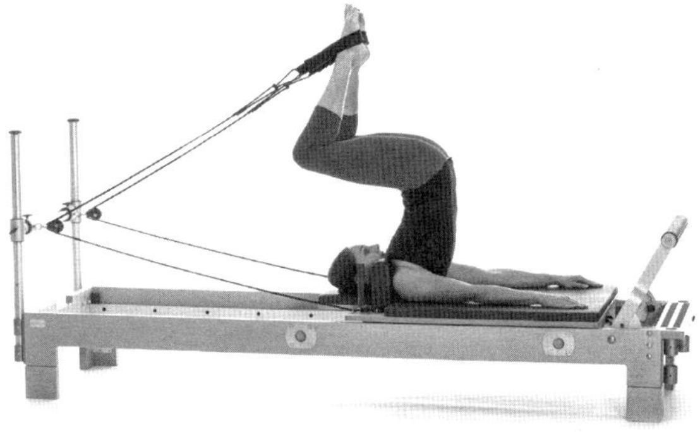

Inhale. Bend the knees, creating a diamond shape with the legs.

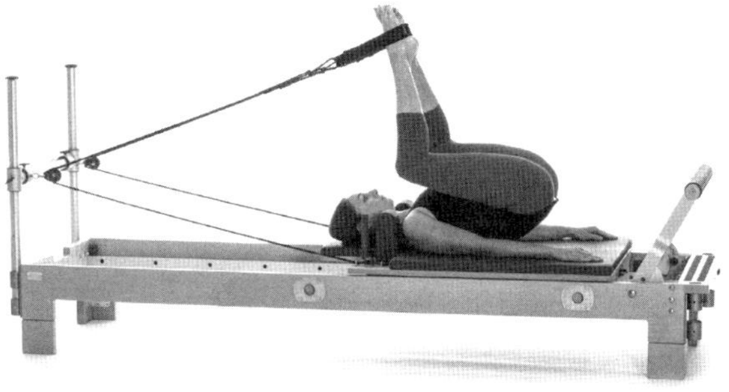

Exhale. Articulate the spine downward, keeping the feet above the eyes, allowing the knees to adapt to the roll-down by straightening slightly and hugging the sides of the chest.

Inhale. Dorsiflex the feet, extend the hips to bring the legs across the body, and place the pelvis on the carriage. Return to the start position. Repeat 5 times.

Long Spine

Muscle Focus

- Abdominals
- Hamstrings

Objectives

- To develop spinal articulation
- To improve abdominal and hip extensor control

RESISTANCE

Light — Medium — Heavy

This version of the Reformer: Long Spine differs from the classic Pilates exercise, in which the carriage is stationary against the stopper during the roll-up onto the shoulders and the straps are lengthened to accommodate this position. In this version, the focus is on balance and stabilization during the roll-up and the roll-down phases. The carriage is still, but not against the stopper, with the springs in a tensioned state. Performing the exercise in this way demands tremendous control of the ISS and the hip extensors, with assistance from the back extensors and shoulder extensors.

Maintaining the straight, upright position of the legs, perpendicular to the floor, requires great control on the way up and even more on the way down. In the down phase, the eccentric contraction of the hip extensors and back extensors allows smooth articulation of the spine without any movement of the carriage. This is a formidable challenge, particularly when the resistance is light.

I recommend that you start with medium resistance. As you gain proficiency, lower the resistance to make it more challenging. The Reformer: Long Spine can only be performed well once you have achieved a high level of competence in other, less challenging spinal articulation exercises. It is important to be aware of the risks of this exercise—if you lose control while up on the shoulders, the springs will pull you onto the neck, placing great stress on the cervical spine and possibly resulting in injury. Note that the potential load placed on the cervical spine precludes those with neck problems—particularly if discs are involved—from performing this exercise.

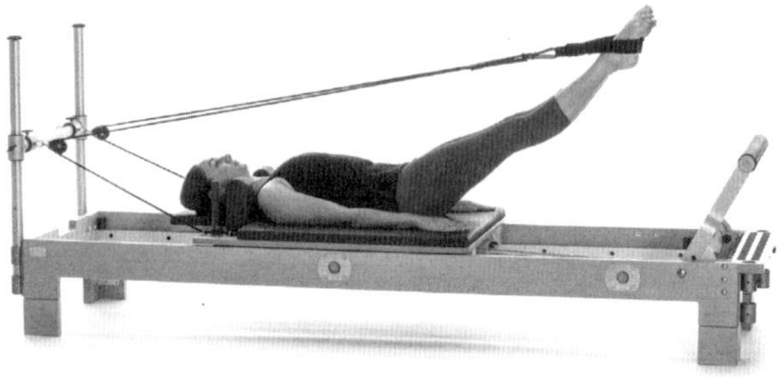

Setup. Lie supine on the carriage, with the feet in the straps and the legs straight and together, forming a diagonal line of approximately a 45-degree angle to the carriage. The headrest must be down (flat).

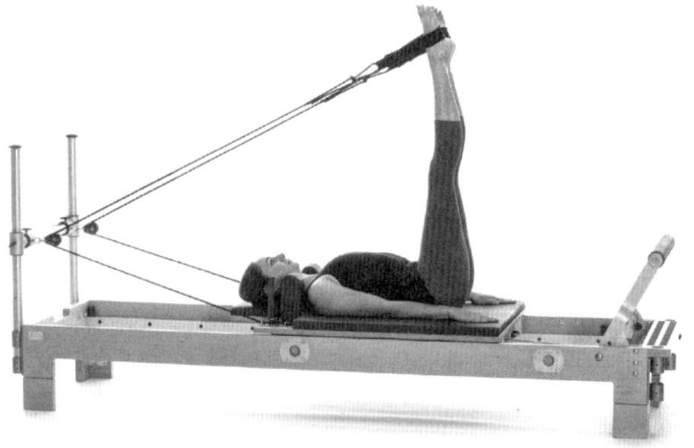

Inhale. Lift the legs to a perpendicular position, keeping the sacrum anchored on the carriage.

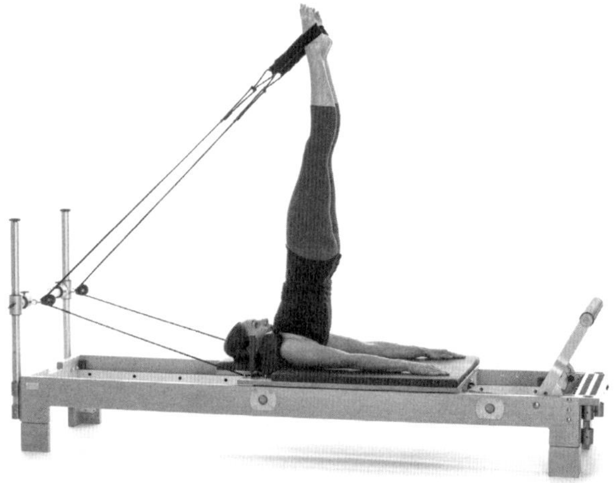

Exhale. Roll up onto the shoulder girdle, articulating the spine. Keep the carriage still during this phase.

Imagery

Imagine the legs being pulled up toward the ceiling like a sail being pulled up a boat's mast. Once at the top, the body remains as straight as the mast. The body is then lowered, like a sail being lowered down the mast.

- Keep the carriage still while articulating the spine up and down, the body in a state of complete balance.
- Use the hip extensors eccentrically during the roll-down phase.
- Place the pelvis down firmly, anchoring the sacrum on the carriage, before returning to the start position.

VARIATION

Reverse the movement pattern by starting with the legs slightly open (abducted). Lift them to perpendicular and roll up onto the shoulder girdle. At the top, adduct the legs, bringing them together, and roll down to the sacrum. Once the pelvis is anchored, lower the legs to a 45-degrees angle. When doing the original version and this variation, repeat 3 times each.

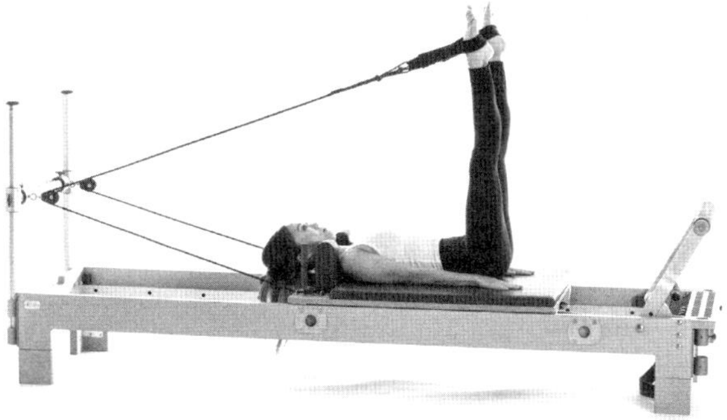

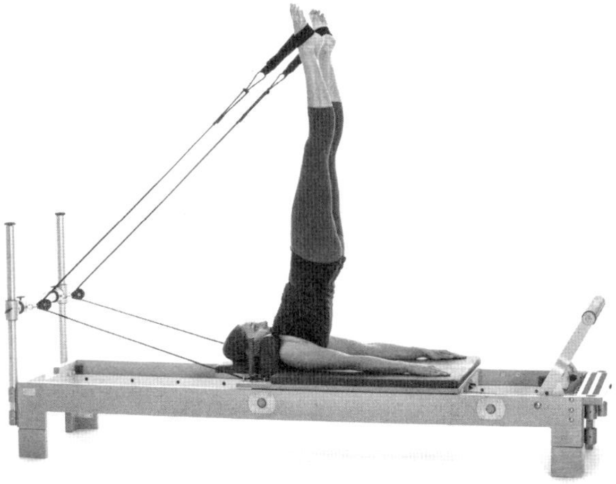

Inhale. Abduct the legs to shoulder width, maintaining the upright position of the body.

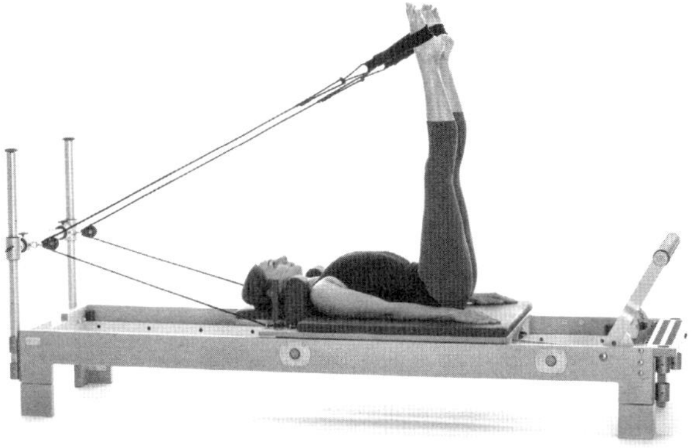

Exhale. Roll down to the carriage, articulating the spine. Keep the carriage still during this phase.

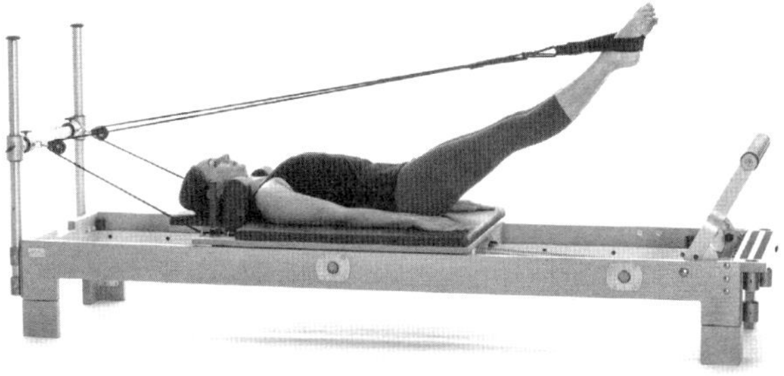

Anchor the sacrum, lower the legs to a 45-degree angle, and bring them together. Return to the start position. Repeat 5 times.

Stretches

Flexibility is an important aspect of any fitness and conditioning regimen. Therefore this block should always be included in a well-balanced session. Although it is up to you to decide what part of the body should be emphasized in terms of flexibility, I suggest that a stretch for the hip flexors and hamstrings be included. These two muscle groups tend to be tight for many people, and they have a profound effect on the alignment and function of the pelvis, which in turn has far-reaching implications on gait and other common daily functions. Balance in the pelvic area is crucial. Even if a person is hypermobile, there tends to be an imbalance between the hamstrings and the hip flexors, although in this case the focus may shift from flexibility to control.

Of course, flexibility of the spine is addressed in the spinal articulation block. Flexibility in general deteriorates with age, making this an element of fitness that must be addressed. For optimum function at any level of activity, flexibility and functional range of motion are key.

Stretches need to be held for a relatively long period of time to allow the muscle (or group of muscles) being stretched to release tension and for the body in general to relax while still maintaining stability where required. Stability is important to assure that there is an anchor point from which the muscle can be stretched. If the attachment points of the muscle are not stable, the muscle cannot stretch effectively. The optimal duration of a stretch is debatable, but in general I prescribe holding the stretch for 3-5 breath cycles. Using visual imagery of the muscle elongating like an elastic band can be extremely advantageous. In addition, focusing on long and deep breaths is invaluable in achieving relaxation and a sensation of a deep stretch in the muscle or muscles.

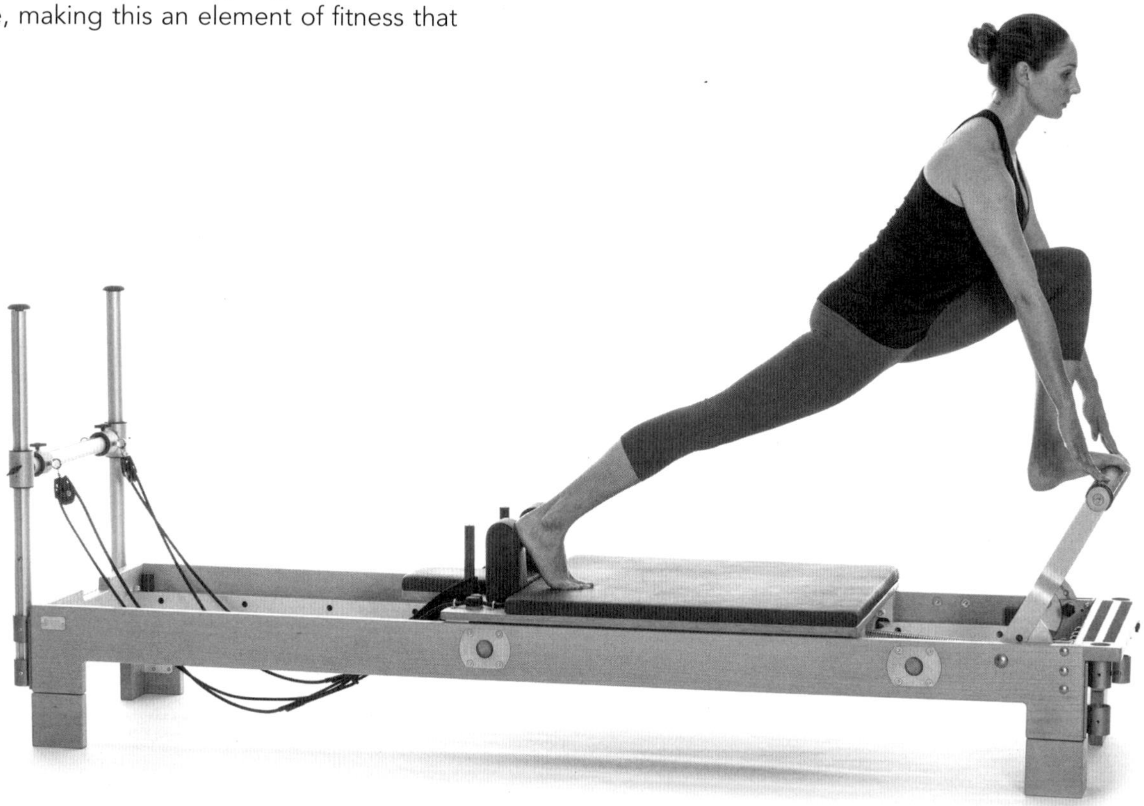

Lunge—Standing

This is the first in a series of hip flexor–hamstring stretches. The primary focus of this exercise is flexibility, which is accomplished in two distinct phases: a hip flexor stretch and a hamstring stretch. Coordinated action of these two muscle groups helps create a balance in pelvic alignment and function.

The basis of every stretch is a stable anchor point. For the hip flexors and the hamstrings, this point is the pelvis, which is anchored in a position that opposes the direction of the stretch in order to maximize the stretch. During the hip flexor stretch, bias the pelvis toward a posterior tilt by contracting the abdominals (to lift the pubic symphysis) and the hamstrings (to lower the ischial tuberosity). The posterior tilt of the pelvis increases the stretch of the hip flexors and helps alleviate pressure on the lower back.

During the hamstring stretch, maintain contraction of the back extensors, which draws the pelvis in an anterior direction and creates a deeper stretch of the hamstrings. It also activates (and potentially strengthens) the muscles of the back, particularly the mid-back, which are so important for healthy posture and yet are so often neglected. Note that, throughout this series of lunge stretches, the front knee never advances beyond the ankle while in the hip flexor stretch position, and the pelvis travels along a consistent horizontal plane without dropping or lifting as the front leg straightens and the hamstrings are stretched.

Imagery

For the hip flexor stretch, imagine the feeling of a strong force pulling the pelvis up the front of the body and resulting in an arc shape of the trunk. For the hamstring stretch, a straight energy line emanates from the back of the pelvis, running up through the spine and out the top of the head, creating a flat back.

- Tilt the pelvis posteriorly and extend the upper back during the hip flexor stretch.
- Travel along a horizontal plane with the pelvis when straightening the front leg for the hamstring stretch.
- Tilt the pelvis anteriorly, keeping the back flat and the head aligned with the spine, during the hamstring stretch.

Muscle Focus

- Hip flexors
- Hamstrings

Objectives

- To improve hip flexor and hamstring flexibility
- To improve hip flexor, hamstring, and back extensor control
- To develop lumbopelvic stabilization

RESISTANCE

Light Medium Heavy

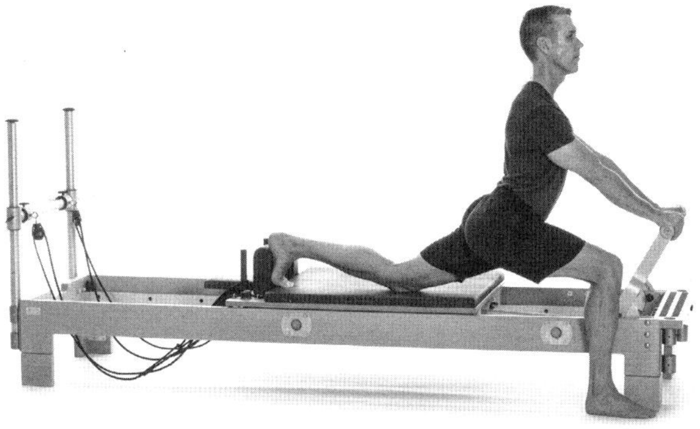

Stand beside the reformer with the hands on the footbar, arms straight. Place the outside foot on the floor in line with the footbar, and place the other leg on the carriage, with the foot pressed against the shoulder rest and the knee resting on the carriage. Bend the knee of the standing leg so that it is directly over the ankle, and maintain an upright position of the trunk. Focus on the hip flexor stretch of the kneeling leg and hold the position for 3-5 breath cycles.

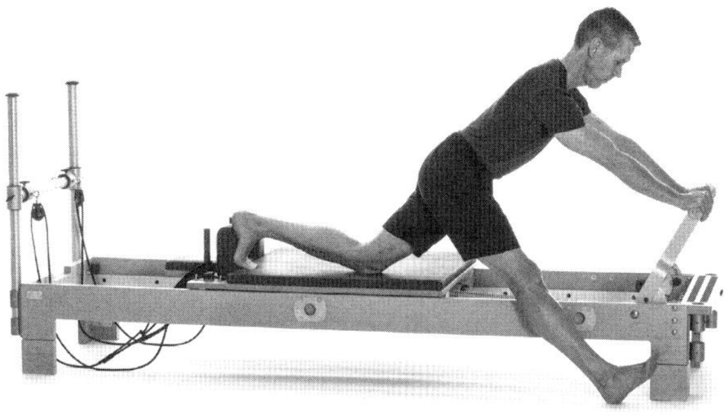

Dorsiflex the foot of the standing leg, pushing the heel into the floor. Straighten the knee, keeping the pelvis on the same horizontal plane as it travels back, and hinge the trunk forward. Keep the back as flat as possible and the back extensors engaged. Focus on the hamstring stretch and hold the position for 3-5 breath cycles.

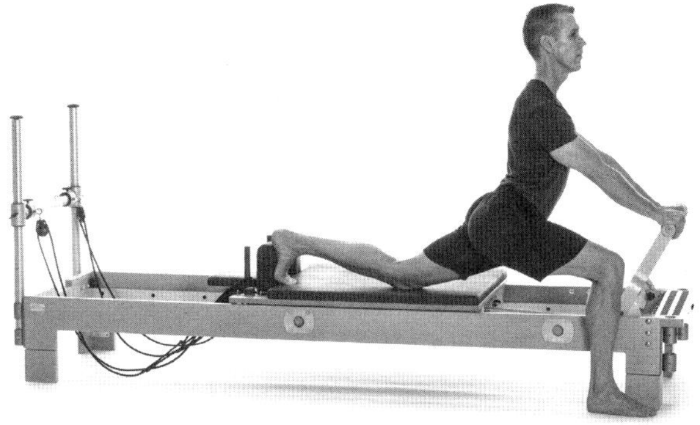

Bend the front knee and lift the trunk, with the pelvis traveling forward along the horizontal plane. Return to the start position. Repeat before switching to the other side.

Lunge—Kneeling

Muscle Focus

- Hip flexors
- Hamstrings

Objectives

- To improve hip flexor and hamstring flexibility
- To improve hip flexor, hamstring, and back extensor control
- To develop lumbopelvic stabilization

RESISTANCE

Light Medium Heavy

The key principles of the hip flexor–hamstring stretches are consistent throughout the series. To maximize the stretch of the hip flexors, focus on activating the abdominals and tilting the pelvis posteriorly, activating the upper back extensors, extending the thoracic spine, and creating an arc shape from the back knee through the thigh, pelvis, trunk, and head. To maximize the stretch of the hamstrings, focus on activating the lower back extensors, tilting the pelvis anteriorly and keeping the pelvis and trunk square. Maintaining the alignment of the spine along a centerline is important. There is a tendency to align the spine over the straightening leg, which results in a lateral curve of the trunk. This is counterproductive.

In the initial position the front knee is aligned directly above the ankle, which is consistent in all the variations in this series. As the body transitions into the hamstring stretch, the pelvis travels along a consistent horizontal plane and does not drop toward the carriage; at the same time, the angle between the kneeling leg and the carriage also remains consistent. This kneeling lunge position necessitates even greater pelvic stabilization and more flexibility than the standing lunge position. A misaligned, unstable pelvis compromises its effectiveness as an anchor and subsequently compromises the stretch itself.

Imagery

The pelvis is the anchor of the stretch, whether stretching the hip flexors or the hamstrings. Align the pelvis to maximize the stretch and feel it pulling on the muscle, stretching it like a rubber band.

- Tilt the pelvis posteriorly and extend the upper back during the hip flexor stretch.
- Travel along a horizontal plane with the pelvis when straightening the front leg.
- Tilt the pelvis anteriorly, engaging the back extensors, and establish a flat back position (or as close as possible) during the hamstring stretch.
- Keep the spine centered and the head aligned with the spine during the hamstring stretch.

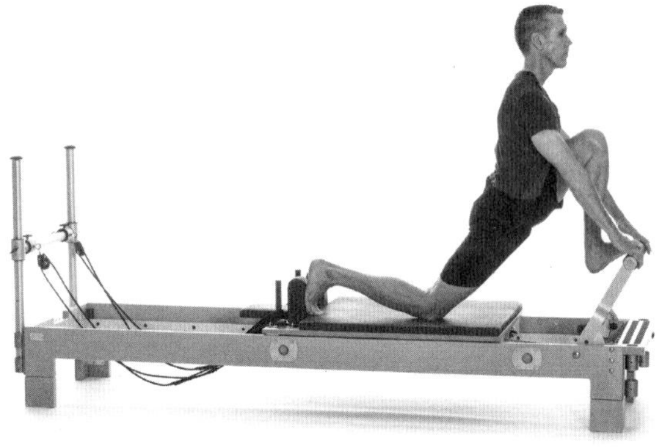

Kneel on the carriage with one foot against the shoulder rest, toes tucked under the foot (extended), and the knee on the carriage. Place the other foot on the footbar, with the knee directly over the ankle. Place the hands on the footbar, shoulder width apart, and maintain an upright position of the trunk. Focus on the hip flexor stretch of the kneeling leg and hold the position for 3-5 breath cycles.

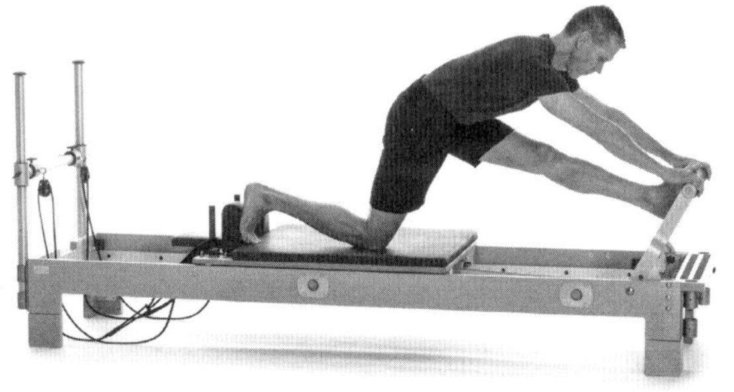

Straighten the leg on the footbar, moving the pelvis along a consistent horizontal plane. Hinge forward with the trunk to create a "crease" between the back leg and the pelvis at the hip joint. The angle of the back leg to the carriage should remain consistent. While keeping the back extensors engaged, focus on the hamstring stretch and hold the position for 3-5 breath cycles.

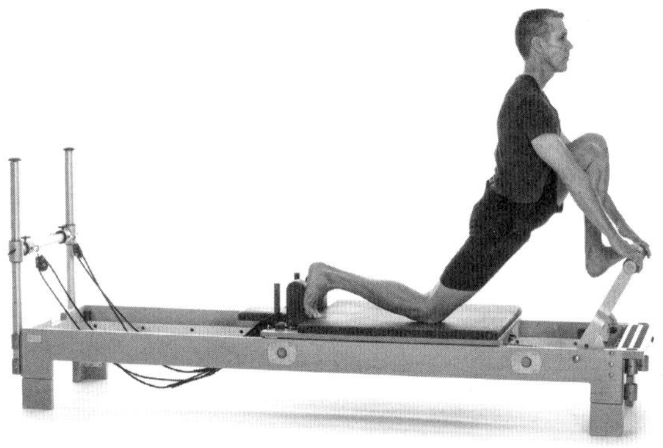

Bend the front knee and lift the trunk, with the pelvis traveling forward along the horizontal plane. Return to the start position. Repeat before switching to the other side.

Lunge—Forward

This third stretch of the series is very challenging because over and above the stretch it includes the elements of balance and immense control. The front knee is again aligned above the ankle, but in this version the back leg is completely straight without the support of the carriage. The back heel is pressing against the shoulder rest with the toes (forefoot) forward of the shoulder rest. As the body transitions from the hip flexor stretch into the hamstring stretch, the pelvis travels along a consistent horizontal plane. Both inflexible and extremely flexible people have a hard time with this stretch. The Reformer: Lunge—Forward develops strength and flexibility concurrently, resulting in a healthy balance between the two.

Maximize the stretch and protect the lower back during the hip flexor stretch by activating the abdominals and tilting the pelvis posteriorly. Emphasize engagement of the back extensors during the hamstring stretch and tilt the pelvis anteriorly to maximize the stretch.

The added steps described in the Progression section further develop control, heightened awareness of the core, functional strength and flexibility of the hamstrings and hip flexors, and, of course, balance.

Imagery

This position is a very powerful one, particularly when the trunk is upright and you are balancing in the lunge position. I like to relate it to the warrior pose in yoga; although the position is slightly different, the sense of strength and power is quite similar. As with all Pilates exercises, the powerhouse is important, yet in this position there is also a tremendous sense of strength emanating from the legs.

- ○ Press the heel of the back leg against the shoulder rest with the toes (forefoot) forward of the shoulder rest.
- ○ Keep the knee of the back leg straight.
- ○ Align the front foot with the hip joint on the same side.

PROGRESSION

For added challenge, establish a strong start position, take the arms out to the sides, and balance with the trunk upright. In this balanced position, straighten and bend the front leg 3-5 times before placing the hands back on the footbar and proceeding with the hamstring stretch.

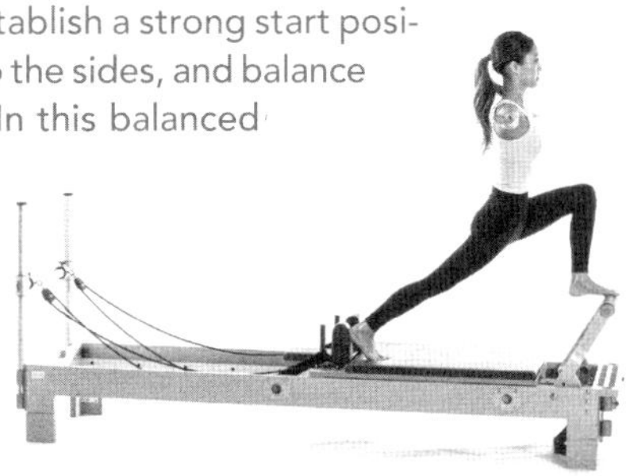

Muscle Focus

- Hamstrings
- Hip flexors

Objectives

- To improve hip flexor and hamstring flexibility
- To improve hip flexor, hamstring, and back extensor control
- To develop lumbopelvic stabilization

RESISTANCE

Light (marked) | Medium | Heavy

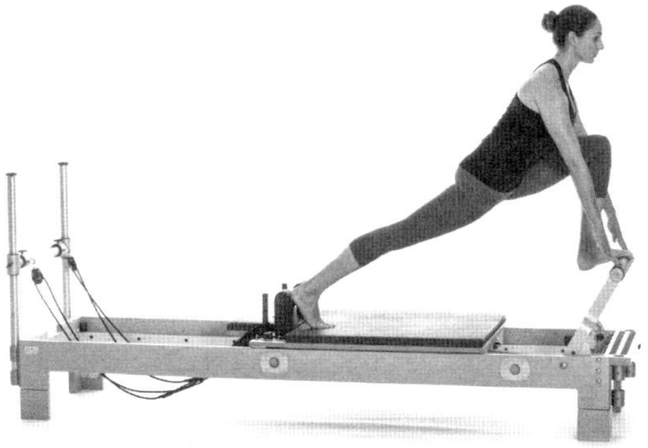

Stand on the carriage with the hands on the footbar, shoulder width apart. Press the heel of one foot against the shoulder rest, with the toes forward of the shoulder rest. Place the toes of the other foot on the footbar, with the front knee directly over the ankle. Keep the back leg straight and focus on the hip flexor stretch. Hold for 3-5 breath cycles.

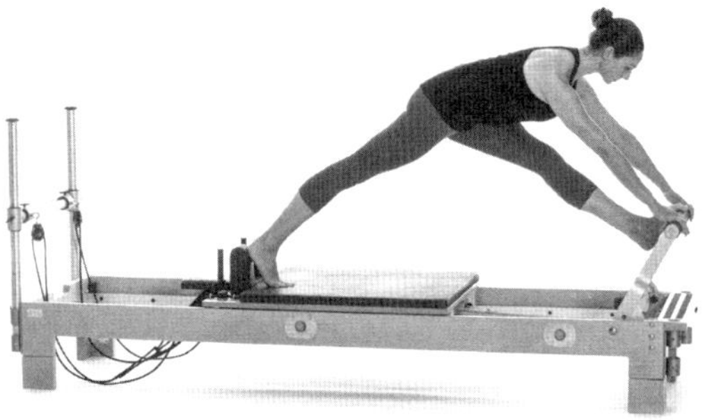

Straighten the front leg, hinging the trunk forward. Tilt the pelvis anteriorly, maintaining the back extensor engagement. Keep the head aligned with the spine on the centerline of the body and focus on the hamstring stretch. Hold for 3-5 breath cycles.

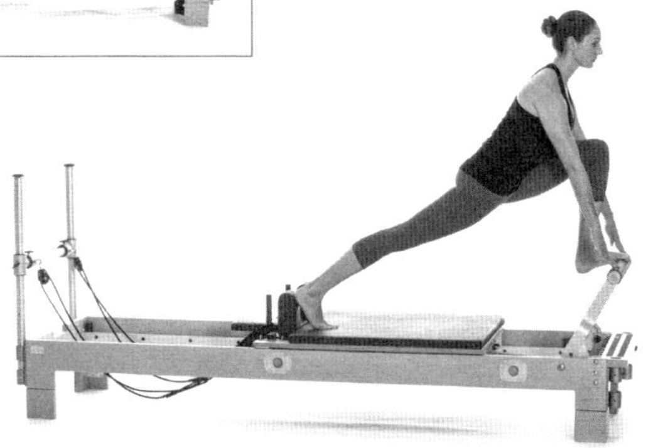

Bend the front knee and lift the trunk, with the pelvis traveling forward along the horizontal plane. Return to the start position. Repeat before switching to the other side.

Full Body Integration (FBI)

This block possibly exemplifies the Pilates philosophy better than any other. It is about the body working as an integrated, well-lubricated, and well-calibrated machine. In essence, all Pilates exercises are about the body working as an integrated unit; however, the exercises in this block are those that defy categorization by region, relying entirely on the integration of the whole body for their performance and a successful outcome.

The many exercises in this block have been further categorized according to level of difficulty and complexity. Full body integration I includes the fundamental- to intermediate-level exercises. Full body integration II includes the advanced- and master-level exercises. All exercises in FBI I should be mastered before proceeding to the higher-level exercises of FBI II. In fact, many of the exercises in FBI II are a progression of those learned in FBI I. However, bear in mind that Pilates is not about learning the higher-level work and then never again doing the more fundamental exercises. Sessions should include a wide variety of exercises from the different levels, which are appropriate for each individual. All FBI exercises demand a high level of body awareness; the better the understanding of the work, the deeper and more profound the results.

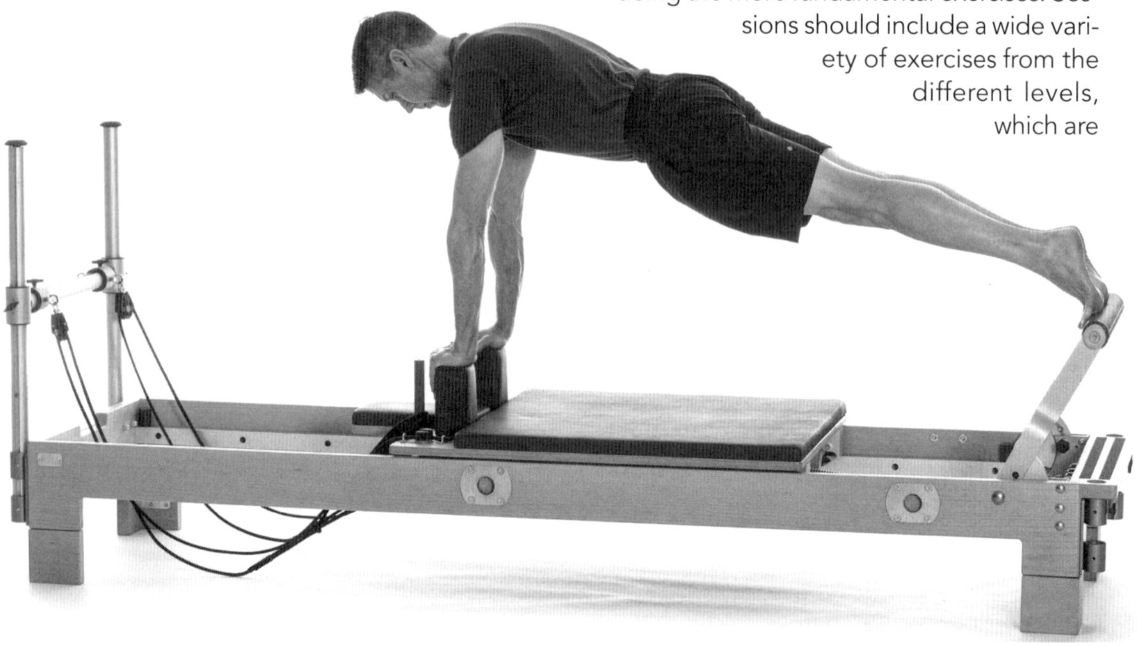

Several of the FBI exercises, such as the Reformer: Scooter, Knee Stretch—Round Back, Knee Stretch—Flat Back, Elephant, and Up Stretch emphasize the *in* (forward) phase of the movement. In these instances, this will occur as the spring is shortening and the resistance decreasing. However, the breath pattern dictates that you exhale, which we typically do on the exertion (the resistance increasing). In these cases, I regard the leg going back as a *windup* for the leg coming forward, which is the *action*. When working with a medium resistance, you resist the pull of the spring as the leg comes forward (hip flexion), working the hip extensors eccentrically. When working on a light setting, the hip flexors play a prominent role, contracting concentrically to draw the legs in (together with minimal assistance from the springs). However, whether lighter or heavier, keep the dynamic of the exercise consistent, emphasizing the power of the movement during the exhale and the slower windup during the inhale. In some of the exercises, such as the Reformer: Knee Stretch—Reverse, there is an increase in the resistance during the exhale as the legs move toward the trunk, with the hip flexors working concentrically. In these exercises, the abdominals and back extensors work as stabilizers of the trunk and pelvis to facilitate efficient movement of the legs (disassociation).

The resistance of the springs must correspond with the objectives of the exercise, whether the emphasis is on strength or stability. Differing tensions will result in very different outcomes. Increasing the tension of the springs offers more support and at the same time focuses on developing strength in the musculature of the limbs, whereas decreasing the tension highlights pelvic and trunk stabilization. I typically recommend starting with an emphasis on stabilization, working with relatively light resistance.

Scooter

The Reformer: Scooter highlights the concept of disassociation, in which one region of the body remains stable, supporting another part of the body that is moving. In this exercise, the trunk, supporting leg, and pelvis remain stable while the other leg moves back and forth. The intention is to extend the moving leg as close to the point of full hip extension as possible without compromising pelvic stabilization. Given the positioning of the pelvis in a posterior tilt, this may mean that the knee does not straighten completely, depending on the flexibility of the hip flexors.

In establishing the position of the trunk, the first step is to draw in the abdominals and round the back. The flexion is focused in the lumbar spine, although clearly the entire spine is in flexion. Initiating the flexion from the lumbar region and allowing the pelvis, upper back, and head to respond to this action creates the desired shape (large C curve) and elicits the desired muscle activation.

There is a tendency to focus on recruiting the gluteals. This will often result in excessive posterior tilt of the pelvis (tucking) and inhibit the unobstructed movement of the hip joint. There is also a tendency to exaggerate the rounding of the upper back, which is due in part to the natural direction of the curve of the thoracic spine. This should be avoided. It diminishes the focus on engaging the abdominals and stretching the lumbar region, plus it often results in shoulder elevation. Furthermore, it reinforces round-shoulder (kyphotic) posture, which is undesirable.

Imagery

The position should resemble a sprinter pushing back into the starting block before a race. It exemplifies power about to be unleashed. The power surges as the leg comes forward.

- ○ Maintain a consistent C curve through the spine, including the head.
- ○ Avoid elevating the shoulders.
- ○ Focus on hip disassociation and lumbopelvic stabilization.
- ○ Keep the wrists neutral and firm, with thumbs and fingers together and straight (or gently wrapped around the footbar).

Muscle Focus

- Abdominals
- Back extensors
- Hip extensors
- Knee extensors

Objectives

- To develop lumbopelvic and trunk stabilization
- To develop hip disassociation
- To improve hip extensor and knee extensor control
- To improve hip extensor and knee extensor strength (use medium-heavy resistance)

RESISTANCE

Light — Medium — Heavy

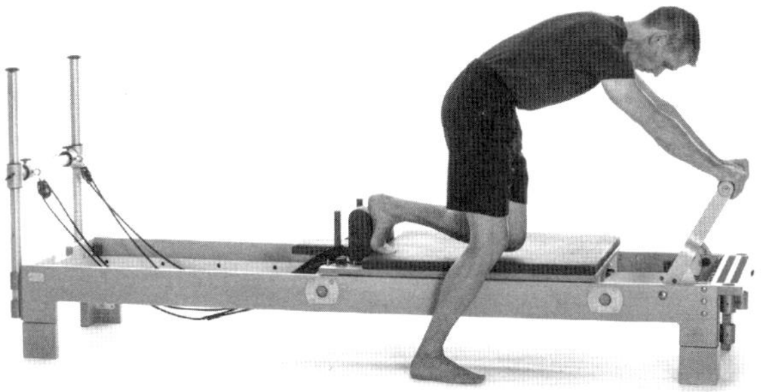

Setup. Place the hands on the footbar, with the arms straight. Note that the inside hand is opposite the shoulder; however, in order for the outside hand to be on the footbar, it cannot be directly opposite the shoulder. Press one foot against the shoulder rest, with the knee slightly off the carriage. Place the other foot on the ground alongside the reformer. Bend the knee of the standing leg. Draw in the abdominals and round the trunk.

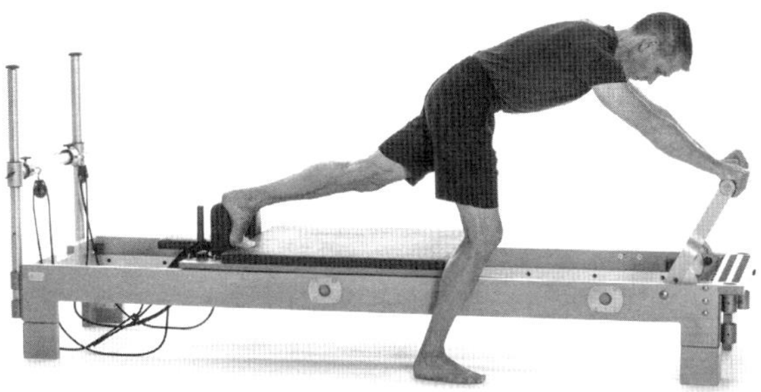

Inhale. Extend the leg that is on the carriage, moving the carriage away from the stopper. Pause before the point at which the pelvis would start to move in an anterior direction.

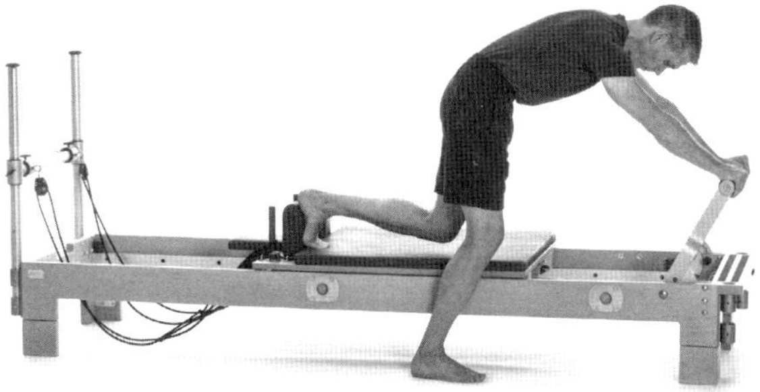

Exhale. Draw the leg forward, bringing the carriage toward the stopper. Emphasize the inward motion, maintaining stability of the shoulders, trunk, and pelvis. Pause before the point at which the pelvis would start to move in a posterior direction. Repeat 10 times before switching to the other side.

Knee Stretch—Round Back

Muscle Focus

- Abdominals
- Back extensors
- Hip extensors
- Knee extensors

Objectives

- To develop lumbopelvic and trunk stabilization
- To develop hip disassociation
- To improve hip extensor and knee extensor control
- To improve hip extensor and knee extensor strength (use medium-heavy resistance)

RESISTANCE

Light | Medium | Heavy

This exercise also uses the concept of disassociation, with the trunk in the same position as the Reformer: Scooter, except that now you are kneeling on the carriage with both knees, and both legs are moving. This makes for a much less stable position, significantly increasing the level of difficulty of the exercise. Maintaining stability of the trunk, including the pelvis, as the legs move is crucial. Note that the range of the extension of the legs in this exercise is smaller than in the Reformer: Scooter.

Achieving the desired alignment of the spine involves rounding (flexing) the lumbar spine and allowing the upper back and pelvis to respond, resulting in a gentle curve of the entire spine (including the head). I advise not tucking the pelvis or contracting the gluteals excessively; doing so restricts the movement of the hip joints, which in turn transfers the pivot point of the movement from the hips to the lumbar spine.

Imagery

Imagine the legs swinging back and forth like a pendulum that is placed on a slight diagonal. As the pendulum swings against gravity, the movement is slightly slower, and as it returns (with gravity assisting), the movement becomes more dynamic.

- ○ Maintain a consistent C curve through the spine, including the head.
- ○ Emphasize the inward phase of the movement.
- ○ Draw the carriage forward, as close to the stopper as possible (without tucking the pelvis).
- ○ Keep the wrists neutral and firm, with thumbs and fingers together and straight (or gently wrapped around the footbar).

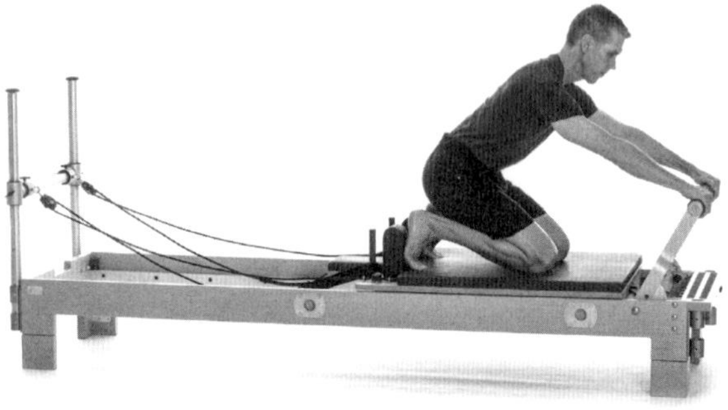

Setup. Kneel on the carriage and sit on the heels, with the feet against the shoulder rests. Place the hands on the footbar, shoulder width apart, with the arms straight. Draw in the abdominals, round the trunk, and lift the pelvis off the heels.

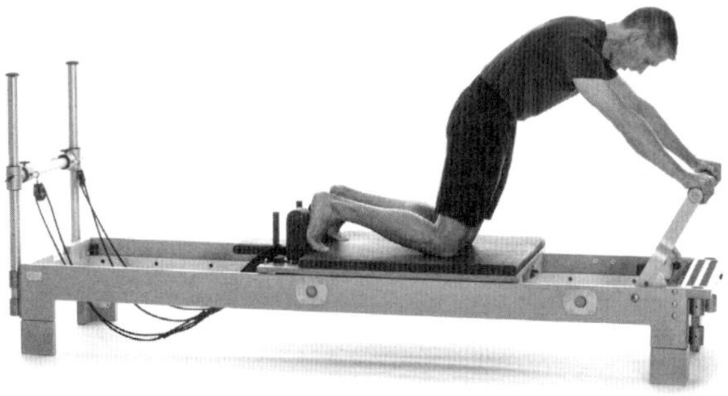

Inhale. Extend the hips, moving the carriage away from the stopper and keeping the arms and trunk stable.

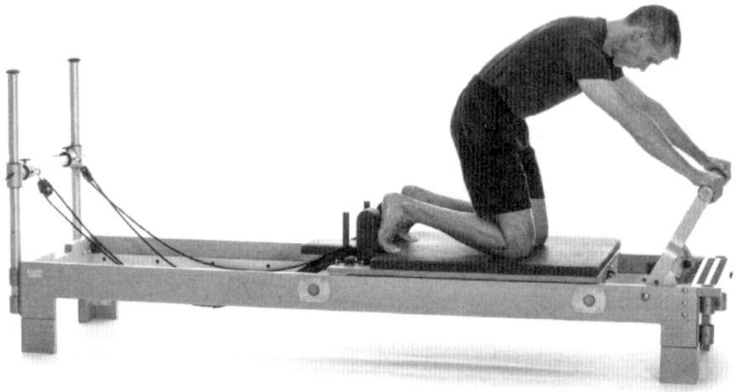

Exhale. Flex the hips, drawing the legs forward, and bring the carriage toward the stopper. Emphasize the inward motion, and maintain stability in the shoulders, trunk, and pelvis. Repeat 10 times.

Knee Stretch—Flat Back

As in the Reformer: Short Box—Flat Back exercise, *flat back* here means a neutral spine position (as opposed to an actual flat back, in which the natural lumbar curve of the spine would be eliminated). A balanced co-contraction of the abdominals and the back extensors keeps the spine in this neutral position. In fact, there is a co-contraction of the abdominals and back extensors in the Reformer: Knee Stretch—Round Back as well. It is the nuanced use of the back extensors that moderates the degree of C curve found in many Pilates exercises. All the other elements, aside from the shape of the spine, are the same between the two knee stretch exercises, particularly the emphasis on trunk stabilization and hip disassociation. A strong sense of an energy line extending from the tailbone through the trunk to the head helps maintain stability and alignment of the spine.

Imagery

Imagine a donkey kicking its hind legs while balancing on its front legs and keeping the upper body stationary, then drawing the legs in vigorously to prepare to kick again.

- ○ Maintain a neutral spine position.
- ○ Emphasize the hinging action of the legs from the hip joints.
- ○ Keep the wrists neutral and firm, with thumbs and fingers together and straight (or gently wrapped around the footbar).

PROGRESSION

To add additional challenge to this exercise in terms of shoulder girdle stability, back extensor control, and hip disassociation, lower the trunk so it is parallel to the floor (the arms should also be parallel). This position will also accommodate a larger range of motion for the legs.

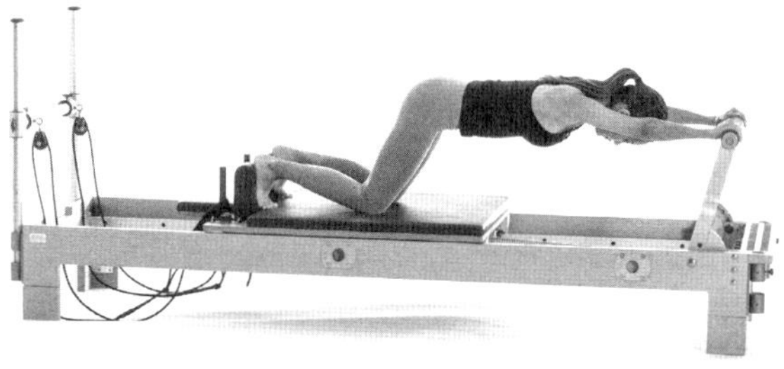

Muscle Focus

- Abdominals
- Back extensors
- Hip extensors
- Knee extensors

Objectives

- To develop lumbopelvic and trunk stabilization
- To develop hip disassociation
- To improve hip extensor and knee extensor control
- To improve hip extensor and knee extensor strength (use medium-heavy resistance)

RESISTANCE

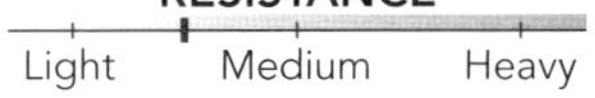

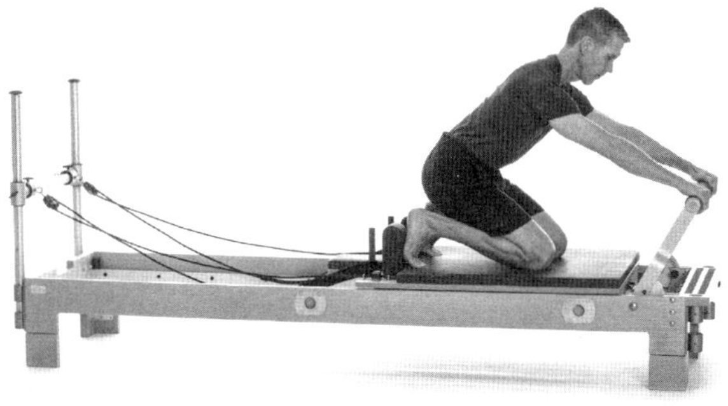

Setup. Kneel on the carriage, sitting on the heels with the feet against the shoulder rests. Place the hands on the footbar, shoulder width apart, with the arms straight. Stabilize the shoulders, maintain a neutral spine, and lift the pelvis off the heels.

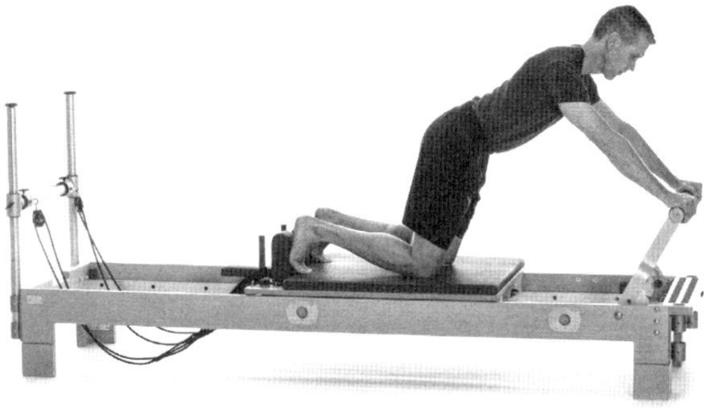

Inhale. Extend the hips, moving the carriage away from the stopper and keeping the arms and trunk stable.

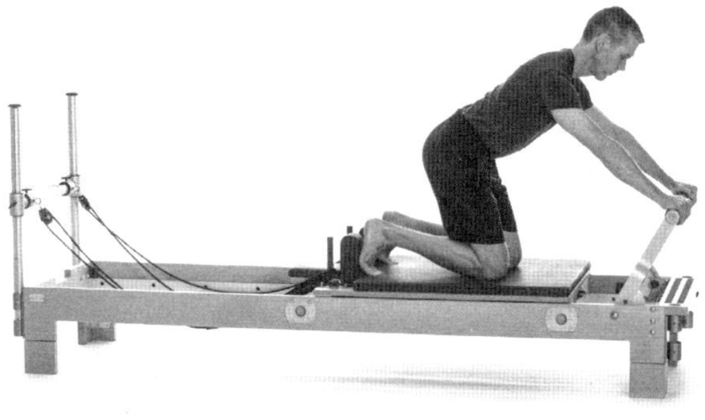

Exhale. Flex the hips, drawing the legs forward, and bring the carriage toward the stopper. Emphasize the inward motion, and maintain stability in the shoulders, trunk, and pelvis. Repeat 10 times.

Knee Stretch—Reverse

Muscle Focus

- Abdominals
- Hip flexors
- Shoulder extensors

Objectives

- To develop lumbopelvic and scapular stabilization
- To improve abdominal and hip flexor strength

RESISTANCE

Light — Medium — Heavy

This exercise focuses on three core principles: lumbopelvic stabilization, scapular stabilization, and hip disassociation. The abdominal support is crucial to keep the pelvis and trunk stable and prevent excessively loading (and potentially straining) the lower back. The juxtaposed actions—the legs moving forward and back while the upper body and the pelvis remain still—facilitate effective hip disassociation. As with most Pilates exercises, this one can be broken down to the stabilization of one area by way of isometric contractions and the movement of another through the use of both concentric and eccentric contractions.

Achieving good form during the concentric phase of the hip flexor contraction (in which the legs come forward toward the chest) is easier than during the eccentric phase (in which the legs move backward and the hip flexors elongate). Both phases demand strong abdominal support to maintain lumbopelvic stabilization while counteracting the pull of the hip flexors. However, in the eccentric phase, there is a tendency for the hip flexors to not elongate but rather remain in an isometric contraction (static). In this case the back will begin to arch as the legs move backward, particularly if the abdominals are not strong enough to counter the pull of the hip flexors on the spine.

Use caution when executing this exercise; the hip flexors are being loaded with resistance, which can potentially place stress on the lower back. For this reason I prefer to do this exercise in spinal flexion, as opposed to a neutral spine position, giving a mechanical advantage to the abdominals in protecting the spine.

Imagery

The legs move back and forth like pistons of an engine, with the driving action being on the forward motion and the control on the return. The fuel of the engine is the powerhouse, the core of the body, from which the movement emanates.

- ○ Maintain spinal flexion and scapular stabilization.
- ○ Place the arms on a slight diagonal, with the shoulders forward of the hands.
- ○ Use the shoulder extensors to counter the pull of the hip flexors.

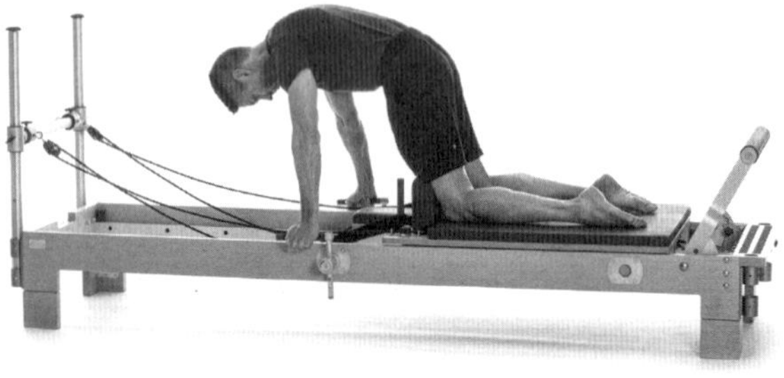

Setup. Kneel in a quadruped position, knees slightly back from the shoulder rests, placing the lower thighs against the shoulder rests and the hands on the frame of the reformer with the fingers on the outside of the rail (use the F2 handles on the BASI Systems reformer). Position the shoulders slightly forward of the hands. Stabilize the shoulder girdle, and round the trunk.

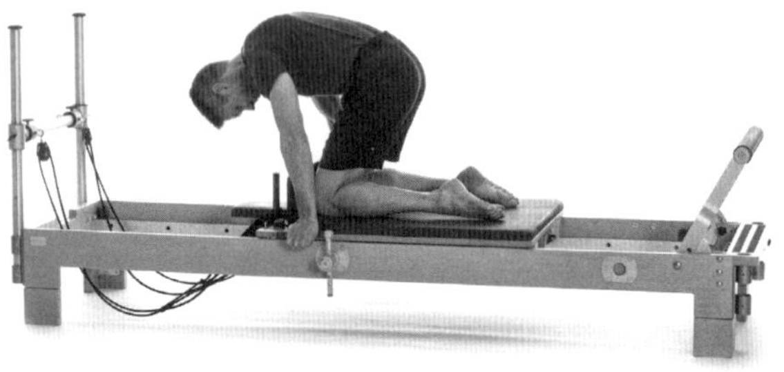

Exhale. Flex the hips, drawing the knees toward the chest, and keep the pelvis stable, maintaining the C curve of the trunk.

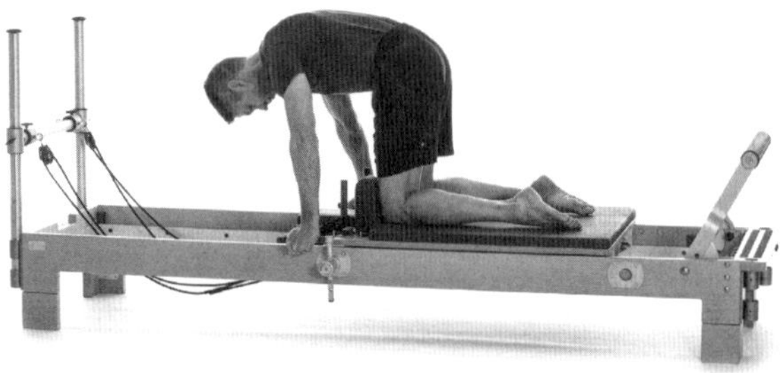

Inhale. Extend the hips without changing the position of the spine or pelvis. Return to the start position. Repeat 10 times.

Stomach Massage—Round Back

This exercise features vigorous, intense work of the legs (including the feet) while the trunk remains stable. In contrast to the supine position used for the foot work, the sitting position intensifies the demand on the muscles of the trunk, particularly the back extensors, and increases the challenge exponentially. With the trunk in an upright position rather than supine, the exercise is more functional—the muscles are used in a way that more closely simulates common upright alignment and movements and enhances postural muscle development. Daily activities such as sitting in a chair, walking, and running are frequently performed without adequate attention to proper muscle activation and support, resulting in misalignment of the trunk and possible muscle imbalance and strain. Proper execution of this exercise develops the stabilizers of the trunk and creates awareness of correct spinal alignment.

Imagery

Push against the footbar as if you were pushing a heavy box away from you or, if you were lying supine, catapulting a heavy load into the air with your legs.

- Press the hands against the front of the carriage.
- Maintain a C curve of the trunk, with the head following the line of the spine.
- Keep the shoulders above the hips.

MODIFICATION

The greatest challenge in this exercise is maintaining a stable trunk. In order to assist, place the reformer box or a large ball behind you. The ball offers good support and due to the round back position, it is more comfortable on the spine. The box offers a more solid support but may not be as comfortable as the ball. However, both will work well.

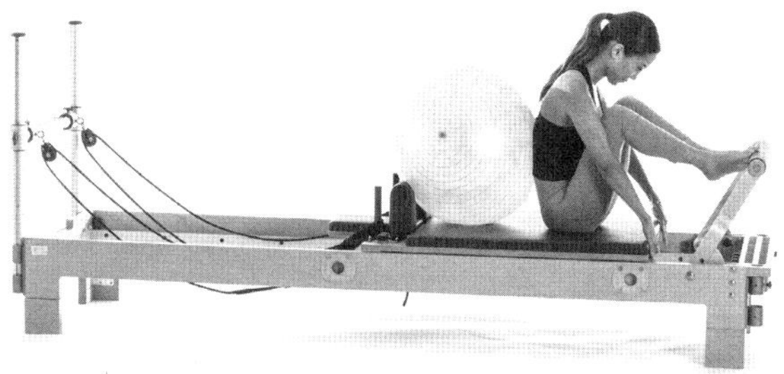

Muscle Focus

- Abdominals
- Back extensors
- Knee extensors
- Ankle–foot plantarflexors

Objectives

- To develop trunk stabilization
- To improve knee extensor and ankle–foot plantarflexor strength

RESISTANCE

Light — **Medium** — Heavy

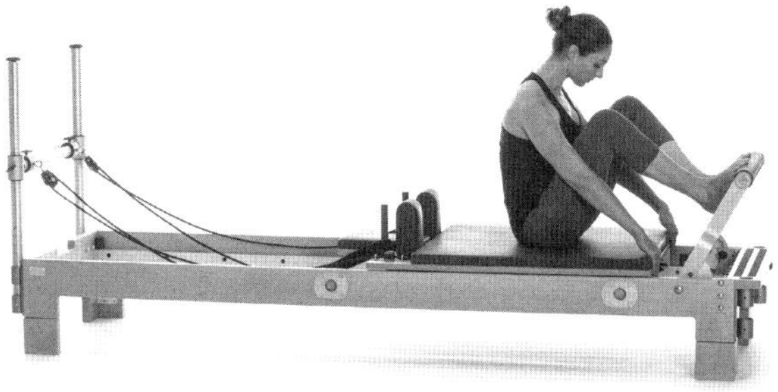

Setup. Facing the footbar, position yourself on the sit bones in the center of the carriage. Place the toes on the footbar, feet in a V position, with the heels together. Press the hands against the front of the carriage and round the trunk, positioning the shoulders directly above the hips. If you have short arms, move closer to the footbar in order to press the hands against the front edge of the carriage.

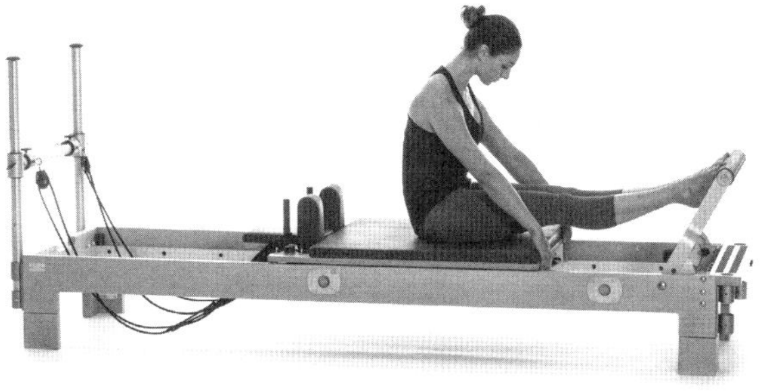

Exhale. Straighten the legs completely. Dorsiflex and then plantarflex the feet.

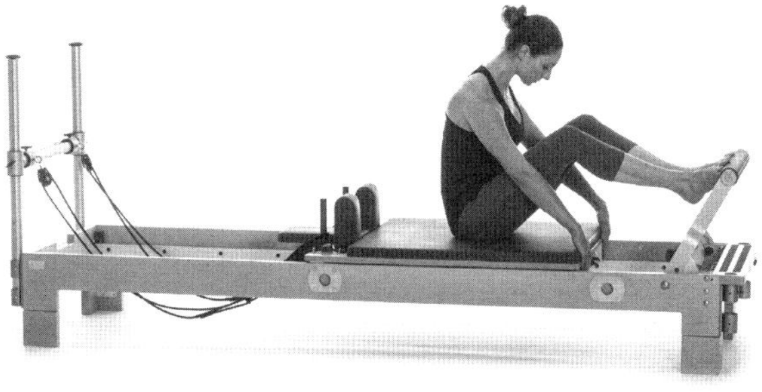

Inhale. Bend the knees. Return to the start position. Repeat 10 times.

Stomach Massage—Flat Back

Muscle Focus

- Abdominals
- Back extensors
- Knee extensors
- Ankle–foot plantarflexors

Objectives

- To develop trunk stabilization
- To improve knee extensor and ankle–foot plantarflexor strength
- To improve thoracic flexibility

RESISTANCE

Light — Medium — Heavy

This exercise shares the movement sequence of the Reformer: Stomach Massage—Round Back. The key difference is that the trunk is in a flat back position, which in this context translates to a neutral spine position (or as close as possible). The trunk should be largely supported by the musculature; the arm position simply creates a supporting frame for the body, like the flying buttresses of a bridge, and adds a stretch across the front of the chest (also felt in the anterior aspect of the shoulder). Keep the elbows pointing directly back, parallel to each other and slightly bent.

Imagery

Similar to the Reformer: Stomach Massage—Round Back, the movement can be likened to leaning against a wall and pushing a large load away or lying on the floor and catapulting a heavy load into the air with your legs.

- ○ Maximize the co-contraction of the back extensors and abdominals.
- ○ Keep the elbows parallel, slightly bent, and reaching backward.
- ○ Keep the trunk stable and upright.

PROGRESSION

Perform the movement pattern as described, but rather than placing the hands on the shoulder rests, reach them forward on an upward diagonal line, arms slightly wider than shoulder width apart. This increases the challenge of the exercise because the arms no longer offer any support, which in turn places greater demand on the stabilizers of the trunk.

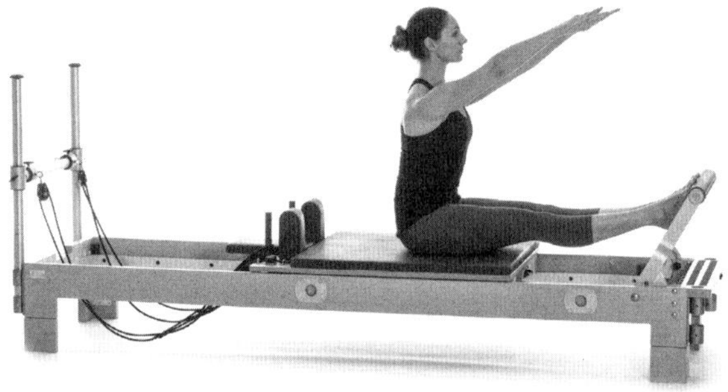

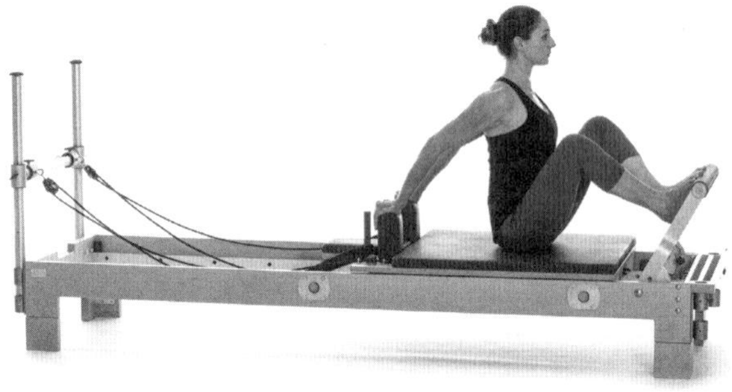

Setup. Facing the footbar, position yourself on the sit bones in the center of the carriage. Make adjustments, if need be, so that the hands sit comfortably on the shoulder rests with the fingers facing back, elbows slightly bent, and the trunk upright in a neutral spine (or as close as possible). Note that those with short arms and short legs may need to place a small box in front of the shoulder rests to achieve the desired position. Place the toes on the footbar, feet in a V position, heels pressing together.

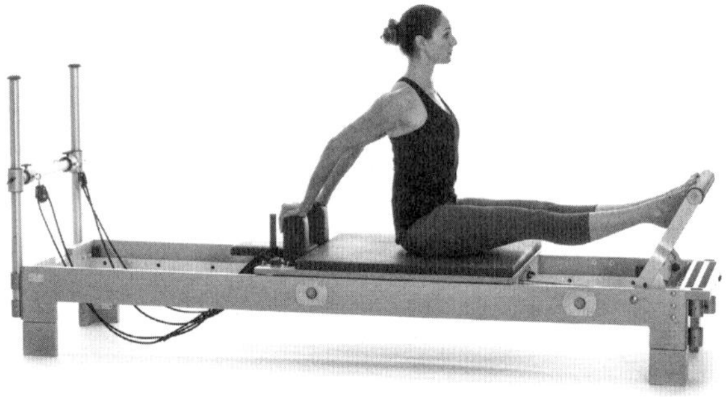

Exhale. Straighten the legs completely. Dorsiflex and then plantarflex the feet.

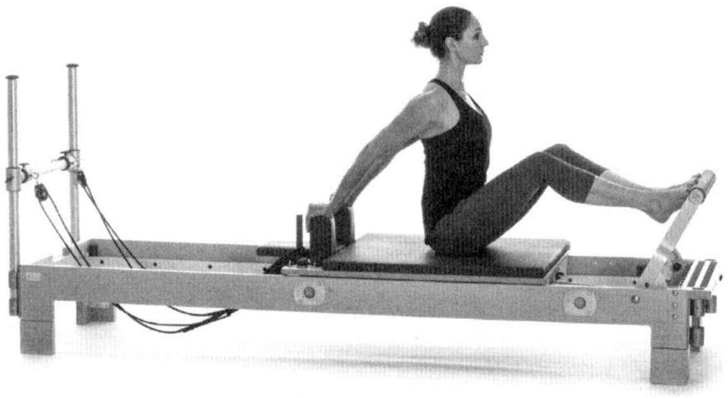

Inhale. Bend the knees. Return to the start position. Repeat 10 times.

Down Stretch

Although this exercise appears relatively simple, it demands considerable control and strength. It highlights the concept of stabilization occurring in several key areas at once: the trunk, lumbopelvic region, and scapulae. The thoracic spine is in extension as are the hips. The abdominals (which draw the pubic symphysis upward) work together with the hamstrings (which draw the sit bones downward) to keep the pelvis stable with a bias toward a posterior tilt. The stable position of the pelvis, together with strong abdominal work, protects the lumbar spine from excessive pressure and amplifies the hip flexor stretch.

The shoulder joint acts as a pivot point for the movement. The shoulder flexors, together with gravity, move the carriage out. The shoulder extensors, with the assistance of the springs, lift the body from the downward phase back to the stopper. Emphasize extension of the thoracic spine as the body rises in the upward phase. Note that the lighter the resistance, the more challenging the exercise becomes.

Imagery

An image I have used in this exercise for many years is the figurehead of an old, wooden ship. Imagine it rolling up and down as the ship sails over huge swells in the ocean. I also like to visualize a fishing line connected to the sternum during the up phase of the movement. As the line is reeled in from above, it helps lift the body, particularly the chest.

- Maintain a slight arc shape of the body.
- Bias toward a posterior tilt of the pelvis.
- Keep the back, hip, and shoulder extensors working.
- Press the heels against the shoulder rests, keeping the legs parallel.

Muscle Focus

- Abdominals
- Back extensors
- Shoulder extensors

Objectives

- To develop trunk and scapular stabilization
- To improve shoulder extensor and upper back extensor control

RESISTANCE

Light — Medium — Heavy

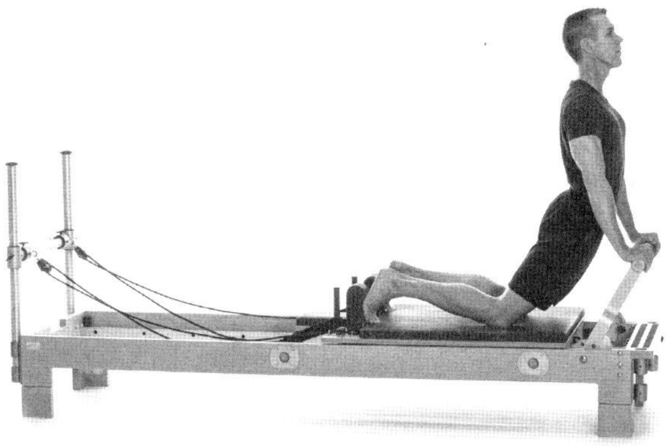

Setup. Kneel on the carriage facing the footbar. Place the hands on the footbar, shoulder width apart, with arms straight. Place the feet against the shoulder rests, with the legs parallel. Establish a line that runs from the knees through the thighs, hips, trunk, and shoulders and out the top of the head.

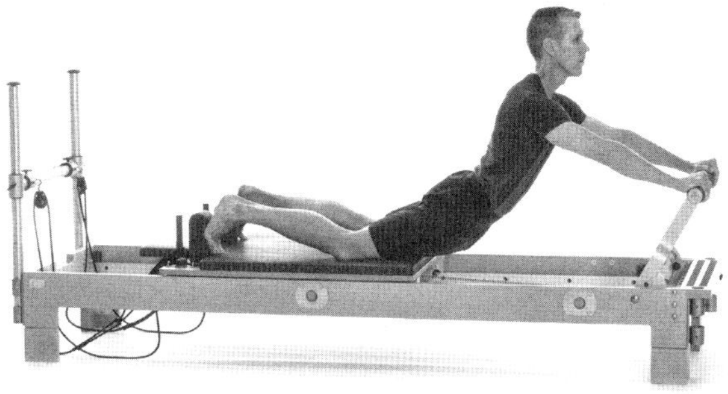

Exhale. Push the carriage back, pivoting from the shoulders and maintaining the arc shape of the body.

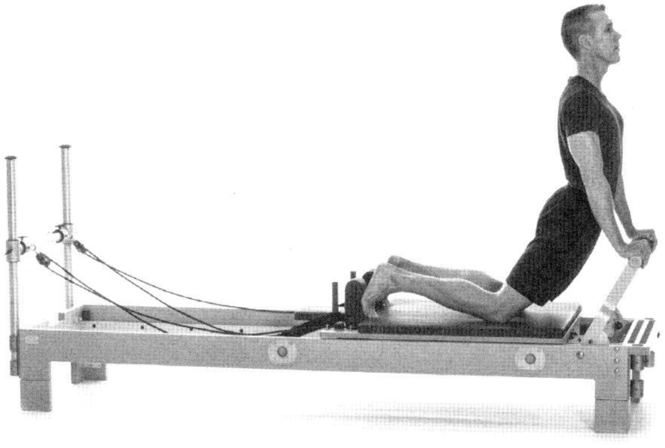

Inhale. Extend the shoulders, pressing down onto the footbar to bring the body up to the start position. Hold the carriage against the stopper momentarily before pushing back. Repeat 10 times.

Elephant

Muscle Focus

- Abdominals
- Back extensors
- Hip flexors
- Scapular stabilizers

Objectives

- To develop trunk and scapular stabilization
- To improve hamstring and shoulder flexibility
- To improve hip flexor control
- To improve core strength

RESISTANCE: Light — Medium — Heavy

The Reformer: Elephant and the Reformer: Up Stretch are almost identical, except that the Reformer: Elephant is performed with the feet flat. This adjustment increases the stretch down the back of the legs, which can be further magnified by lifting the toes. Although this exercise is sometimes performed with a round back, my preference is to keep the back flat, establishing one long line from the hip joints through the trunk, shoulders, arms, and hands. This ensures strong work of the back extensors (in co-contraction with the abdominals), particularly those of the mid- and upper back. Keeping the back flat accommodates a deep stretch of the shoulders and, in addition, by activating the back extensors, the pelvis is pulled in an anterior direction, accentuating the hamstring stretch.

The legs should move back and forth fluidly, pivoting from the hip joint and emphasizing the inward phase. The legs are pulled in by the springs and hip flexors, depending on the resistance. When the resistance is medium, the springs pull the carriage in and not only do the hip flexors not do the work, their antagonist, the hip extensors, work eccentrically to control the movement and resist the pull of the springs. However, when the resistance is light, the focus is on stabilization. In this case, the hip flexors will work to draw the carriage in. The lighter the resistance, the more demand there is on the hip flexors. The range of motion of the movement and the distance the carriage travels should be relatively small.

Imagery

The legs move like pendulums swinging from the hip joints. The movement should be disassociated from the pelvis and the trunk. The image of using the abdominals to pull the legs in deepens the abdominal work (although physiologically, of course, the abdominals do not pull the legs in). Two energy lines are present throughout: One runs from the hips through the trunk, shoulders, and arms; the other runs from the hips down the legs and through the heels. Together they form a pyramid, with the tailbone as the top point. The carriage forms the solid base of the pyramid.

- ○ Maintain stability of the arms, shoulders, and trunk.
- ○ Align the head with the spine and maintain the pyramid shape.
- ○ Keep weight on the heels to maximize the stretch down the back of the legs.
- ○ Distribute the weight evenly between the upper body and the legs.

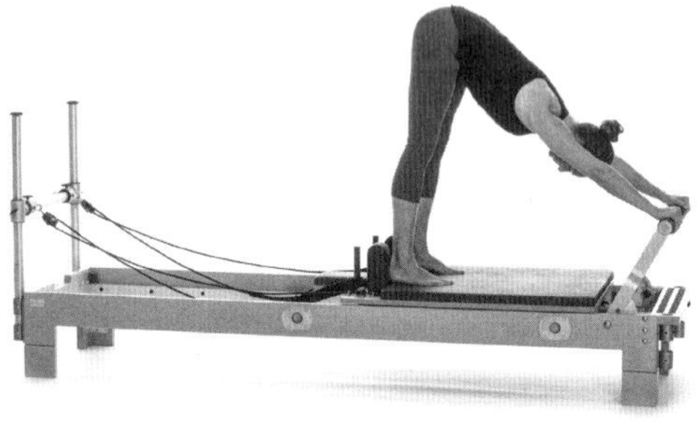

Setup. Stand on the carriage. Place the hands on the footbar shoulder width apart, wrists neutral and firm, with thumbs and fingers together and straight (or gently wrapped around the footbar). The feet should be flat on the carriage with the heels against the shoulder rests. (Optional: Lift the toes slightly.) The pelvis should be high in the air, creating a pyramid shape with the body.

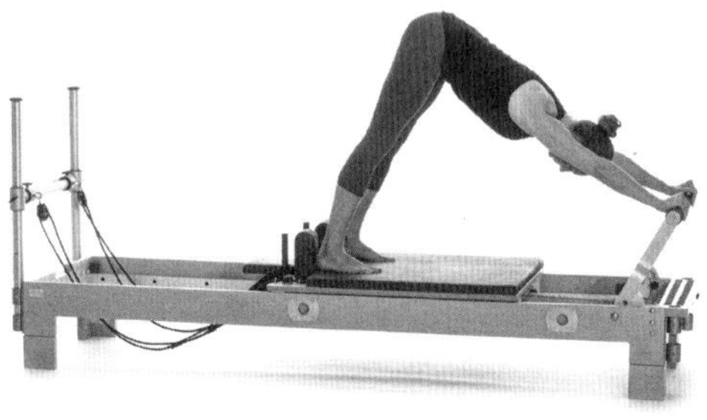

Inhale. Extend the hips, hinging at the hip joint and moving the carriage back.

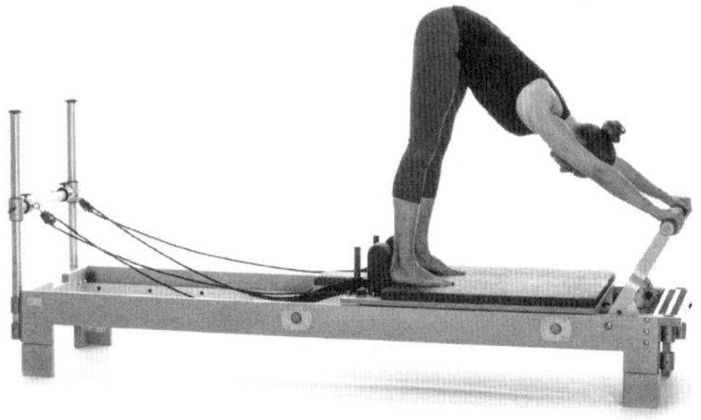

Exhale. Flex the hips, moving the carriage forward toward the stopper. Return to the start position. Repeat 10 times.

Note in this exercise and the Reformer: Up Stretch, there is no need to actually touch the stopper. Certainly if flexibility and control allow, then you should do so; however, the goal is to bring the carriage as close to the stopper as possible while maintaining perfect alignment.

Up Stretch

This exercise and others that are based on the pyramid position are about creating straight lines and pivoting from specific joints. The line of the body extends from the hips through the trunk, shoulders, arms, and hands. With this line serving as a solid foundation, the legs merely move in and out like a pendulum, creating a second straight line. Trunk stabilization and core strength are the essence of this exercise, with a coordinated contraction of the abdominals (which prevent hyperlordosis as the carriage moves out) and the back extensors (which prevent spinal flexion as the carriage returns toward the stopper). The shoulders should remain firm and stable, establishing a strong connection to the trunk. There are several variations of the Reformer: Up Stretch; this exercise forms the foundation for the more complex and advanced versions.

As with many of the FBI exercises, using less resistance increases the level of difficulty, particularly challenging the body's core strength and stabilization.

Imagery

As with the Reformer: Elephant, there is a sense of pulling the legs in with the abdominals, although it is important to reiterate that the abdominals serve as stabilizers and play no part in the movement of the legs. I like to visualize a pyramid, with the tailbone as its tip and the feet and hands as the ends of its base. The size of the base changes as the legs move back and forth, but the pyramid shape remains consistent, with the tailbone reaching skyward.

- ○ Maintain stability of the arms, shoulders, and trunk.
- ○ Align the head with the spine.
- ○ Press the heels into the shoulder rests.

Muscle Focus

- Abdominals
- Back extensors
- Hip flexors
- Scapular stabilizers

Objectives

- To develop trunk and scapular stabilization
- To improve hamstring and shoulder flexibility
- To improve hip flexor control
- To improve core strength

RESISTANCE

Light — Medium — Heavy

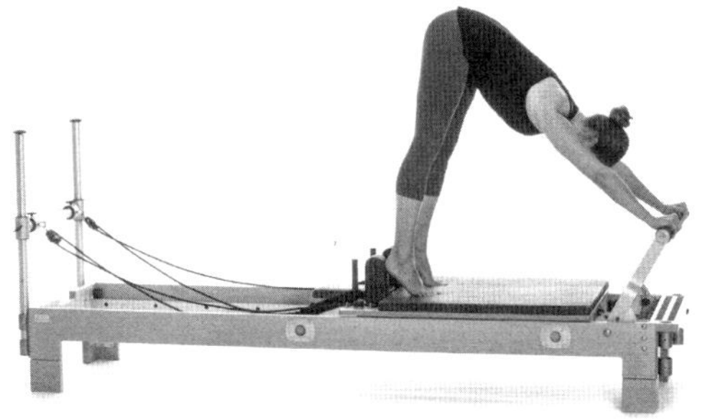

Setup. Stand on the carriage. Place the hands on the footbar shoulder width apart, wrists neutral and firm, with thumbs and fingers together and straight (or gently wrapped around the footbar). Press the heels into the shoulder rests about halfway up. The pelvis should be high in the air, creating a pyramid shape with the body.

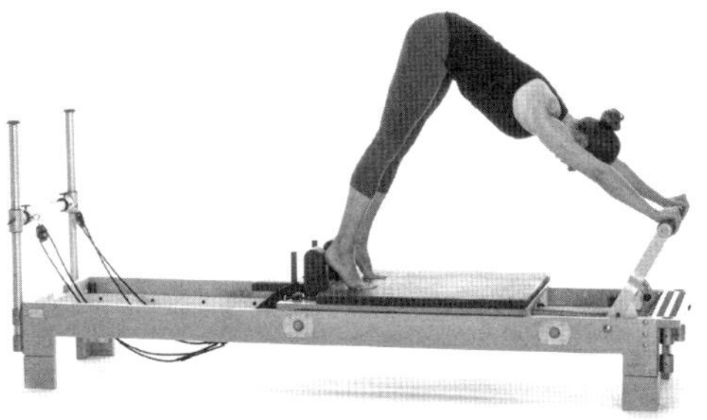

Inhale. Extend the hips, hinging at the hip joint, stabilizing the trunk and shoulders, and moving the carriage back.

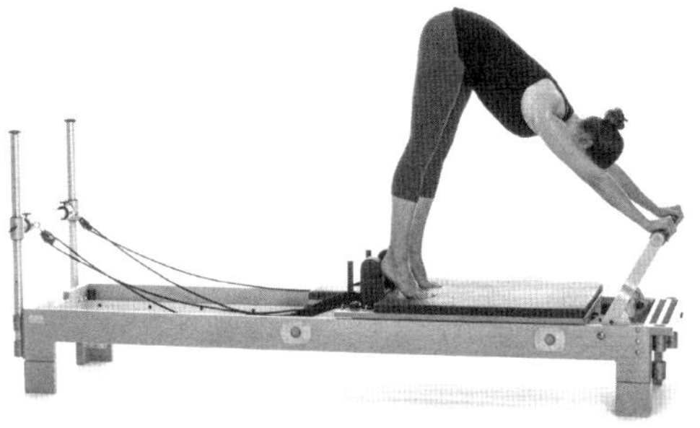

Exhale. Flex the hips, hinging at the hip joint, moving the carriage forward toward the stopper. Return to the start position. Repeat 10 times.

Long Stretch

Muscle Focus

- Abdominals
- Scapular stabilizers
- Shoulder flexors

Objectives

- To develop trunk and scapular stabilization
- To improve shoulder flexor and core strength

RESISTANCE

Light | Medium | Heavy

The Reformer: Long Stretch begins in the Reformer: Up Stretch position. The pelvis is lowered from this high point to a front support position, commonly regarded as a push-up position. This is accomplished by keeping the arms stable and pivoting from the shoulder and hip joints. Then, without altering the position of the body and with the arms controlling the movement, the carriage glides toward the stopper (and reaches it if possible) until the shoulders are aligned over the wrists. The arms then push away from the footbar and the body returns to the start position.

Fitness enthusiasts who have grown up doing hundreds of push-ups will soon recognize that this exercise takes the common push-up to a whole new level of difficulty. The precision, control, and core strength achieved in the Reformer: Long Stretch can then be incorporated into all forms of the push-up on all apparatus, including the mat. This will heighten both the integrity of the alignment and the intensity of the exercise.

Imagery

Imagine being catapulted out of a cannon. This powerful image may initially seem frightening. But once you establish a strong, stable platform with the body, your confidence—and your enjoyment of performing this challenging movement—will grow. Visualize bringing the carriage all the way to the stopper, even if body mechanics and height prevent you from actually doing so.

- Maintain trunk and scapular stabilization.
- Avoid scapular elevation and adduction.
- Keep the head aligned with the spine.
- Bias toward a slight posterior tilt of the pelvis to encourage abdominal engagement; this protects the lower back and avoids sinking of the pelvis.

VARIATION

By repeating the first step of the Reformer: Long Stretch—dropping the body from the pyramid position down to the push-up position and then back up to the triangular shape of the pyramid—we essentially create a new exercise. Note that you are hinging at the shoulders and hips, keeping the arms absolutely stable. It should feel like a seesaw going up and down.

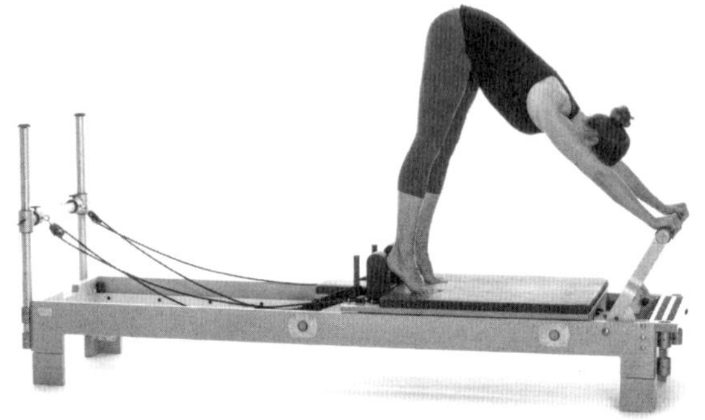

Setup. Stand on the carriage and place the hands on the footbar, shoulder width apart. Hold the pelvis high in the air, and press the heels into the shoulder rests about halfway up.

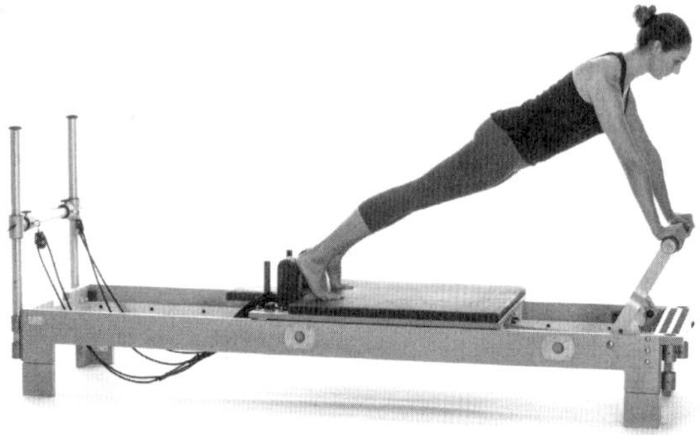

Lower the body to a push-up position without altering the angle of the arms or shifting the shoulders. Establish a 90-degree angle in the shoulder joints.

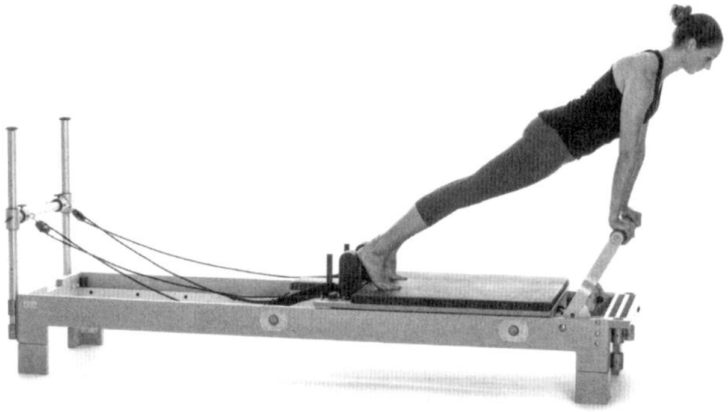

Inhale. Glide the body forward over the footbar until the carriage reaches the stopper (or as close as possible) and the shoulders are above the wrists, arms perpendicular to the footbar.

Exhale. Push the carriage back to a 90-degree angle in the shoulder joints. Repeat 5-10 times.

Balance Control Front

This exercise is reminiscent of the classic push-up position and resembles the Reformer: Long Stretch. However, it places the body in a more unstable and somewhat precarious position, which raises the level of difficulty considerably. Co-contraction of the abdominals and the back extensors creates the necessary stabilization of the trunk and pelvis plus support for the movement, exemplifying the meaning of core strength. In addition, proper form in this exercise requires scapular stabilization and immaculate control of the shoulders.

I recommend orienting the pelvis toward a posterior tilt, which provides a mechanical advantage to the abdominals and helps prevent the pelvis from sinking. This would compromise the stability of the entire structure, potentially placing pressure on the lower back and risking injury. Likewise, a bias toward scapular depression and abduction reinforces the stability of the shoulder girdle. Allowing this area to collapse may also result in strain or injury. I have added plantarflexion of the feet to the positioning of this exercise, which is classically performed with the feet either in a neutral position or dorsiflexed. The plantarflexed position gives the exercise a beautiful line as well as adding an additional dimension of challenge. As with most of the exercises oriented toward stabilization, the lighter the resistance, the more challenging the exercise becomes.

Imagery

Visualize the body suspended like a drawbridge. The movement of the arms, like the mobile section of the bridge, occurs independently of the rest of the body. There should be a sensation of floating—the more relaxed you feel, the better. In addition, visualize one strong energy line running through the body from the tips of the toes to the top of the head, and a second line running from the shoulders through the arms, hands, and fingers.

- ○ Maintain trunk and scapular stabilization.
- ○ Avoid scapular elevation and adduction.
- ○ Align the head with the spine.
- ○ Bias toward a slight posterior tilt of the pelvis to encourage abdominal engagement; this protects the lower back and avoids sinking of the pelvis.
- ○ Keep the feet plantarflexed.

Muscle Focus

- Abdominals
- Scapular stabilizers
- Shoulder flexors

Objectives

- To develop trunk and scapular stabilization
- To improve shoulder flexor and core strength

RESISTANCE

Light (marked) — Medium — Heavy

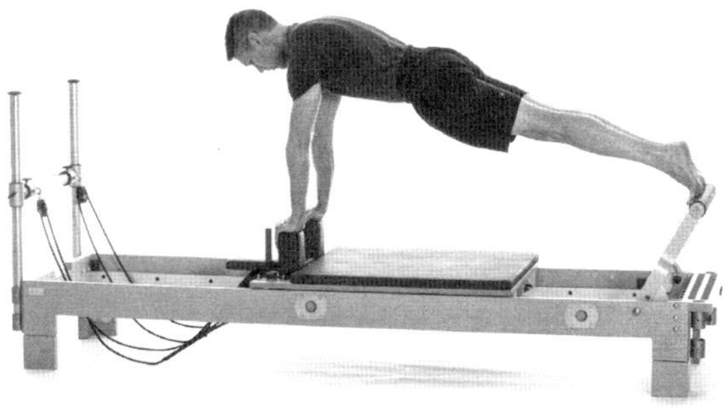

Setup. Stand on the carriage facing the back of the reformer. Place the hands on the shoulder rests and align the shoulders directly above the wrists. Place one foot on the footbar in a plantarflexed position, straighten the leg, and lower the body into a plank position, establishing stability and support. Lift the other leg and place the foot, also plantarflexed, on the footbar with minimal shifting of weight. Ensure that the body is in one straight line.

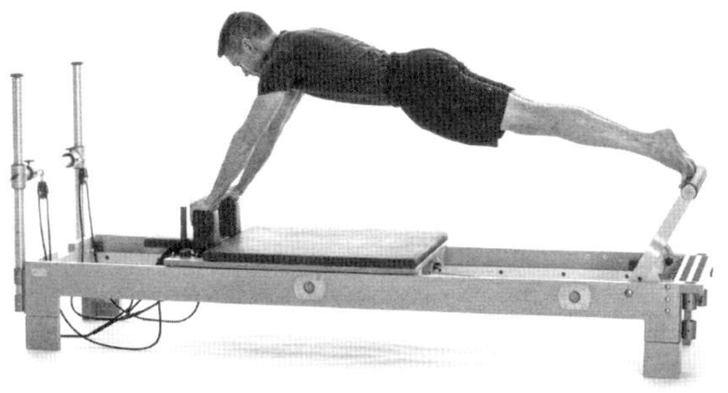

Exhale. Flex the shoulders, pushing the carriage toward the back of the reformer while maintaining a stable, plank-like position of the body. The movement is isolated to the hinging action of the shoulder joints.

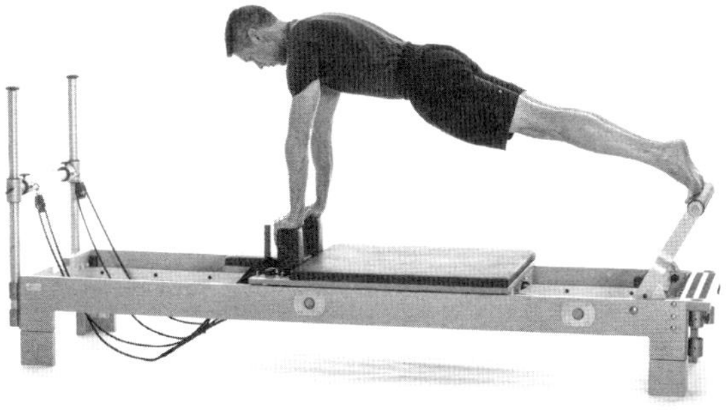

Inhale. Extend the shoulders, controlling the carriage as it moves toward the footbar. Return to the start position. Repeat 5 times.

Balance Control Back Prep

Muscle Focus

- Shoulder extensors
- Triceps
- Hamstrings
- Back extensors

Objectives

- To develop trunk and scapular stabilization
- To improve shoulder extensor and elbow extensor strength
- To improve hip extensor control

RESISTANCE

Light Medium Heavy

This exercise divides the body into two separate and distinct units in terms of function: the trunk is the upper section and the legs are the lower section. The hinging action occurs at the hip and shoulder joints. The movement is relatively small and the focus is primarily on maintaining an L shape, formed by the trunk and legs. The L shape opens slightly as the shoulders extend and the carriage is moved back, then closes as the carriage moves forward toward the stopper.

The back extensors and scapular stabilizers, fortified by the abdominals, support the upper body. The hip extensors play an important role in supporting the lower body and keeping the entire structure elevated; they should remain engaged throughout the exercise. The movement is initiated by the shoulder extensors. A common tendency, particularly when the pectorals are tight, is to round the shoulders and upper back, which eliminates the L shape and the upright trunk position. Avoid rounding, even if it means minimizing the degree of movement.

Imagery

The letter L provides a good image for the initial position. Visualize two spring hinges: one in the shoulder joint and one in the hip joint. These points open slightly and then spring back to position.

- ○ Maintain a neutral spine position.
- ○ Keep the back extensors activated.
- ○ Maintain scapular stabilization, with a bias toward scapular depression and abduction.

PROGRESSION

By taking the movement further you can do the Mat: Back Support on the reformer. This movement is often referred to as balance control back, a very challenging and advanced Pilates exercise. Initiate the movement as described, with the shoulder, hip, and back extensors. Rather than coming back to the L shape immediately, continue the movement until the body is in a long, straight line, suspended like a bridge. To allow more movement in the shoulders, which is particularly helpful for people with tight pectoral muscles, assume a more neutral (open) shoulder position by placing the hands on the sides of the shoulder rests, palms facing inward.

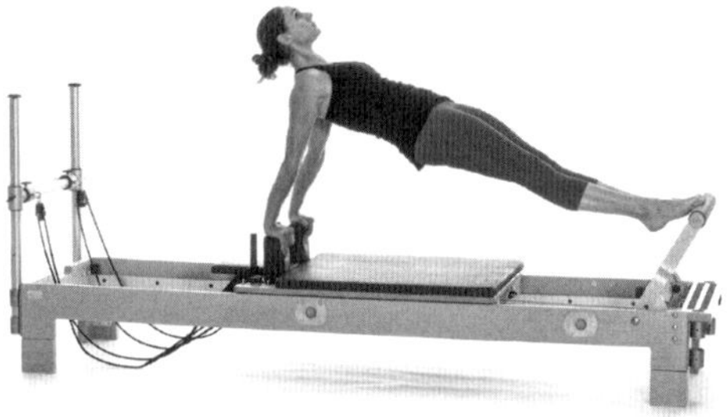

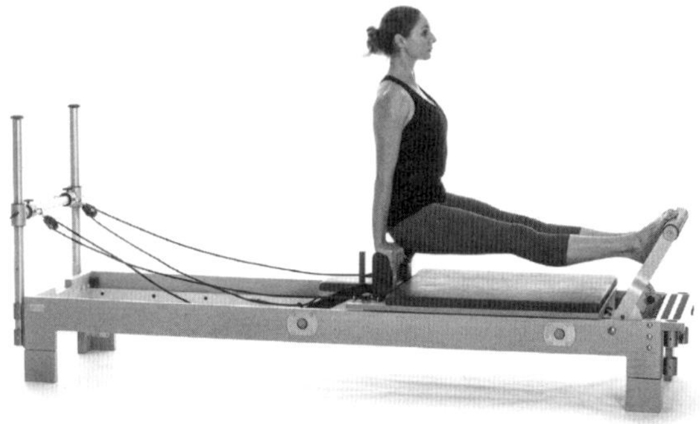

Setup. Sit on the carriage facing the footbar, hands on the shoulder rests, palms facing back. Place the toes on the footbar, feet plantarflexed and hip width apart, legs straight and parallel. Straighten the arms and lift the body up, establishing an L shape with the legs and the trunk.

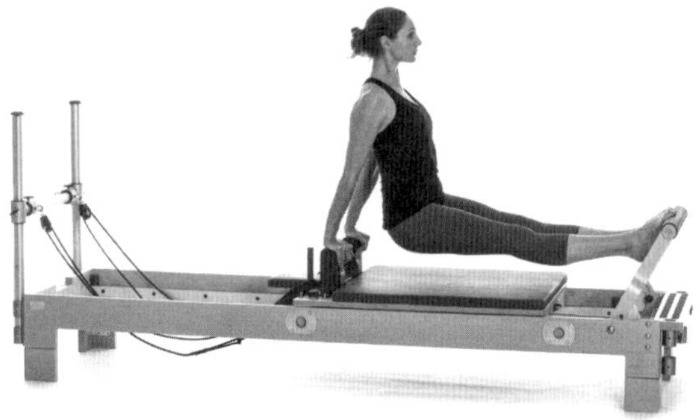

Exhale. Extend the shoulders as you push the carriage back, keeping the back straight.

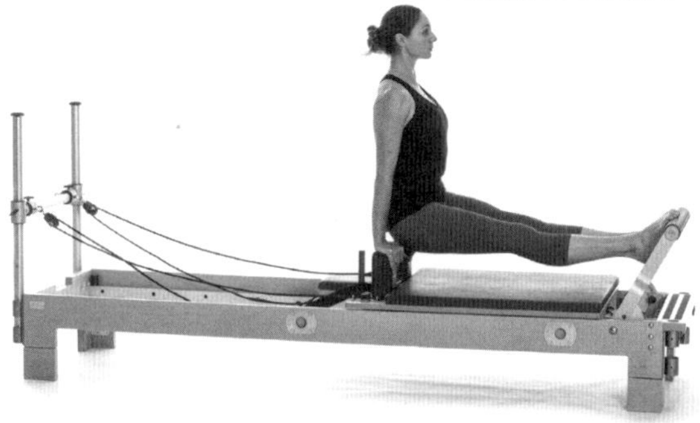

Inhale. Flex the shoulders, controlling the carriage as it comes forward toward the footbar. Return to the start position. Repeat 5 times.

Arm Work

There are myriad upper body exercises in Pilates, and many are initiated or accomplished through specific movements of the arms. I have arranged the many arm work exercises into series, or groupings, to simplify the organization of the session. This in turn maximizes flow from one exercise to the next and enhances the effect of the exercises. Rather than choose an array of individual exercises, you can choose an entire series. Each series offers a well-balanced upper body workout that challenges the body in different ways and offers variety in both execution and effect.

A crucial element in arm work is clearly the shoulder joint. The shoulder is a wonderfully mobile joint, but at the same time it is potentially very unstable. It relies primarily on the musculature for support, as opposed to bone structure and tendon and ligament support, and thus is often called a *muscle-dependent joint*. Immaculate control of the shoulder mechanism is required to reap the benefits of the arm work. As you enter into the advanced- or master-level repertoire and the movements become more difficult and complex, this fact becomes increasingly pertinent.

Correct shoulder mechanics involves a coordinated, linked movement of the humerus and scapula termed the *scapulohumeral rhythm*. Many of the movements of the arm require intricate coordination of the scapular muscles to prevent undesired actions. The scapula provides a stable base on which the arm can move. In addition, coordinated use of the rotator cuff when elevating the arm is essential to prevent undesired upward motion of the head of the humerus into the overlying structures (impingement). Without correct mechanics, it is likely that at some point problems will occur in the shoulder, the neck, or even the back.

The scapulae provide the base of support for the arms and should move in relation to the movement of the arms; however, the amount and direction of the movement must be proportional and controlled. The image used in the hip work of a spoon stirring a pot of porridge or syrup can also be used with the shoulder. The movement of the arms should be smooth and uninterrupted, with the scapulae making small, intricate adjustments to accommodate this movement. When using straps or handles, the hands can either be in a relaxed fist position or an open-hand position with the fingers straight and together. Either way, there should not be tension in the hands and the wrists should be in a neutral position.

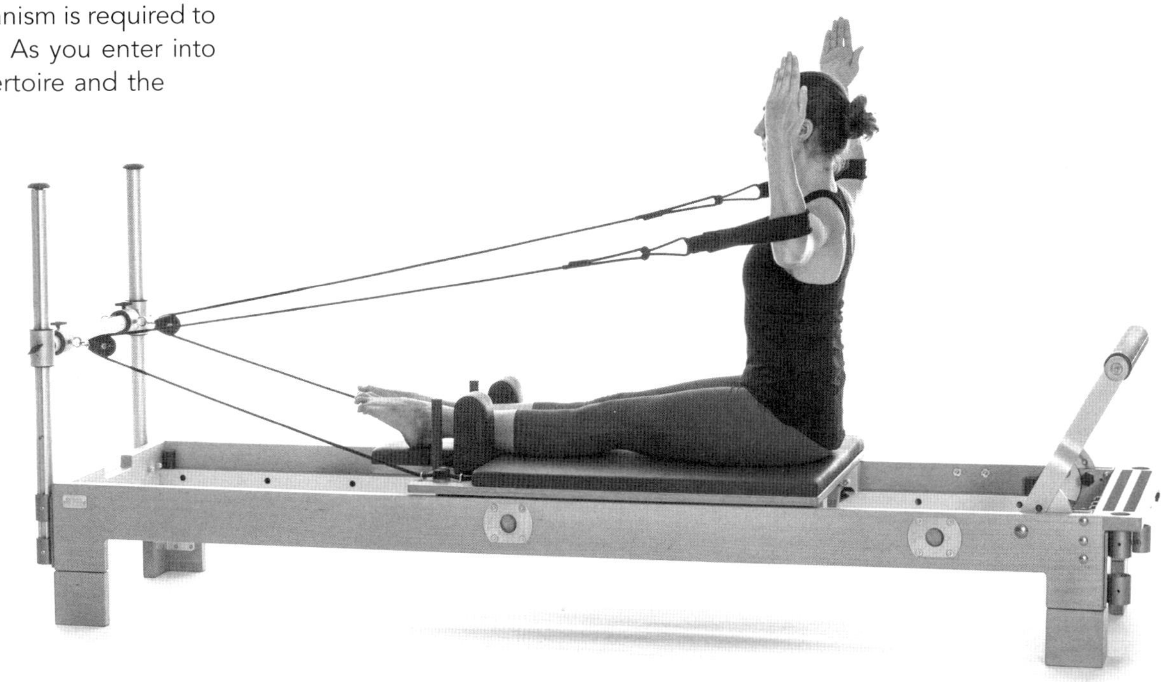

Shoulder Extension—Supine

Muscle Focus

- Shoulder extensors
- Abdominals
- Hip flexors

Objectives

- To improve shoulder extensor strength
- To improve hip flexor control
- To develop trunk and scapular stabilization

RESISTANCE
Light Medium Heavy

Performed with the spine in a neutral position, this arm work supine series requires extensive use of the core stabilizers. The emphasis is on developing a rhythmic coordination of the scapular stabilizers—specifically the lower trapezius (which helps maintain scapular depression) and the serratus anterior (which helps maintain scapular abduction)—with the muscles that move the arm, in this case primarily the latissimus dorsi. Healthy scapulohumeral rhythm facilitates smooth and unencumbered movement while preventing excessive elevation and adduction of the scapulae during movement of the arms.

The supine series is particularly valuable because it places the body in a safe, comfortable, non-weight-bearing position, developing arm and shoulder strength together with trunk stabilization. All of the work occurs in a range of motion below shoulder height, which is valuable for people who have painful conditions such as shoulder impingement, for which lifting the arm higher than the shoulder is often contraindicated.

Imagery

Imagine that you are swimming on your back and your arms are like large flippers, propelling the body through the water with each movement. Keep the movement smooth and integrated, with the body remaining stable. I always tell my students, "The better the stabilization, the better the mobilization." In essence, when movement is performed with a stable base the result will be more effective. In this case, the focus of the movement is in the glenohumeral joint and the stabilization is in the trunk and scapulae.

- Maintain lumbopelvic and scapular stabilization.
- Use a smooth and even rhythm during both the concentric and eccentric phases of the arm movement.
- Keep the arms straight, without placing excessive force on the elbows.

MODIFICATION

One of the most challenging elements of this series is holding the legs in a tabletop position for an extended period. The quadriceps and hip flexors fatigue, as do the abdominals, risking pressure on the lower back—and certainly ineffective arm work. One of the simplest solutions is to cross the legs. This is a more comfortable position than tabletop and puts less load on the hip flexors and therefore the back. Make sure to switch legs with each exercise in the series.

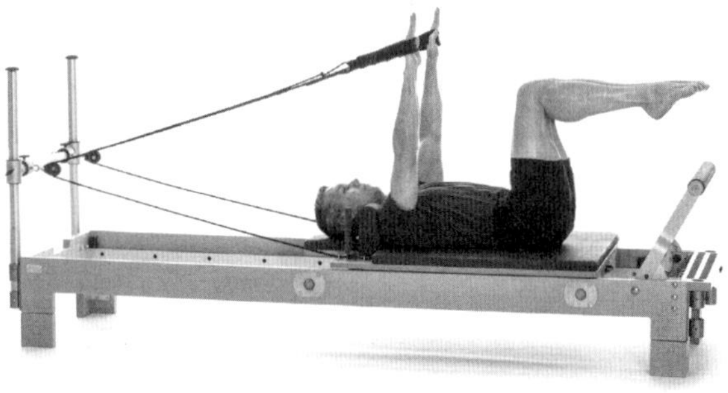

Setup. Lie supine on the reformer in a neutral spine position, knees and hips in tabletop position. Hold the arms perpendicular to the carriage, with the shoulders stable and the hands in the straps. Maintain slight tension in the straps, with the palms facing the knees.

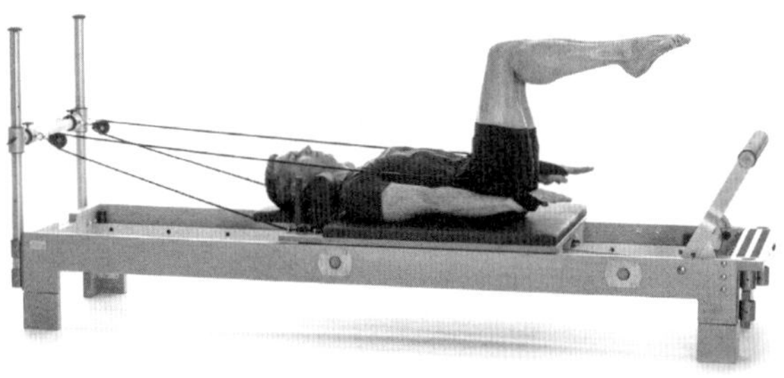

Exhale. Extend the shoulders, lowering the arms down toward the carriage. Pause when they reach the sides of the body, in line with the shoulders and parallel to the carriage.

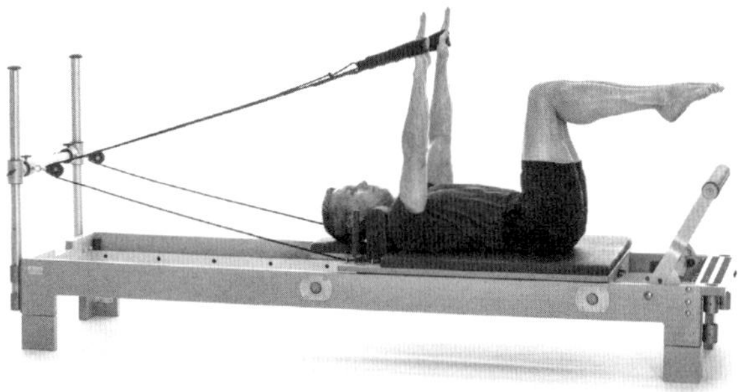

Inhale. Flex the shoulders, lifting the arms. Return to the start position. Repeat 10 times.

Shoulder Adduction—Supine

This exercise is similar to the Reformer: Shoulder Extension—Supine, except that the shoulders adduct, and the arms move to the sides of the trunk. Emphasize the same points as in the previous exercise, including rhythmic coordination of the arms and scapulae, a neutral spine, trunk stabilization, and scapular stabilization. In this exercise, the scapulae naturally tend to adduct, or squeeze together. Being in a supine position enables you to feel the scapulae against the carriage and dynamically stabilize them.

Imagery

Use the image of swimming on your back described in the previous exercise. As the arms, like large flippers, move toward the body, the body is propelled through water or soft gel.

- Maintain lumbopelvic and scapular stabilization.
- Avoid elevating and adducting the scapulae.
- Keep the arms straight, with the biceps activated, to avoid placing excessive force on the elbows (keep a micro-bend in the elbows).

PROGRESSION

An effective progression that can be used with this exercise as well as Reformer: Shoulder Extension—Supine is to lift the head and shoulder girdle into forward flexion as the shoulders extend (or in the case of Reformer: Shoulder Adduction—Supine, adduct) and lower the body as the arms return to the start position. This progression adds more movement and coordination to the exercise, as well as additional challenge for the abdominals. In the original versions of the exercises, the abdominals are certainly active as stabilizers; however, in the progression they become both stabilizers and movers.

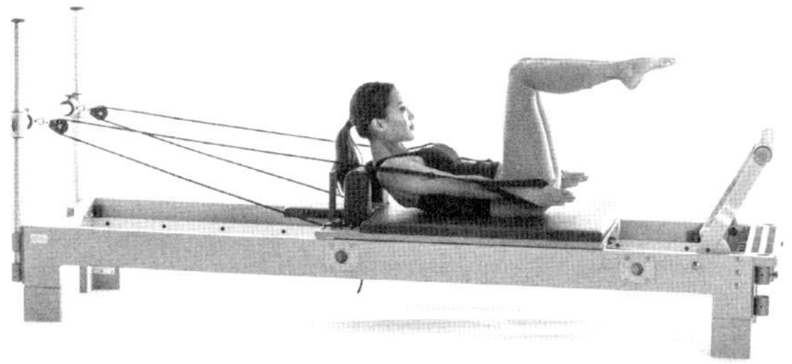

Muscle Focus

- Shoulder adductors
- Abdominals
- Hip flexors

Objectives

- To improve shoulder adductor strength
- To improve hip flexor control
- To develop trunk and scapular stabilization

RESISTANCE

Light — Medium — Heavy

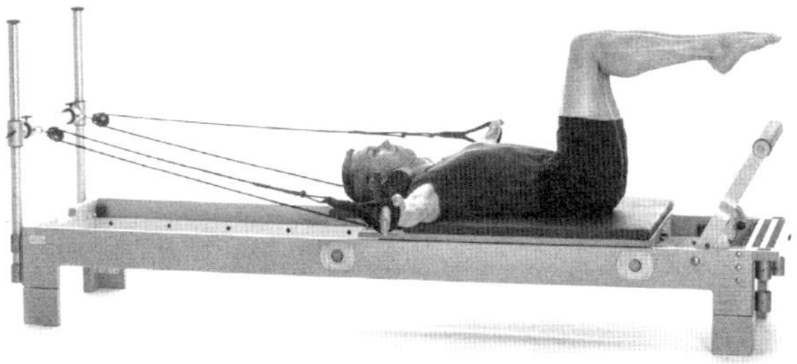

Setup. Lie supine on the reformer in a neutral spine position, with legs in a tabletop position. Hold the arms out to the sides in a T position, with the shoulders stable and the hands in the straps. Maintain slight tension in the straps, with the palms facing forward.

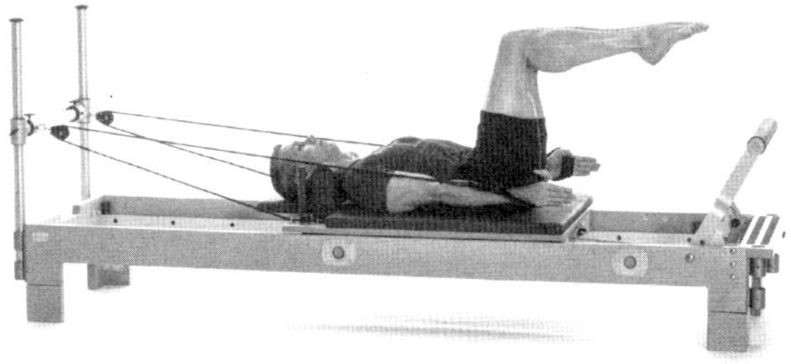

Exhale. Adduct the shoulders, pressing the arms against the sides of the body.

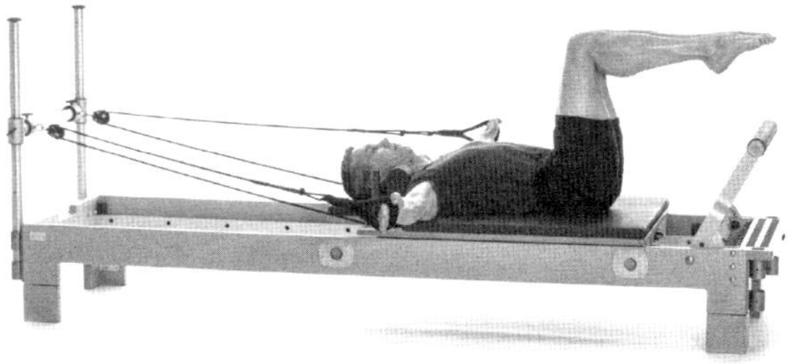

Inhale. Abduct the shoulders, opening the arms. Return to the start position. Repeat 10 times.

Arm Circle Up—Supine

Muscle Focus

- Shoulder adductors
- Shoulder extensors
- Abdominals
- Hip flexors

Objectives

- To improve shoulder adductor and shoulder extensor strength
- To improve shoulder mobility
- To improve hip flexor control
- To develop trunk and scapular stabilization

RESISTANCE
Light — Medium — Heavy

The Reformer: Arm Circle Up—Supine is a combination of the previous two exercises. The name can be misleading. Rather than tracing a true circle, the arms draw two semi-circles, drawing a straight line up the center together and then parting to draw semi-circles in opposite directions. The arm movement should be fluid and as large as possible, reaching each point of the semi-circle and rotating the shoulder accordingly.

Imagery

The feeling is like moving through gel, providing a sense of resistance. There should be no difference in sensation or presentation between the concentric and eccentric phases. The dynamic is smooth and constant.

- Do not raise the arms above shoulder height.
- Maintain flowing movement.
- Pause when the arms are alongside the body to rotate the arms, and pause again momentarily when they are perpendicular to the floor.

VARIATION

This movement is also performed in reverse. Begin the movement with Reformer: Shoulder Extension—Supine, pressing the arms down toward the carriage. When they are alongside the body, parallel to the carriage, externally rotate the shoulders so the palms face the body. Take them out to the T position, and finally bring them back to the perpendicular start position. Observe the same principles of maximizing the range of motion of the shoulders and using the movement patterns learned from the extension and adduction exercises.

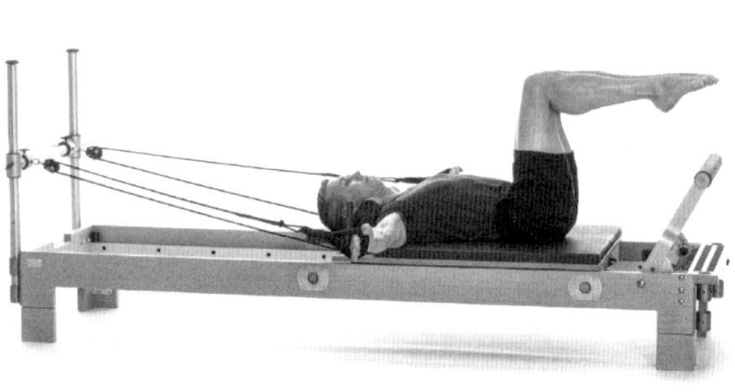

Setup. Lie supine on the reformer in a neutral spine position, legs in a tabletop position. Hold the arms out to the sides in a T position, keeping the shoulders stable, and place the hands in the straps. Maintaining slight tension in the straps, with the palms facing forward.

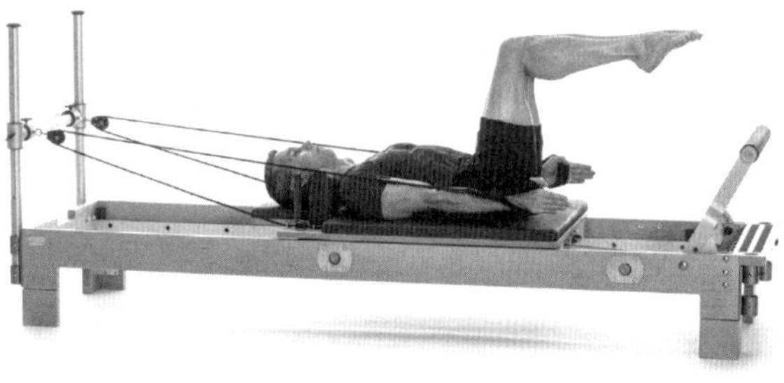

Exhale. Adduct the shoulders and press the arms against the sides of the body. Internally rotate the shoulders so that the palms face the carriage.

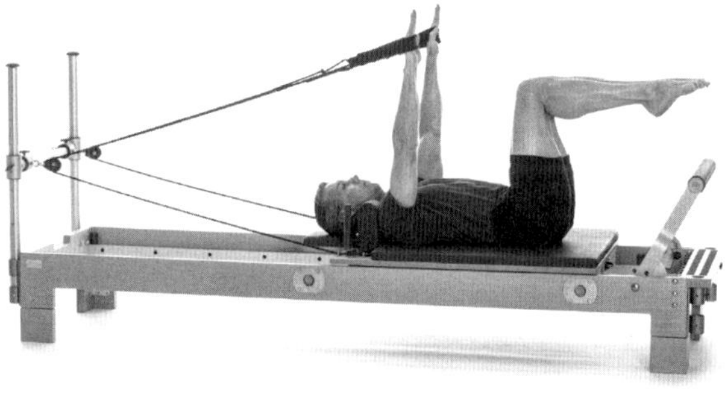

Inhale. Flex the shoulders, lifting the arms up to a perpendicular position. Open the arms out to the T position. Return to the start position. Repeat 10 times.

Triceps—Supine

The motion in this exercise focuses solely on the triceps, isolating the movement of the elbow. The wrist must remain straight and firm, creating a line from the elbow through the hand and fingers. The upper arms are parallel to the carriage, aligned with the shoulders. Press the upper arms into the sides of the body to assist in keeping them stable and maintaining correct alignment. The movement commences with the elbows at a 90-degree angle and the fingers (or fist) pointing straight up toward the ceiling. It ends with the elbows at 180 degrees, with the arms forming a straight line from the shoulders to the fingers. The upper arms remain parallel to the carriage throughout and do not push down onto the carriage. (Pushing down onto the carriage with the elbows, a common mistake, often results in adduction and elevation of the scapulae and thrusting the ribs forward.)

Imagery

Imagine pushing through water and propelling yourself with your forearms only, like an upside-down dog paddle.

- ○ Hold the upper arms parallel to the carriage.
- ○ Press the upper arms against the sides of the body and keep them stable.
- ○ Keep the wrists firm, in a neutral position (straight line with the arms).

PROGRESSION

It is possible to use the same progression for this exercise as for Reformer: Shoulder Extension—Supine and Shoulder Adduction—Supine; that is, to lift into forward flexion as the arms straighten and to lower the body as the arms bend. It is important to maintain the integrity of the arm work despite the added movement of the trunk and increased abdominal challenge.

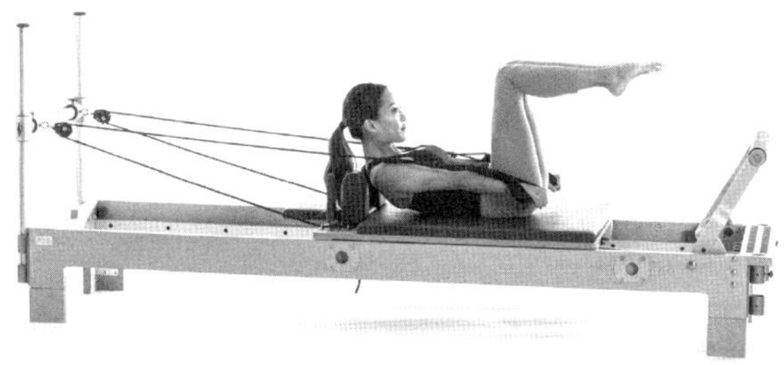

Muscle Focus

- Triceps
- Abdominals
- Hip flexors

Objectives

- To improve elbow extensor strength
- To improve hip flexor control
- To develop trunk and scapular stabilization

RESISTANCE

Light — Medium — Heavy

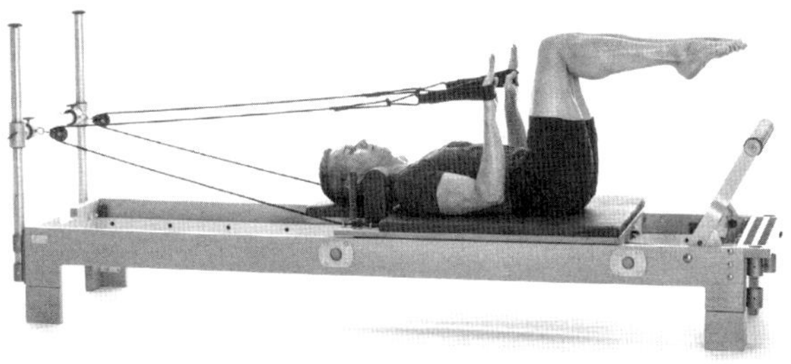

Setup. Lie supine on the reformer in a neutral spine position, with the legs in a tabletop position. Place the arms by the sides of the body, with the hands in the straps and the elbows at a 90-degree angle. Maintain slight tension in the straps, with the palms facing the footbar.

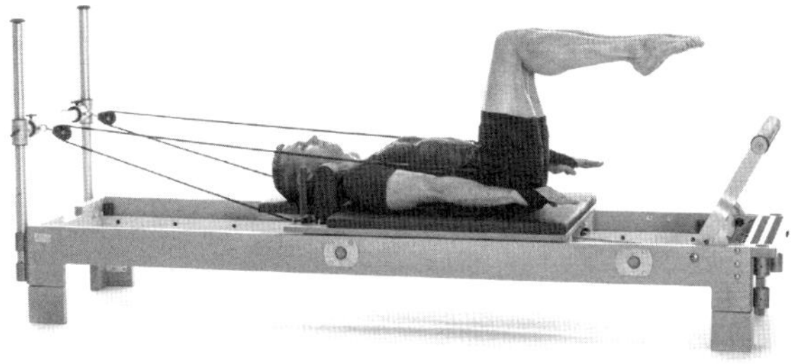

Exhale. Extend the elbows, straightening the arms and pressing the hands down toward the carriage. Pause when the arms are in a straight line, parallel to the carriage.

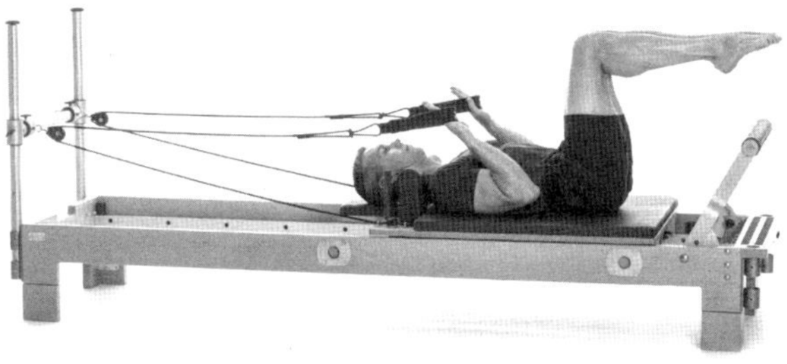

Inhale. Flex the elbows, bending the arms beyond the 90-degree angle and working the full range of motion of the elbow. Repeat 10 times.

Chest Expansion—Seated

Muscle Focus

- Shoulder extensors
- Triceps
- Back extensors

Objectives

- To improve shoulder extensor and elbow extensor strength
- To develop trunk and scapular stabilization

RESISTANCE

Light Medium Heavy

The key to this series, and debatably the most challenging aspect, is keeping the trunk upright and as close to neutral alignment as possible. This demands co-contraction of the abdominals and back extensors throughout the series. Avoid the common tendency to round the upper body or, conversely, to thrust the ribs forward. As the arms move toward the footbar, the shoulders extend beyond the centerline of the body. Precisely how far beyond the centerline the shoulders extend is dictated by strength, flexibility, and the ability to maintain correct trunk alignment. Once alignment is compromised, the exercise has exceeded its functional range of motion. Any further shoulder extension will likely cause compensations, including scapular elevation, rounding of the shoulders, and incorrect muscle recruitment.

Imagery

Many people visualize a horizontal back-and-forth motion of the arms in this exercise. I prefer to imagine the fingertips reaching down and drawing a line along the floor while the head simultaneously reaches up toward the ceiling. This image gives more of a vertical feeling.

- Keep the trunk upright and stable.
- Keep the arms straight.
- Reach the fingertips (fists) toward the floor.
- Avoid thrusting the ribs forward.

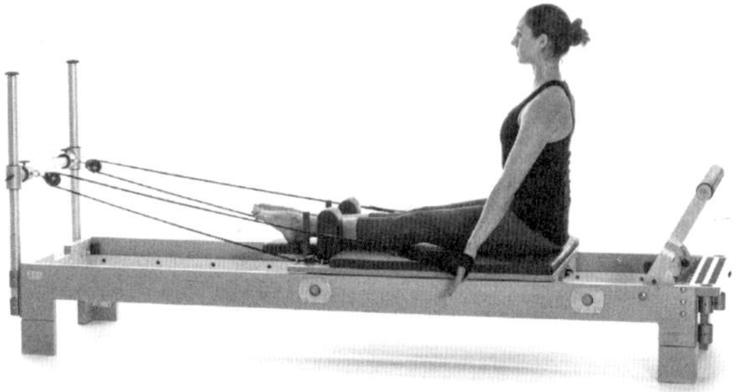

Setup. Sit upright facing the back of the reformer at the edge of the carriage closest to the footbar, with the legs straight and between the shoulder rests. Hold the straps with the palms facing back and fingertips (fists) reaching toward the floor. Keep the arms close to the sides of the body, approximately 20 degrees forward of the plumb line.

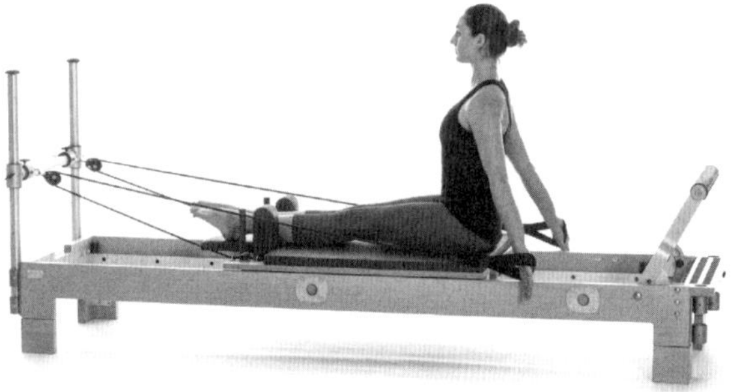

Exhale. Extend the shoulders as far back as possible without compromising the upright alignment of the trunk (10-20 degrees past the plumb line).

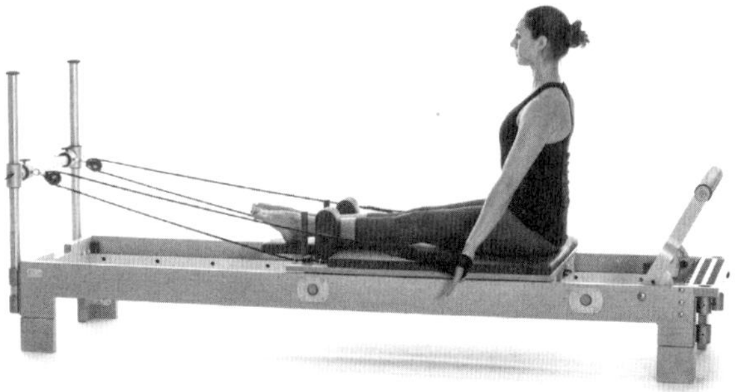

Inhale. Flex the shoulders, bringing the arms forward. Return to the start position. Repeat 10 times.

Biceps—Seated

Muscle Focus

- Biceps
- Shoulder flexors
- Back extensors

Objectives

- To improve elbow flexor strength
- To improve shoulder flexor control
- To develop trunk stabilization

RESISTANCE

Light — Medium — Heavy

As with the Reformer: Chest Expansion—Seated, maintain strong, balanced, upright alignment of the trunk, as close to a neutral spine position as possible. You should feel all the trunk stabilizers working. Avoid leaning back, which is a common mistake in this exercise.

The upper arms play a crucial role in the proper execution of the Reformer: Biceps—Seated. They are the stable foundation that remains immobile as the lower arms move. Straighten the arms directly forward of the shoulders, parallel to each other and to the carriage. Keep them absolutely stable. The arms should neither drop nor lift as they bend and straighten. Any deviation involves improper muscle recruitment and possible undesired elevation of the scapulae, which in turn compromises the isolated movement of the elbows and contraction of the biceps. Feel free to hold the straps or handles with a fist rather than an open hand, which can be challenging, particularly in this exercise.

Imagery

The trunk and upper arm should create a stable platform for the lower arm to move on. The sensation should be like the upper arms are resting on a table; the movement of the lower arms is completely disassociated from the upper arms. This image counters the tendency to lift the arms, which results in shoulder flexion as opposed to the desired isolated flexion of the elbows.

- ○ Keep the upper arms parallel to each other and to the carriage.
- ○ Straighten the elbows completely after each repetition.
- ○ Maintain the upright alignment of the trunk.

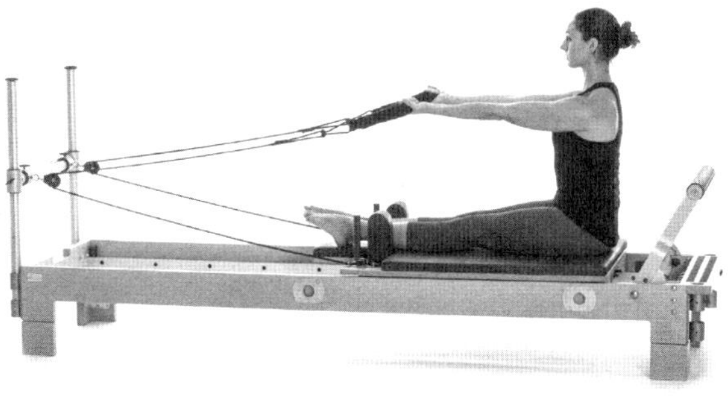

Setup. Sit upright facing the back of the reformer at the edge of the carriage closest to the footbar, with the legs straight and between the shoulder rests. Straighten the arms forward at shoulder height, parallel to the carriage, and hold the straps with the palms facing up.

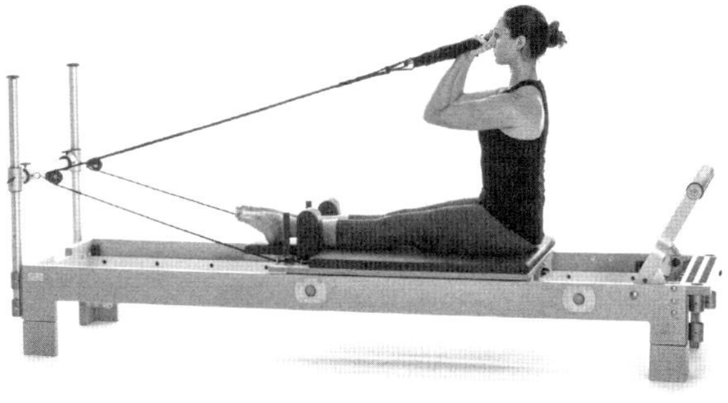

Exhale. Flex the elbows, bending the arms beyond a 90-degree angle and working the full range of motion of the elbows. Keep the upper arms stable.

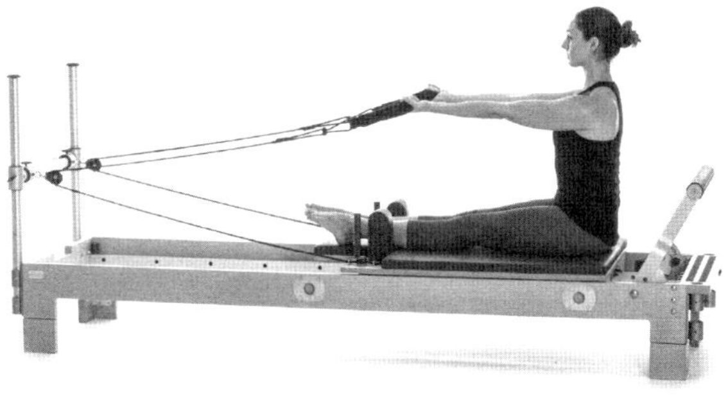

Inhale. Extend the elbows, straightening the arms completely. Return to the start position. Repeat 10 times.

Rhomboids—Seated

Muscle Focus

- Deltoids
- Rhomboids
- Back extensors

Objectives

- To improve shoulder horizontal abductor strength
- To improve scapular adductor strength
- To develop trunk stabilization

RESISTANCE

Light Medium Heavy

Although the name of this exercise singles out the rhomboids, the emphasis is initially on scapular stabilization and horizontal abduction of the shoulders. As in the Reformer: Biceps—Seated, focus on keeping the upper arms at a right angle to the body, parallel to each other and to the carriage, but with the elbows at a 90-degree angle. Horizontally abduct the shoulders to the point where the scapulae are about to adduct (retract), but do not adduct them, then bring the arms forward, returning to the start position. Be aware of the rhomboids, which are located between the scapulae, and focus the energy there.

Imagery

The palms are like two spotlights shining beams of light toward the face. The more stable the arm position is, the more isolated the movement in the glenohumeral joint will be.

- ○ Externally rotate the shoulders slightly to avoid internal rotation.
- ○ Maintain a 90-degree angle in the elbows.
- ○ Keep the upper arms parallel to the floor.
- ○ Avoid elevating the shoulders.

PROGRESSION

At a later stage, when good form and control have been achieved, you can add scapular adduction. The adduction occurs once you have reached the end range of shoulder horizontal abduction. Adduct the scapulae while continuing to take the arms back. It is as if the scapulae and arms lock together. This will load the rhomboids with resistance. After the scapular adduction, the scapulae then abduct (protract) and are stabilized before the arms return to the start position.

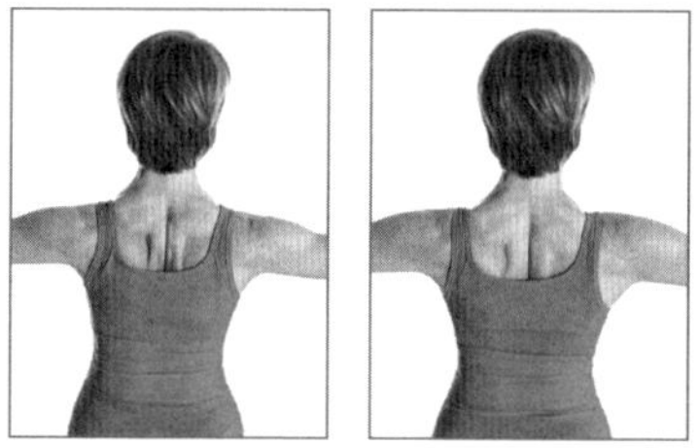

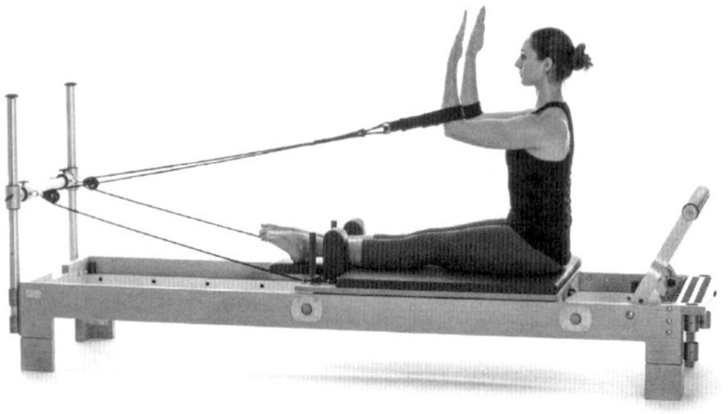

Setup. Sit upright facing the back of the reformer at the edge of the carriage closest to the footbar, with the legs straight and between the shoulder rests. Thread the arms through the straps, bend the elbows to a 90-degree angle, and place the straps on the forearms close to the elbows. Make sure the upper arms are at shoulder height, parallel to both the carriage and each other, with the palms facing the body.

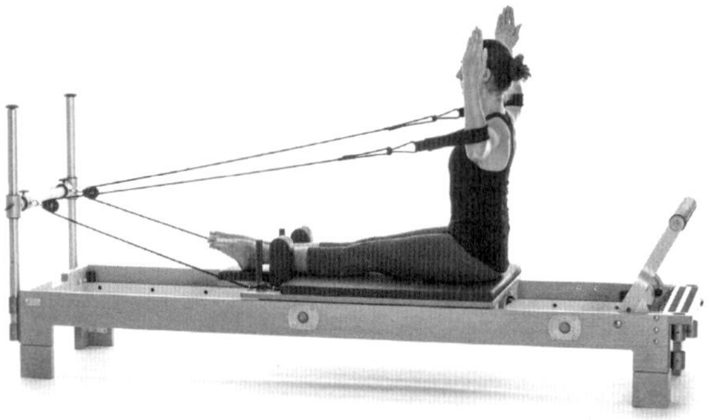

Exhale. Horizontally abduct the shoulders, keeping the upper arms on a consistent horizontal plane and maintaining the 90-degree angle in the elbows.

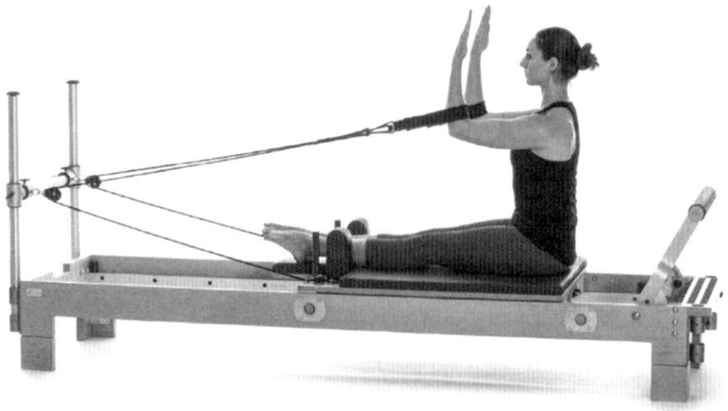

Inhale. Horizontally adduct the shoulders, bringing the arms forward. Return to the start position. Repeat 10 times.

Hug-a-Tree—Seated

The image of hugging a tree often results in rounding the arms and shoulders excessively, which is contrary to the goal of this exercise. As the shoulders horizontally adduct, I advise focusing on mid- and upper back extension and scapular stabilization, which helps prevent flexion and rounding of the upper thoracic spine and abduction of the scapulae. Elongating the arms out to the sides, rather than rounding them, encourages correct muscle recruitment, keeps the resistance engaged throughout the range of motion, and creates a long lever arm, which makes the exercise more challenging. I cannot emphasize enough the importance of a strong upright position and a stable trunk. Focus the work on the chest, as opposed to the arms, and feel the wonderful stretch across the chest as the arms open.

Imagery

Imagine spreading your wings, like an eagle with a large wingspan. The trunk of the body should feel like a strong, sturdy tree trunk.

- ○ Keep the back and shoulders broad and the scapulae stable.
- ○ Keep the arms straight, with a micro-bend in the elbows (slight flexion) and the hands within your peripheral vision when the arms open.
- ○ Maintain slight external rotation of the shoulders, leading the movement with the small finger.

PROGRESSION

Once a good grasp of the Reformer: Hug-a-Tree—Seated has been achieved, add this progression for additional challenge. The shoulders are biased toward external rotation, which in turn promotes good placement of the scapulae. This progression also introduces a higher level of coordination. Start the exercise with the arms in a T position, palms facing upward. Bring the arms forward so they are in line with the shoulders, parallel to each other and to the carriage. Bend the elbows and take them directly backward so the hands are alongside the trunk, palms still facing upward. Straighten the arms opposite the shoulders and open them to the T position.

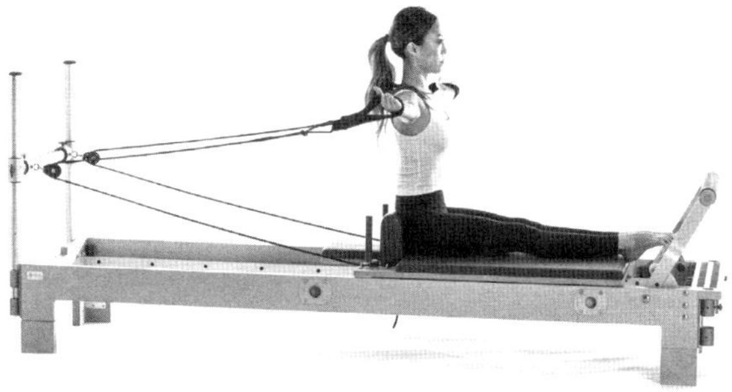

Muscle Focus

- Pectorals
- Back extensors

Objectives

- To improve shoulder horizontal adductor strength
- To develop trunk and scapular stabilization

RESISTANCE

Light — Medium — Heavy

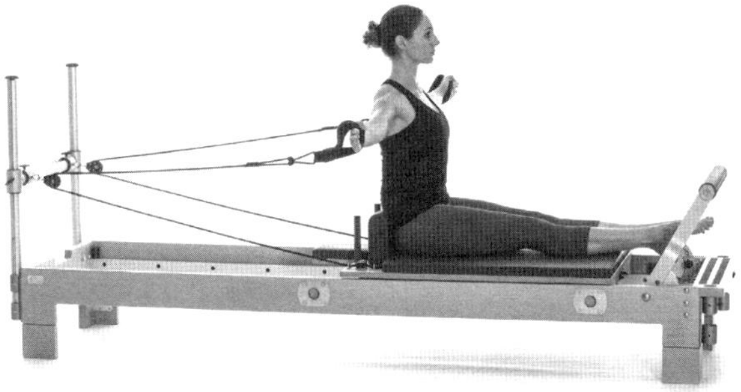

Setup. Sit upright on the carriage facing the front of the reformer (footbar), with the back of the pelvis against the shoulder rests and the legs directly forward. Hold the arms out to the sides in a T position, parallel to the floor, arms elongated with a micro-bend in the elbows.

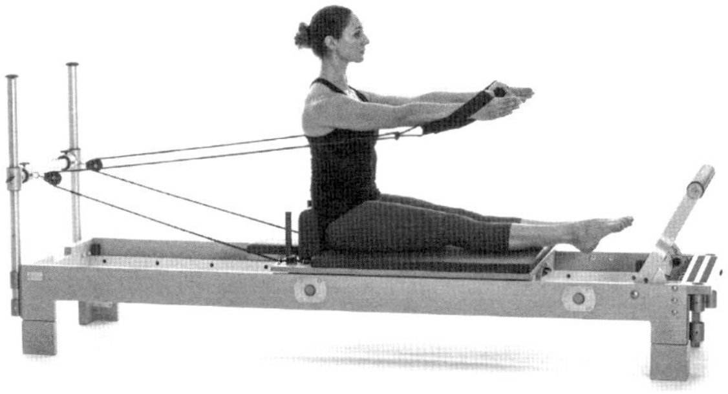

Exhale. Horizontally adduct the shoulders, moving along a horizontal plane, until the arms are parallel to each other and in line with the shoulders.

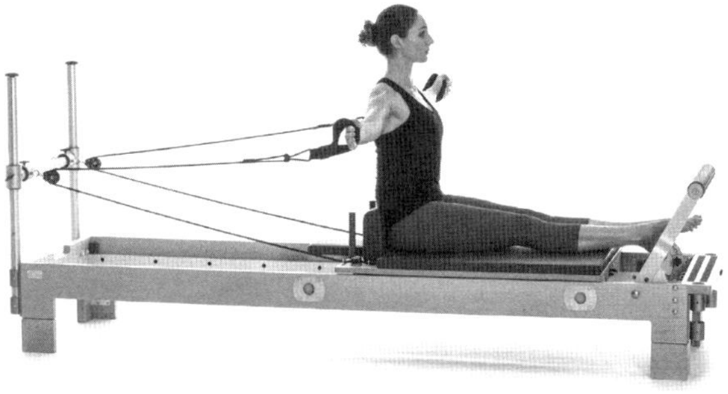

Inhale. Horizontally abduct the shoulders, maximizing the eccentric contraction of the muscles of the chest. Reach the T position without moving the scapulae. Return to the start position. Repeat 10 times.

Salute—Seated

Muscle Focus

- Triceps
- Deltoids
- Back extensors

Objectives

- To improve elbow extensor and shoulder horizontal adductor strength
- To develop trunk and scapular stabilization

RESISTANCE

Light — Medium — Heavy

Although the focus of this exercise is the triceps, the entire arm work seated series emphasizes trunk stabilization and correct positioning of the scapulae. In this exercise in particular, there is a tendency to round the upper body and elevate the shoulders. A good indication of the correct height of the arms from the outset is for the hands to be alongside the temples and the ropes slightly above the shoulders, but not touching them. The fingers (fists) should be directed forward to guide the arms traveling on a diagonal line.

Imagery

Imagine the arms gliding along a ramp slightly above the horizon. Envisioning the horizon encourages a long, seemingly infinite line.

- Maintain scapular stabilization.
- Keep the elbows lifted and reaching out to the sides when bent.
- Direct the fingers (fists) along the line of the movement.

PROGRESSION

To add challenge to this exercise, lean forward with the trunk. This will accentuate the back work exponentially, as well as make the work of the triceps and shoulders more demanding. The hands begin from the same position, alongside the temples, however the angle of the diagonal line will be higher. As the elbows straighten and the arms reach up and forward, create a long line with the trunk and the arms.

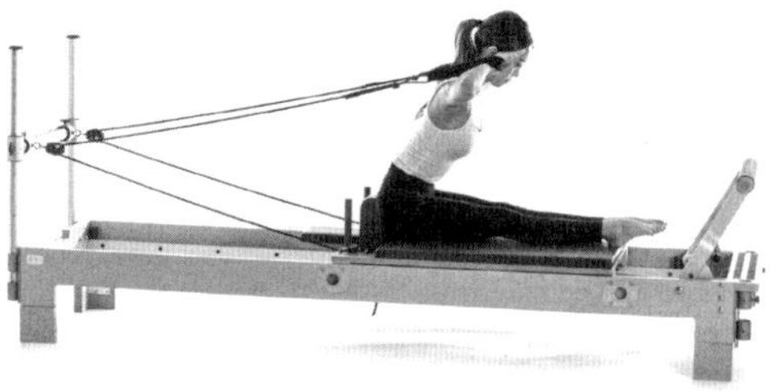

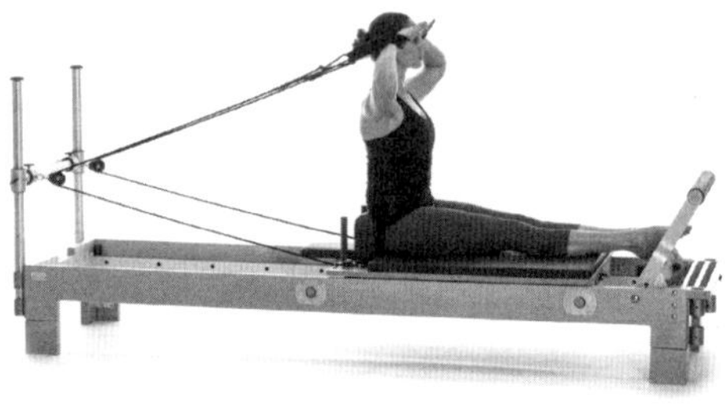

Setup. Sit upright on the carriage facing the front of the reformer (footbar), with the back of the pelvis against the shoulder rests and the legs directly forward. Place the hands in the straps, alongside the temples, with the elbows out to the sides. The fingers face forward and slightly upward, in the direction of the movement.

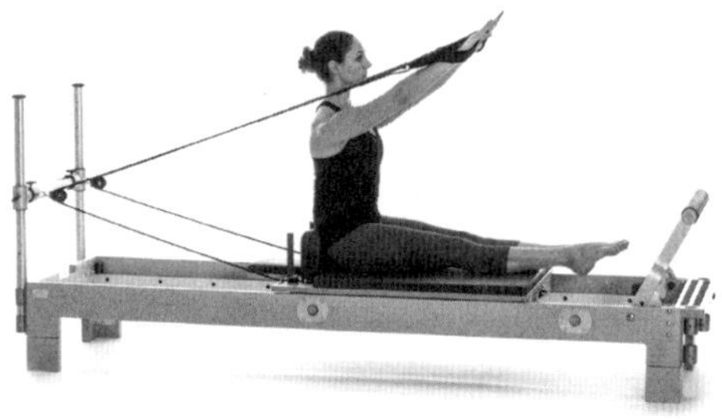

Exhale. Extend the elbows, straightening the arms on a diagonal line, 20-30 degrees above horizontal.

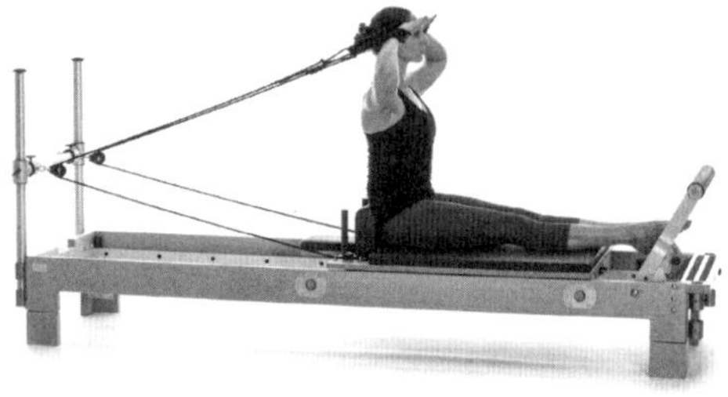

Inhale. Flex the elbows, moving them out to the sides as the arms bend, with the fingers still facing forward (the direction of the movement). Return to the start position. Repeat 10 times.

Chest Expansion—Kneeling

Muscle Focus

- Shoulder extensors
- Triceps
- Abdominals
- Back extensors

Objectives

- To improve shoulder extensor and elbow extensor strength
- To develop trunk stabilization

RESISTANCE

Light | Medium | Heavy

This exercise is more challenging, and certainly more precarious, than the seated version on the reformer, the standing version on the cadillac, and the seated version on the F2 chair. This is primarily due to the element of instability. It requires a very high degree of trunk stabilization, balance, control, and focus. The control is particularly required as the arms return to the start position in the eccentric phase of the exercise. If this phase is done too quickly, the carriage will slide back toward the stopper rapidly and the body will likely fall forward.

This potential instability offers immediate feedback when and if the body is out of alignment, or the arms are returned to the start position too rapidly, indicating that the eccentric contraction is not being utilized.

Although a neutral spine is ideal, I often recommend a slight posterior tilt of the pelvis, which encourages abdominal and hamstring activation. This in turn counters the tendency to flex at the hips, tilt the pelvis anteriorly, thrust the ribs forward, and hyperextend the back.

Many people, particularly those with tight hamstrings, find achieving good alignment and correct form in the kneeling version more accessible than the Reformer: Chest Expansion—Seated.

Imagery

The trunk should feel like the trunk of a tree: tall, upright, and able to adapt to the subtle shifts as the arms move back and forth. As with the Reformer: Chest Expansion—Seated, imagine the hands reaching down to the floor while the head simultaneously reaches up toward the ceiling.

- ○ Keep the trunk upright and stable.
- ○ Maintain co-contraction of the abdominals and back extensors.
- ○ Keep the hip flexors elongated, feeling a stretch through the front of the thighs.
- ○ Avoid thrusting the ribs forward.

PROGRESSION

At the point that the shoulders are in full extension, you can add a rotation of the head, first to one side and then to the other, before bringing the head back to center and moving the arms forward to the start position. Alternate the side the head turns to first with each repetition. Add the head rotation only after the movement of the arms and stabilization of the trunk have been mastered and the exercise can be done without tension in the shoulders or neck.

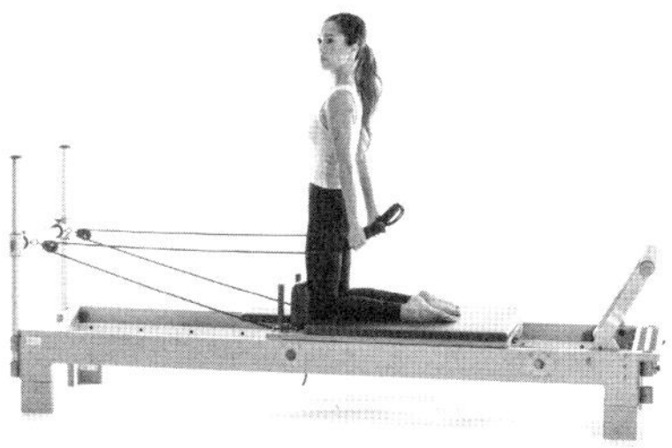

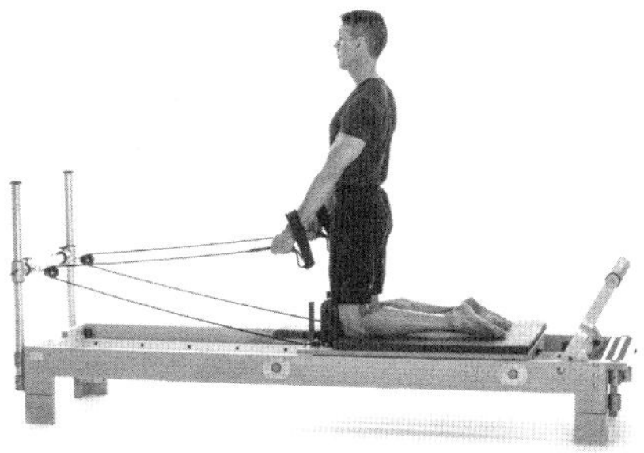

Setup. Kneel facing the back of the reformer, with the knees against the shoulder rests and the body upright. Hold the ropes just above the straps (or fold the straps over the ropes), with the palms facing each other. Place the arms in front of the body, approximately 20 degrees forward of the plumb line.

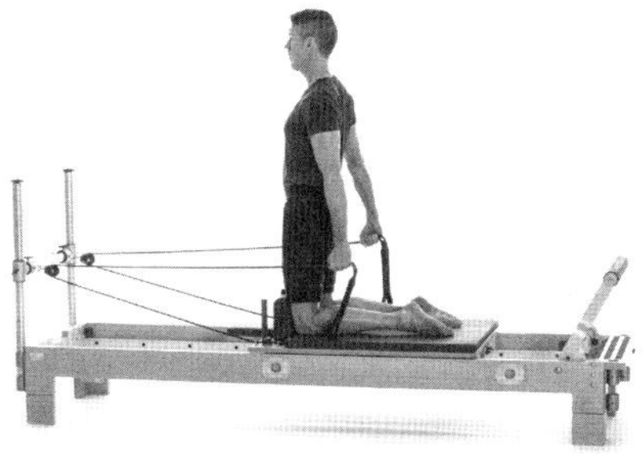

Exhale. Extend the shoulders, taking the arms back as far as possible without compromising the upright alignment of the trunk (10-20 degrees past the plumb line).

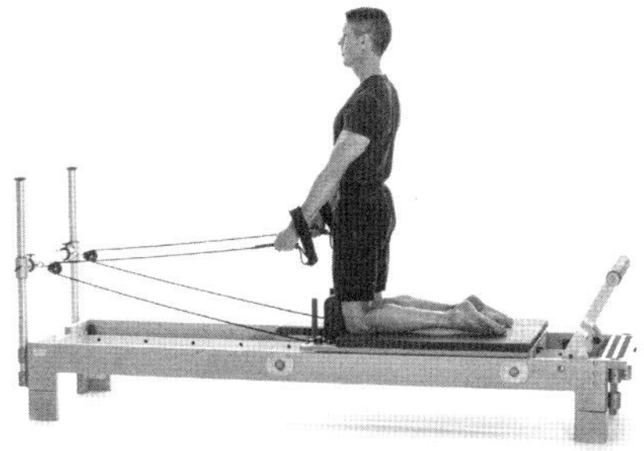

Inhale. Flex the shoulders, bringing the arms forward. Return to the start position. Repeat 10 times.

Arm Circle Up—Kneeling

Muscle Focus

- Deltoids
- Abdominals
- Back extensors

Objectives

- To improve shoulder flexor and shoulder abductor strength
- To develop trunk and scapular stabilization

RESISTANCE

Light Medium Heavy

Few series of exercises challenge the upper body and the trunk as profoundly as the arm work kneeling series. Athletes of many disciplines find the exercises challenging and extremely beneficial. Swimmers in particular can benefit from these exercises because they address muscle patterns fundamental to swimming.

There is a tendency to overuse the quadriceps and often the legs fatigue more than the arms. As you learn to utilize the muscles of the core and the trunk becomes more stable, there will be less of a tendency to rely on the legs for support. As with the Reformer: Chest Expansion—Kneeling, maintain a slight posterior tilt of the pelvis and focus on elongating the hip flexors and thighs. Avoid elevating the arms higher than the flexibility of the shoulders allows, which will result in scapular elevation and tension in the neck. At the same time, maximize the range of motion of the shoulders by aiming to reach the arms completely overhead.

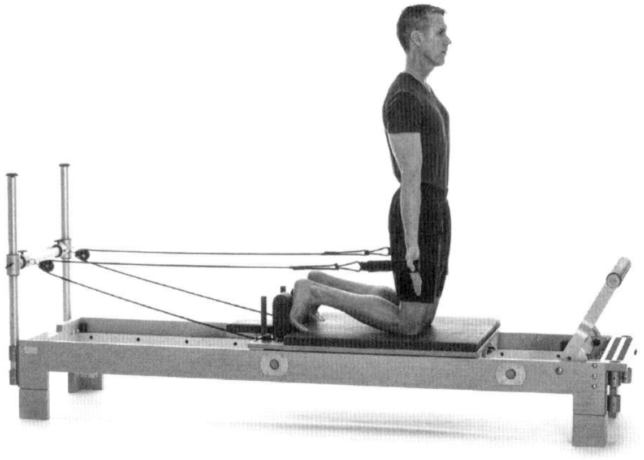

Setup. Kneel facing the front of the reformer (footbar), with the feet against the shoulder rests and the trunk upright. Place the hands in the straps, with the palms facing forward and the arms by the sides of the body.

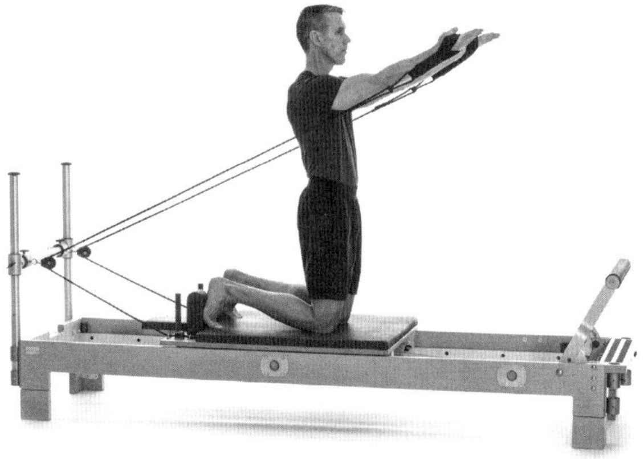

Exhale. Flex the shoulders, reaching the arms forward and upward, the palms continuing to face up.

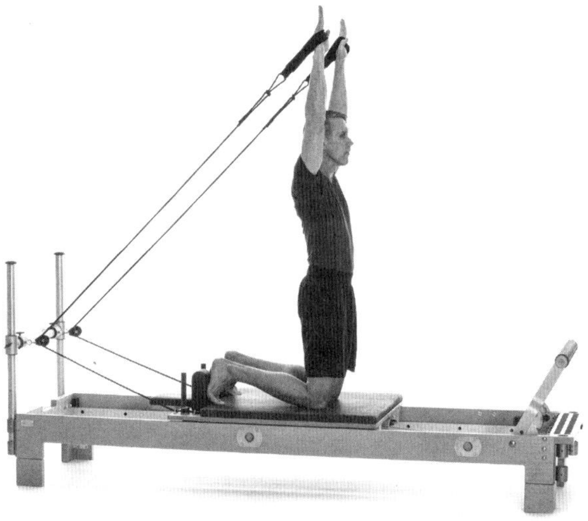

Inhale. Rotate the arms as they reach overhead so the palms face forward.

Imagery

In the initial phase, I like to imagine that I am lifting a large, light beach ball in each hand, as if to toss it high into the air. This encourages a light and effortless feel in the arms. The arms then float down to the sides of the body to repeat the toss of the ball.

- Face the palms forward and upward during shoulder flexion.
- Rotate the shoulders at the top (overhead) so the palms face forward, and the small finger leads the way down to the sides of the body.
- Keep the arms within peripheral vision as they circle around to the sides.
- Avoid elevating the scapulae as the arms rise above shoulder height.

PROGRESSION

This movement can also be performed in reverse. Abduct the shoulders and reach the arms out to the sides and overhead, palms facing forward. When the arms are overhead, rotate the shoulders so the palms face up, and then lower the arms to the sides of the body. Maximize the range of motion of the shoulders. The reverse direction is more challenging in terms of scapular stabilization and the demand on the shoulder abductors; reduce the resistance, if necessary.

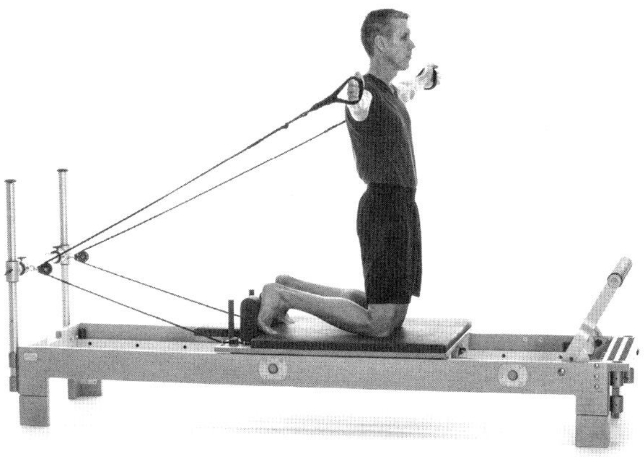

Continuing to inhale, circle the arms out to the side.

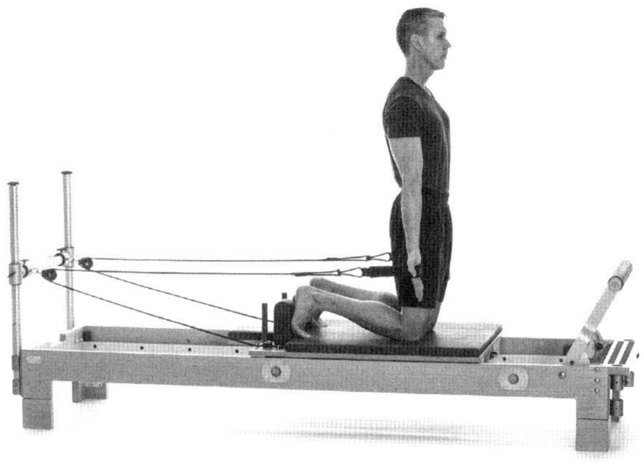

Continuing to inhale, bring the arms down to the sides of the body. Return to the start position. Repeat 10 times.

Triceps—Kneeling

Muscle Focus

- Triceps
- Deltoids
- Abdominals
- Back extensors

Objectives

- To improve elbow extensor and shoulder abductor strength
- To develop trunk and scapular stabilization

RESISTANCE

Light Medium Heavy

The focus of this exercise is the triceps and is similar to the Reformer: Salute—Seated and the Arm Chair: Salute. But, given the unstable position, the high center of gravity, and the hands traveling upward rather than forward, it is a great deal more challenging. There is a strong tendency to round the upper body, elevate the shoulders, and reach the hands forward as opposed to upward. All these tendencies should be avoided. Lower the resistance if necessary.

The feel of this exercise should be extremely upright. There is a straight energy line traveling from the knees, through the trunk, and finally through the arms as they straighten, fingers reaching toward the ceiling.

Imagery

Imagine the hands shaving the back of the head as the arms straighten and bend. Think of the triangular shape created by the fingers as a spearhead, leading the movement as the arms straighten.

- ○ Maintain trunk and scapular stabilization.
- ○ Keep the elbows facing outward.
- ○ Direct the fingers upward along the line of movement.

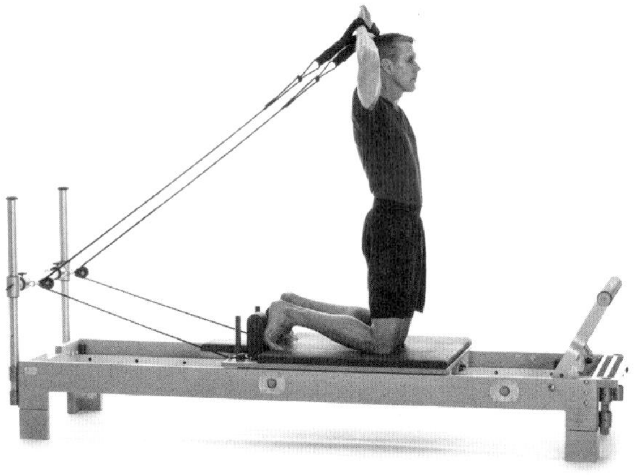

Setup. Kneel facing the front of the reformer (footbar), with the feet against the shoulder rests and the trunk upright. Hold the straps with the hands behind the head, pressing the thumb and index finger of each hand together to create a triangle. The elbows remain wide, reaching out to the sides.

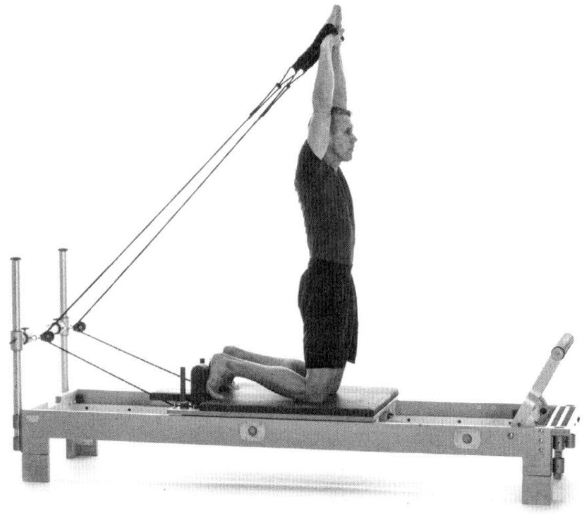

Exhale. Extend the elbows, straightening the arms and abducting the shoulders. Keep the fingers touching while reaching up to the ceiling.

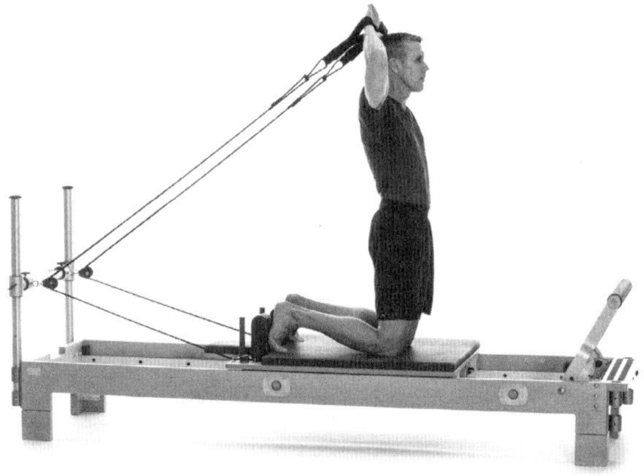

Inhale. Flex the elbows, bending the arms. Return to the start position. Repeat 10 times.

Biceps—Kneeling

This is an exercise I added to the original arm exercises created by Joseph Pilates. The fully stretched position of the biceps is unique and very effective for developing strength and flexibility of the biceps specifically, and the shoulder and chest region in general. Men in particular are often tight in the biceps and across the chest, which tends to limit range of motion and interfere with normal function of the shoulders.

Imagery

Imagine the body as the figurehead of a majestic, old, wooden ship. With each bend of the arms, the chest should open more, reaching the chest forward. It is important to keep the abdominals engaged so that the chest can open without the lower ribs thrusting forward and the lower back hyperextending.

- Keep the upper arms stable.
- Keep the arms parallel to each other (or as close as possible).
- Maintain scapular stabilization, avoiding adduction of the scapulae.

Muscle Focus

- Biceps
- Abdominals
- Back extensors

Objectives

- To improve elbow flexor strength
- To improve thoracic and shoulder flexibility
- To develop trunk and scapular stabilization

RESISTANCE

Light Medium Heavy

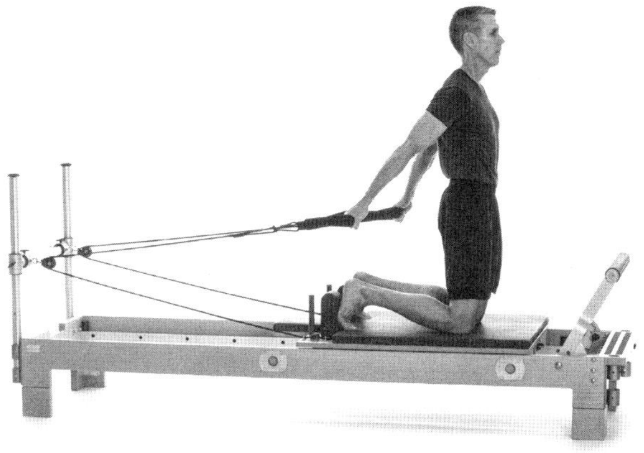

Setup. Kneel facing the front of the reformer (footbar), with the feet against the shoulder rests and the trunk upright. Reach the arms back, extend the shoulders, and hold the straps.

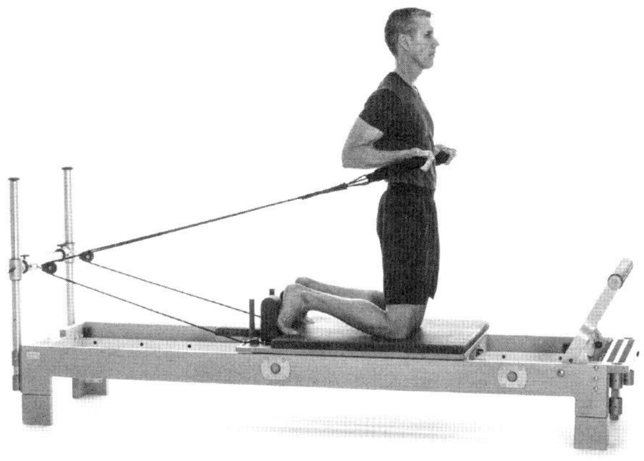

Exhale. Flex the elbows, bending the arms while keeping the upper arms stable.

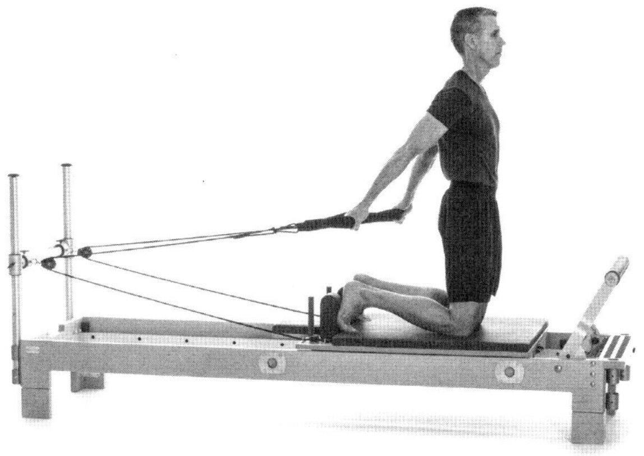

Inhale. Extend the elbows, straightening the arms. Return to the start position. Repeat 10 times.

Rowing Back 1

Muscle Focus

- Deltoids
- Abdominals
- Back extensors

Objectives

- To improve shoulder abductor and shoulder horizontal abductor strength
- To improve shoulder mobility
- To improve abdominal and back extensor control

RESISTANCE
Light — Medium — Heavy

The rowing series, which begins with this exercise, highlights many of the wonderful elements of Pilates. Understanding this series will offer insight into the intricacies of the method itself. Coordinated muscle activation is key, with the entire body working as an integrated unit. The combination of shoulder mobility, together with upper body and trunk support, illuminates the principle of functional movement and range of motion. Avoid neck tension and shoulder elevation, which often occur as a result of the enormous demands placed on the upper body.

Due to the complexity of the exercises in the rowing series, laying a good foundation before attempting them is highly recommended. Mastering related arm work exercises that are performed in a seated position on the reformer, as well as the Mat: Roll-Up and Neck Pull, will assist in achieving this goal. Once the elements of these exercises have been learned and practiced, pay attention to the seamless flow of movement. In the roll-down phase, the sacrum and even part of the lower back imprints into the carriage, with a bias toward a posterior pelvic tilt.

Imagery

Rowing a boat is a good visual image of the action in this exercise: Imagine a long, sleek boat gliding across smooth water, propelled by the long, dynamic strokes of the arms.

- Bring the hands to the chest before rolling down in the first phase of the exercise.
- Keep the carriage still when moving from the supine position to forward flexion.
- Circle the arms around to the front, keeping them as high as possible, as if swimming the butterfly, before rolling the spine up to a sitting position.

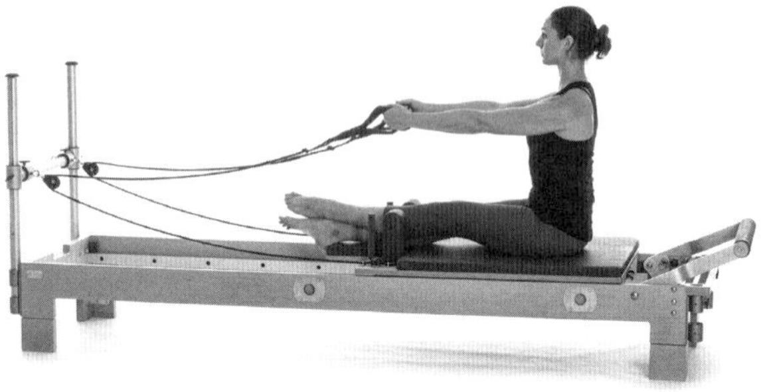

Setup. Place the footbar down. Sit upright on the carriage facing the back of the reformer, approximately one-third of the way down the carriage. (Leave enough space behind you to support the sacrum and part of the lower back when in the supine position.) Keep the legs straight between the shoulder rests (you may need to cross them) and the arms straight out in front, parallel to each other and to the floor. Hold the straps with the hands facing each other.

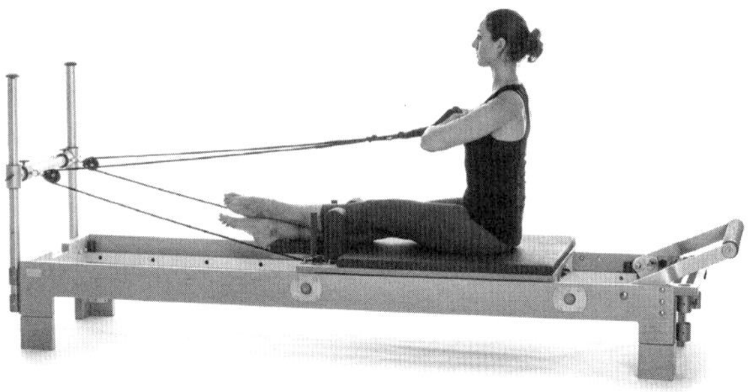

Inhale. Flex the elbows, bending the arms and bringing the hands to the sternum, with the elbows wide.

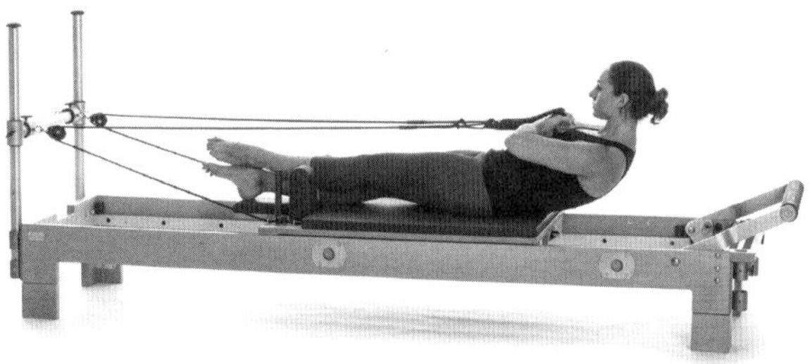

Exhale. Roll down into a supine position, keeping the hands in front of the sternum and maintaining flexion of the trunk.

PROGRESSION

To add an element of challenge to this already difficult exercise, when supine and the arms are out to the sides in the T position, move the arms even farther back toward the footbar (closer to a true T position) prior to hinging the body forward and taking the arms back. Once the hands touch, the remainder of the exercise remains the same.

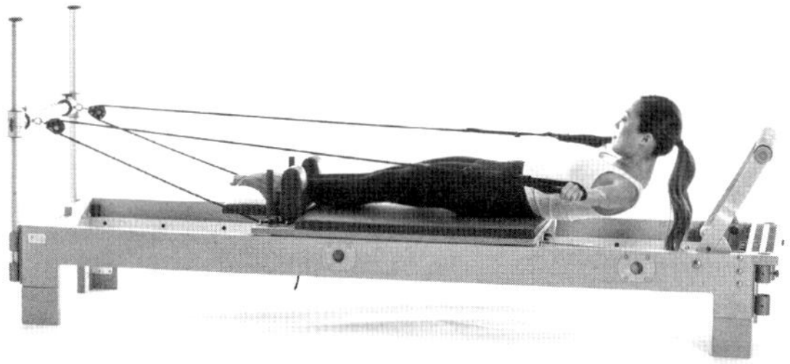

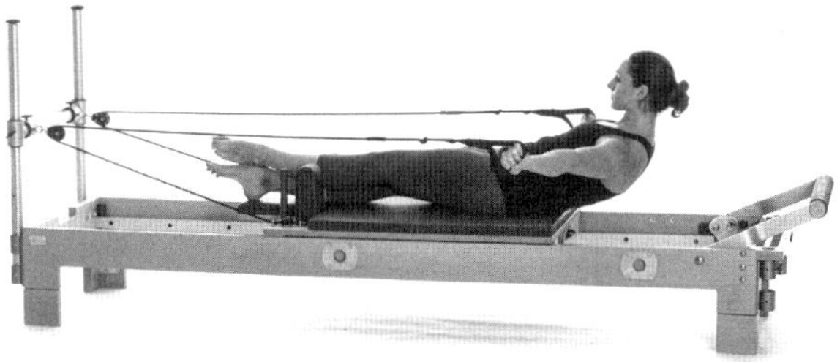

Inhale. Remain in the supine position. Internally rotate the shoulders and straighten the arms out to the sides, creating a T position (or as close as possible) with the arms. Pause.

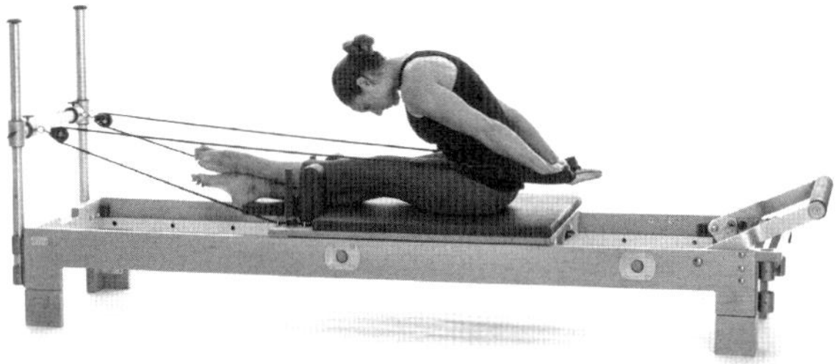

Exhale. Transfer the trunk over the legs, flexing at the hip joints, while reaching the arms behind the body and touching the hands together. Elongate the trunk with the back extensors while staying as close to the legs as possible. Keep the carriage still and maintain tension in the straps throughout this phase.

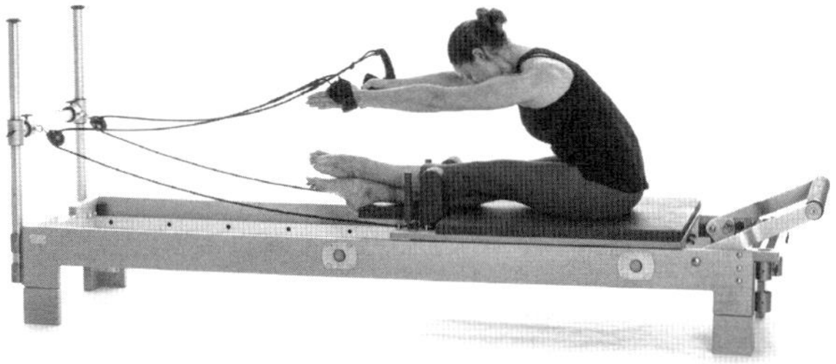

Inhale. Remain forward with the trunk over the legs, stretching the hamstrings. Circle the arms around to the front, reaching over the legs, as if swimming the butterfly. Note that at this point there will be no tension in the straps.

Exhale. Roll the trunk up to an upright position. Return to the start position. Repeat 5 times.

REFORMER
Arm Work
INTERMEDIATE

Muscle Focus

- Biceps
- Deltoids
- Abdominals
- Back extensors

Objectives

- To improve elbow flexor and shoulder flexor strength
- To improve abdominal and back extensor control

RESISTANCE

Light Medium Heavy

Rowing Back 2

The emphasis on full body integration and flow continues in this exercise. In terms of arm work, the focus is now directed to the biceps. The Reformer: Biceps—Seated is an excellent preparation for this exercise, and I consider it a prerequisite. The elbows are held at a 90-degree angle for much of the exercise, with the biceps in an isometric contraction. Keeping this angle consistent adds greatly to the challenge of the exercise, together with the coordination and high level of body awareness involved in the movement.

Focus on the coordinated contraction of the abdominals and the back extensors, particularly when lifting from supine into a sitting position. There is a tendency to throw the pelvis forward at this point, resulting in an anterior tilt of the pelvis and hyperlordosis, which can put strain on the lower back. This exercise is often performed with the trunk in extension throughout the movement, including when lowering to the carriage. I prefer to roll down, reinforcing the familiar pattern of spinal articulation and reducing the possibility of strain on the lower back.

Imagery

I enjoy feeling the undulating, circular motion of the entire trunk as it rolls down and then unwinds to roll up like a wave. Coordinating the arm movement with that of the trunk accentuates the rolling sensation and the strong connection between the movement of the trunk and the arms. Visualizing this flowing, rhythmic motion will assist in achieving the desired dynamic in this exercise.

- ○ Keep the elbows at a 90-degree angle when rolling down to the supine position.
- ○ Hold the elbows firmly by the sides of the body when supine.
- ○ Begin the lift with slight lumbar flexion before transitioning into spinal extension.

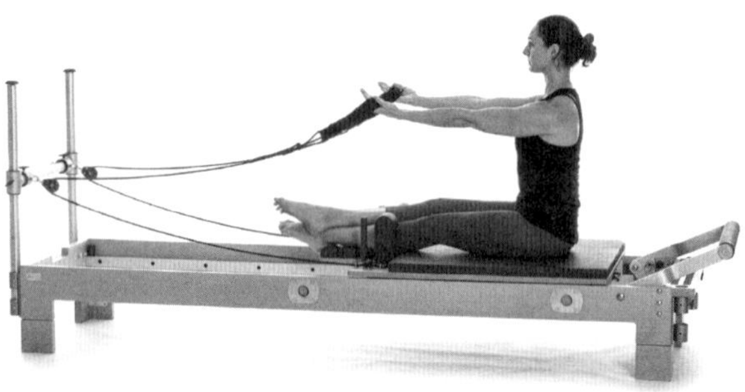

Setup. Place the footbar down. Sit upright on the carriage facing the back of the reformer, approximately one-third of the way down the carriage. (Leave enough space behind you to support the sacrum and part of the lower back when in the supine position.) Keep the legs straight between the shoulder rests (you may need to cross them) and the arms straight out in front at shoulder height, parallel to each other and to the carriage. Hold the straps in the hands, with the palms facing upward.

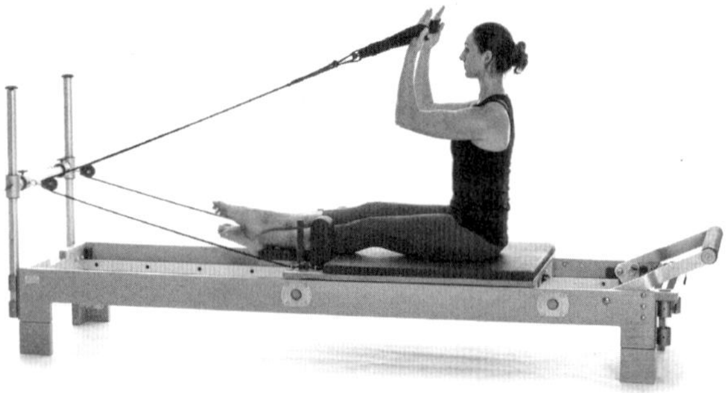

Inhale. Flex the elbows, bending the arms to a 90-degree angle.

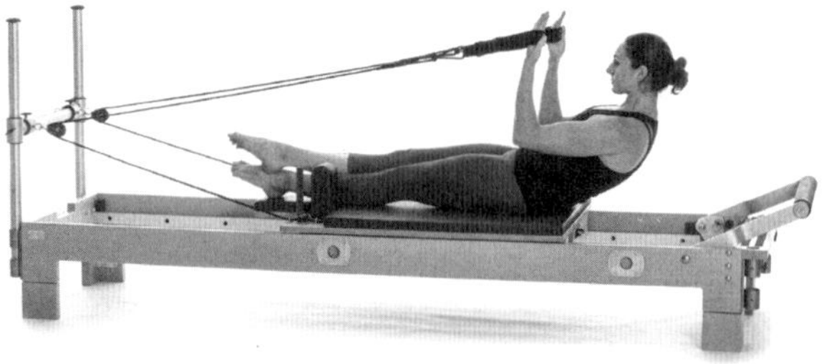

Exhale. Roll down into a supine position and lower the arms to the sides of the body, maintaining the 90-degree angle in the elbows.

PROGRESSION

Once the movement has been mastered and stability of the trunk has been achieved, establishing neutral spine alignment on the way up, you can expand the movement to be larger and more extreme. When lifting from the supine position, rather than extending the trunk to a neutral spine position and reaching the arms up and forward on a diagonal line, reach the arms directly up to the ceiling and extend the upper back into an arch. Continue to move the arms forward, establishing neutral alignment of the spine in the upright sitting position.

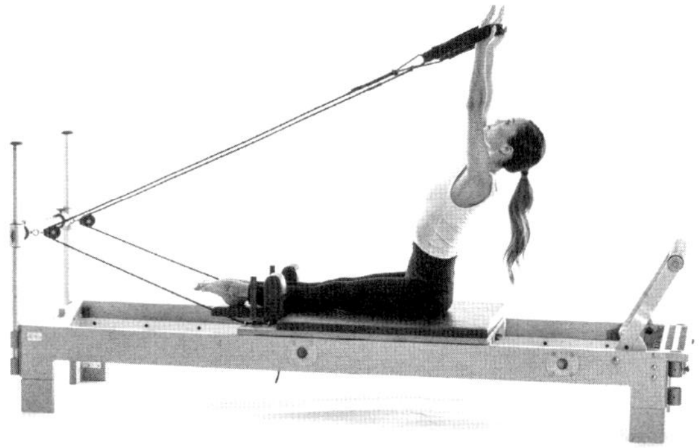

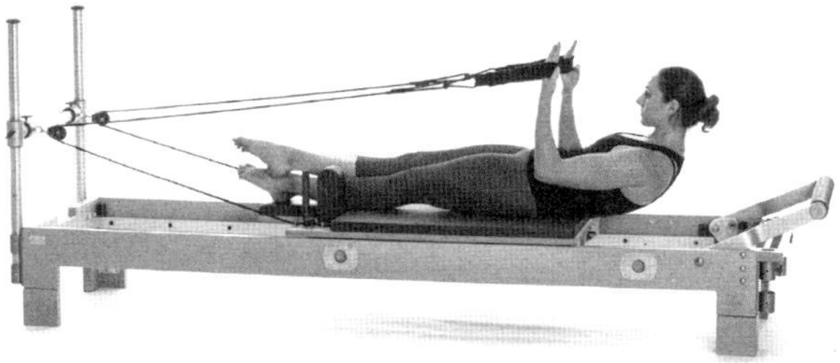

Inhale. Pause in the supine position, maintaining a stable trunk and arm position.

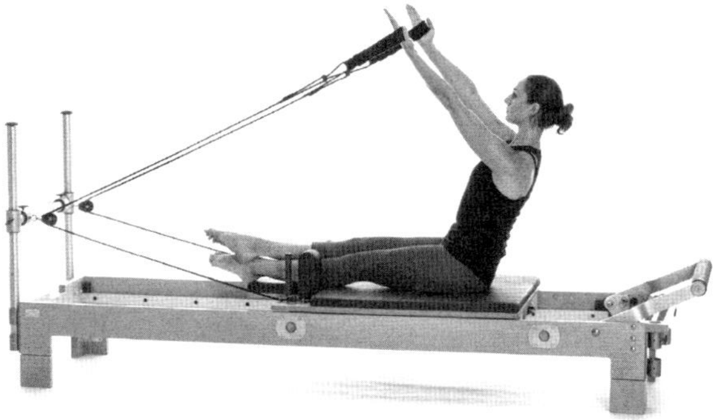

Exhale. Lift the body, initiating the movement by drawing in the abdominals and deepening the spinal flexion. Extend the spine through coordinated contraction of the back extensors and abdominals to reach a straight diagonal line of the trunk. Simultaneously straighten the arms, reaching forward and upward. Continue lifting the trunk to the upright sitting position without changing the relationship of the arms to the trunk. Lower the arms to the start position. The arm motion should feel like it grows out of the movement of the trunk as the trunk goes from the supine position, through the diagonal line, to the upright sitting position. Repeat 5 times.

REFORMER
Arm Work
INTERMEDIATE

Muscle Focus

- Deltoids
- Triceps
- Abdominals
- Back extensors

Objectives

- To improve shoulder flexor and elbow extensor strength
- To develop trunk and scapular stabilization

RESISTANCE
Light Medium Heavy

Rowing Front 1

In this exercise, the trunk is upright and facing the front of the reformer (footbar). The trunk should feel as sturdy as the trunk of a huge tree, similar to the Reformer: Hug-a-Tree—Seated. I recommend being very familiar with the arm work seated series before embarking on the rowing exercises. The sensation of a strong, solid trunk is achieved by co-contracting the abdominals and the back extensors.

The focus is on stability of the trunk and mobility of the shoulders. Having the resistance pulling from behind makes the movement more challenging.

If the hamstrings are tight and the back muscles are weak, the hip flexors will tend to work excessively and become fatigued. Sitting on a pad or small box to elevate the body is advisable; this takes the strain off the hamstrings and hip flexors and allows the focus to shift to the back extensors. It also allows you to establish the upright position of the trunk required in this exercise. Avoid leaning back, and do not allow the arms to go behind the body at any point. This can be achieved by keeping the arms in your peripheral vision as they circle from overhead to the sides of the body.

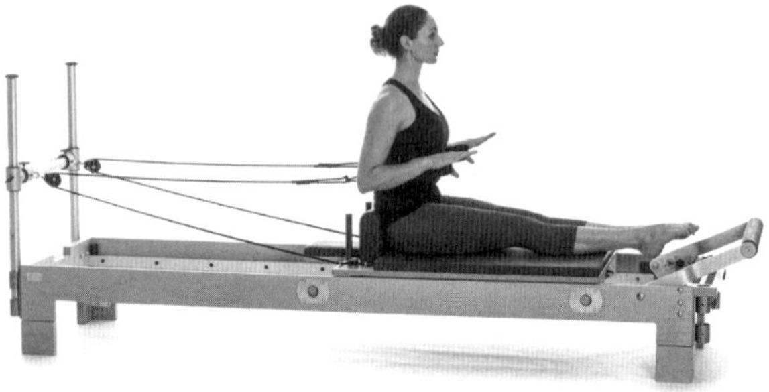

Setup. Sit upright facing the front of the reformer (footbar), with the back of the pelvis against the shoulder rests and legs straight forward. Place the thumbs in the straps, with the rope running under the armpits. Bend the arms, bringing the hands to the sides of the chest, palms facing down, fingers reaching forward, and elbows reaching out to the sides.

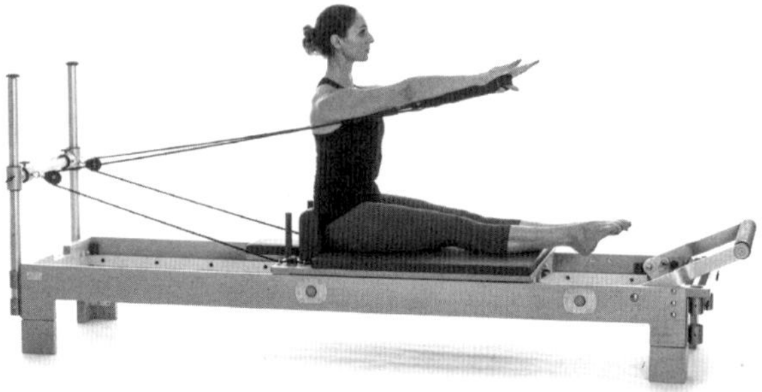

Exhale. Extend the elbows, straightening the arms forward and upward on a slight diagonal line.

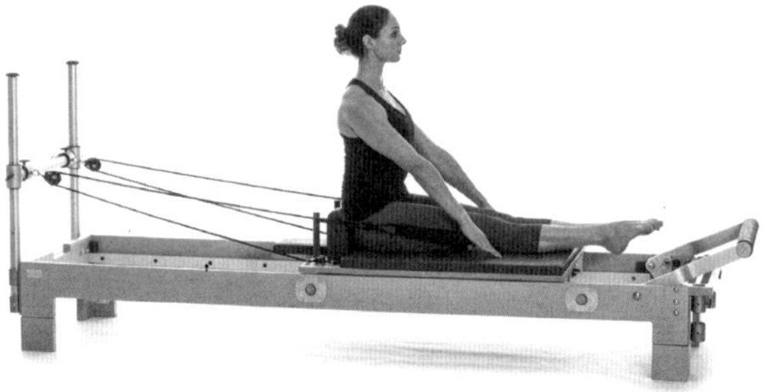

Inhale. Lower the arms to the carriage, reaching as far forward as possible, and touch the carriage with the fingertips.

Imagery

Visualize laser beams shooting out from the fingertips as you maximize the range of motion in all directions. When in the start position, imagine that there is air under the arms, as if they are floating. This will allow the rope to pass comfortably under the arms.

- ○ Maintain upright alignment of the trunk.
- ○ After straightening the arms on a slight diagonal and lowering them, reach as far forward as possible on the carriage before lifting them to accentuate the feeling of length.
- ○ Maintain trunk and scapular stabilization.

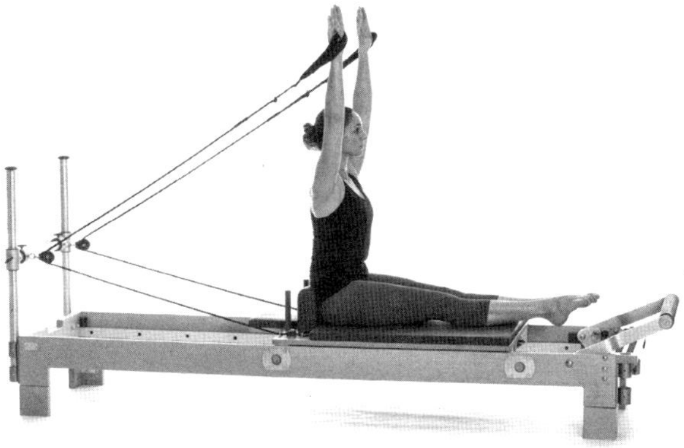

Exhale. Lift the arms overhead, internally rotating the shoulders so that the ropes pass the arms unobstructed.

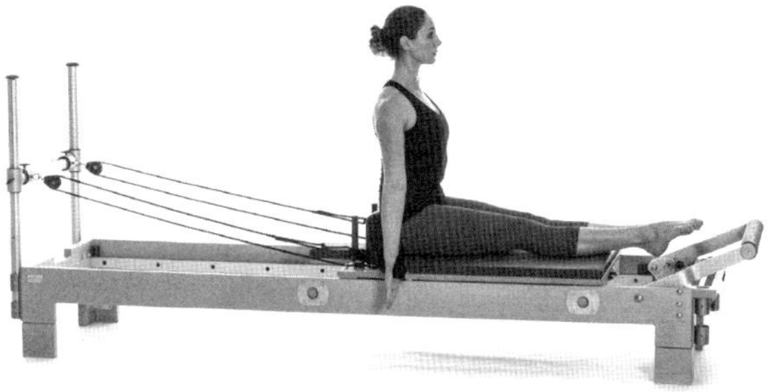

Continuing to exhale, externally rotate the shoulders so the palms face forward. Circle the arms around to the sides of the body, continuing to keep the palms facing forward, leading with the small finger.

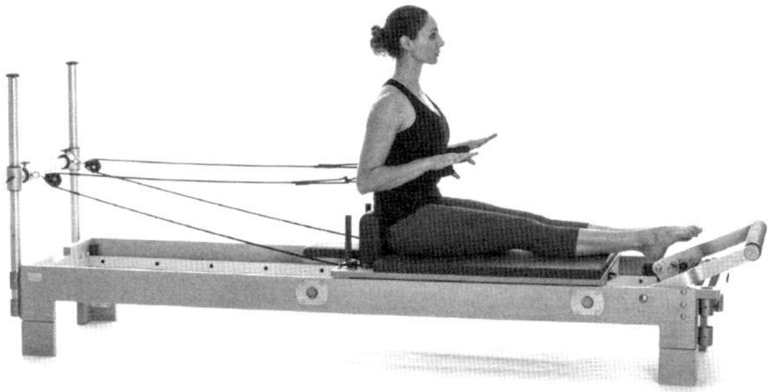

Inhale. Bend the arms, bringing the hands to the sides of the chest, palms facing down, fingers reaching forward, and elbows reaching out to the sides. Return to the start position. Repeat 5 times.

Rowing Front 2

Muscle Focus

- Deltoids
- Triceps
- Abdominals
- Back extensors

Objectives

- To improve back extensor, elbow extensor, and shoulder flexor strength
- To improve hamstring flexibility
- To develop trunk and scapular stabilization

RESISTANCE

Light Medium Heavy

This exercise is particularly valuable due to the profound involvement of the trunk and the coordinated movement of the trunk and arms required to do it well. Proper execution involves not only trunk strength and stability but also hamstring flexibility. The transition from flexion to extension of the trunk should be initiated from the lower back, with the energy flowing up through the trunk, head, arms, and all the way to the fingers. By focusing on extending the spine and achieving a straight diagonal line with the trunk immediately prior to straightening the arms, you will likely avoid common mistakes such as scapular elevation and inadequate extension of the trunk. I recommend pausing momentarily at the moment when the trunk and arms have created a powerful diagonal line, prior to sitting upright. In the first movement, bringing the hands forward (under the shoulders) and placing the arms by the sides of the body as the trunk rounds into forward flexion is a small but very important movement that is often minimized or even ignored. This movement places the trunk and arms in a strong position to then straighten on the diagonal line.

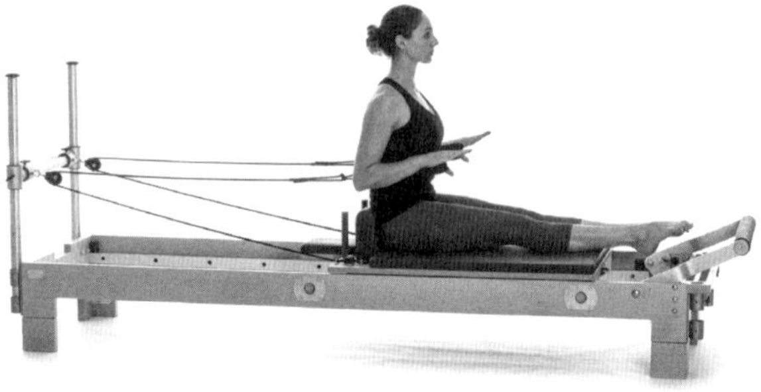

Setup. Sit upright facing the front of the reformer (footbar), with the back of the pelvis against the shoulder rests and legs straight forward. Place the thumbs in the straps, with the rope running under the armpits. Bend the arms, bringing the hands to the sides of the chest, palms facing down, fingers reaching forward, and elbows reaching out to the sides.

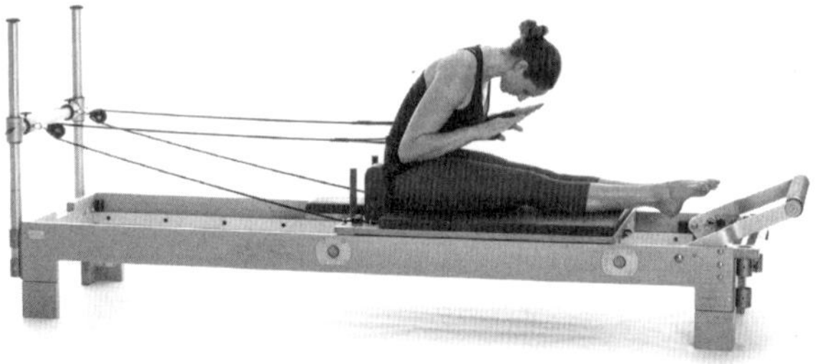

Exhale. Round the trunk into forward flexion over the thighs, keeping the arms close to the sides of the body and bringing the hands under the shoulders.

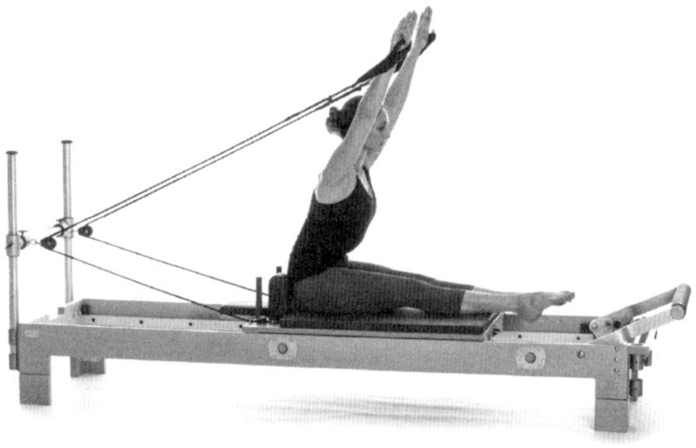

Inhale. Extend the back on a diagonal, straightening the arms to complete the line. Simultaneously internally rotate the shoulders so the ropes pass the arms unobstructed, similar to Reformer: Rowing Front 1 when circling the arms.

Imagery

Imagine a surge of energy, like an electrical current, moving sequentially up the back through the arms and fingers. Alternatively, think of colored ink rising up the back, like litmus paper changing color.

- Initiate the extension from the lumbar spine and then move through the mid- and upper spine before starting the arm movement.
- Pause in the diagonal extended back position before lifting to sitting upright.

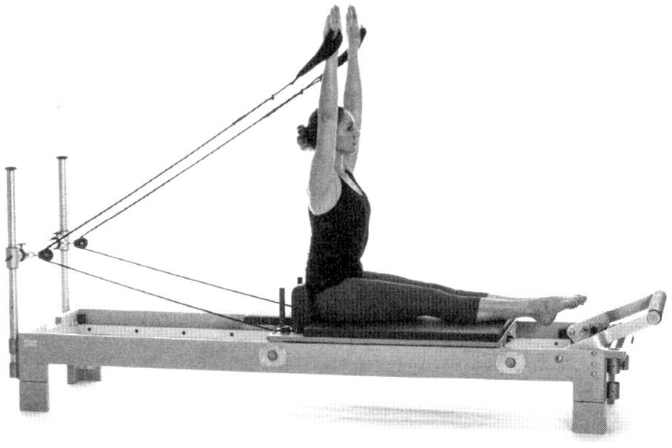

Exhale. After a momentary pause, lift the body to the upright position, arms overhead, keeping the shoulders internally rotated.

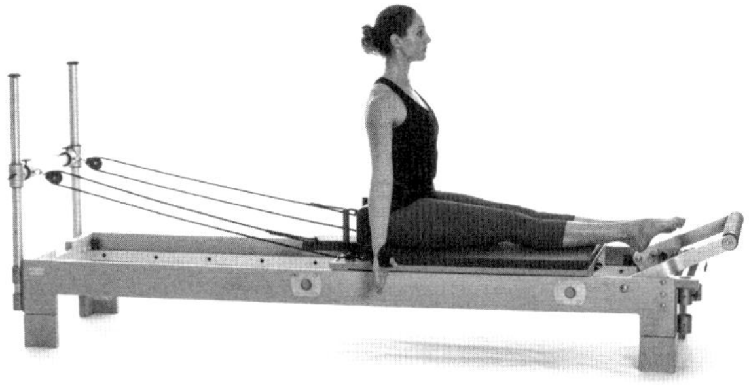

Continuing to exhale, externally rotate the shoulders so the palms face forward. Circle the arms around to the sides of the body, keeping the palms facing forward, leading with the small finger.

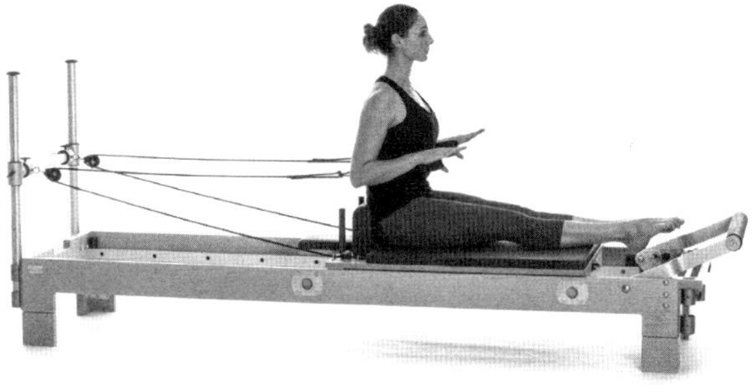

Inhale. Flex the elbows, bending the arms and lifting the hands up. Return to the start position. Repeat 5 times.

Leg Work

This block of exercises supplements the foot work block and offers an opportunity to augment the work of the lower limbs and address the demands on the musculature of the lower body. The specific agenda for this block depends on the goals of the individual. Each population has specific as well as general needs, and each activity demands specialized skills that correlate with the recruitment of certain muscles and muscle groups.

Typically we use this block to work the hip adductors and abductors (with emphasis on the gluteus medius), which tend to be weak in relation to the larger muscles of the leg, the quadriceps and hamstrings. This imbalance can lead to diminished performance, dysfunction, and even injury. Exercises to develop the legs may involve resistance, balance, specific skills, or a combination of all three.

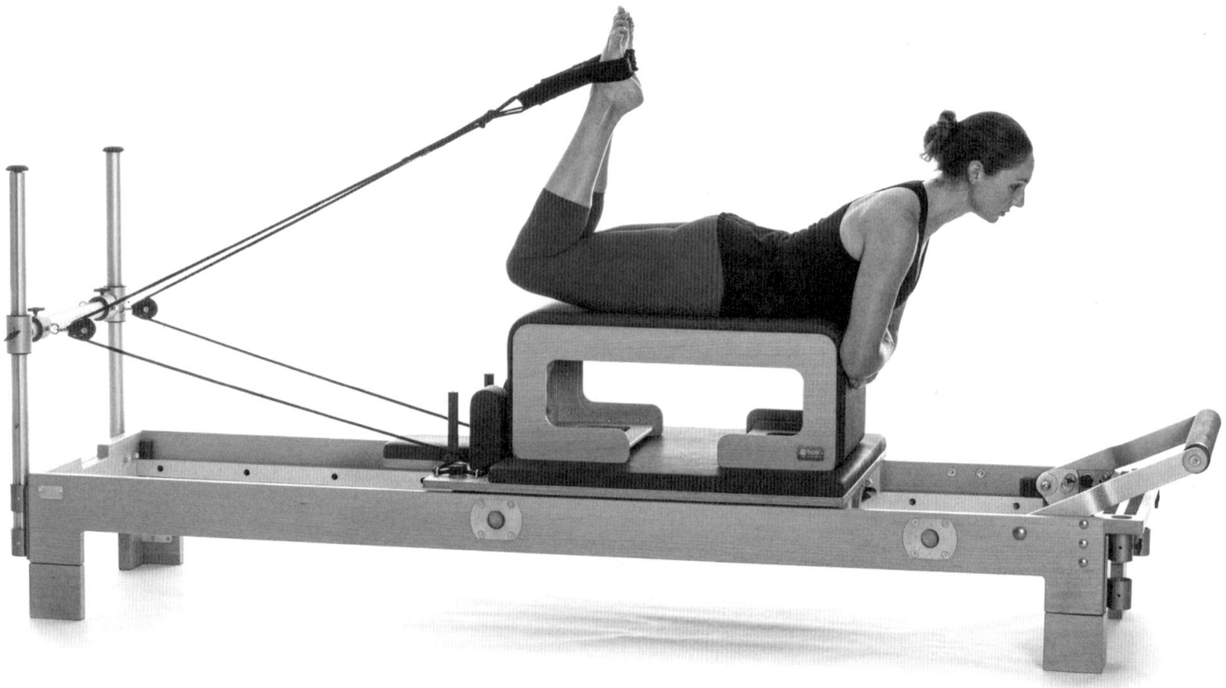

Split—Side

Functional range of motion can be defined as the maximum range of the joint, or joints, while maintaining the integrity of the body's alignment. Once the alignment has been compromised, the functional range of motion has been exceeded. Perhaps no other exercise demonstrates this concept as well as the Reformer: Split—Side, which demands an intricate balance of strength and flexibility. A lack of either will potentially affect the integrity of the exercise.

Both phases require coordinated muscle activation of the hip adductors, abdominals, and back extensors: The "out" phase involves an eccentric contraction of the hip adductors, and the "in" phase involves a concentric contraction of the same muscles. The abdominal engagement prevents hyperlordosis and anterior tilting of the pelvis, which are particularly common at the point where the hips are in maximum abduction. The back extensors assist in maintaining upright alignment and avoiding posterior tilt of the pelvis. The resistance should be challenging (meaning light).

Imagery

I like the image of a puppet being controlled by a string that runs from the base of the pelvis, through the body, and out the top of the head. There should be a sense of controlled release as the legs open and the puppet string is lowered, and then a sense of suction as the string is lifted and the legs come together.

- Bias the pelvis toward a slight posterior tilt until you can achieve, and maintain, a neutral pelvic position.
- Press down into the feet, particularly as the carriage is drawn back toward the stopper.
- Keep the trunk upright.
- Use both legs equally, keeping the weight of the body centered.

MODIFICATION

Initially, as you acquire control, it is best to be safe and place the foot in the middle of the carriage rather than against the shoulder rest. To prevent the foot from sliding, I suggest placing a rubber pad under the outside portion of the foot that is on the carriage (alternatively, place a small box between the side of the foot and the shoulder rest). Progressively move the foot closer to the shoulder rest as you become more proficient. Placing the hands behind the head simplifies the arm position.

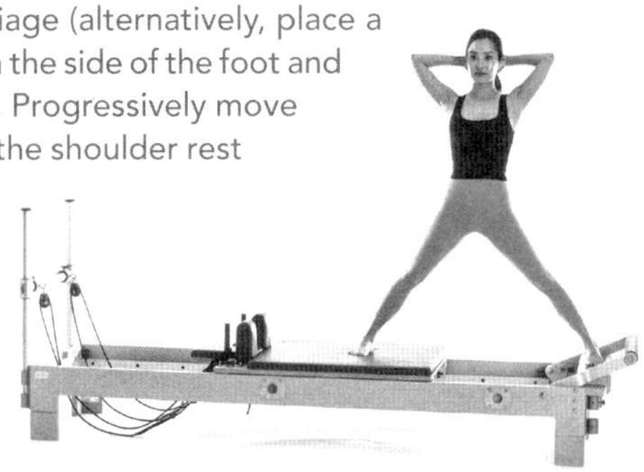

Muscle Focus

- Hip adductors
- Abdominals
- Back extensors

Objectives

- To improve hip adductor flexibility and strength
- To develop lumbopelvic stabilization

RESISTANCE

Light — Medium — Heavy

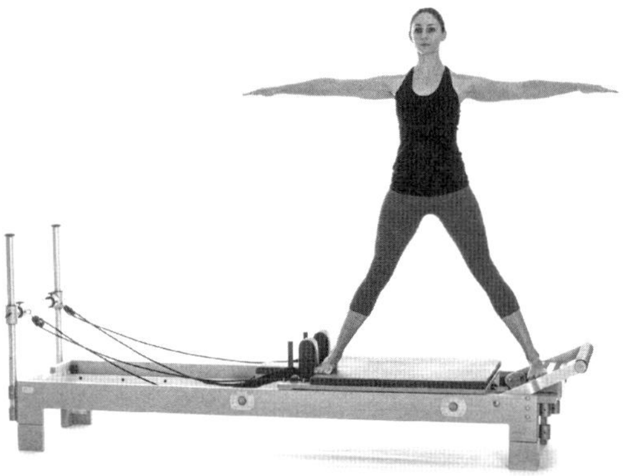

Setup. Stand on the foot platform with one foot. Place the other foot against the shoulder rest. Hold the arms in a T position.

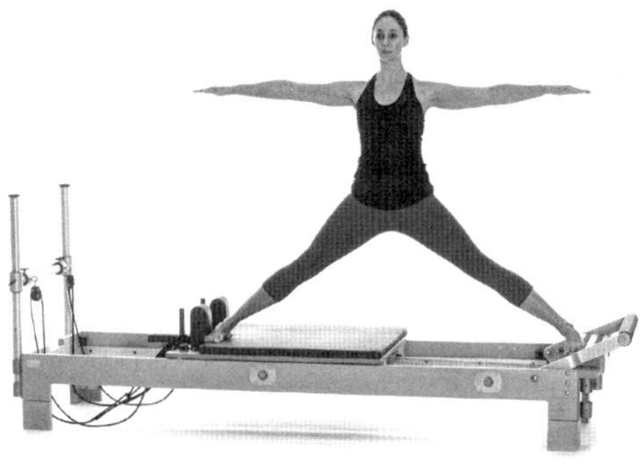

Inhale. Abduct the hips, opening the legs and allowing the carriage to move outward. Control the movement with the hip adductors. Pause at the end of the range of motion.

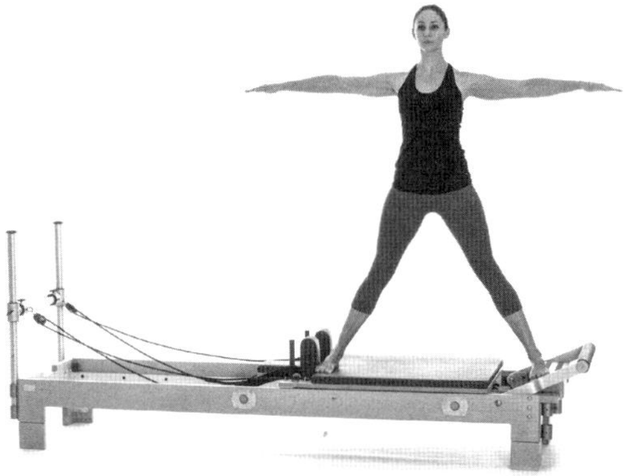

Exhale. Adduct the hips, bringing the legs together and pausing with the carriage against the stopper. Return to the start position. Repeat 5 times.

REFORMER

Leg Work

INTERMEDIATE

Muscle Focus

- Hip abductors
- Knee extensors
- Abdominals
- Back extensors

Objectives

- To improve hip abductor strength
- To improve knee extensor control
- To develop lumbopelvic stabilization

RESISTANCE

Light | Medium | Heavy

Skating—Single Leg

This is an excellent hip abductor exercise. Specific focus is placed on the gluteus medius, which is an important muscle for healthy hip function and plays a prominent role in everyday movements such as walking, running, sitting down, and climbing stairs.

It is important to distinguish between the standing leg and the moving leg, which perform very different functions. The standing leg creates the solid foundation. The moving leg performs the action, relying on a stable platform to push off from. Although the moving leg creates the movement, an equal amount of attention must be allocated to the standing leg, which remains stable along with the pelvis. Avoid the common mistake of pushing with the standing leg at the same time as the working leg and shifting the weight toward the carriage. This often indicates that the resistance is too high, the leg is weak, or both. Another indication that the resistance is too high is if the body lifts as the working leg straightens. It is important to straighten the moving leg completely and not stop short of full extension. It is in the final 5-10 degrees of knee extension that the hip abductors work the hardest; also, the resistance at this point is the highest. Finally, maintain upright alignment and avoid leaning forward in a squat position. This is a common tendency, particularly for those with tight calves.

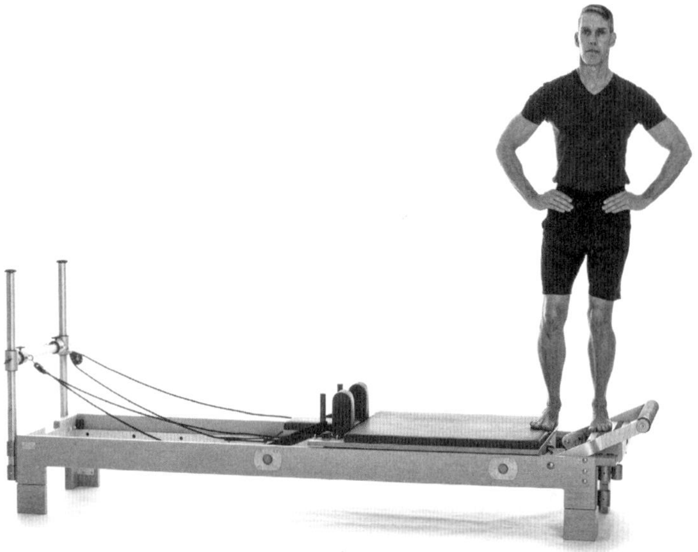

Setup. Place one foot on the foot platform and the other foot on the front edge of the carriage in a wedge position, keeping the weight entirely on the standing (outside) leg. Place the hands on the hips or behind the head and keep the trunk upright. Bend the standing leg as deep as possible (maximum knee flexion) while keeping the heel down and maintaining upright alignment. Keep the moving (inside) leg weightless at this point. Make sure to focus the pressure on the instep of both feet, particularly the foot on the carriage.

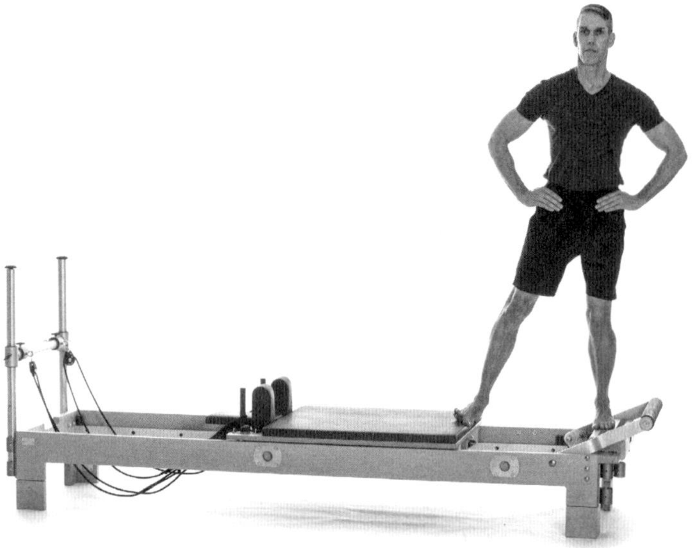

Exhale. Extend the inside knee, straightening the leg completely and pushing the carriage away from the footbar.

Imagery

For this exercise, I like to use the image of a side kick in karate: powerful and directed.

- Keep the weight on the standing leg and avoid pushing with it.
- Keep the trunk upright.
- Maintain a neutral and stable pelvis.
- Straighten the working leg completely and control its return to the start position.

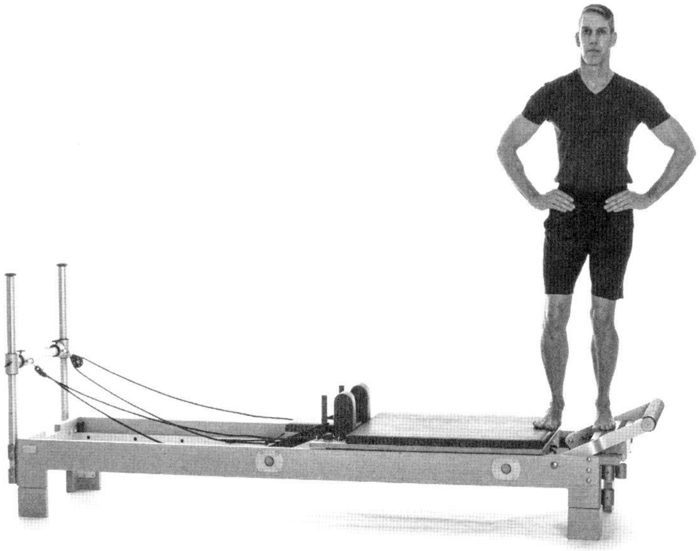

Inhale. Flex the inside knee, bending the leg. Return to the start position. Repeat 10 times before switching to the other side.

PROGRESSION

This exercise can be performed with both legs pushing out simultaneously and the body hinged forward. This allows for increased range of motion and provides a greater challenge for the back extensors. Place the foot about one-third of the way down the length of the carriage, rather than on the edge. The arms reach out to the sides. It is important in this version to move both legs simultaneously. Keep the back flat and the head aligned with the spine. The pelvis should remain at the same height throughout, and not bob up and down. Visualize the fluid lateral force of a speed skater smoothly gliding at high velocity across the ice. I highly recommend becoming proficient at the Reformer: Skating—Single Leg before attempting this progression. Each has unique and valuable benefits.

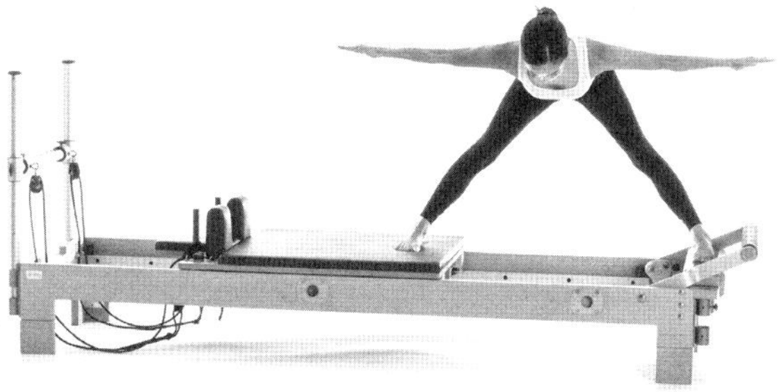

Hamstring Curl

Muscle Focus

- Hamstrings
- Abdominals
- Back extensors

Objectives

- To improve knee flexor and hip extensor strength
- To develop lumbopelvic stabilization

RESISTANCE

Light Medium Heavy

As its name implies, this exercise focuses primarily on knee flexion. By adding hip extension, we maximize the work of the hamstrings by using their functions as a hip extensor and knee flexor. Engaging the hip extensors also helps inhibit the action of the hip flexors, which often become involved when the knee bends, particularly if the rectus femoris is tight. This may result in the pelvis being pulled into an anterior tilt as the knee bends, creating hyperlordosis. Of course, this should be avoided. Recruitment of the abdominals also helps prevent hyperlordosis, and engagement of the back extensors counters rounding of the thoracic spine. The pelvis, together with the abdominals and the back extensors, creates a stable foundation for the exercise. Hugging the front of the box offers additional, and very welcome, support.

Imagery

Prior to the actual curl (knee bend), the body should assume the shape of an archer's bow. The bending of the knees can then be viewed as pulling the twine and placing tension on the bow. However, this image should not result in excessive extension of the back, particularly the lower back. Focus the extension in the mid- and upper back.

- ○ Maintain hip extension, particularly as the knee bends.
- ○ Keep the mid- and upper back extended.
- ○ Use the abdominals to protect the lower back and prevent hyperlordosis.

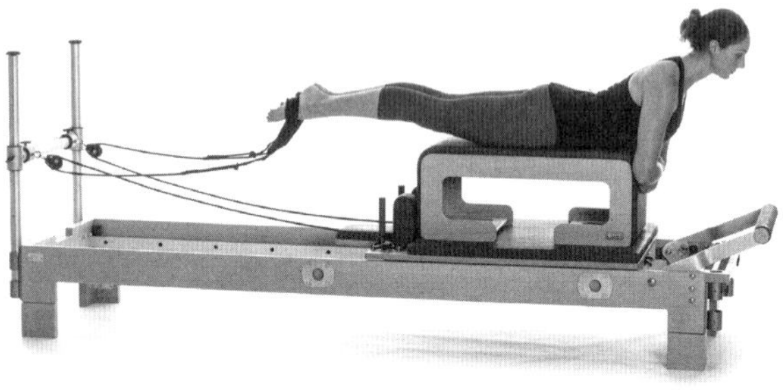

Setup. Lie prone on the long box facing the front of the reformer (footbar). Hug the front of the box with the arms. Extend the mid- and upper back and engage the abdominals. Place the feet in the straps, with the hips extended and the legs straight and lifted slightly off the box. (Note that the straps will need to be shortened for this exercise.)

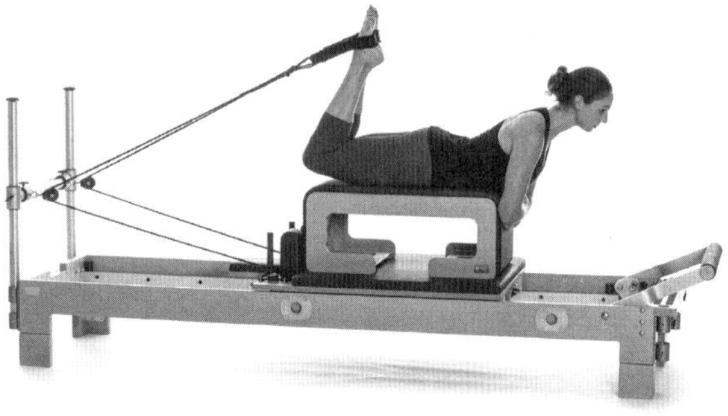

Exhale. Flex the knees, bending the legs and keeping the hips extended (there is a tendency to drop them as the knees bend). Press the pubic symphysis into the box to avoid anterior tilt of the pelvis.

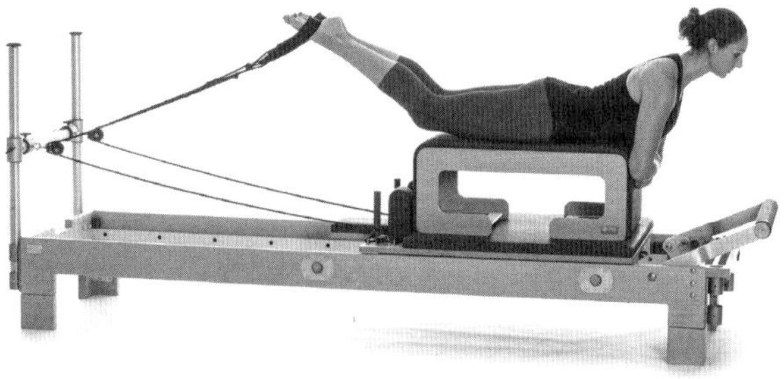

Inhale. Extend the knees, straightening the legs. Return to the start position. Repeat 10 times.

Lateral Flexion and Rotation

Lateral flexion and rotation are important in both everyday activities and athletic pursuits, yet they are often neglected in many fitness programs. When it comes to training the abdominals, the predominant action used is forward flexion. This is only a small part of a very big picture. Training the abdominals fully involves addressing all facets of this important muscle group. Abdominals that are well conditioned in all ranges of motion contribute significantly not only to the many actions initiated by the trunk (for instance, that elusive golf swing) but also to the stabilization mechanism that protects the spine. Without including lateral flexion and rotation exercises, the abdominals are not being trained to their full capacity. This may result in less-than-optimal performance and could eventually lead to ailments and injury.

Every conditioning program should include lateral flexion and rotation movements, at whatever level is appropriate. The muscles must be addressed in terms of both strength and flexibility. Often, in recreational activities, like golf, tennis, volleyball, and many more, the arms and shoulders compensate for lack of range of motion and strength in the trunk; this results in compromised performance and excessive wear and tear on the shoulders. When strong and flexible abdominals, working in concert with the other muscles of the trunk, drive the movement, it is more powerful, efficient, and safe.

Circular energy forms the basis of the imagery for lateral flexion, often an arc rather than a full circle. When performing rotation, the energy is more of a spiral. In either case, these energy trails promote smooth and flowing movement. When doing lateral flexion, I like to visualize a circle and try to touch every point on the circle as I go through the range of motion. When doing rotation, I view it as a spiral that gathers energy along the way, like a spring winding up. There is infinite energy to be found as the spiral unwinds.

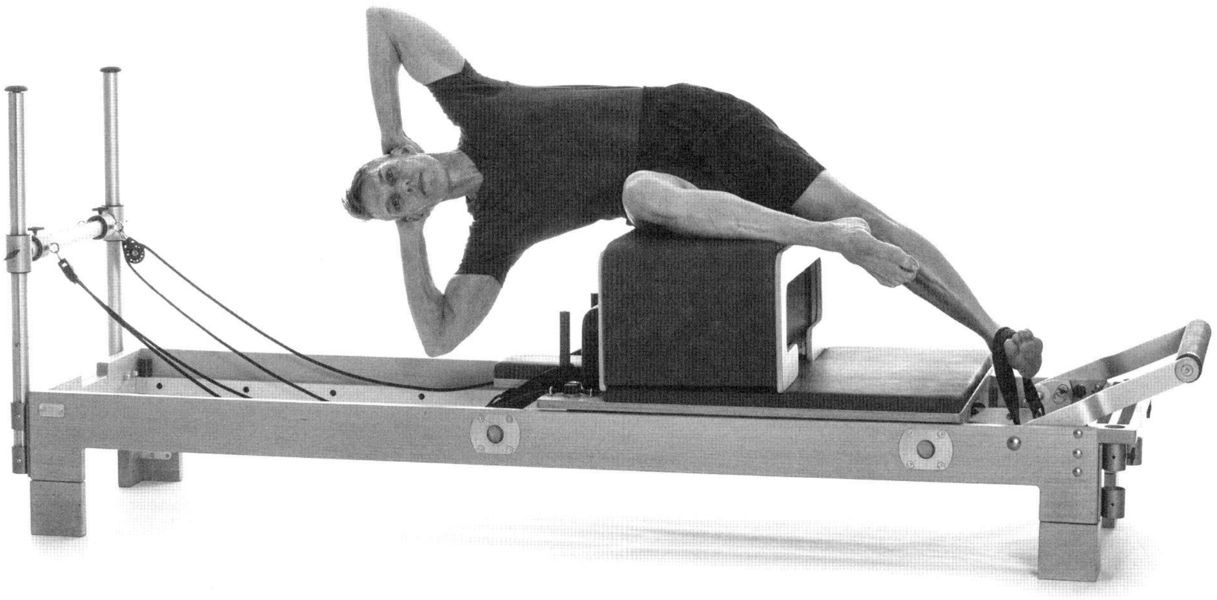

Muscle Focus

- Abdominal obliques
- Back extensors

Objectives

- To improve abdominal oblique flexibility and control
- To develop lumbopelvic stabilization

RESISTANCE

Light — Medium — Heavy

Short Box—Tilt

This exercise is part of the short box series. Although it is not a particularly challenging exercise, it prepares the body for more difficult exercises by teaching correct alignment and muscle recruitment for lateral flexion. An important aspect of this exercise is initiating the lateral motion from the region of the waist while keeping the pelvis stable and the weight evenly distributed on the sit bones.

The movement begins from the crown of the head (which remains aligned with the spine), creating as large an arc as possible without thrusting the ribs forward or displacing the rib cage laterally. Aim to achieve maximum range of motion, creating a continuous arc shape, while keeping the pelvis anchored on the box and equal weight on the sit bones. When lifting back up, begin the movement from the lower spine, with the final piece being the head. The lower body provides the foundation for this exercise and remains stable.

Imagery

The image of a young, green tree trunk being pulled over from the top and springing back to an upright position illustrates the elongated, gentle curve that is desired. The movement occurs in the coronal plane, so the image of movement between two panes of glass is also helpful.

- ○ Co-contract the abdominals and back extensors.
- ○ Keep both sit bones in contact with the box.
- ○ Avoid thrusting the ribs forward and arching the back.
- ○ Avoid shifting the rib cage laterally to the opposite side of the movement.

PROGRESSION

To add intensity to the movement and challenge the lateral flexors, open the arms into a T position when in lateral flexion. One arm will be reaching upward on a diagonal and the other downward on a diagonal. Direct your gaze up to the top hand. Bring the hands back behind the head and gaze forward before lifting and returning to the start position. Alternate sides.

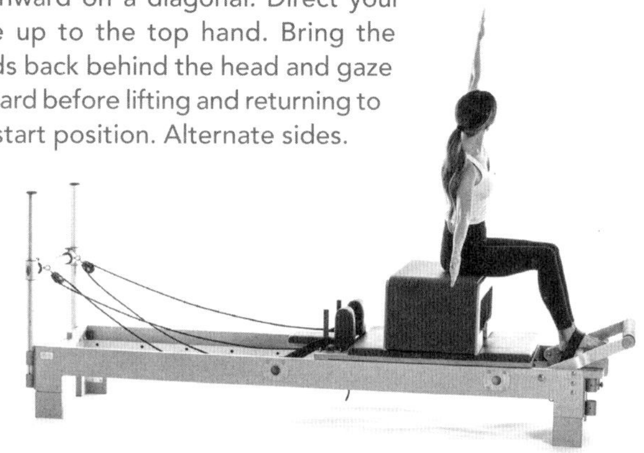

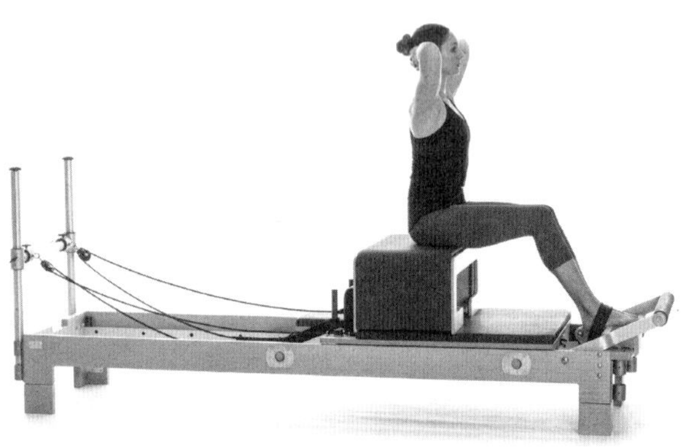

Setup. Sit upright on the box, close to the front. Place the feet hip width apart under the foot strap on the foot platform. Firmly anchor them on the front end of the reformer and bend the knees. Interlace the fingers behind the head.

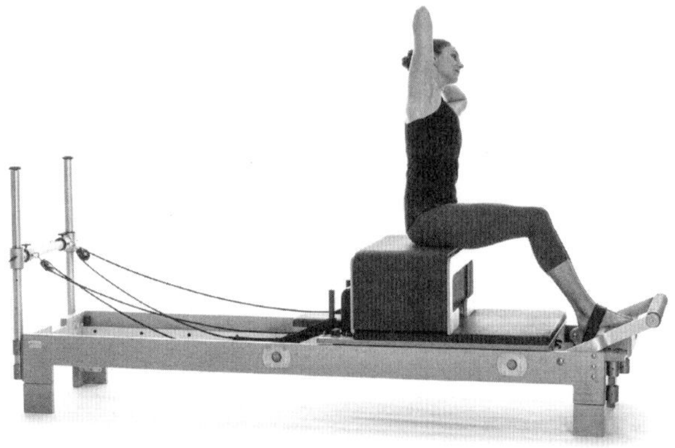

Inhale. Lower the trunk over to one side, reaching out and over, moving from the waist and keeping the pelvis stable.

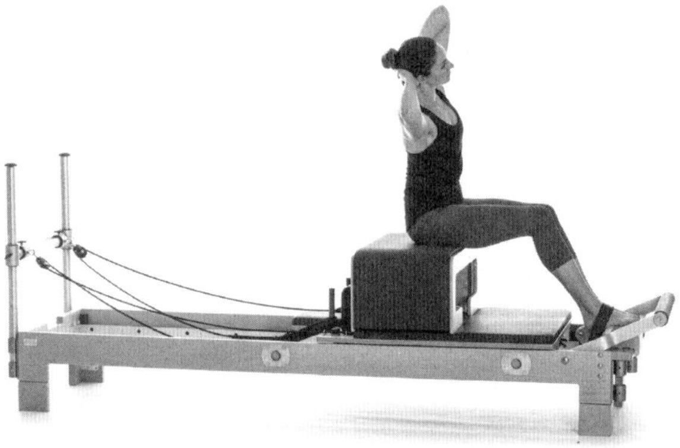

Exhale. Lift the trunk to the upright position, again moving from the waist. Return to the start position. Alternate sides with each repetition. Repeat 5 times to each side.

Short Box—Twist

REFORMER

Lateral Flexion and Rotation

INTERMEDIATE

Muscle Focus

- Abdominal obliques
- Back extensors

Objectives

- To improve abdominal oblique strength
- To develop trunk and lumbopelvic stabilization

RESISTANCE

Light Medium Heavy

Also from the short box series, this exercise has two distinct phases: first the trunk rotates around the longitudinal axis, and then the trunk hinges diagonally back from the hips as one unit. This sequence is repeated in reverse as you return to the start position.

During the second phase, focus on a coordinated contraction of the abdominals and the back extensors to prevent the common error of hyperextending the back. The range of motion is dictated by the ability to keep the sit bones anchored on the box. The pelvis hinges back together with the trunk. Once the pelvis has reached its maximum range, the upper trunk should stop moving in order to avoid hyperlordosis and excessive pressure on the lower back.

Imagery

Rotation around the longitudinal axis—in the initial and final phases—is key to executing this exercise correctly. I use the image of a revolving door. When the body has rotated and then lunges back on a diagonal path, I visualize the entire door being tilted on its side. Then the door returns to upright alignment before revolving to face front.

- ○ Co-contract the abdominals and back extensors.
- ○ Rotate around the longitudinal axis before hinging back.
- ○ Lift the trunk back onto the longitudinal axis before turning to face forward again.

PROGRESSION

The Pilates exercises are like building blocks; they are built on one another, and at times two or more are combined to form another exercise. By combining the Reformer: Short Box—Flat Back (abdominal work) and Reformer: Short Box—Twist (lateral flexion and rotation), we create a very challenging new movement. Twist and lower to one side, transition through the center by doing the flat back position, and then twist to the opposite side before lifting to the center and rotating to face forward. Repeat in the opposite direction. The entire exercise demands a high level of control and core strength, particularly the transition through the center with the trunk on a diagonal. At this point, maintain a flat back and avoid both spinal hyperextension and spinal flexion. Keeping the arms overhead, holding a pole, will make this exercise even more challenging.

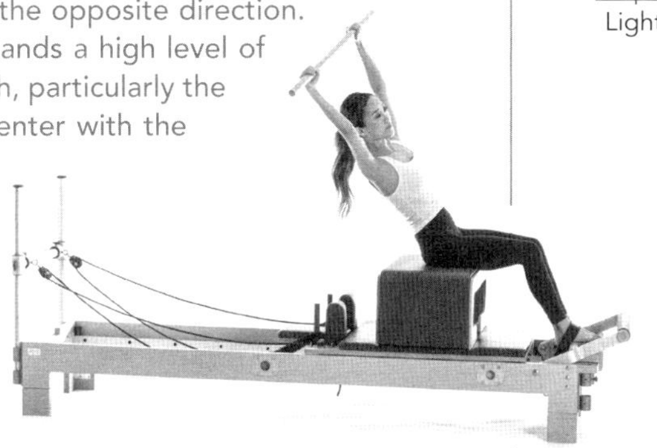

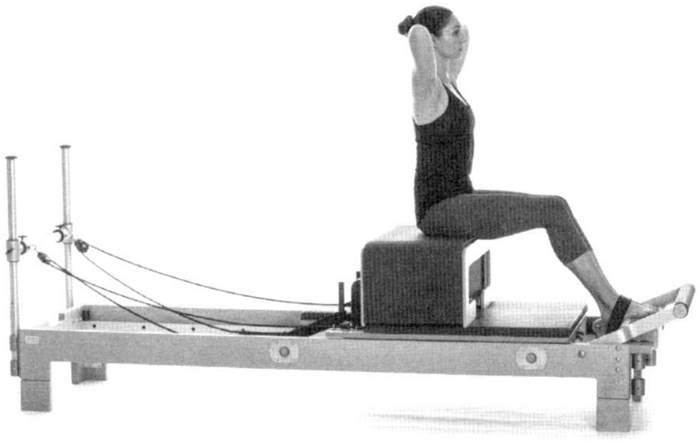

Setup. Sit upright on the box, close to the front. Place the feet hip width apart under the foot strap on the foot platform. Firmly anchor them on the front end of the reformer and bend the knees. Interlace the fingers behind the head.

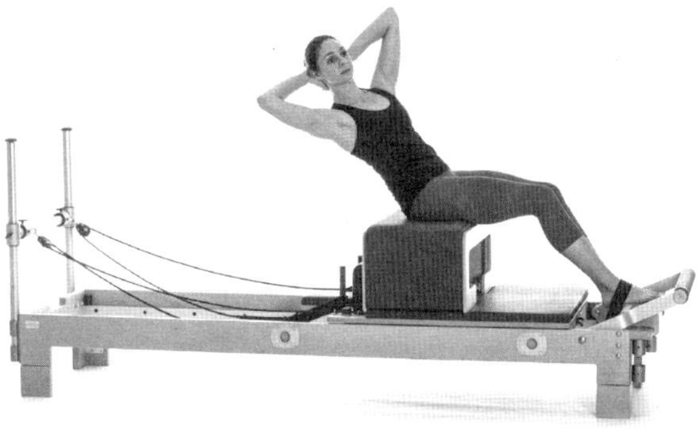

Inhale. Rotate around the longitudinal axis, focusing on elongation of the spine; then hinge from the hip joints, lowering the pelvis and trunk backward on a diagonal.

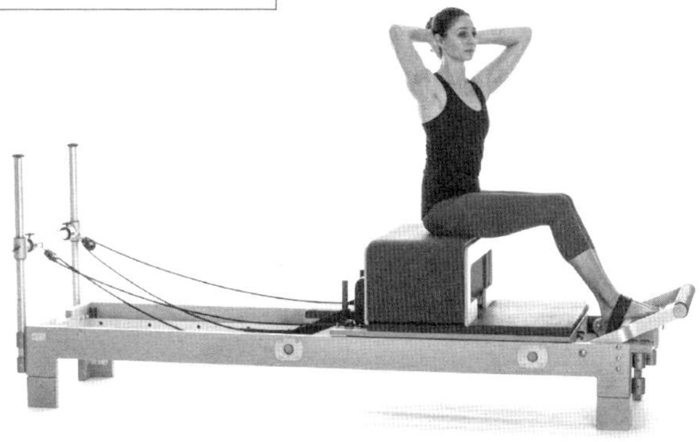

Exhale. Lift the trunk and return to the upright position while maintaining the rotation, and then face forward. Alternate sides with each repetition. Repeat 5 times to each side.

Side Over

Muscle Focus

- Abdominal obliques
- Back extensors

Objectives

- To improve abdominal oblique strength
- To develop trunk and lumbopelvic stabilization

RESISTANCE

Light — Medium — Heavy

I consider this to be the "bread and butter" of lateral flexion exercises—it is my favorite! The idea of an energy line that stretches from the feet through the leg, spine, and out the top of the head is particularly pertinent in this movement. The start position is a stable, diagonal line. As the trunk lowers, it reaches over as if it is being pulled from the top of the head. The diagonal energy line is now curved while the pelvis and lower body remain stable. The pull is then released, and the trunk returns from a curve to a diagonal line.

Be mindful that the head is a continuation of the spine and extends the line of the body. When the body is in lateral flexion, avoid the common tendency to try to lift back up with the head, which creates tension in the neck and certainly does not achieve the desired result. Similarly, avoid pulling with the anchored leg to lift the trunk. The lift must emanate from the lateral flexors of the trunk. As with many of the lateral flexion exercises, co-contracting the abdominals and back extensors helps maintain the body alignment and keeps the movement in the coronal plane. The abdominals prevent hyperextension and the back extensors prevent trunk flexion; working together they encourage activation of the correct muscles in a well-balanced manner. Keep the pelvis anchored and as stable as possible. Tipping the pelvis *slightly* forward or back may be necessary to achieve optimal activation of the abdominal obliques and to overcome compensations. In addition, be aware of the abdominal obliques on the underside of the body, which are important in achieving the elongated alignment of the spine during the lowering and lifting.

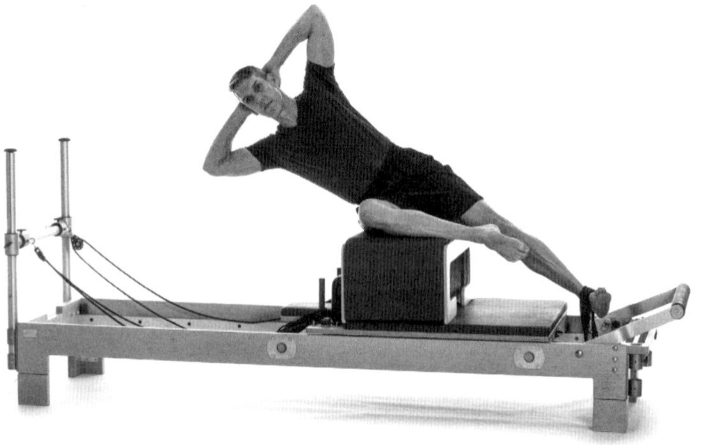

Setup. Place the box in the short box position on the carriage. Sit sideways on the box and adjust for individual body height by placing the box closer to, or farther from, the footbar. For those who are very tall, it may prove advantageous to move the stopper out so the entire carriage is farther from the footbar (if possible). A guideline is that the anchored leg should be straight and able to reach the foot strap while you sit comfortably on the box. Place the foot, dorsiflexed, under the foot strap with the leg straight in neutral hip alignment (minimize hip external rotation). Bend the other leg on top of the box in front of you. Loosely interlace the fingers behind the head. Establish a diagonal line running from the foot that is under the strap to the head.

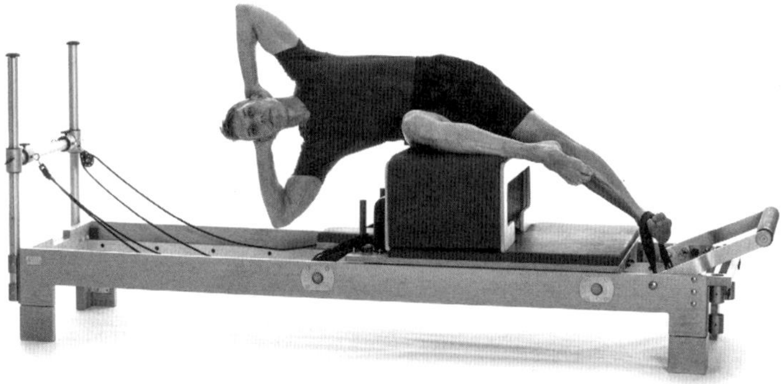

Inhale. Lower the trunk over the box, creating a large arc. Keep the pelvis and both legs stable.

Imagery

The previously used image of a tree trunk being pulled over and then allowed to return to its upright position represents the correct dynamic and shape for this exercise. Cultivating a sense of movement between two panes of glass is also appropriate for this exercise.

- Co-contract the abdominals and the back extensors.
- Avoid lifting the trunk higher than the diagonal line established with the straight leg in the start position.
- Distribute the lateral flexion throughout the spine, creating an arc shape with the body.
- Maintain stability of the pelvis and lower limbs.

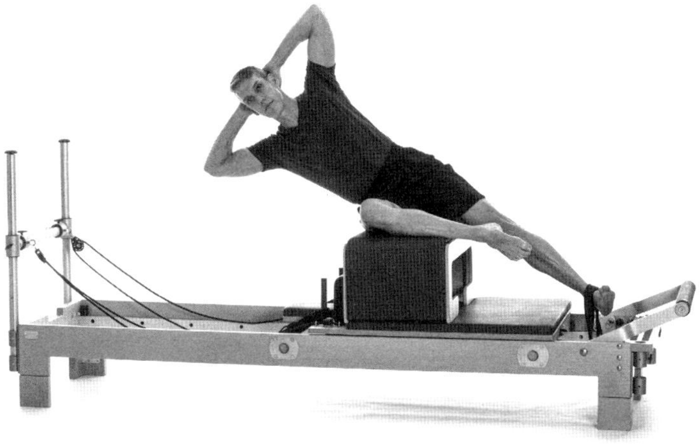

Exhale. Lift the trunk to the diagonal line. Return to the start position. Repeat 5 times before switching sides.

PROGRESSION

If you wish to elevate the intensity of the exercise (seldom necessary), reach both arms overhead to increase the length of the lever arm. I often recommend holding a pole in the hands to encourage good positioning of the arms. Following the exercise, I suggest resting the forearm on the headrest of the carriage and reaching the upper arm overhead to enjoy a stretch of the lateral flexors of the trunk and shoulder adductors before switching to the other side.

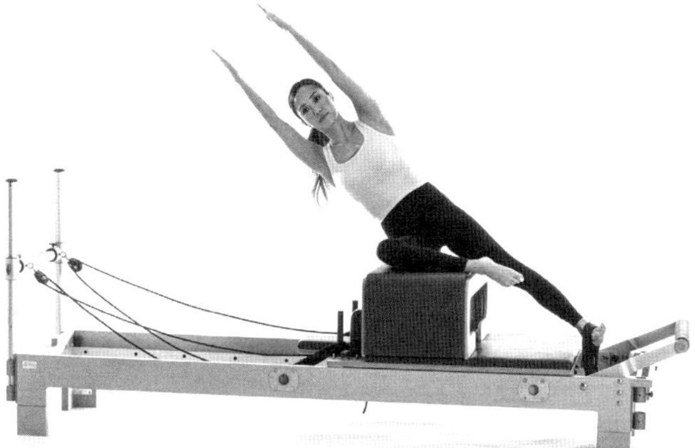

REFORMER

Lateral Flexion and Rotation

INTERMEDIATE

Muscle Focus

- Abdominal obliques
- Back extensors
- Scapular stabilizers

Objectives

- To improve spinal mobility
- To improve abdominal oblique and back extensor control
- To improve shoulder flexibility and stability
- To develop trunk and scapular stabilization

RESISTANCE

Light Medium Heavy

Mermaid

The Reformer: Mermaid has a beautiful flow and exemplifies the choreographic intricacies involved in Pilates. This version differs significantly from the classical exercise, with a different focus and objectives. It can be viewed as a movement sequence with three distinct positions. First, a stable position of the trunk is established with the sit bones resting on the carriage (if someone has tight hips, both sit bones may not be completely on the carriage), the shoulders square, and both arms straight. Second, the carriage is pushed out as the trunk, moving as one stable unit, is lowered toward the springs. The carriage continues moving out until the arm holding the footbar is parallel to the floor and the trunk close to parallel. The movement should feel as fluid as possible. Although the shoulder abductors initiate the movement, there should be a sense that the movement emanates from the underside of the body. The supporting arm follows the movement of the trunk and lifts to form a diagonal line (90-degree angle in the shoulder joint). Note that the outer sit bone will naturally lift off the carriage as the trunk and pelvis move together. Third, the body rotates around the shoulder of the working arm so that the trunk faces the floor. The supporting arm follows the rotation of the trunk and slices through the air to rest on the footbar. The shoulders are now square to the footbar, in line with each other and parallel to the floor. During this phase, the back extensors should remain engaged and the trunk elongated; there should be a feeling of disassociating the trunk from the pelvis and rotating the trunk around a pole.

The return from the third position back to the second position should be precise and clear, with the trunk pivoting around the shoulder joint and the supporting arm returning to the diagonal line. Finally, lift the trunk to the start position, lowering the pelvis so the sit bones are anchored on the carriage (or as close as possible depending on hip flexibility). Both arms remain straight throughout the exercise and the scapulae remain stable. When the carriage moves back toward the start position it does not need to reach the stopper—in fact, in most cases it will not. The transition between positions should be clear and controlled. Avoid excessive movement with the upper arm. I call it the "breathing" or "floating" arm; it should float weightlessly, responding to the breath and the movement of the trunk.

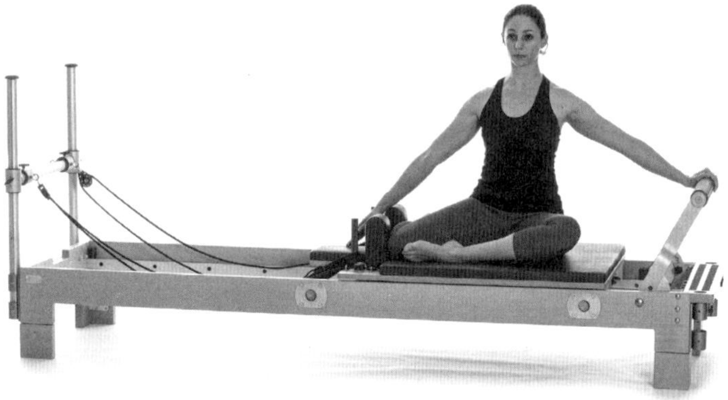

Setup. Sit sideways on the carriage so that the shin of the back leg is placed against the shoulder rests, and the leg closest to the footbar is bent in front of the pelvis. Place the hand of the arm closest to the footbar on the footbar, directly opposite the shoulder, and straighten the arm. Place the other arm down by the side, with the fingers reaching toward the headrest.

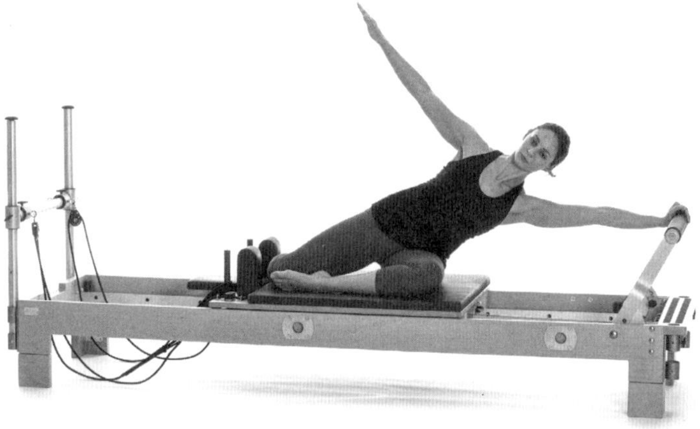

Inhale. Push the carriage away from the footbar until the pushing arm is parallel to the floor. Simultaneously lower the trunk as one unit toward the springs, allowing the outside sit bone to lift with the movement. Lift the other arm, allowing it to move with the trunk, creating a 90-degree angle in the shoulder joint.

Imagery

Imagine the body as a spring being wound up and then unwinding with control and precision.

- Keep both arms straight.
- Pivot around the working shoulder during the rotation.
- Allow the breathing arm to move weightlessly with the movement of the trunk.

VARIATION

To cap off the enjoyment of this flowing and intricate movement, bend the arm on the footbar to bring the carriage in to the stopper. Laterally flex the trunk in the opposite direction of the footbar, reaching the arm overhead. Rest the forearm of the other arm on the headrest. Hold for 3-5 breaths before switching to the other side. Enjoy this wonderful stretch of the lateral flexors of the trunk and the shoulder adductors.

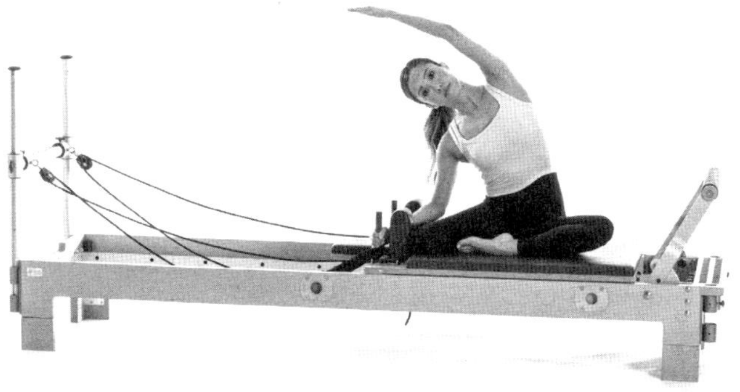

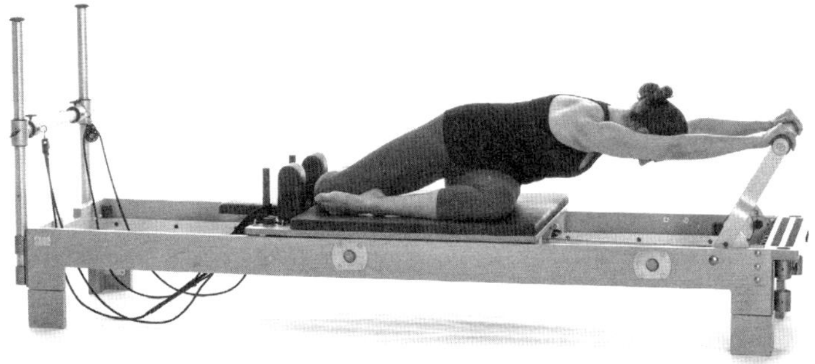

Exhale. Rotate the trunk, keeping it as elongated as possible and pivoting around the shoulder, while bringing the breathing arm around to rest on the footbar. The trunk and shoulder girdle should now be square and parallel to the floor. Keep the carriage stable during this transition.

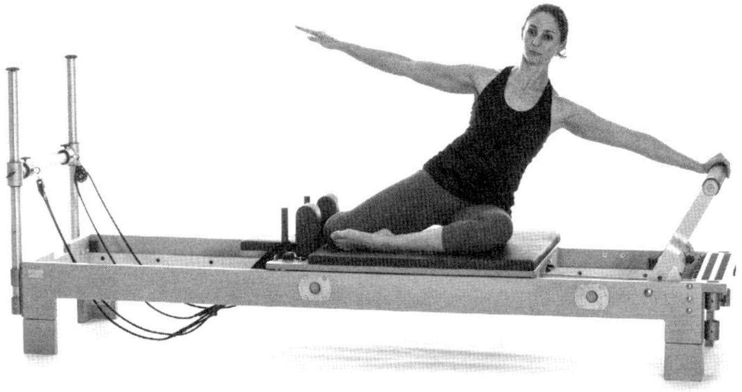

Inhale. Return to the previous position, pivoting around the shoulder and moving the breathing arm back to the diagonal line. Keep the carriage stable during this transition.

Exhale. Begin lifting the trunk and lowering the sit bone to the carriage. Simultaneously lower the breathing arm while keeping the working arm straight and moving the carriage in toward the stopper. Return to the start position. Repeat 5 times before switching sides.

Back Extension

I suppose I may be regarded as somewhat of a back extension fanatic! There are many reasons I qualify for this title, the most apparent being that I virtually never forgo back extension in a session. I am all too aware that our modern lifestyle, coupled with the inevitable and unavoidable pull of gravity and the natural inclination of the spine to fold forward, predisposes us to a forward-leaning posture and an eventual loss of range of spinal extension. I will add that as a somewhat tight, male dancer, my back extension always paled in comparison to my peers, so I was determined to milk every drop of extension I could out of my spine—safely! Now, as I suddenly find myself in my mid-60s galloping toward 70, I experience daily the toll aging takes on spinal extension, a phenomenon I observed countless times with clients over the past four decades. While in my early career, I was an outside observer, I currently find myself deeply immersed in the very same group that has always inspired me to no end.

Pilates places a great deal of focus on the abdominals and hence on spinal flexion, often at the expense of spinal extension. At the very least, the ratio of abdominal work to back extension work is often disproportionate. We must not forget that it is the extensors that hold us upright all day, every day. Although the abdominals are certainly important in offering additional support, the extensors do the primary work. The back extensors, particularly the deeper-lying, intervertebral extensors, also offer support to the ever-important and vulnerable spine. They work in concert with the other muscles of the ISS to protect this central pillar of our bodies.

It is important to recognize that there are distinct regions in the back, and that the many back extension exercises target different areas and different muscles. Typically, when teaching fundamental-level back extension movements, I focus on bracing and stabilizing the lower back and concentrating the movement in the mid- and upper back. The main reason for this is that most people automatically extend from their lumbar region, because the natural curve of the lower spine is in the direction of extension. The upper back, which has a natural curve in the direction of flexion, is therefore often neglected. This results in a weakening of the mid- and upper back extensors, coupled with a tightening of their antagonists, the flexors of the thoracic region. These tendencies are exacerbated by a modern lifestyle: working on computers, driving, cycling, even golfing, which all involve (or certainly have a propensity toward) flexion of the upper body, round shoulders, and kyphotic posture. It takes time to become reacquainted with the often-neglected mid- and upper back muscles while learning to stabilize the lumbar region. To facilitate activation of the mid- and upper back, the program must be augmented by exercises that stretch the muscles of the chest and the abdominals—if the chest muscles are tight, thoracic extension and scapular adduction (retraction) are restricted, and if the abdominals are tight, extension of the entire spine is restricted. Once you become accomplished in doing fundamental back extension exercises, you can move on to exercises with more extreme ranges of motion that require the participation of the lumbar extensors and often the hip extensors as well.

Three distinct images relate to extension exercises, and each result in the recruitment of a different region of the back, different muscles, and a different outcome. The first is used when the goal is to emphasize the mid- and upper back, with the height of the extension being low to moderate. *Elongation* is the pertinent image, reaching out from the top of the head. Keeping the legs stable and engaging the gluteals only enough to assist in stabilizing the pelvis, and no more, will help achieve this in exercises like Reformer: Breaststroke Prep.

The second image is used when one of the primary goals is height. In this case I use the image of an archer's bow ready to unleash its power. This image works well for exercises that move in and out of extension as well as those in which holding an arched, stable position is important, such as the Reformer: Pulling Straps 1. In these exercises, the entire posterior aspect of the body will be active: the mid- and upper back extensors, the lower back muscles, and the hip extensors.

The third image requires very intricate control. The goal is seamless movement that uses the deep intervertebral muscles that are integral to the movement and stabilization of the spine. *Spinal articulation* is used to meet this goal. Achieving this is much more challenging than spinal articulation in flexion, such as in the Mat: Pelvic Curl. I often refer to it as *reverse spinal articulation*. Reverse spinal articulation can be used when doing exercises from both groups previously described: elongation and high arch.

Finally, I must emphasize the role of the breath. I prefer to use an inhale as the trunk extends in all the back extension exercises, on the mat and on the various apparatus, whether there is external resistance or not. This is for two reasons: first, the inhale conceptually assists in elevating the body, and second, certain muscles that assist in the inhalation process also assist in spinal extension. This does not mean that an exhale is never used during an extension. The prescribed breath pattern should be learned, but once an exercise is mastered, it is possible, and encouraged, to change the breath pattern without compromising the quality of the movement.

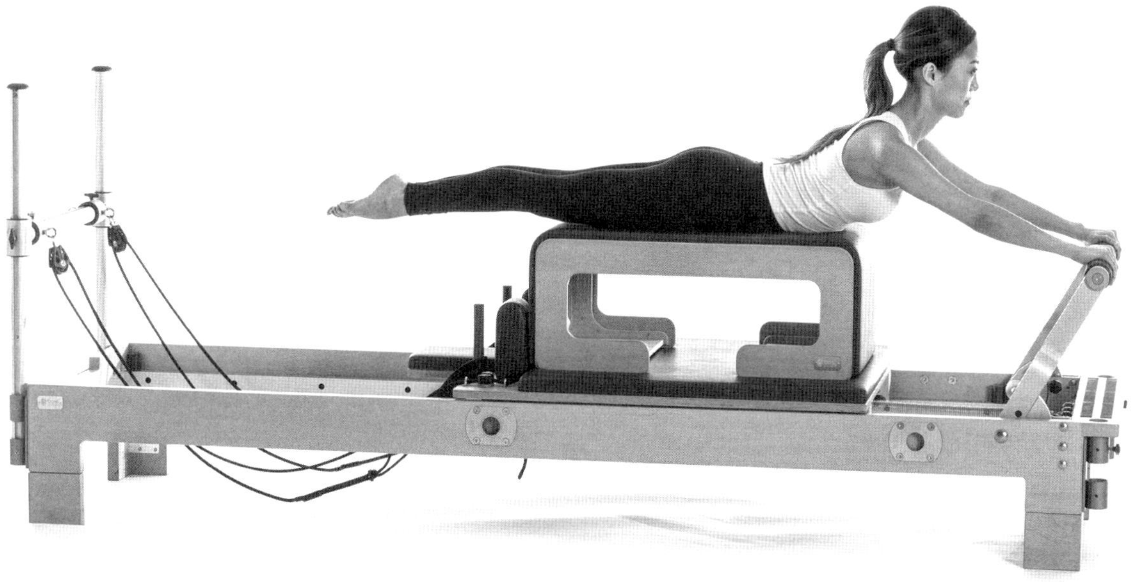

Breaststroke Prep

Muscle Focus

- Back extensors
- Abdominals
- Hip extensors
- Scapular stabilizers

Objectives

- To improve back extensor strength
- To improve abdominal and hip extensor control
- To develop scapular stabilization

RESISTANCE

Light — Medium — Heavy

This is an excellent back extensor exercise for people of all age groups and fitness levels. It uses relatively low resistance and has a large base of support, making it safe and user friendly. It works the arms and shoulders together with the back extensors. The degree of extension can be easily moderated, depending on the individual and the objectives.

Imagery

The image of effortlessly gliding across smooth ice as you push away from the footbar gives a flowing quality to the exercise. When doing the progression with added extension, the same gliding quality should be achieved; however, in this case, the energy lines will move both horizontally and vertically as the body arches.

- ○ Engage the back extensors prior to moving the carriage.
- ○ Keep the wrists firm and the fingers pointing forward (or gently wrapped around the footbar).
- ○ Keep the head aligned with the spine.

PROGRESSION

Once you have achieved correct muscle activation and good form, extend the trunk into a moderate arch while simultaneously straightening the arms. You should reach the arched position of the trunk and the fully straightened position of the arms at the same time. Then lower the body and bend the arms.

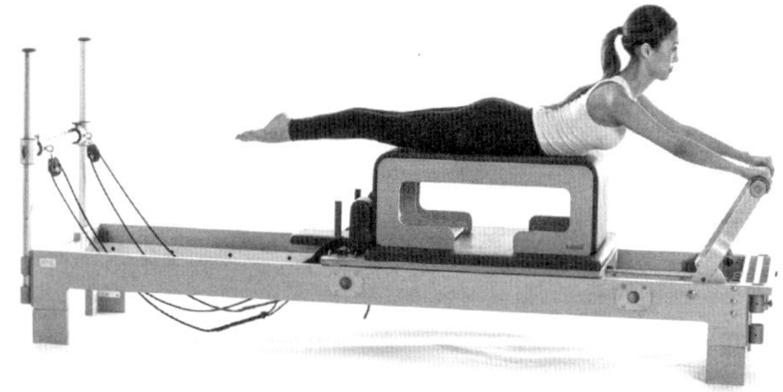

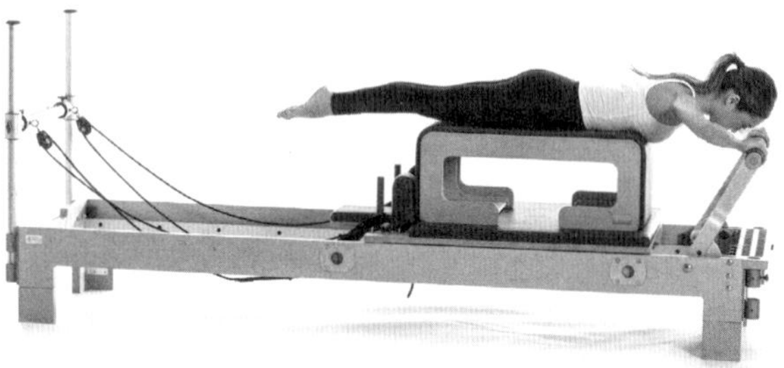

Setup. Lie prone on the long box, facing the front of the reformer (footbar), with the sternum at the front edge. Place the hands on the footbar, shoulder width apart.

Direct the elbows out to the sides as if the arms were on a flat surface, and keep the body horizontal (parallel to the floor) with the back extensors and hip extensors engaged.

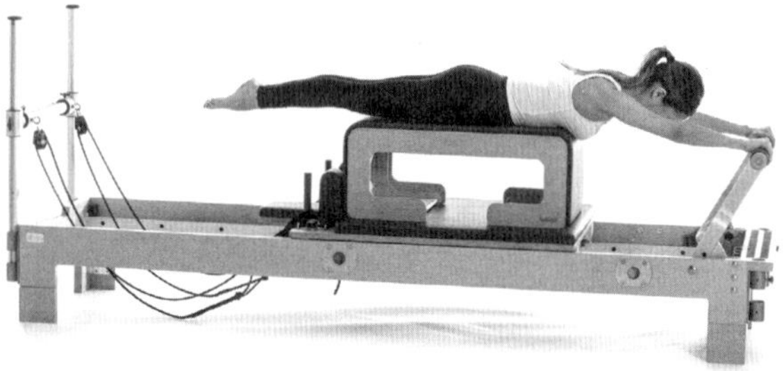

Inhale. Straighten the arms while elongating the entire body and moving horizontally.

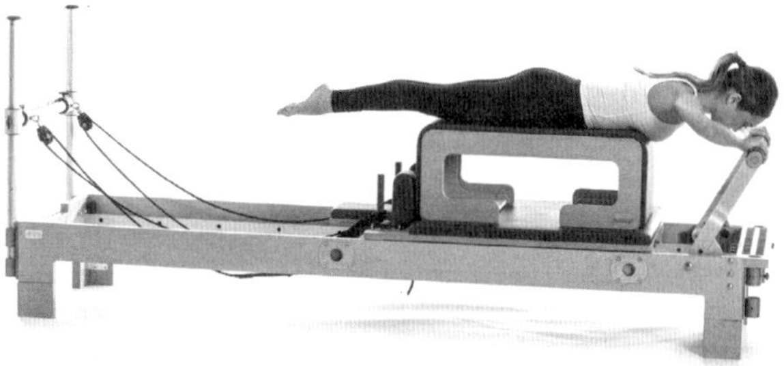

Exhale. Bend the arms, reaching the elbows out to the sides, and bring the carriage in toward the footbar. Return to the start position. Repeat 5-10 times.

Breaststroke

This exercise emphasizes coordinated movement of the shoulders and arms together with the back extensors. The movement emanates from the back and should flow up the spine sequentially, leading into the shoulders and through the arms. There is a tendency to begin the movement with the arms, which is incorrect and does not facilitate effective back work. The degree of extension should initially be small to moderate and evenly distributed throughout the back.

Following the extension of the back and straightening of the arms, the arms remain straight and the back extended until the arms have circled around to the sides of the body; avoid bending the elbows during this phase. As the arms reach the sides of the body, the arms bend, and the trunk is lowered. Keep the upper arms as still as possible and maximize shoulder external rotation as the elbows bend, bringing the hands to the shoulders; the forearms should move as if sliding across a flat surface. The legs should remain parallel to the floor and stable.

Everyone can benefit from this exercise. The height of the back extension should be determined by the specific objective. The mid- and upper back extensors work harder if the trunk is kept low and the movement has a horizontal orientation. The lower back is activated more when the trunk lifts into a higher arch. I often work people outside of their comfort zone. For instance, dancers tend to immediately lift into extreme spinal extension—this is within their comfort zone and their lower backs love it! Therefore, I keep them lower and emphasize even distribution of the extension throughout the back.

Imagery

I encourage the use of the image of swimming the breaststroke in a very shallow pool of water, keeping the movement of the arms almost two-dimensional in the coronal plane. This exercise promotes the concept of a strong horizontal component in back extension work, keeping the trunk relatively low and avoiding the tendency to immediately lift as high as possible.

- ○ Begin the movement with the back and follow with the arms.
- ○ Keep the head in line with the spine and between the arms when the arms are reaching forward during the back extension.
- ○ Maintain external rotation of the shoulders as the elbows bend in the final phase.
- ○ Focus on back extension without excessive hip extension; keep the legs parallel to the floor.
- ○ Keep the palms facing the floor (down).

Muscle Focus

- Back extensors
- Abdominals
- Elbow extensors
- Shoulder abductors
- Hip extensors

Objectives

- To improve back extensor, shoulder abductor, and elbow extensor strength
- To improve hip extensor control

RESISTANCE

Light — Medium — Heavy

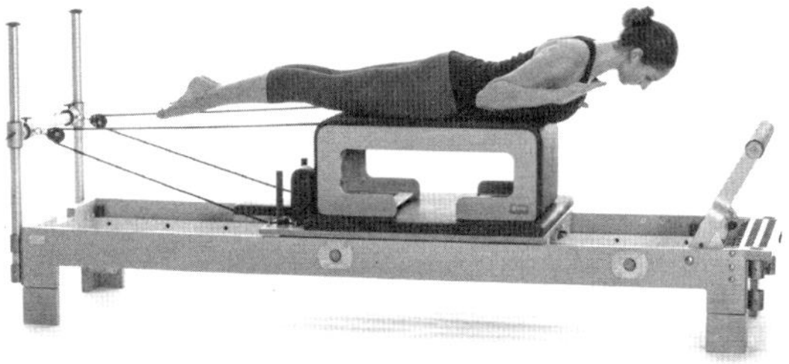

Setup. Lie prone on the long box, facing the front of the reformer (footbar), with the sternum at the front edge. Place the thumbs in the straps so that the ropes run under the arms. The elbows are bent by the sides with the shoulders biased toward external rotation. Face the fingers forward, with the hands slightly higher than the elbows and aligned with the shoulders (or as close as possible).

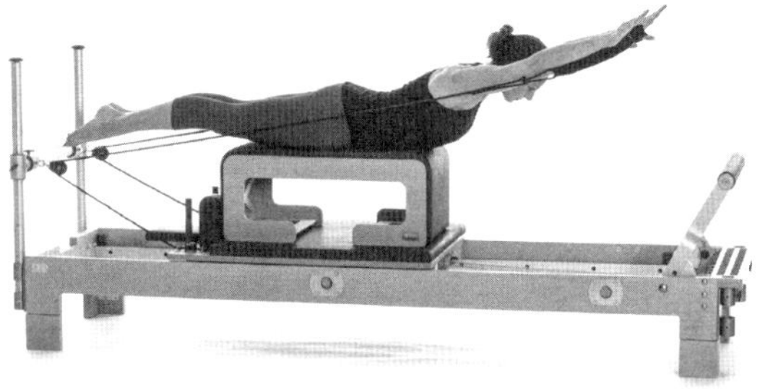

Inhale. Extend the trunk, then immediately straighten the arms forward and upward along a diagonal line, head in between the arms.

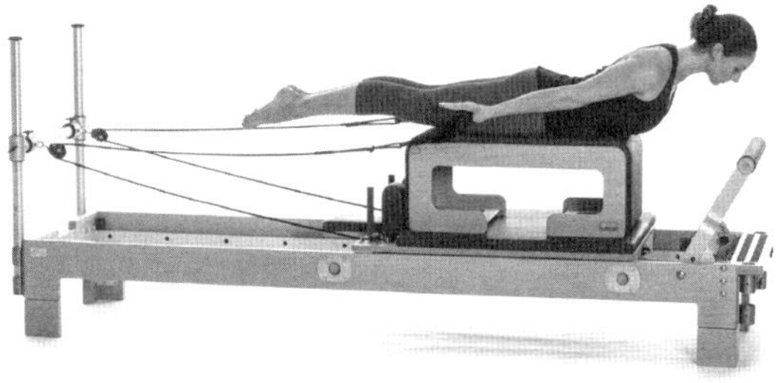

Continuing to inhale, circle the arms around to the sides of the body while holding the trunk stable in extension.

Exhale. Bend the elbows, keeping the upper arms hugging the sides of the body. Maintain external rotation of the shoulders and move the forearms as if they are gliding over a flat surface. Simultaneously lower the body. Return to the start position. Repeat 5 times.

Pulling Straps 1

Muscle Focus

- Back extensors
- Shoulder extensors
- Abdominals
- Hip extensors

Objectives

- To improve back extensor and shoulder extensor strength
- To improve hip extensor control

RESISTANCE

Light Medium Heavy

The next two exercises highlight the back extensor complex and correct muscle activation, together with arm and shoulder work. Starting from the top of the head, the muscles are sequentially recruited toward the lower back. The back extension is accompanied by extension of the shoulders as the straps are pulled back—a powerful combination. As the extension occurs, the legs remain in a stable position, parallel to the floor. The degree of back extension depends on which area of the back you wish to target. The higher the arch, the more the lower back extensors will be activated. Keep the palms facing the reformer throughout, avoiding internal rotation of the shoulders and the temptation to round the chest, particularly as the arms approach the end of the extension alongside the legs. Focus first on arching the thoracic spine and opening the chest as the arms pull back, followed, if you wish, by increasing the back extension as the arms reach their end range.

Imagery

Being a surfer, I find it difficult to resist using the image of paddling a surfboard, which combines back, shoulder, and arm strength in a coordinated pattern. No exercise will better prepare surfers for that elusive perfect wave!

- ○ Engage the back extensors from the outset.
- ○ Keep the arms straight and the palms facing the reformer.
- ○ Press the hands against the thighs at the conclusion of the shoulder extension.

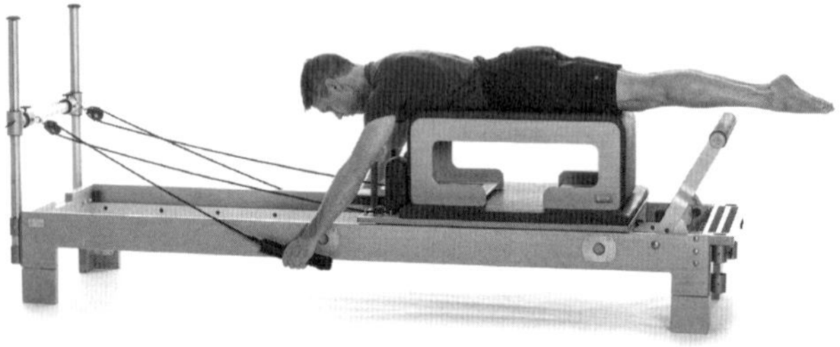

Setup. Lie prone on the long box, facing the back of the reformer, with the sternum at the edge of the box. Hold the ropes with the arms straight, approximately 20 degrees forward of a perpendicular line drawn down from the shoulders. (It may be necessary to shorten the straps or simply fold each strap over and hold the strap and rope together.)

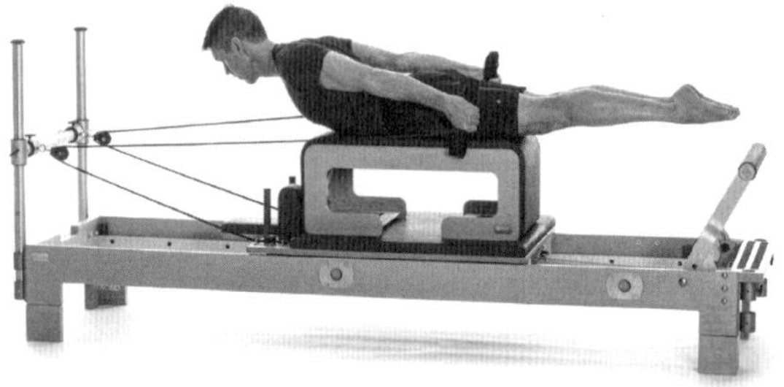

Inhale. Extend the back, lifting the trunk, and simultaneously extend the shoulders, keeping the arms straight. Take them back to the sides of the legs, with the palms facing the body.

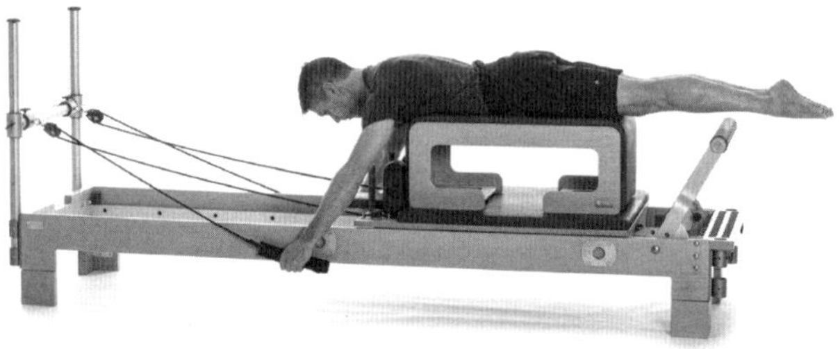

Exhale. Lower the body and bring the arms forward. Return to the start position. Repeat 5 times.

Pulling Straps 2

Like the Reformer: Pulling Straps 1, this exercise emphasizes the importance of the back extensor complex and focuses on coordinated muscle activation of the back and the shoulders. In this case, however, back extension is accompanied by shoulder adduction, rather than shoulder extension. This is a more complex and difficult movement, demanding tremendous strength of the back extensors, which serve as a platform for the arms to move on.

Both exercises demand strong recruitment of the latissimus dorsi, which extends the shoulders in the previous exercise and adducts the shoulders in this one. However, the latissimus dorsi is also a strong internal rotator of the shoulder, an action that is undesired in both exercises. This action is neutralized by the shoulder external rotators, which function as synergists here and in the Reformer: Pulling Straps 1. The close relationship of the shoulder external rotators and the back extensors, particularly the mid- and upper extensors, is highlighted in this exercise. By keeping the palms facing the floor, recruitment of these muscles is encouraged. Move the arms along a horizontal plane.

In addition, the posterior aspect of the shoulder, particularly the posterior deltoid, must work very hard to keep the arms lifted and able to move along a horizontal plane parallel to the floor. It may be necessary to work with very light resistance in order to achieve this.

Imagery

Imagine pulling the body forward along two rails or cables, one on either side of the body, with the arms never rising above or dropping below shoulder level. Although the motion of the horizontal energy line is very powerful, a vertical energy line appears as the trunk lifts into extension.

- Maintain external rotation of the shoulders.
- Hold the arms at the same height as the shoulders when in the T position.
- Pause in the T position after each repetition.
- Keep the hands facing the floor (down).

Muscle Focus

- Back extensors
- Deltoids
- Shoulder adductors
- Abdominals
- Hip extensors

Objectives

- To improve back extensor strength
- To improve shoulder adductor and shoulder horizontal abductor strength
- To improve back extensor control

RESISTANCE

Light Medium Heavy

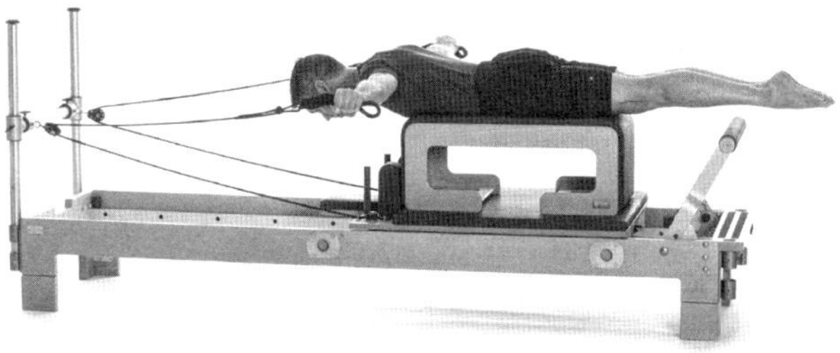

Setup. Lie prone on the long box, facing the back of the reformer, with the sternum at the edge of the box. Hold the ropes with the arms in a T position, parallel to the floor and with the palms facing the floor.

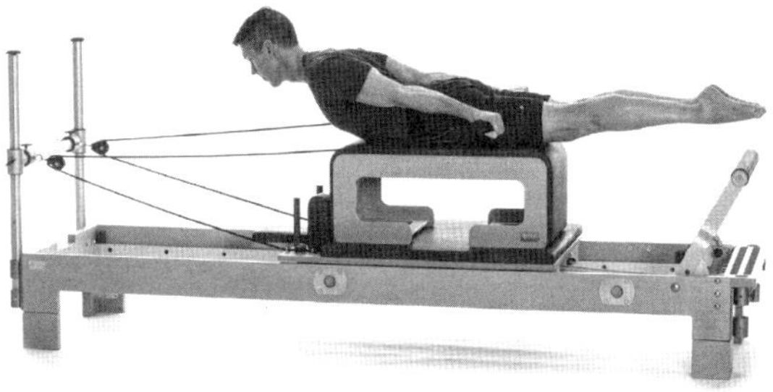

Inhale. Extend the back and pull the arms to the sides of the legs, palms continuing to face the floor. Lead the movement of the arms with the small finger.

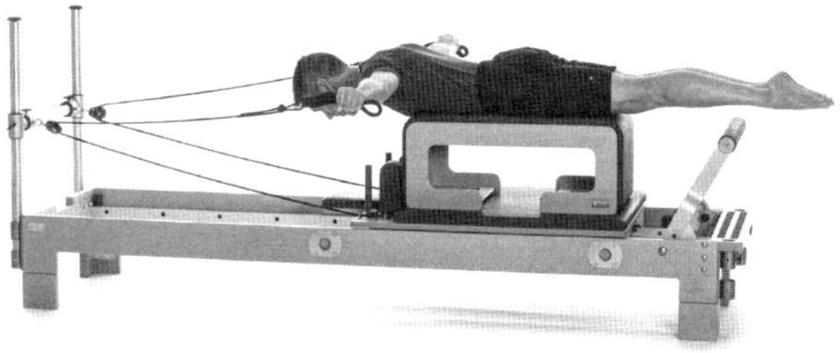

Exhale. Lower the body, moving the arms forward along a horizontal plane parallel to the floor. Return to the start position. Repeat 5 times.

6

Cadillac

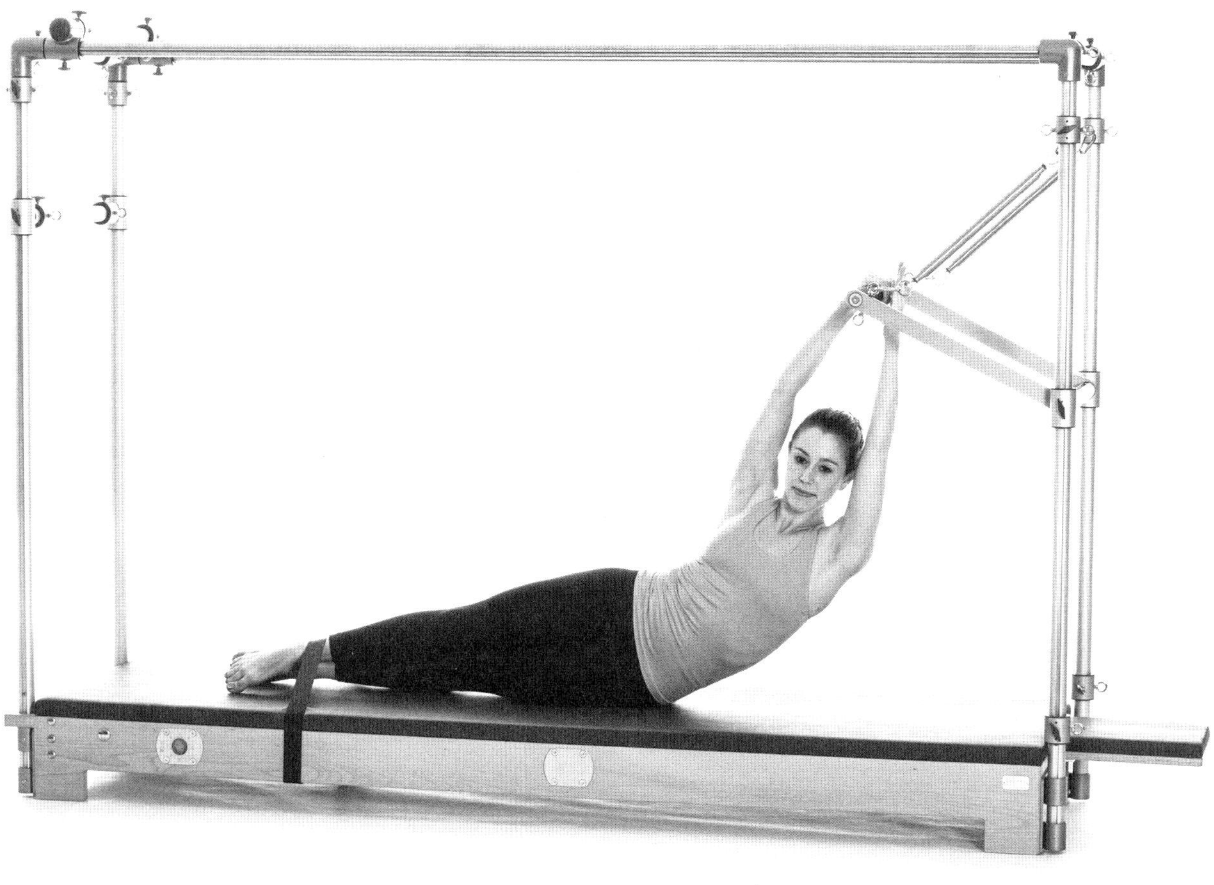

Much has been written about Joseph Pilates' work helping to rehabilitate the ill and the injured. When viewing the cadillac (also called the *trap* or *trap table*), it seems clear that the inspiration for this piece of apparatus was a hospital bed.

Like all the Pilates apparatus, the cadillac is unique and versatile. The foot work on the cadillac, for instance, highlights the work of the hamstrings in terms of both flexibility and strength. This is quite different from the foot work on the reformer and offers many benefits, as long as you maintain the correct position and are careful not to compromise alignment. The cadillac's structure also permits hanging exercises, opening up tremendous possibilities for the upper and lower body. These exercises develop balance, coordination, flexibility, and strength through acrobatic-like movements—and they are a lot of fun to do!

The fact that the cadillac does not move, but instead provides a stable base of support, is an advantage for people who lack balance and stability, such as older adults and those with injuries. In addition, it is relatively high off the ground, making it easier for those with limited mobility to mount and dismount. These characteristics also make it comfortable for the teacher to work closely with students and provide physical support.

The cadillac facilitates ranges of motion that surpass even those of the reformer, particularly in the leg spring work, which can be performed supine, side-lying, prone, and standing while facing in all directions. The cadillac is a three-dimensional piece of apparatus in every sense of the word. Finally, just as the reformer offers exercises that are not easily duplicated on the other apparatus, the cadillac offers unique movements that can only be performed on the cadillac.

Safety is a major issue generally in Pilates, but all the more so on the cadillac. When the springs are bottom-loaded on the push through bar, it is important to always first place the safety strap in position prior to loading the springs. When holding any of the bars, the fingers and thumb must be wrapped around the bar to form a closed ring and establish a secure grip. Make sure that you are standing at a safe distance from any bar or spring that could accidentally be released. All other safety protocol must be observed.

Now it is time to enjoy this intriguing piece of equipment—it always makes me feel like a kid again, spending hours on my favorite jungle gym!

Parallel Heels and Toes

Muscle Focus

- Hamstrings
- Quadriceps

Objectives

- To improve hip extensor and knee extensor strength
- To improve hamstring flexibility
- To develop lumbopelvic stabilization

RESISTANCE

Light Medium Heavy

The foot work on the cadillac duplicates that done on the reformer and all the same cues and directives apply. Although the foot positions are identical, the positioning of the legs is different: On the reformer, the legs move horizontally on the same plane as the trunk; on the cadillac, they move on a vertical line perpendicular to the trunk. This translates to approximately 90 degrees of hip flexion when the legs are straight. People with tight hamstrings who are unable to maintain the recommended position may lie with the head facing the opposite direction; rather than the hip joints being directly under the crossbar of the footbar, they can be further back. This will decrease the angle of hip flexion as well as significantly decrease the stretch on the hamstrings. In turn, this will allow better alignment.

The foot work positions on the cadillac require a smaller degree of knee flexion than those on the reformer. This can be an advantage when knee flexion greater than a 90-degree angle is contraindicated, particularly when performing weight-bearing exercises. This range of knee flexion (greater than a 90-degree angle) is also within the "power range" of the knee when jumping. In short, we are training in a more functional and advantageous range of motion for the knee.

Although the heel position amplifies the stretch and work felt in the hip extensors, the toe position generates greater resistance. It also works the ankle–foot plantarflexors and foot alignment. As with the reformer, the degree of dorsiflexion is established by achieving maximum dorsiflexion when the knees are bent and then keeping the angle of the foot relative to the footbar consistent. The degree of plantarflexion is established by achieving maximum plantarflexion when the legs are straight and then keeping the angle of the foot relative to the footbar consistent. In both dorsiflexion and plantarflexion, the respective positions ensure that the movement occurs around the ankle joint.

Imagery

Imagine that the legs are like pillars holding up the ceiling of a large building. Lift the ceiling a little higher with each

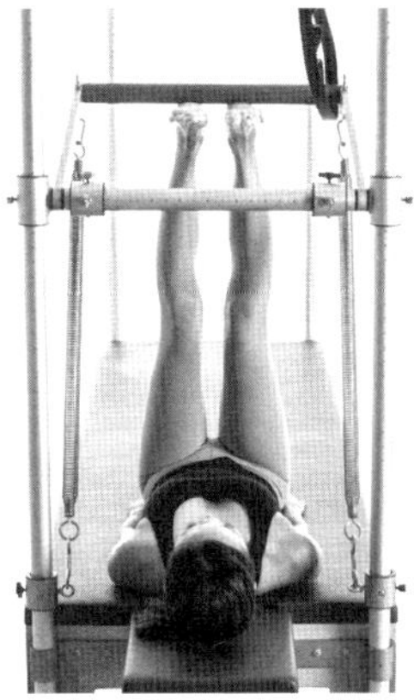

Parallel heels position.

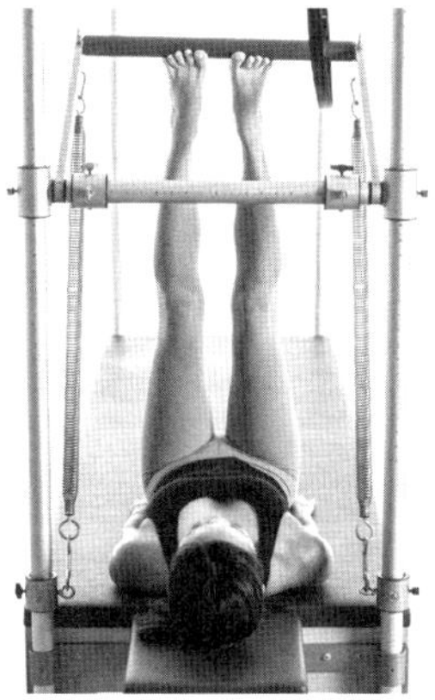

Parallel toes position.

extension of the knees and then lower it as the knees bend, feeling tremendous power in the legs.

- ○ Bend the knees without tucking the pelvis.
- ○ Keep the sacrum anchored on the mat (as close as flexibility allows).
- ○ Keep the hip extensors engaged as the legs straighten and bend.
- ○ Extend the knees and straighten the legs completely with each repetition.

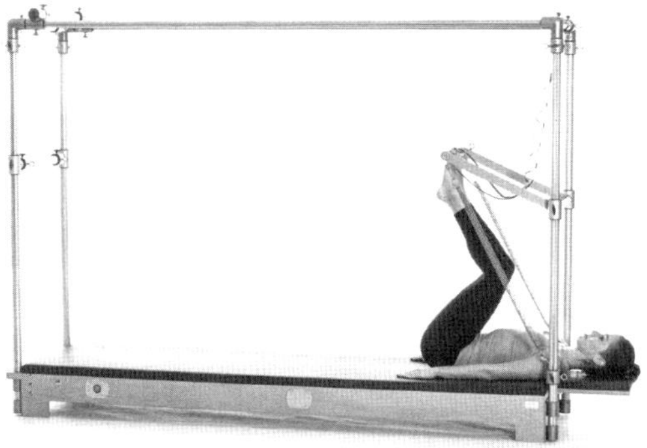

Setup. Lie supine, arms by the sides of the body, knees bent, and legs parallel, with either the heels or toes on the bar.

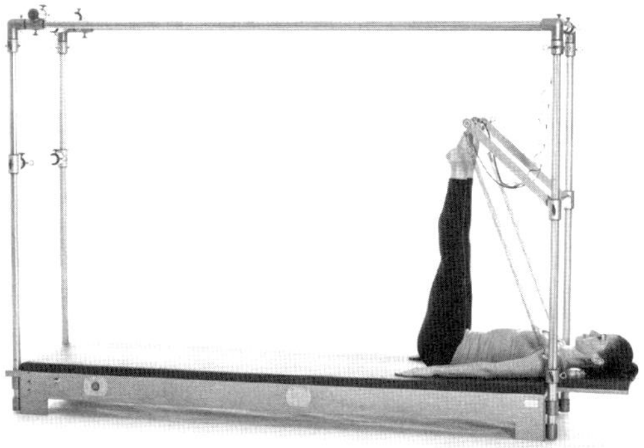

Exhale. Straighten the legs completely, extending the hips and knees while maintaining stability in the pelvis and trunk.

Inhale. Bend the knees and flex the hips. Repeat 10 times.

V Position Toes

Muscle Focus

- Hamstrings
- Quadriceps
- Hip adductors

Objectives

- To improve hip extensor, hip adductor, and knee extensor strength
- To improve hamstring flexibility
- To develop lumbopelvic stabilization

RESISTANCE

Light Medium Heavy

Create the small V position by simply bringing the heels together from the parallel toes position. In this position, the thighs hug the sides of the chest as the knees bend, therefore the knee flexion can be slightly greater than in the parallel position. At the same time, the pelvis must remain stable with the sacrum anchored.

It is important to keep the heels actively pressing together. This will in turn engage the hip external rotators and adductors. Maintaining plantarflexion of the feet is important in order to keep the resistance constant. Although the footbar is typically narrower on the cadillac than on the reformer, it is still important to try to keep all the toes engaged with the footbar, although this will depend on an individual's foot shape.

An advantage of the foot work on the cadillac is that the nature of the position minimizes the possibility of hyperlordosis and, in fact, stretches the lower back. However, you must avoid the common tendency to allow the pelvis to curl up (tilt posteriorly). The pelvis should serve as a stable platform from which the legs can move. Compromising the position of the pelvis will in turn reduce the impact of the foot work exercises, in particular the profound work of the hamstrings.

Imagery

The image of a frog leaping works well in this position. Keep the shape of the V moderate; resist externally rotating the hips excessively and opening the legs too wide.

- ○ Bend the knees without tucking the pelvis.
- ○ Avoid the knees opening wide or bending beyond 90 degrees.
- ○ Keep the heels pressing together.
- ○ Maintain plantarflexion.

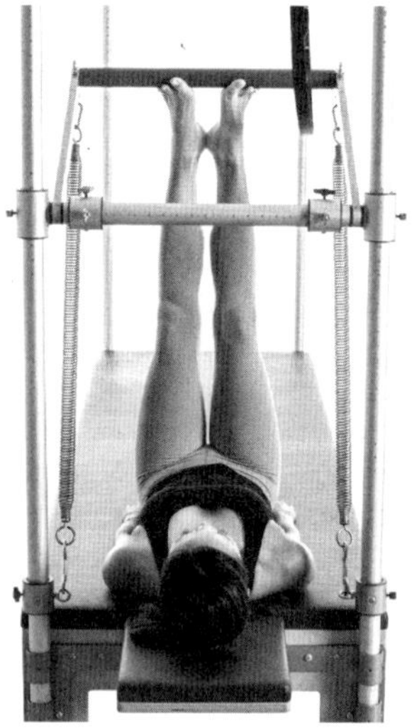

Toes in the V position.

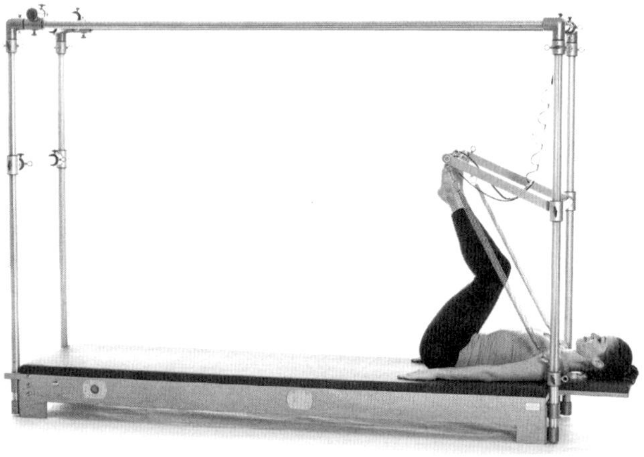

Setup. Lie supine, arms by the sides of the body, knees bent, toes on the footbar, and feet in a V position with the heels together.

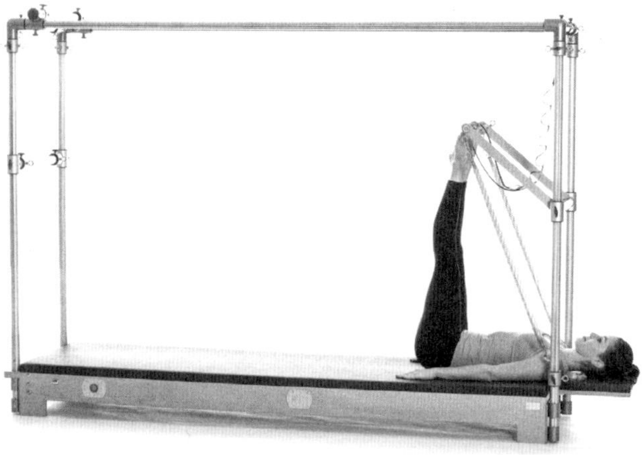

Exhale. Straighten the knees and extend the hips.

Inhale. Bend the knees and flex the hips. Repeat 10 times.

Open V Position Heels and Toes

In the two open V positions, the degree of hip external rotation remains the same as the V position, except the legs are now apart. In this position the knees can bend further without the restriction of the chest, allowing a tremendous stretch for the hips. At the same time remember to keep the pelvis anchored, which in turn will help facilitate the stretch.

The open V heel position has two options. The first option, which is the preferred one, demands flexibility of the calf muscles and the Achilles tendon. The heels are placed on the footbar and the toes are placed under the respective sidebars. If the stretch is too intense in this position, place the toes above the sidebars. The open V toes position provides the deepest stretch of all the positions for the hip joint. Maintain plantarflexion throughout the movement to ensure consistent resistance.

Imagery

The image of a frog leaping used in the V position works well here too. In this position the legs open out wide, so you can take advantage of a deeper stretch as long as the pelvis is anchored.

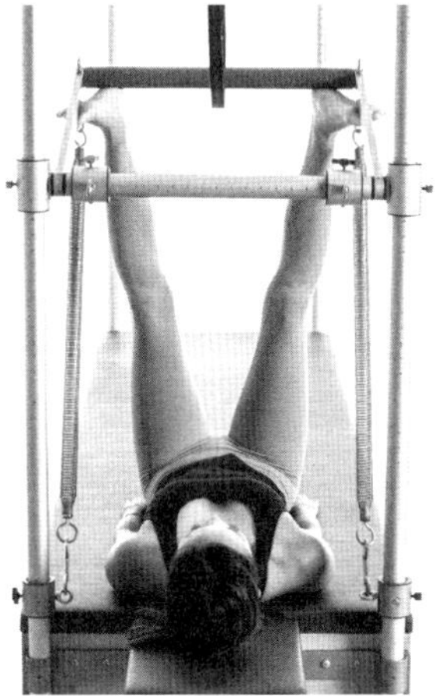
Heels in the open V position.

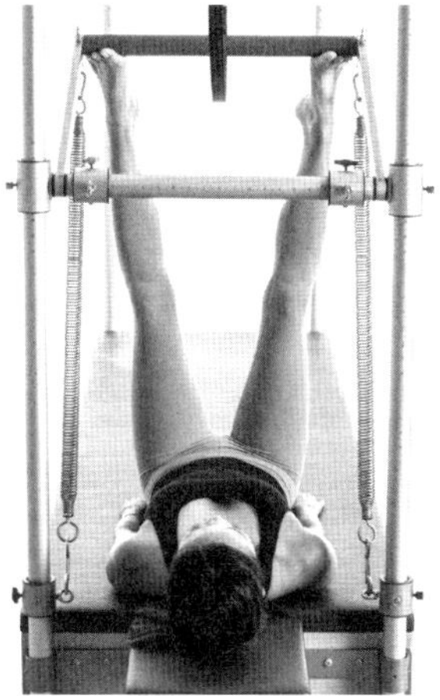
Toes in the open V position.

- ○ Bend the knees without tucking the pelvis.
- ○ Keep the heels pressing into the bar (in the heel position).
- ○ Maintain plantarflexion with a consistent angle of the foot relative to the footbar.

Muscle Focus

- Hamstrings
- Quadriceps
- Hip adductors

Objectives

- To improve hip extensor, hip adductor, and knee extensor strength
- To improve hamstring flexibility
- To develop lumbopelvic stabilization

RESISTANCE
Light Medium Heavy

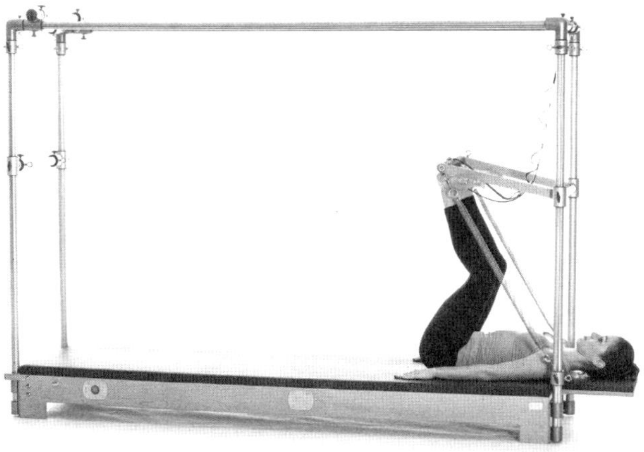
Setup. Lie supine, arms by the sides of the body, knees bent, and feet in an open V position with either heels or toes on the bar.

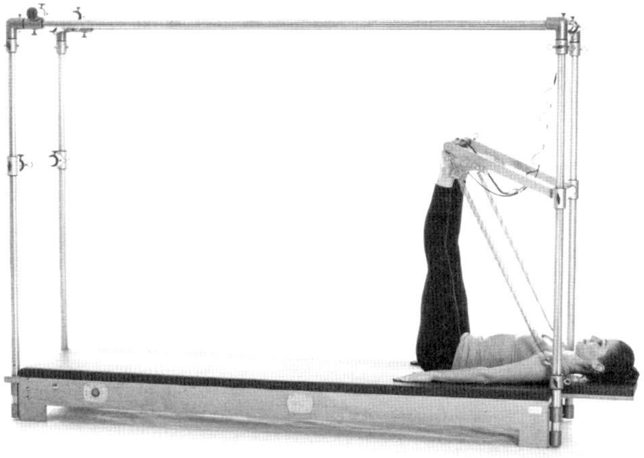
Exhale. Straighten the knees and extend the hips.
Inhale. Bend the knees and flex the hips. Repeat 10 times.

Calf Raises

Muscle Focus

- Ankle–foot plantarflexors

Objectives

- To improve ankle–foot plantarflexor strength
- To improve ankle–foot plantarflexor and hamstring flexibility
- To develop foot and ankle alignment

RESISTANCE
Light Medium Heavy

The Cadillac: Calf Raises is more intense than the version performed on the reformer because of the upright position of the legs, which is particularly helpful (and challenging) for those with tight calves and hamstrings. Another advantage of this position is the opportunity to observe the feet during the exercise, which assists in correcting alignment.

Imagery

I try to imagine lightness in the feet, as if I were tossing and catching a balloon with the feet.

- ○ Use the full range of motion of the ankle and foot.
- ○ Actively dorsiflex the feet at the end range, not only relying on the pull of the springs.
- ○ Keep the knees straight.

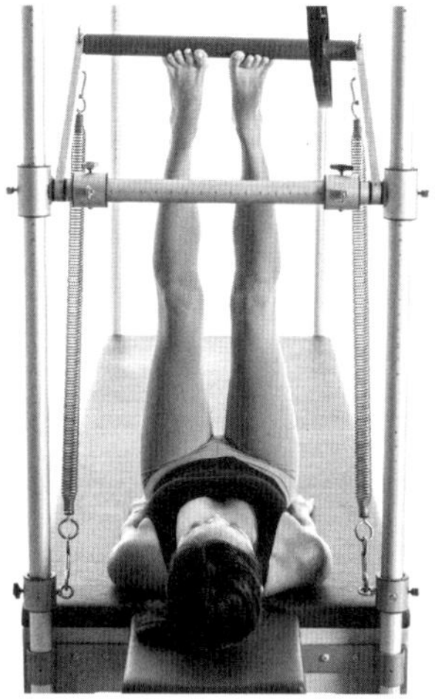

Feet in the calf raises start position.

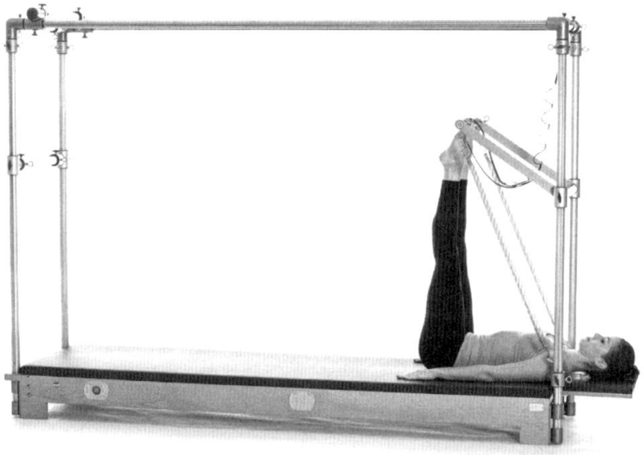

Setup. Lie supine, arms by the sides of the body, toes on the bar, legs parallel and hip width apart, knees straight, and feet plantarflexed.

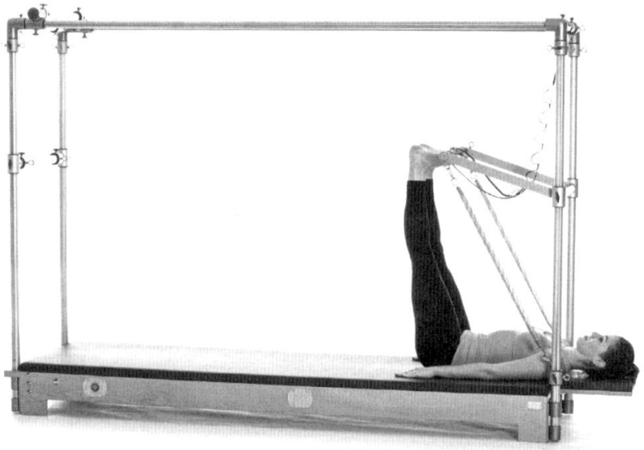

Inhale. Dorsiflex both feet.

Exhale. Plantarflex both feet. Repeat 10-20 times.

Prances

When performing the Cadillac: Prances, the same flow and smooth transitions that are required on the Reformer: Prances should prevail. The anchored position of the pelvis helps stabilize it, reducing the tendency to tilt the pelvis from side to side.

Imagery

As with the Cadillac: Calf Raises, I try to imagine lightness in the feet, as if I were tossing and catching a balloon with the feet.

- Use the full range of motion of the ankle and foot.
- Keep equal pressure on both feet.
- Actively dorsiflex one foot while maximizing the plantarflexion of the other.
- Transition through straight legs and full plantarflexion after each repetition.

VARIATION

In order to amplify the stretch of the calf muscles, allow a double pulse to deepen the stretch on the leg that is dorsiflexed before changing to the other side and repeating. Continue this pattern of a double pulse on the dorsiflexed foot.

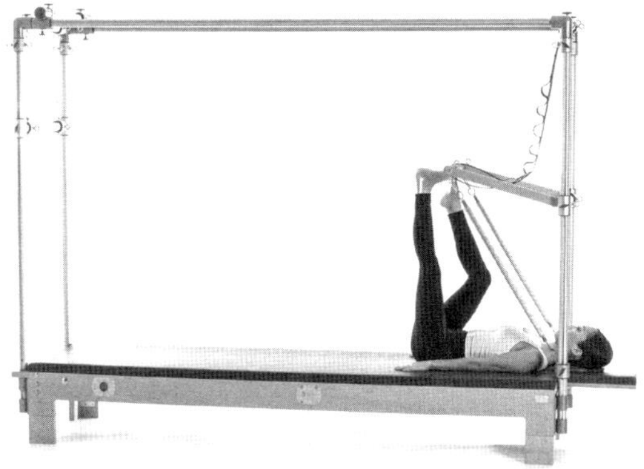

Muscle Focus

- Ankle–foot plantarflexors

Objectives

- To improve ankle–foot plantarflexor strength
- To improve ankle–foot plantarflexor and hamstring flexibility
- To develop foot and ankle alignment
- To develop coordination

RESISTANCE

Light — Medium — Heavy

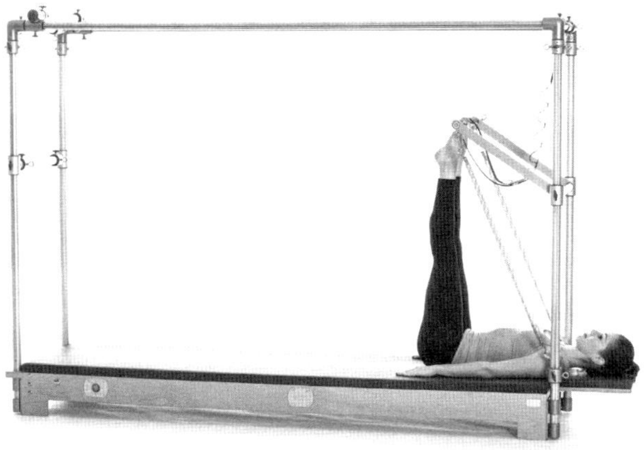

Setup. Lie supine, arms by the sides of the body, toes on the bar, legs parallel and hip width apart, knees straight, and feet plantarflexed.

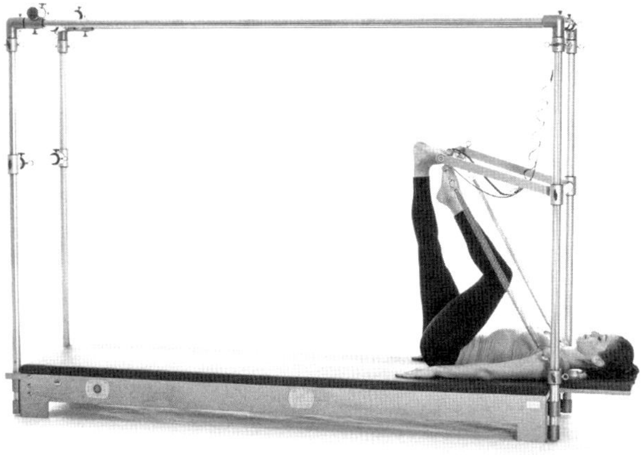

Inhale. Plantarflex one foot while bending the knee and dorsiflexing the other foot. Straighten the bent leg and plantarflex the foot that is dorsiflexed so that both legs are straight and both feet are plantarflexed before transitioning to the other leg. Repeat on the other side.

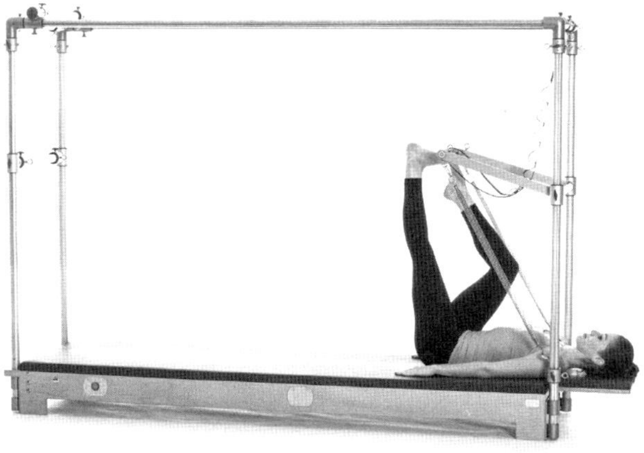

Exhale. Plantarflex one foot while bending the knee and dorsiflexing the other foot. Straighten the bent leg and plantarflex the foot that is dorsiflexed so that both legs are straight and both feet are plantarflexed before transitioning to the other leg. Repeat on the other side.

Alternate; one full cycle while exhaling and one full cycle while inhaling. Repeat 10 times.

Single-Leg Heel

Muscle Focus

- Hamstrings
- Quadriceps

Objectives

- To improve hip extensor and knee extensor strength
- To improve hamstring flexibility
- To develop lumbopelvic stabilization

RESISTANCE
Light — Medium — Heavy

The single-leg positions place the body in optimal alignment to stretch the hamstrings of the working leg and to stretch the hip flexors of the supporting leg. The interplay between strength and flexibility of the working leg underscores the principle of *balance* in Pilates. In this heel position, you can readily feel the stretch in the back of the leg and the work of the hip extensors. The supporting leg should lie flat on the mat, aligned with the hip joint. There is a tendency for the supporting leg to "drift" laterally and for the knee to bend, especially if the hip flexors are tight. If this tendency cannot be controlled, bend the knee of the supporting leg and place the foot firmly on the mat. This releases the stretch on the hip flexors of the supporting leg and less stretch will be felt on the hip extensors of the working leg. It will also be easier to align the pelvis in a neutral position (or as close as possible) if tightness is an issue.

Imagery

Energy lines offer a profound image for this position. One line shoots from the hip joint of the working leg out through the heel. The other shoots down from the hip joint of the supporting leg out through the toes, as well as up through the trunk and out through the head. This image helps maintain optimum alignment.

- Keep the pelvis stable.
- Maintain dorsiflexion of the foot of the working leg and plantarflexion of the foot of the supporting leg.
- Bend the supporting leg if the hamstrings and hip flexors are tight.

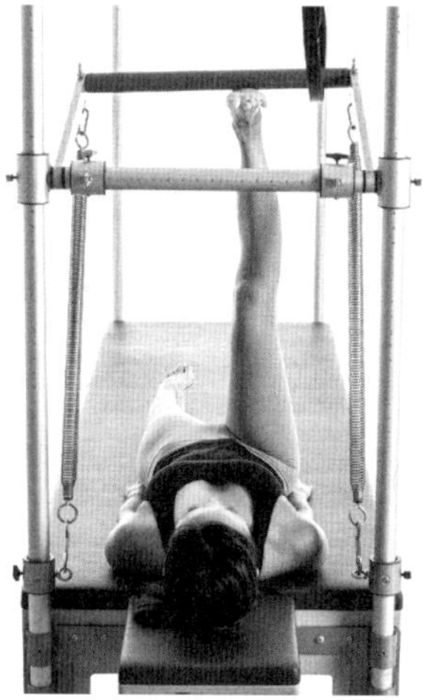

Knee and hip extended with heel on the bar.

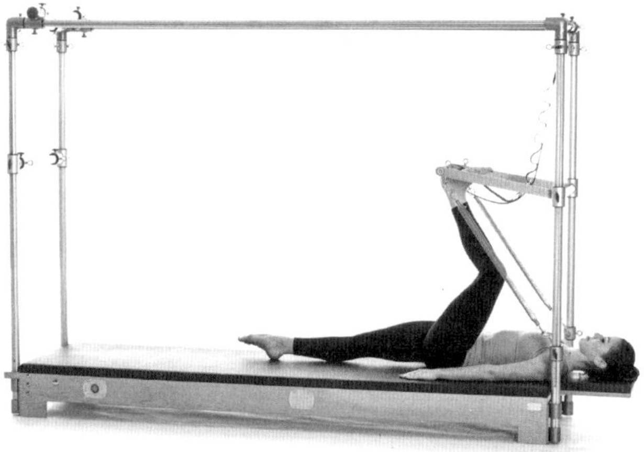

Setup. Lie supine, arms by the sides of the body. Place the heel of one foot on the bar and bend the knee. The supporting leg remains straight and anchored on the mat, foot plantarflexed.

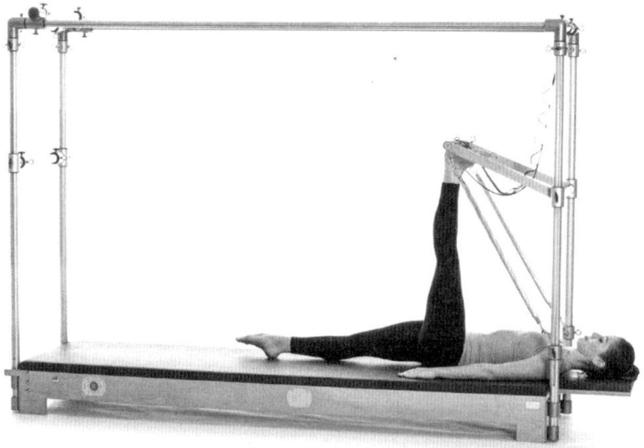

Exhale. Straighten the knee and extend the hip.

Inhale. Bend the knee and flex the hip. Repeat 10 times before switching to the other leg.

Single-Leg Toes

As with all toe positions, the increased stretch of the springs creates a slight increase in resistance. It may be necessary to lower the resistance if you did not lower it for Cadillac: Single-Leg Heel. The ankle–foot plantarflexors, as well as the muscles that control supination and pronation, play a prominent role in this position of the foot work. Observe the alignment of the foot and correct as needed. As with the Cadillac: Single-Leg Heel, there is a tendency for the supporting leg to drift laterally and for the knee to bend. If this tendency cannot be controlled, bend the knee of the supporting leg and place the foot firmly on the mat.

Imagery

The energy lines used to maintain alignment in Cadillac: Single-Leg Heel are also useful here. One line shoots from the hip joint of the working leg out through the toes. The other shoots down from the hip joint of the supporting leg out through the toes, as well as up through the trunk and out through the head.

- Keep the pelvis stable.
- Maintain plantarflexion throughout the movement.
- Bend the supporting leg if the hamstrings and hip flexors are tight.

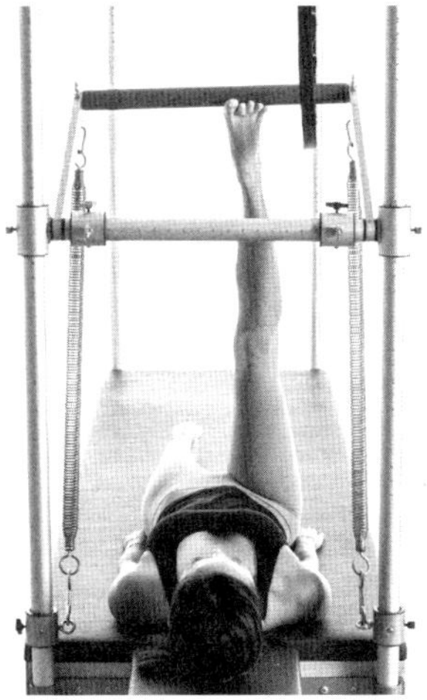

Knee and hip extended with toes on the bar.

Muscle Focus

- Hamstrings
- Quadriceps

Objectives

- To improve hip extensor and knee extensor strength
- To improve hamstring flexibility
- To develop lumbopelvic stabilization
- To develop foot and ankle alignment

RESISTANCE

Light — Medium — Heavy

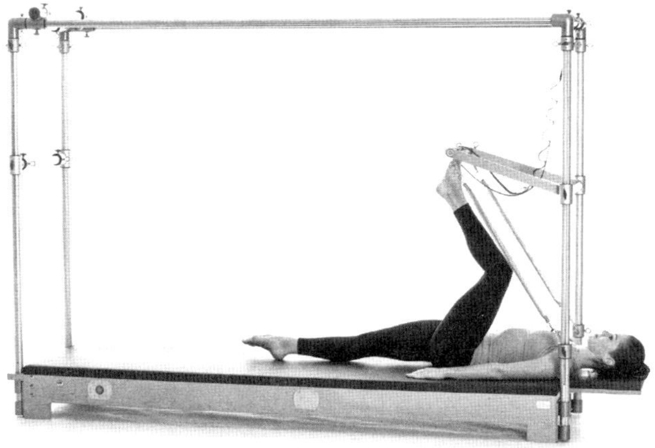

Setup. Lie supine, arms by the sides of the body. Place the toes of one foot on the bar and bend the knee. The supporting leg remains straight and anchored on the mat, foot plantarflexed.

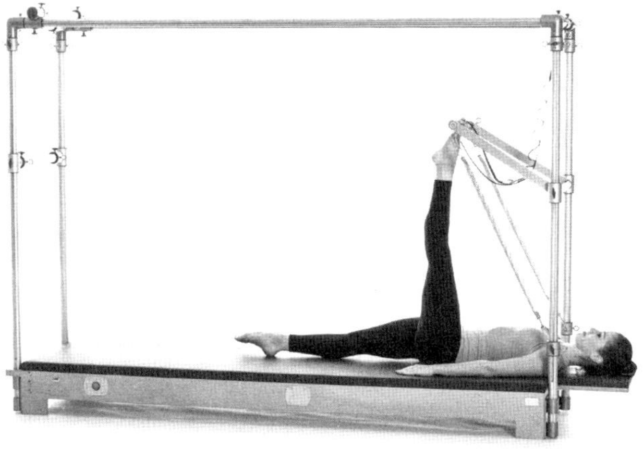

Exhale. Straighten the knee and extend the hip.

Inhale. Bend the knee and flex the hip. Repeat 10 times before switching to the other leg.

Roll-Up

Muscle Focus

- Abdominals

Objectives

- To improve abdominal strength
- To improve back extensor flexibility
- To develop trunk stabilization

RESISTANCE

Light Medium Heavy

This exercise is essentially a spring-assisted Mat: Roll-Up and will prove particularly helpful for people who are experiencing difficulty performing that movement correctly. It is also an excellent option to include in a warm-up on the cadillac. The springs help facilitate the recruitment of the correct muscles in the correct sequence, beginning with the abdominal engagement as the head, shoulders, and thoracic spine are lifted off the mat. Once the C shape is established, the abdominals, together with the back extensors, become stabilizers, and the hip flexors are then activated to lift the trunk and pelvis into a sitting C curve (with the assistance of the springs). There is no change in the shape of the trunk as it is lifted from the supine to the sitting position. The assistance of the springs also helps release excess tension, particularly in the muscles of the lower back, which may be hampering proper execution of this exercise.

Often, it is not lack of strength that hinders the successful execution of the Mat: Roll-Up, but rather the inhibition of certain muscles being recruited for a variety of reasons, such as tightness of the back extensors, a lack of awareness of the abdominals, or the breakdown of the neuromuscular pathways in which the individual does not have a sensation of the muscles and cannot recruit them. This is often the case following surgery in the abdominal area such as a C-section. Finally, body type has a profound effect on the level of difficulty in executing this movement.

Imagery

As with most spring-assisted exercises, you should work with the springs as if they were an integral part of your body and musculature, rather than an external force. Think of them as an extension of the abdominals or an extra abdominal muscle.

- ○ Keep the legs straight and the feet plantarflexed.
- ○ Keep the head aligned with the spine.
- ○ Maintain scapular stabilization and avoid scapular abduction when in the sitting C curve.
- ○ Engage the hip adductors throughout the exercise.

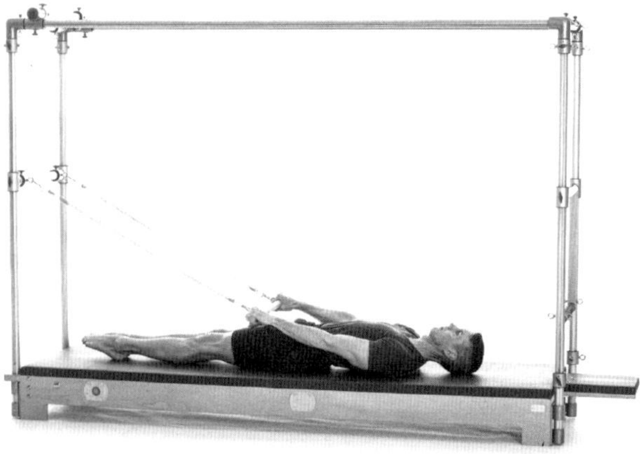

Setup. Lie supine with the legs straight. Hold the roll-up bar with the hands shoulder width apart, placing the body far back enough on the mat of the cadillac that there is tension in the springs.

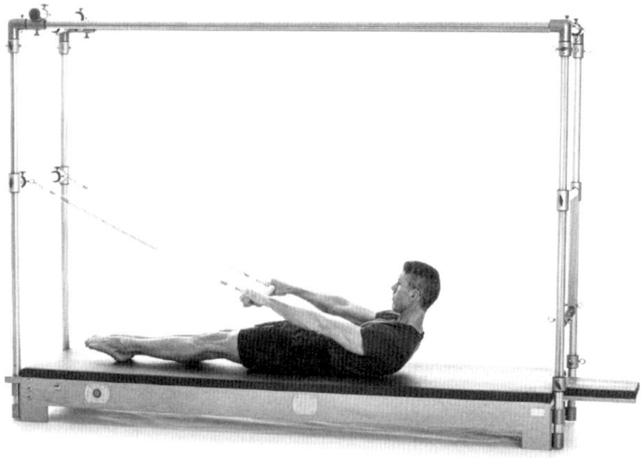

Inhale. Lift the head, shoulders, and chest into spinal flexion, establishing the C curve.

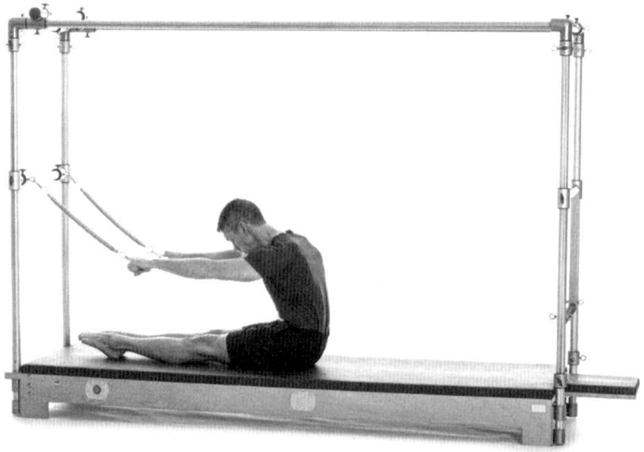

Exhale. Slowly roll up, maintaining the C curve in the trunk.

Inhale. Pause when the shoulders are above the hip joints (err on the side of going a little beyond the hip joints rather than not far enough).

Exhale. Roll back down through each vertebra to the start position. Repeat 5-10 times.

Mini Roll-Up

This exercise is, in essence, a spring-assisted Mat: Chest Lift. I view the springs as an extension of the abdominals, supplementing their strength and making it easier to overcome compensations and achieve perfect form. The springs allow the release of redundant tension in the lower back extensors, which often prevents the trunk from achieving adequate forward flexion and the abdominals from fully contracting. Note that the trunk should remain in forward flexion throughout, and the round shape of the body should remain constant, similar to the Mat: Rolling Like a Ball. The movement occurs between the base of the scapulae and the sacrum, peeling the spine off the mat, vertebra by vertebra, and then lowering back down.

Imagery

Think of a wheel or ball rolling forward and backward in a small arc. Focus on hollowing the abdominal bowl with each roll.

- Focus on maintaining spinal flexion.
- Keep the shoulders relaxed and the scapulae stable.
- Maintain a neutral pelvis at the outset of the exercise. (Allow a posterior tilt of the pelvis if it helps achieve the desired goals of abdominal activation and good form, particularly when hyperlordosis is present.)

CADILLAC
Abdominal Work
FUNDAMENTAL

Muscle Focus

- Abdominals

Objectives

- To improve abdominal strength
- To improve lower back extensor flexibility
- To develop trunk stabilization

RESISTANCE
Light Medium Heavy

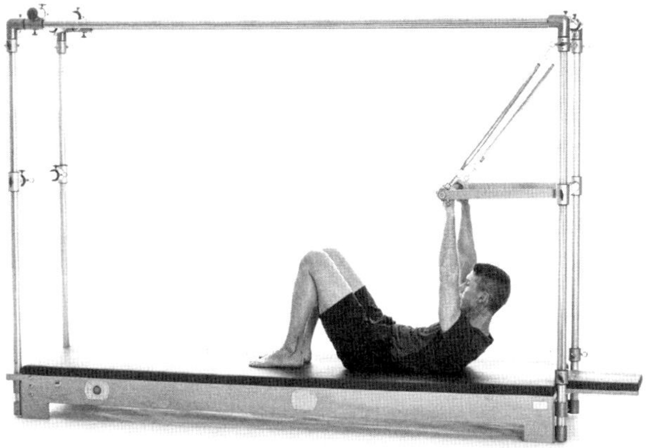

Setup. Lie in a supine position with the knees bent and the feet anchored on the mat, hip width apart. Hold the push through bar with an overhand grip, hands placed in line with the shoulders. Raise the head, shoulders, and chest into spinal flexion, with the shoulders directly under the push through bar.

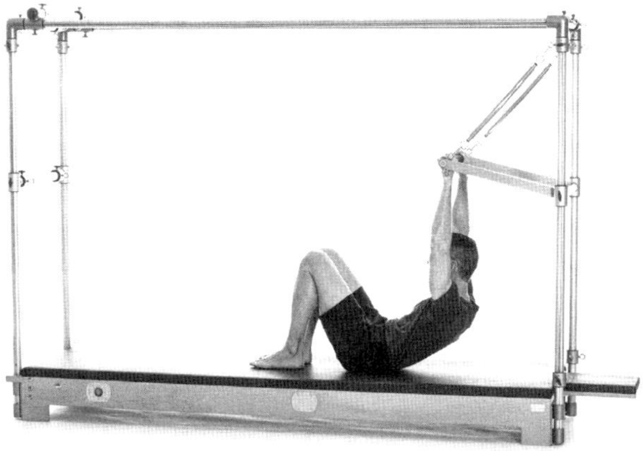

Exhale. Slowly roll up, maintaining the C curve of the trunk. Stop at the point the sacrum begins lifting off the mat or the C curve cannot be maintained.

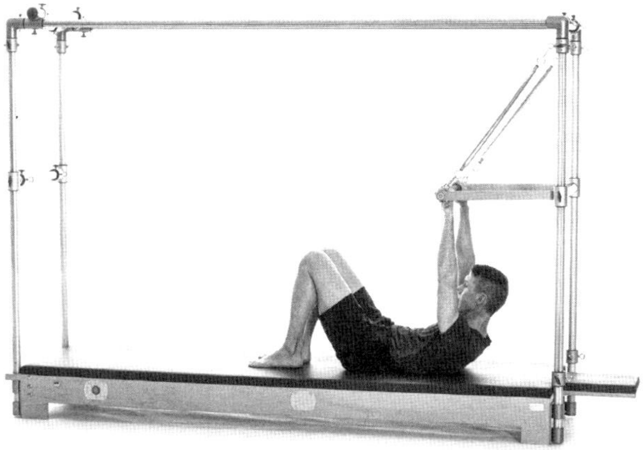

Inhale. Lower to the start position. Repeat 5-10 times before lowering to a supine position.

Mini Roll-Up—Oblique

Muscle Focus

- Abdominal obliques

Objectives

- To improve abdominal strength with an emphasis on the abdominal obliques
- To improve lower back extensor flexibility
- To develop trunk stabilization

RESISTANCE

Light — Medium — Heavy

This exercise uses the same form and positioning as the Cadillac: Mini Roll-Up, but it is made more challenging by adding a rotational component to the spinal flexion. Resist laterally tilting the pelvis by keeping the feet evenly weighted and the pelvis stable. Switch to an underhand grip on the bar, which helps maintain scapular stabilization and prevent the shoulders from elevating. Draw the ribs in on the side you are rotating toward, recruiting the internal obliques, and avoid swiveling (lateral flexion) in favor of rotating. Finally, keep the arm straight and override the strong tendency to bend the elbow and try to pull up with the arm. The arm should function simply as a connecting rod between the trunk and the push through bar.

Imagery

Initiate the movement from the abdominals, consciously straightening the arm and thinking of lifting the bar up to the ceiling. To ensure pure rotation as opposed to lateral flexion, keep the distance between the lower ribs and the iliac crest on both sides equal.

- ○ Engage the internal and external abdominal obliques on both sides of the body.
- ○ Maintain flexion of the spine (prioritize flexion over degree of rotation).

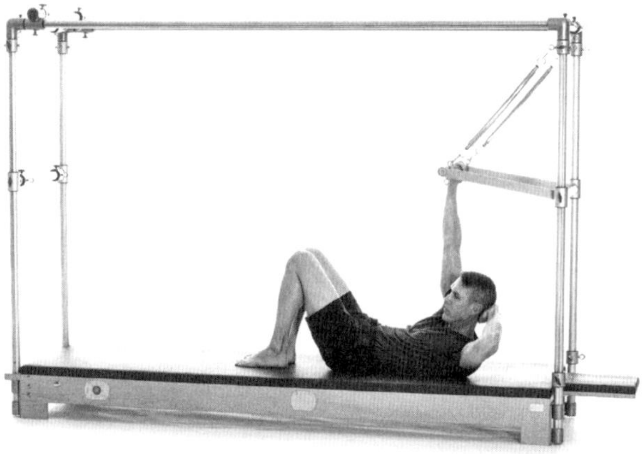

Setup. Lie supine with the knees bent and the feet hip width apart, anchored on the mat. Hold the push through bar with an underhand grip, hands shoulder width apart. Place one hand behind the head. Lift the head, shoulders, and chest into spinal flexion and rotate the trunk away from the arm holding the push through bar.

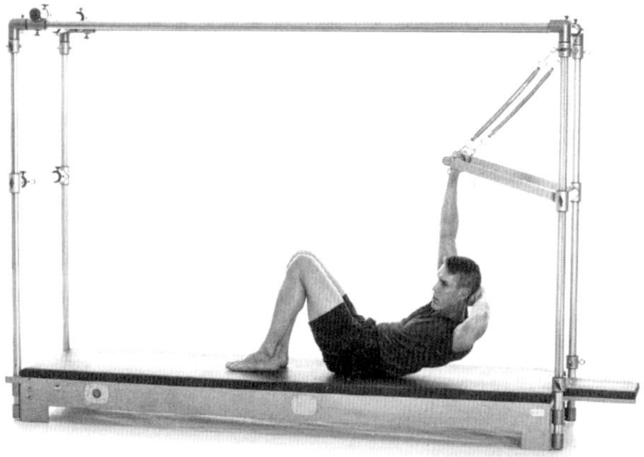

Exhale. Roll up while keeping the C curve position and maintaining rotation of the trunk.

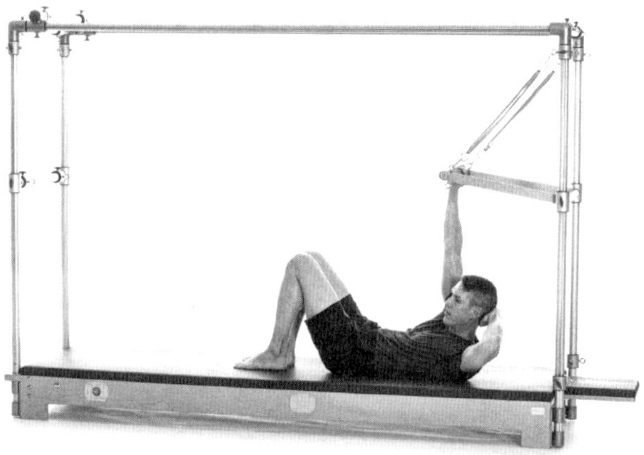

Inhale. Lower to the start position, maintaining rotation of the trunk. Repeat 5-10 times before returning to center and lowering to a supine position. Switch to the other side.

Teaser

This exercise is performed in various forms on nearly all the Pilates apparatus. This version on the cadillac is exceptional in that the push through bar assists the abdominals and back extensors and facilitates refinement of the movement and muscle recruitment. Use higher resistance for more assistance, lower resistance to make it more challenging, and no springs for minimal assistance. As with other versions of the teaser, it would be quite legitimate to categorize the Cadillac: Teaser in the full body integration block.

Imagery

The fact that you are hanging from a spring-loaded bar promotes the feeling of weightlessly floating up and slowly rolling down. Always strive for this quality of movement in this exercise, whether it is performed on the mat, or on any of the other apparatus.

- ○ Articulate through the spine during the roll-up and roll-down phases.
- ○ Extend the back fully in the final V position.
- ○ Keep the legs at a consistent height.

CADILLAC

Abdominal Work

INTERMEDIATE

Muscle Focus

- Abdominals
- Back extensors
- Hip flexors

Objectives

- To improve abdominal strength
- To improve back extensor and hip flexor control
- To develop trunk stabilization

RESISTANCE

Light — Medium — Heavy

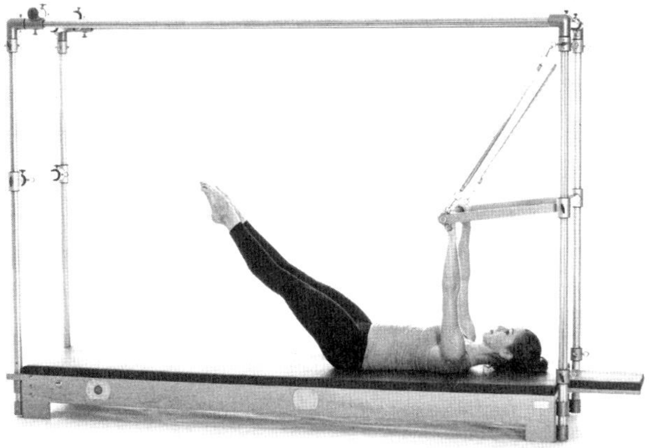

Setup. Lie supine, holding the push through bar. Position the shoulders directly below the hands. Keep the legs straight at an angle of approximately 45 degrees from the mat.

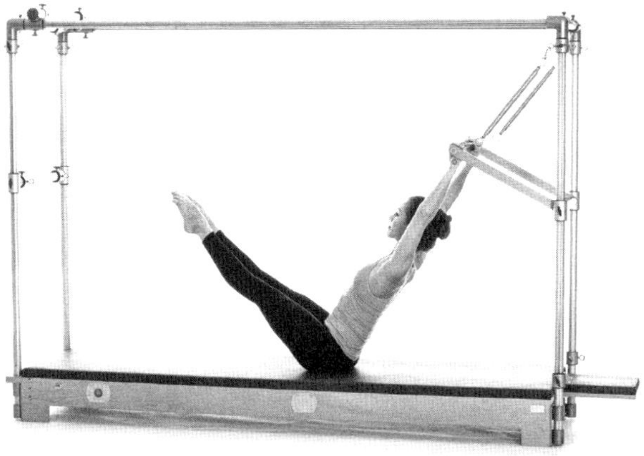

Inhale. Roll up from the head through the spine. Transition from spinal flexion to extension, creating a V shape with the body, arms overhead and diagonally aligned with the trunk.

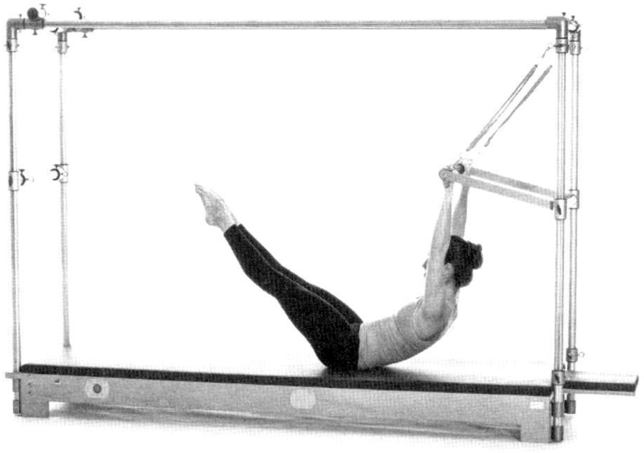

Exhale. Roll down through the spine to the start position, keeping the legs stable. Repeat 5 times.

Roll-Up With Push Through Bar

Muscle Focus

- Abdominals
- Back extensors
- Shoulder flexors

Objectives

- To improve abdominal strength
- To improve back extensor control
- To improve shoulder flexibility

The sequence of this exercise is similar to the spring-assisted Cadillac: Roll-Up; however, this version includes a transition from spinal flexion through spinal extension into an upright seated position. It includes an arm movement to stretch the shoulders and challenge the upright alignment of the trunk. (There is a tendency to thrust the ribs forward when in upright alignment, particularly during the arm movement, which should be avoided.) During the flexion of the elbows, emphasize shoulder external rotation and abduction of the scapulae. When rolling up and down, focus on keeping the arms straight and reaching forward, the bar as far away from the body as possible. This exercise can be done with the springs top-loaded; however, I prefer to do it without springs, which makes it slightly more challenging.

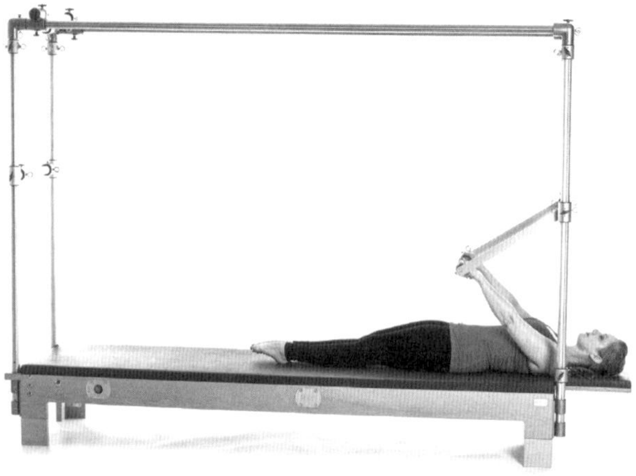

Setup. Lie supine with the legs straight and the head beyond the edge of the cadillac on the headrest. (If your cadillac does not have a built-in headrest, you can make one by placing a stool behind the cadillac with a cushion on top.) Exact placement will be dictated by where the body is when in the upright seated position (determined after the first repetition). With practice you will know where to place the body and will only need to make minor adjustments. Hold the push through bar with the arms straight.

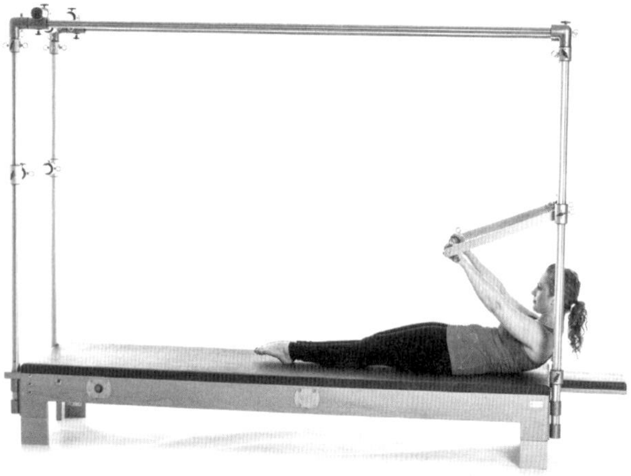

Inhale. Raise the head, shoulders, and chest into spinal flexion.

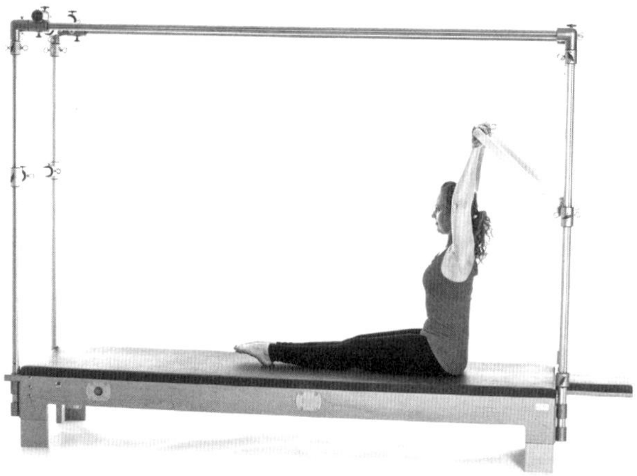

Exhale. Roll up, maintaining the C curve as long as possible. Extend the trunk into an upright seated position and reach the arms overhead, pushing the push through bar up.

Imagery

Imagine pushing the ceiling up and supporting it with the arms, like pillars holding up a building. When the elbows bend, imagine that they are being pulled out to the sides by strong springs. As the elbows draw back in and straighten, imagine that they are working against the pull of the imaginary springs, again pushing the ceiling up.

- Position the body on the cadillac so that when the trunk reaches the final upright position with the arms overhead, it is perpendicular to the mat.
- Maintain the C curve as long as possible before straightening up to the seated position.
- Co-contract the abdominals and back extensors to stabilize the trunk when sitting upright.
- Bias toward shoulder external rotation while bending the elbows.

PROGRESSION

This exercise can be done by loading springs from the bottom (remember to use the safety strap!), in which case the springs resist the movement, generating an increased challenge for the abdominals, back extensors, arms, and shoulders. It is important to first master the Cadillac: Roll-Up With Push Through Bar prior to trying the progression, which is far more difficult.

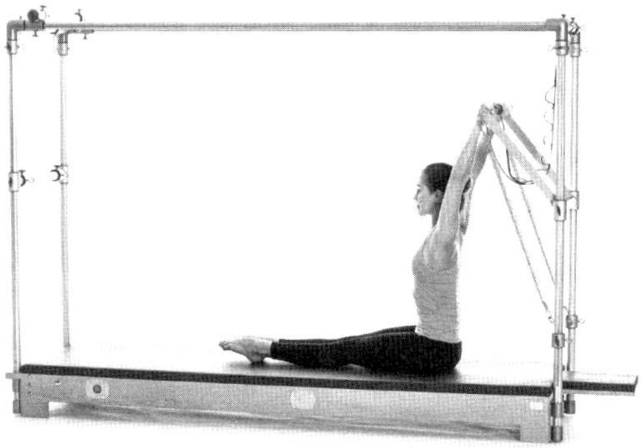

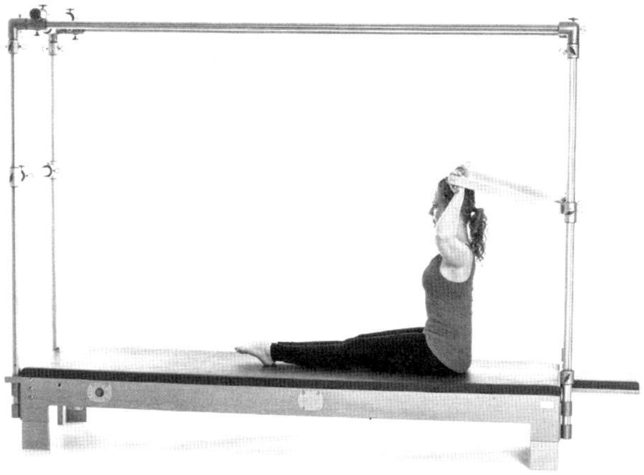

Inhale. Bend the elbows out to the sides and slightly forward (shoulder external rotation), keeping the scapulae stable, then straighten the elbows.

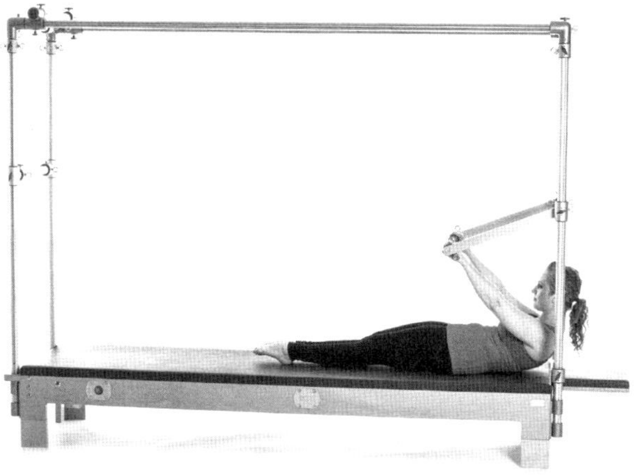

Exhale. Roll down to the start position. Repeat 5-10 times.

Frog

Muscle Focus

- Hip adductors
- Abdominals
- Back extensors

Objectives

- To improve hip adductor and hip extensor strength
- To develop lumbopelvic stabilization

RESISTANCE

Light — Medium — Heavy

Hip exercises performed on the cadillac have several advantages over the same exercises done on the reformer. First, lying on the cadillac promotes a feeling of stability. Second, the height of the cadillac makes mounting and dismounting easier than on the reformer. Finally, each leg uses a separate spring, which facilitates independent leg work, an advantage particularly when an imbalance is present.

Although this exercise is similar to the version done on the reformer, the muscle action is slightly different because of the angle of resistance. In broad terms, a greater load is placed on the hip extensors. Consider the movement of the heels following a horizontal path, as opposed to the diagonal path they tend to follow on the reformer.

Imagery

The image of the jumping frog used for the Reformer: Frog is a good starting point, but the Cadillac: Frog has a distinctly different feel. Visualize pushing a wall away from you with the feet as the legs straighten; the wall then rebounds back as the knees bend.

- ○ Maintain a neutral spine throughout the movement.
- ○ Keep the feet traveling along a consistent horizontal plane.
- ○ Initiate the movement with the hamstrings and adductors.

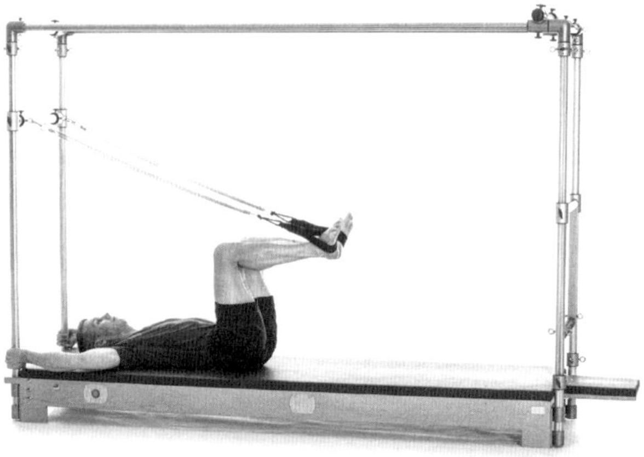

Setup. Lie supine, with the feet in the straps and dorsiflexed in a V position, knees bent. Hold the upright poles with the hands, arms in a "goal post" position, shoulders relaxed.

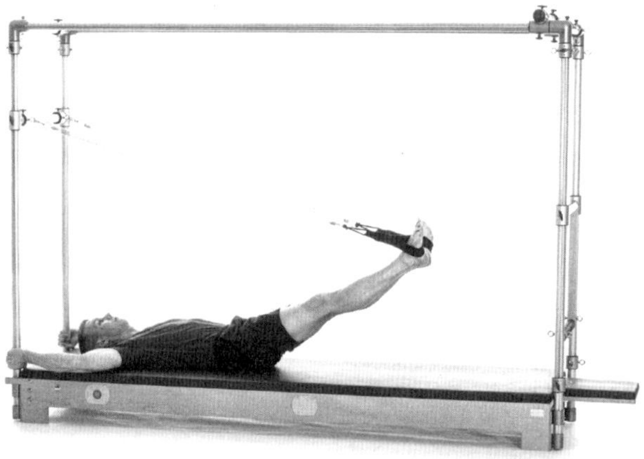

Exhale. Straighten the knees, squeezing the heels together.

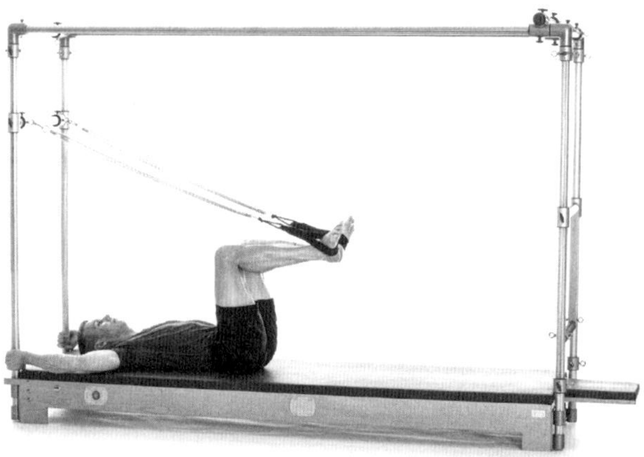

Inhale. Bend the knees. Return to the start position. Repeat 10 times.

Hip Circle

Like the hip work on the reformer, this exercise highlights the principles of hip disassociation and hip mobility. On the cadillac, however, the primary emphasis shifts from the hip adductors to the hamstrings because of the angle of resistance. In addition, as in the Cadillac: Frog, each leg has an individual spring and therefore works independently, preventing a dominant side from doing more of the work (as is sometimes the case on the reformer).

Imagery

As on the reformer, you should work on drawing two back-to-back semi-circles (or D shapes) in the air, increasing the size as your control improves. When moving down the centerline on the cadillac, I imagine the legs not only squeezing together to highlight the hip adductor work but also pressing down, as if pressing against a big ball or balloon.

- ○ Maximize hip disassociation.
- ○ Maintain external rotation of the hip joints.
- ○ Keep the size of the circles within a range that can be comfortably controlled.

Muscle Focus

- Hamstrings
- Hip adductors
- Abdominals
- Back extensors

Objectives

- To improve hip extensor strength
- To improve hip adductor control
- To develop lumbopelvic stabilization
- To develop hip disassociation

RESISTANCE

Light — Medium — Heavy

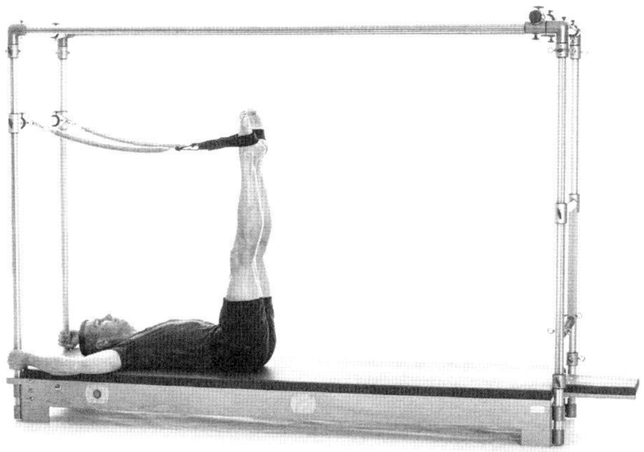

Setup. Lie supine, with the feet in the straps, legs straight and together, perpendicular to the mat (or as close as possible). Externally rotate the hips and plantarflex the feet. Hold the upright poles with the hands, arms in a "goal post" position, shoulders relaxed.

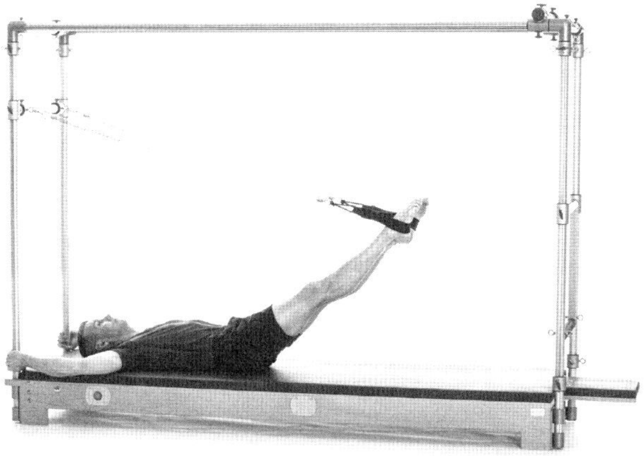

Exhale. Extend the hips, pressing the legs down the centerline and squeezing them together.

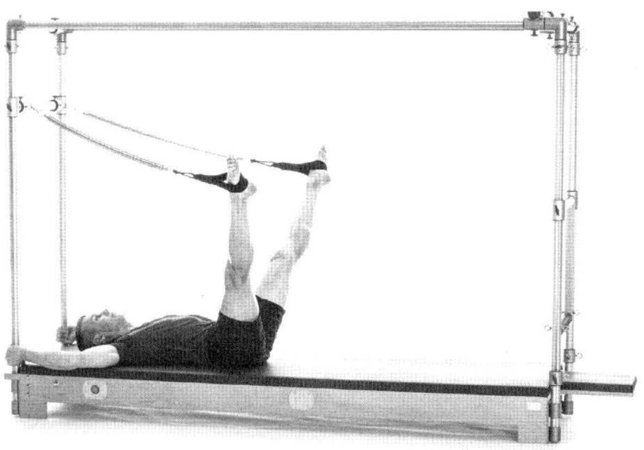

Inhale. Circle the legs around to the sides, up and together. Return to the start position. Repeat 5-10 times before reversing the direction.

Muscle Focus

- Hamstrings
- Abdominals
- Back extensors

Objectives

- To improve hamstring strength
- To develop hip disassociation
- To develop lumbopelvic stabilization

RESISTANCE
Light Medium Heavy

Walking

The emphasis in this exercise shifts from the hip extensors *and* adductors, which were recruited in the Cadillac: Frog and Hip Circle, to the hip extensors only. The action of the hamstrings is the primary focus and therefore the hips change from an externally rotated position to a parallel one. This facilitates a more balanced recruitment of the hamstrings.

Two types of movement occur simultaneously. The first is the continuous switching of the legs, a few inches up and down in opposition to one another. The second is the descent of both legs toward the mat of the cadillac and subsequent ascent to the perpendicular position (90-degree angle in the hip joints). Although neither type of movement is particularly daunting on its own, accomplishing both at the same time demands great coordination and can be quite challenging. The small, vigorous fluttering of the legs continues without interruption as the large movement of lowering and lifting takes place.

Imagery

Rather than thinking of this as walking, I prefer to imagine flutter kicks, as if swimming freestyle: The movement should be small, vigorous, and contained.

- Keep the leg switches small.
- Keep tension in the springs.
- Maintain a stable pelvis.

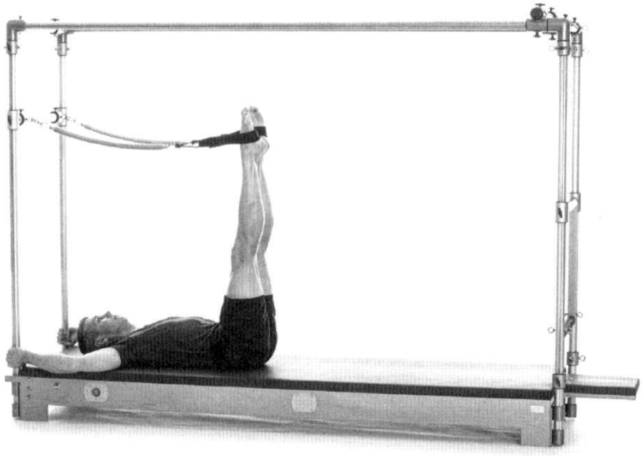

Setup. Lie supine, with the feet plantarflexed in the straps, and the legs straight, together, and perpendicular to the mat (or as close as possible). Hold the upright poles with the hands, arms in a "goal post" position, shoulders relaxed.

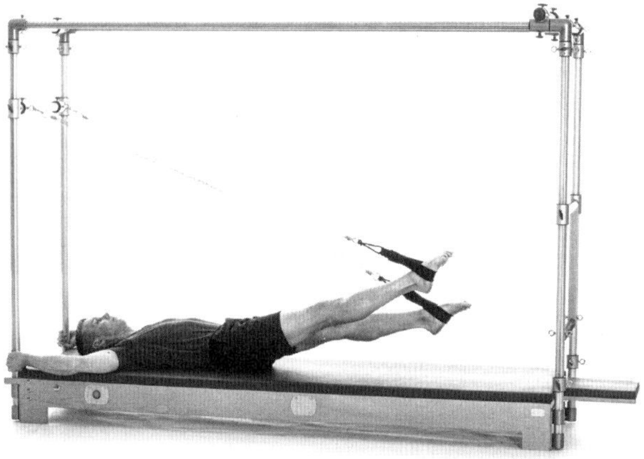

Exhale. Alternately switch the legs up and down in a small scissor-like motion while simultaneously extending the hips and pressing the legs down toward the mat over the course of 5 counts.

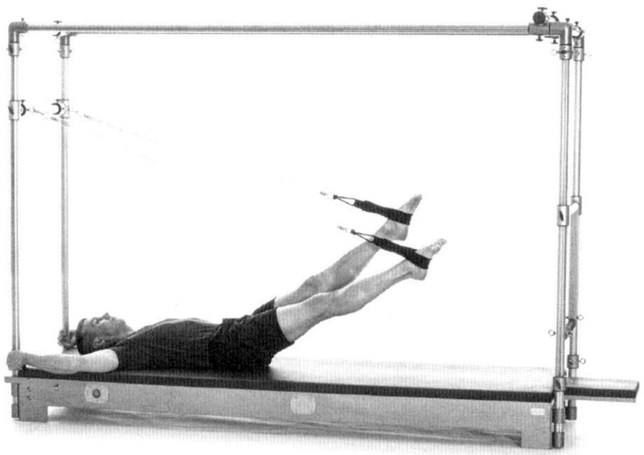

Inhale. Continuing the same scissor-like motion, flex the hips and lift the legs upward until they are perpendicular to the mat while resisting the springs over the course of 5 counts. Return to the start position. Repeat 10 times.

Bicycle

The coordination required for this exercise can be challenging. Focus on making a large cycling motion with the legs. The movement should be fluid, with a sense of elongation. The hip extensors are engaged throughout. Maintain a parallel position of the legs and keep a micro-bend in the knee of the leg that is pressing down toward the mat to promote a strong contraction of the hamstrings, which act as both knee flexors and hip extensors.

During this large movement of the hip and knee joints, the pelvis must remain anchored and provide a stable platform for the legs to move freely.

Imagery

I often use the image of a penny-farthing, an old-fashioned bicycle with a large front wheel and a small back one. The small wheel (the pelvis) stabilizes the bicycle, while the big wheel (the legs) provides the movement.

- ○ Establish an L position, with one leg close to the mat and the other perpendicular to it, before switching.
- ○ Maintain pelvic stabilization and spring tension.
- ○ Keep the movement continuous and flowing.

PROGRESSION

Once you have gained proficiency in the movement pattern, you can reverse the direction, which changes the muscle action and elevates the coordination challenge substantially, making it essentially a different exercise. The feeling is one of stretching the hip extensors, more than strengthening them, as they contract eccentrically.

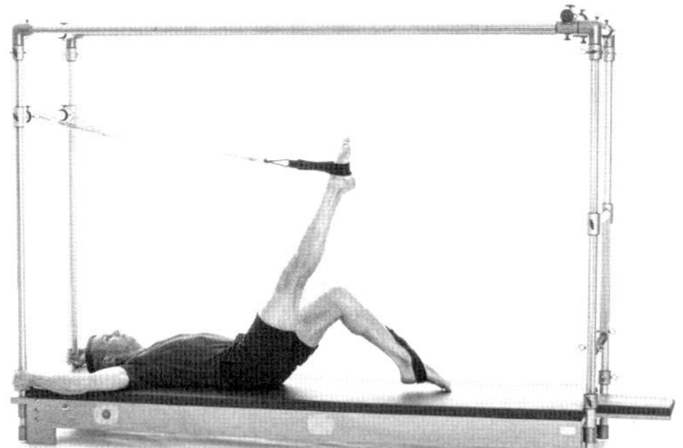

Muscle Focus

- Hamstrings
- Abdominals
- Back extensors

Objectives

- To improve hip extensor strength
- To develop hip disassociation
- To develop lumbopelvic stabilization
- To develop coordination

RESISTANCE

Light Medium Heavy

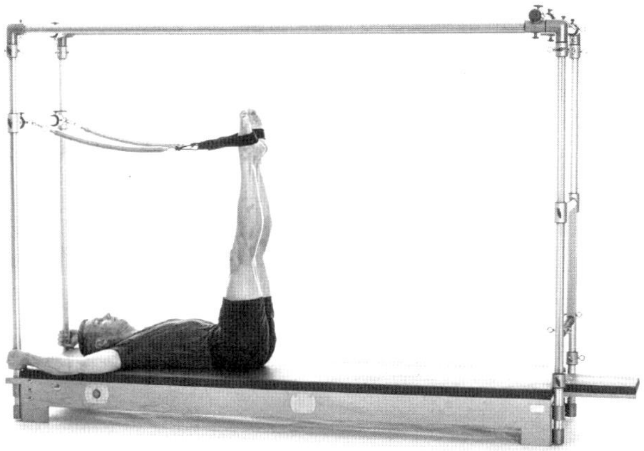

Setup. Lie supine, with the feet plantarflexed in the straps. The legs are straight, parallel and together, and perpendicular to the mat. Hold the upright poles with the hands, arms in a "goal post" position, shoulders relaxed.

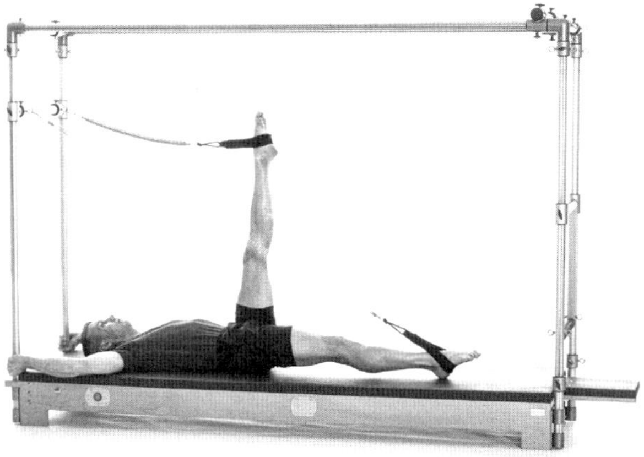

Exhale. Extend one leg, pressing it straight down toward the mat.

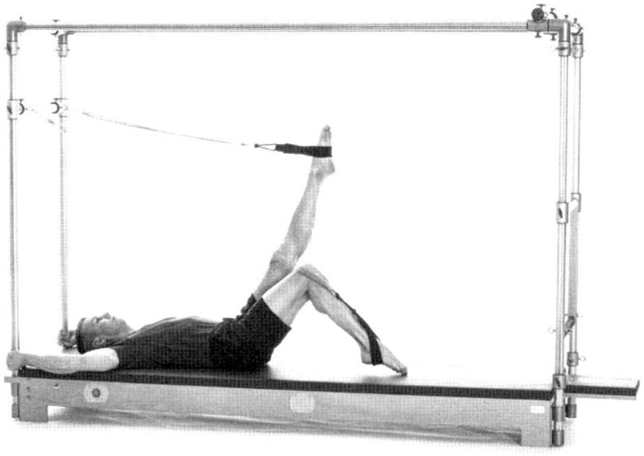

Inhale. Bend the extended leg in toward the chest, sliding the toes on or slightly above the mat, and then straighten the leg toward the ceiling. Simultaneously extend the other leg straight down toward the mat of the cadillac, maintaining tension in both springs. Continue repeating this pattern for 10 cycles.

Monkey

Muscle Focus

- Abdominals
- Back extensors
- Hamstrings

Objectives

- To improve abdominal and back extensor control
- To improve spinal mobility
- To improve hamstring and calf flexibility

RESISTANCE

Light — Medium — Heavy

This exercise, which focuses on spinal articulation and hamstring flexibility, serves as an excellent preparation for the Cadillac: Tower. It also reinforces the deep pike position, which is used in many of the flexion exercises on all the apparatus, particularly on the wunda chair (chapter 7). Note that the term "pike position" is used loosely to describe the body being folded at the waist with the trunk over the thighs. There are exercises or positions in which the trunk is in flexion even though the body is folded, whereas in other exercises, such as this one, the back is extended.

Use the abdominals to create the spinal flexion, followed by recruiting the back extensors for spinal extension, which helps magnify the hamstring stretch. The arms are used only for support, like rods connecting the trunk and the push through bar.

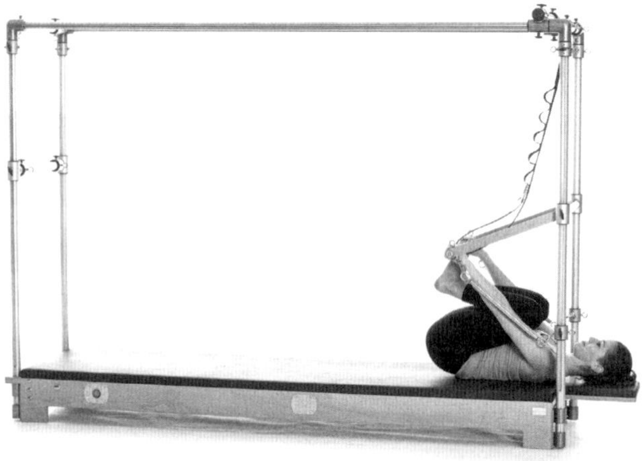

Setup. Lie supine, with the head on the headrest. (If your cadillac does not have a built-in headrest, you can make one by placing a stool behind the cadillac with a cushion on top.) Bend the knees and place the toes on the bar so that the hips are approximately under the plantarflexed feet (placement will vary slightly depending on the height of the individual). Hold the bar with the hands shoulder width apart. Strive to anchor the sacrum on the mat (or as close as possible).

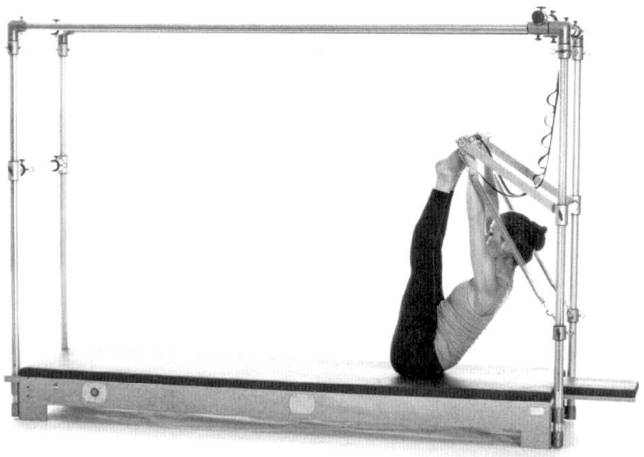

Exhale. Roll up through the spine into a pike position while straightening the knees and maintaining plantarflexion of the feet.

Imagery

The top phase of this exercise is reminiscent of a diver's body folding into a tight pike position in the air (although the chest is not held as close to the thighs as a diver's would be). This powerful image encourages the correct muscle recruitment and dynamic, which in turn establishes a solid foundation for all the exercises that use a similar position.

- Engage the abdominals to lift the trunk into flexion.
- Maintain plantarflexion while articulating up and down through the spine.
- Hold the legs straight and the back flat when dorsiflexing the feet.
- Maintain scapular stabilization with the shoulders relaxed.

VARIATION

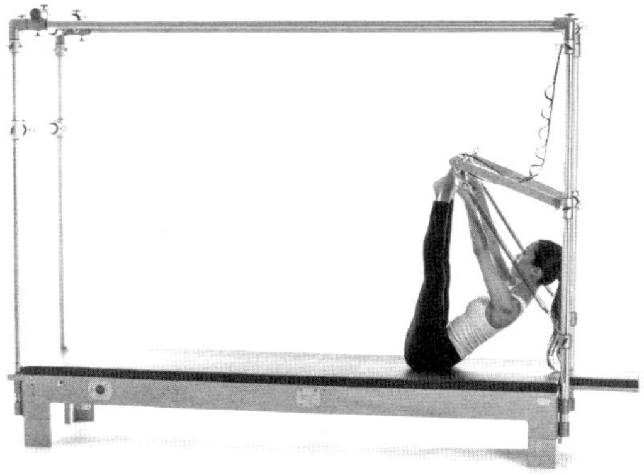

One of the drawbacks of this exercise is that people with short arms, particularly if coupled with a longer trunk and legs, will find it almost impossible to perform simply because they cannot reach the bar. Add to this a lack of flexibility and the challenge becomes insurmountable. In order to assist in overcoming this issue, wrap hand towels or straps around the push through bar, one on each side, and hold on to these rather than the bar itself. The choreography of the exercise and all the cues remain the same.

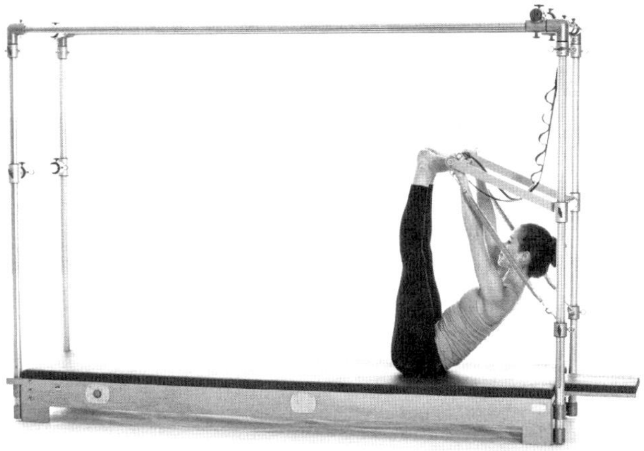

Inhale. Dorsiflex and plantarflex the feet, maintaining the pike position and keeping the shoulders relaxed.

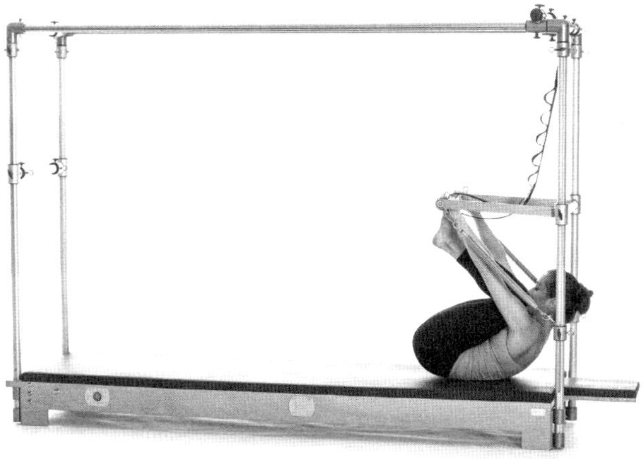

Exhale. Bend the knees and roll down. Return to the start position. Repeat 10 times.

CADILLAC

Spinal Articulation

INTERMEDIATE

Muscle Focus

- Abdominals
- Hamstrings
- Back extensors

Objectives

- To improve abdominal and back extensor control
- To improve hamstring and lower back extensor flexibility
- To develop spinal articulation

RESISTANCE

Light · Medium Heavy

Tower

This exercise addresses spinal articulation as well as back and hamstring flexibility. It is a wonderfully satisfying and enjoyable exercise—however, it must be approached with caution because of the load on the spine. It is important to actively push away from the upright poles with straight arms, which helps alleviate pressure on the spine, particularly the cervical region. Activate the back extensors and the abdominals to support the trunk, especially when rolling up onto the shoulders. At the same time, keep the hip extensors engaged, even as the knees bend when in the top position. All of this assists to prevent sinking into the back and neck, which could potentially result in excessive pressure on the spine. Maximize the stretch of the hamstrings and calves, particularly when the feet are dorsiflexed during the final phase. When rolling down, focus on the eccentric contraction of the back extensors and hip extensors, and aim to anchor the sacrum on the mat (or as close as possible) at the conclusion of each repetition.

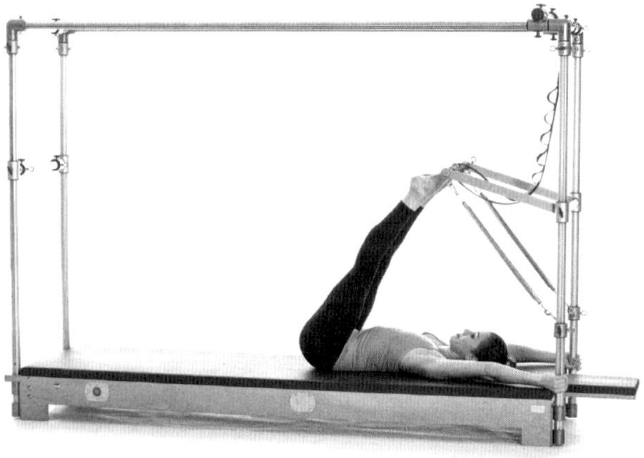

Setup. Lie supine and reach the arms straight overhead to hold the upright poles. Place the toes on the push through bar, with the feet plantarflexed and the legs straight and parallel.

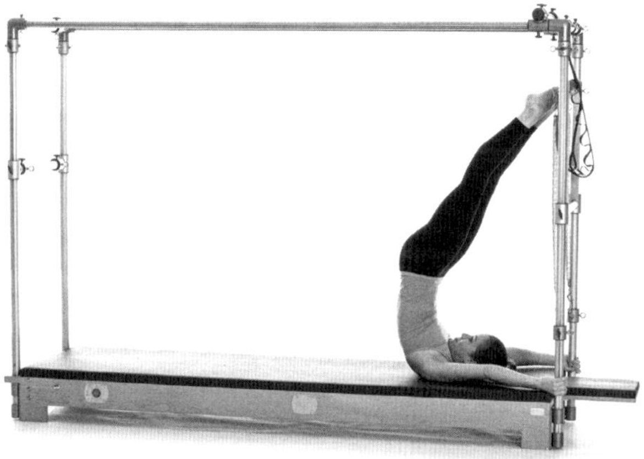

Exhale. Roll up onto the shoulder girdle, articulating the spine.

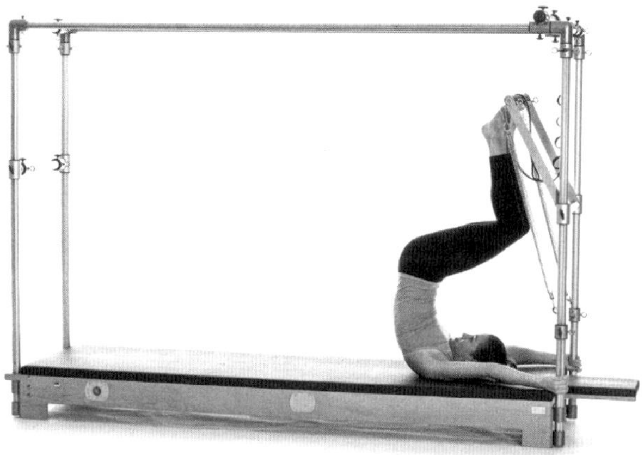

Inhale. Bend and straighten the knees, maintaining hip extensor engagement.

Imagery

The image of an accordion opening and closing captures the rhythm of the opening, folding, and reopening of the body in this exercise. Although the physical positions clearly differ from those of an accordion, the dynamic of the movement is similar.

- Initiate the spinal articulation with activation of the abdominals and deep flexion of the spine.
- Maintain hip extensor and back extensor engagement when up on the shoulders.
- Bend the knees cautiously at the top (no more than 90 degrees), without sinking into the spine and shoulders.

VARIATION

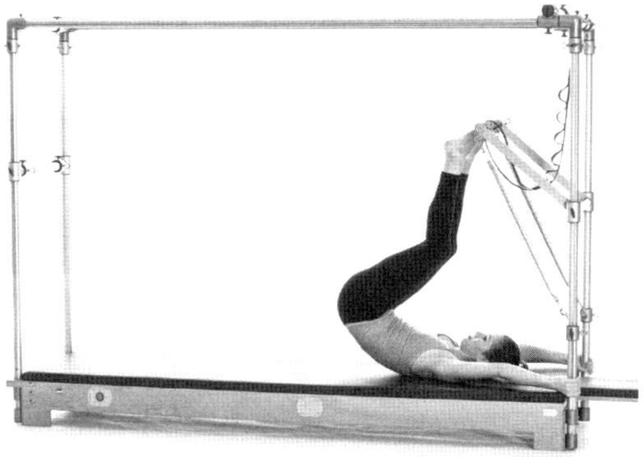

In this variation, begin in the same position as the Cadillac: Tower; however, as you roll up, simultaneously bend the knees. When you reach the top, you are in essentially the same position as when the knees are bent in the top phase of the Cadillac: Tower. It is very important to maintain hip extensor and back extensor engagement as the knees bend to alleviate pressure on the spine. From this top position, roll the spine down to the mat, simultaneously straightening the legs. Once at the bottom, add the dorsiflexion and plantarflexion of the feet as in the Cadillac: Tower. This version has a wonderful circular feel to it.

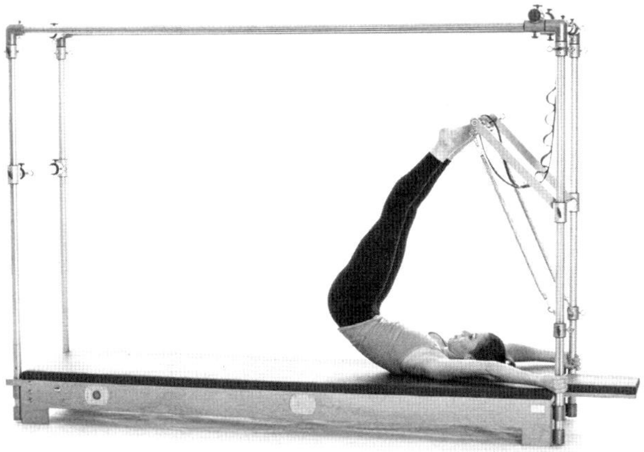

Exhale. Roll down through the spine to the start position, anchoring the sacrum in the final phase.

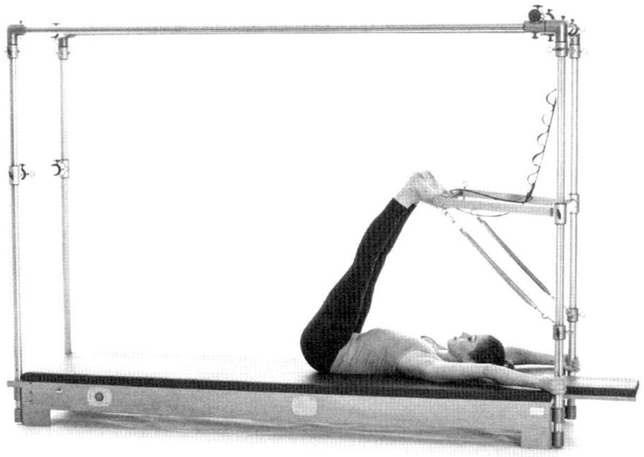

Inhale. Dorsiflex and plantarflex the feet. Return to the start position. Repeat 5 times.

INTERMEDIATE

Push Through—Sitting Forward

Muscle Focus

- Abdominals
- Back extensors
- Shoulder extensors

Objectives

- To improve abdominal, back extensor, and shoulder extensor control
- To improve hamstring flexibility

RESISTANCE

Light Medium Heavy

This exercise demonstrates the transition of the trunk from spinal flexion to spinal extension and vice versa. It also pairs shoulder extension with spinal flexion, a muscle recruitment pattern that appears in many Pilates exercises. Finally, it offers the benefit of a hamstring stretch in tandem with spinal extension using the push through bar. It truly is a full body integration exercise in every sense.

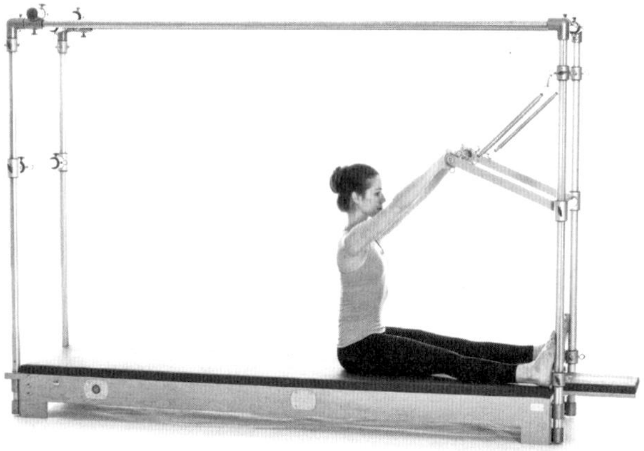

Setup. Sit upright, facing the push through bar, and press the feet against the poles. Hold the bar, arms straight and shoulder width apart.

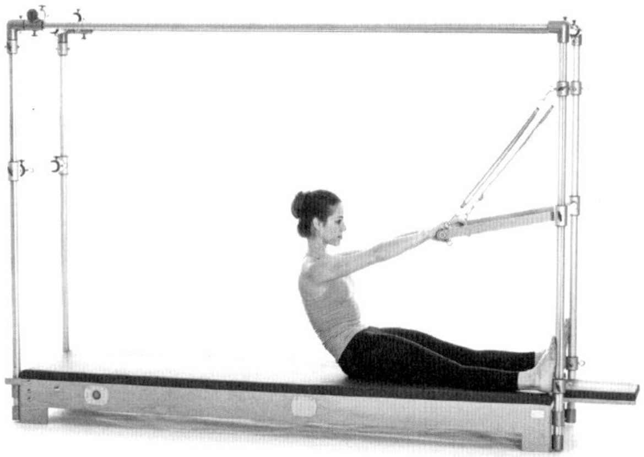

Exhale. Round the trunk and glide the pelvis under into a posterior tilt. Press the push through bar down and then forward, reaching the body over the legs.

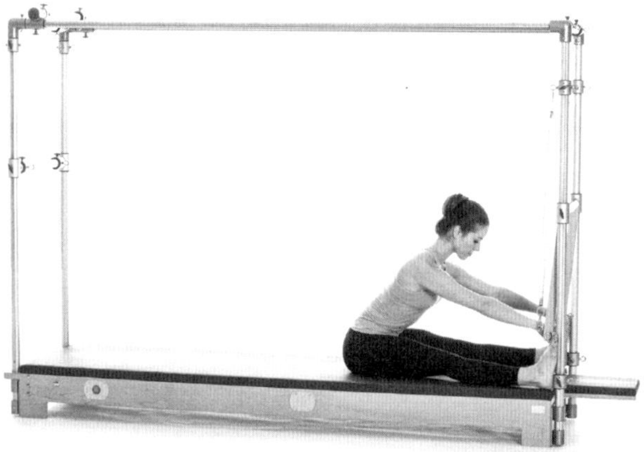

Inhale. Extend the spine, flattening the back on a diagonal.

Imagery

The backward and forward motion of the trunk and the use of the push through bar for control is reminiscent of rowing a boat.

- Keep the arms straight.
- Differentiate between the movement of the trunk and that of the arms.
- Keep the heels pressing against the upright poles of the cadillac.
- Glide the pelvis under during spinal flexion, accentuating the posterior tilt of the pelvis.

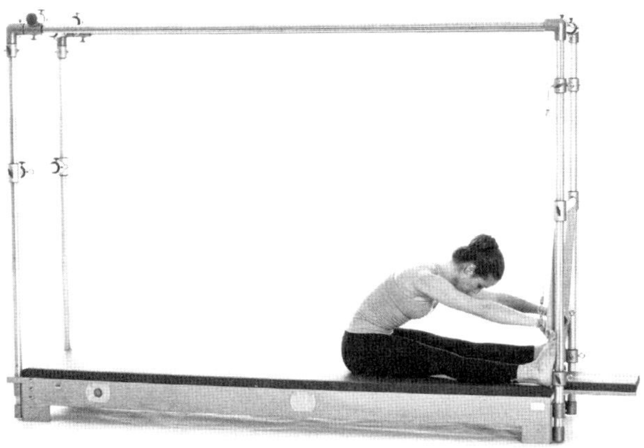

Exhale. Draw the spine back into spinal flexion and then lean back. Control the push through bar while bringing it back and up, maintaining flexion of the trunk.

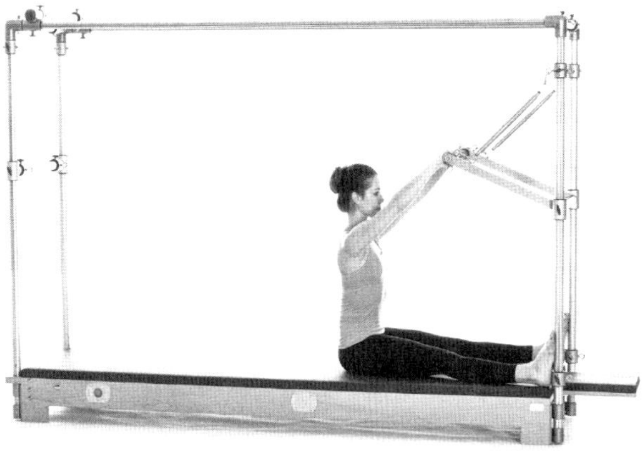

Inhale. Extend the spine and sit upright. Return to the start position. Repeat 5 times.

CADILLAC

Full Body Integration I

INTERMEDIATE

Muscle Focus

- Abdominals
- Back extensors
- Shoulder extensors

Objectives

- To develop spinal articulation
- To develop scapular and trunk stabilization

RESISTANCE

Light Medium Heavy

Cat Stretch

I perform this exercise when I want to spoil myself, because it feels so good! The Cadillac: Cat Stretch fortifies the neutral alignment of the spine, both in an upright position and then in the more demanding forward-leaning position. The exercise requires trunk stability as well as shoulder stability.

When rolling down at the beginning of the exercise and rolling up at the end, articulate the spine and keep the body as close to the plumb line as possible.

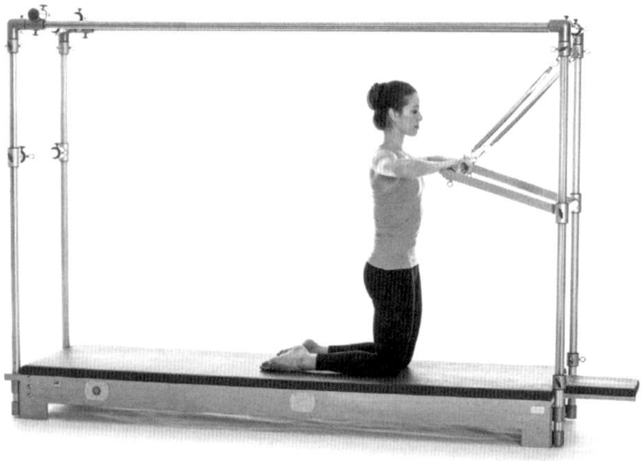

Setup. Kneel facing the push through bar. Hold the bar, with hands shoulder width apart and the arms bent, elbows reaching out to the sides.

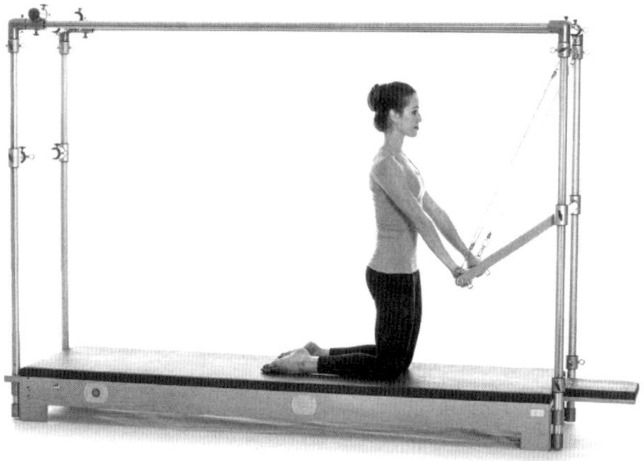

Inhale. Straighten the elbows, pressing the arms down.

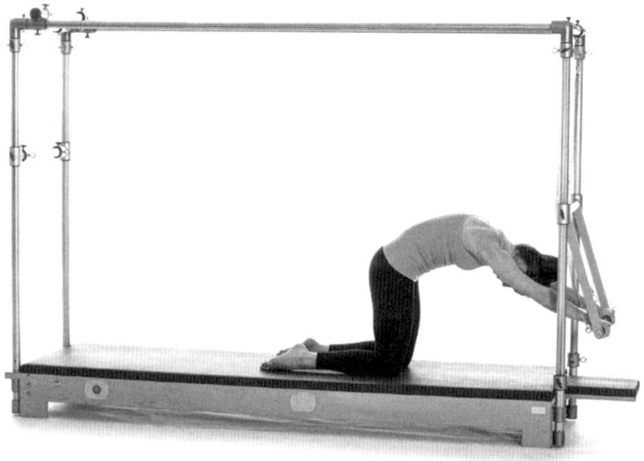

Exhale. Roll down, articulating through the spine.

Imagery

The name says it all—stretch like a cat! A cat exemplifies immaculate spinal articulation and the quality of joyful stretching. It is important to establish control and good alignment before you try to reach the more extreme ranges of cat-like movement found in the progression, but the image helps.

- Maintain abdominal support during all phases of the movement.
- Avoid thrusting the ribs forward, particularly during the forward-leaning position.
- Maintain scapular stabilization, particularly during the forward-leaning position.
- Align the spine in a neutral position in the initial phase and during the forward-leaning position.

PROGRESSION

If you feel secure and stable in the forward-leaning position with the trunk parallel to the floor, press the trunk down toward the mat, stretching the shoulders further into shoulder flexion. Maintain a neutral spine position (or as close as possible) during the stretch. It is important to first be proficient in the original exercise before doing this progression, as tempting as it may be.

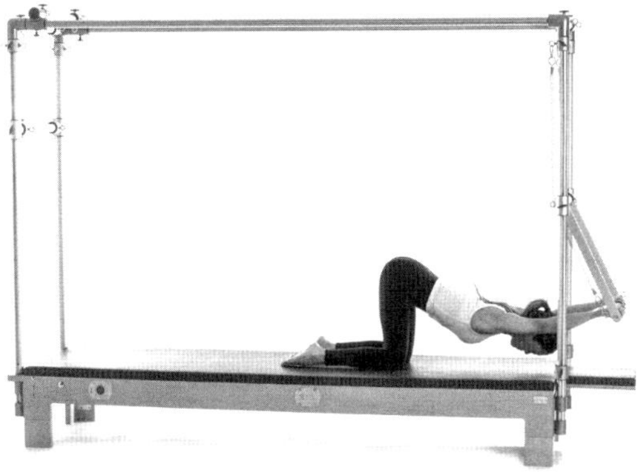

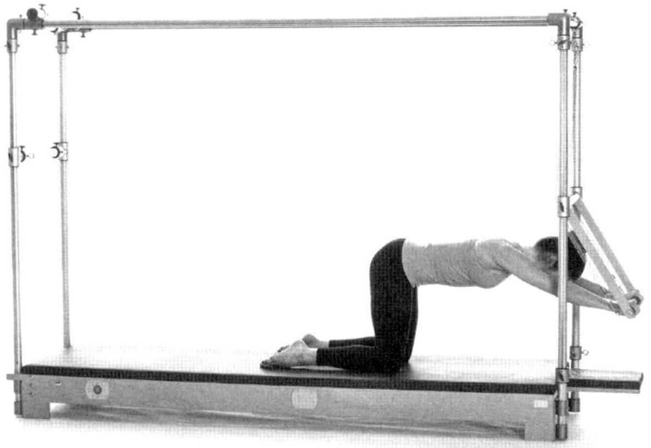

Inhale. Extend the trunk forward into a neutral spine position, parallel to the floor. Maintain trunk and scapular stabilization.

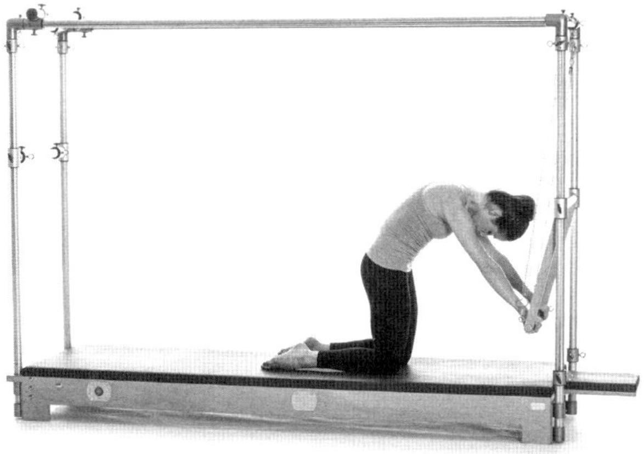

Exhale. Draw the back into spinal flexion, articulating the spine as you return to the upright position. Bend the elbows and lift the arms. Return to the start position. Repeat 5 times.

CADILLAC
Arm Work
INTERMEDIATE

Muscle Focus

- Shoulder extensors
- Triceps
- Abdominals
- Back extensors

Objectives

- To improve shoulder extensor and elbow extensor strength
- To develop trunk stabilization

RESISTANCE
Light Medium Heavy

Chest Expansion—Standing

Relatively few exercises from the classic repertoire are performed in an upright standing position; therefore, the ones that are should be fully utilized in a comprehensive program. The standing arm work exercises are certainly among this group; not only do they develop arm and shoulder strength, flexibility, and control but they also demand core strength and good posture and alignment. To intensify the impact, increase the challenge, and develop balance, these exercises can be performed on an unstable surface, such as a balance board or rotating disc, or even standing on one leg.

Note that the distance from the cadillac is crucial—the farther away you stand, the greater the tension, and vice versa. Adjust accordingly.

Imagery

I like to visualize the body in a stable, upright position with the crown of the head lifting upward. With each pull of the arms the spine straightens up more as if being inflated by a pump.

- Reach the arms down, as if touching the fingertips to the floor (use an open-hand or a fist position).
- Maintain scapular and trunk stabilization.
- Establish correct posture and alignment.
- Keep tension in the springs while moving slowly and deliberately, particularly during the return (eccentric contraction).
- Increase upper back extensor activation as the shoulders extend.
- Straighten the arms completely, reinforcing triceps activation, prior to each repetition.

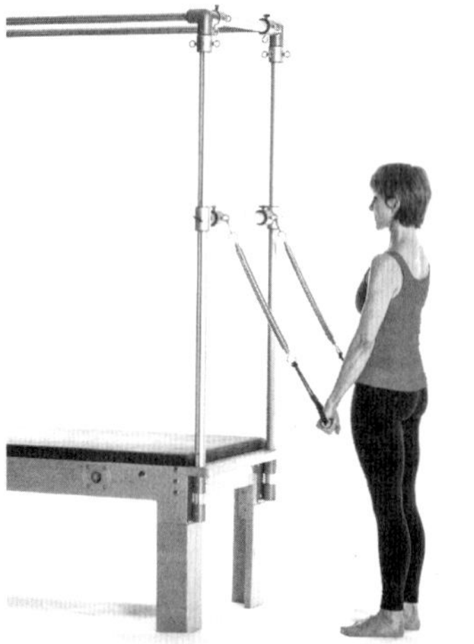

Setup. Stand approximately 24 inches (60 centimeters) away from the cadillac, facing the apparatus, with the crossbar at eye level. Hold the handles, with the palms facing back and slight tension in the springs.

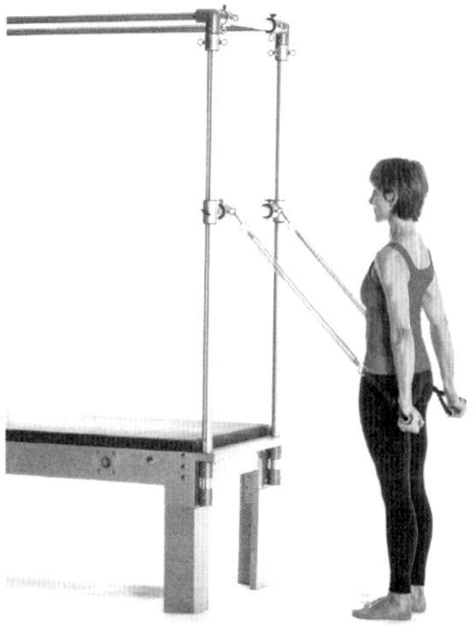

Exhale. Extend the shoulders, pressing the arms back while maintaining the upright alignment of the body.

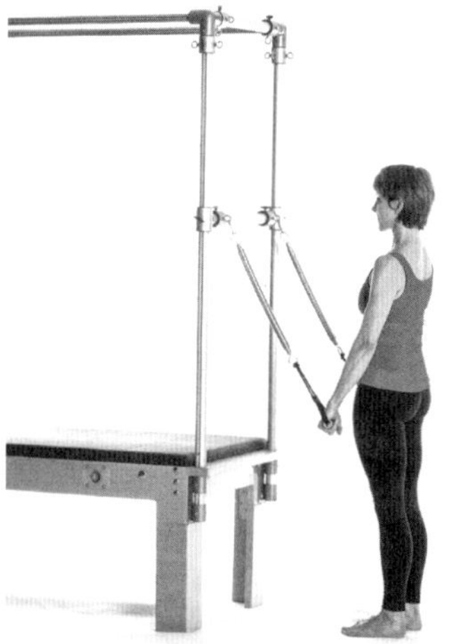

Inhale. Flex the shoulders, bringing the arms forward. Return to the start position. Repeat 10 times.

Hug-a-Tree—Standing

This exercise is similar to the Reformer: Hug-a-Tree—Seated and Arm Chair: Hug-a-Tree. As with those exercises, trunk stabilization is crucial. When standing, however, stabilization is taken a step further by integrating the element of balance, which makes the exercise particularly functional and challenging. Few exercises are better for discovering your center.

As with the Cadillac: Chest Expansion—Standing, the farther you stand from the apparatus, the greater the resistance; adjust the distance accordingly. Although the body is upright on the plumb line in that exercise, in all the exercises facing the opposite direction the body is leaned forward (while still maintaining excellent alignment). The lean, occurring at the ankle joints, should be just enough to counteract the backward pull of the springs, but not enough to rely entirely on the springs for support. Recruiting the ISS, particularly the abdominals, is vital for maintaining ideal alignment; it is the essence of successful execution of this exercise as well as the entire standing arm work series. As you become more proficient, add resistance by stepping farther away from the cadillac and leaning into the springs more. Finding the perfect balance of maximum resistance while still being able to maintain stability is a never-ending challenge.

Imagery

Imagine a large bird spreading its wings. The arms spread to achieve the largest span possible, moving in and out gracefully as if flying. There are few sensations as wonderful as feeling that you are soaring like an eagle—graceful, centered, and stable.

- ○ Keep the back broad and the scapulae stabilized to focus the work on the shoulder horizontal adductors.
- ○ Maximize the stretch across the chest during the eccentric phase (opening the arms).
- ○ Lean forward while maintaining ideal posture and alignment.
- ○ Keep the arms elongated, with a micro-bend in the elbows, the fingers (or fists) reaching out to the sides in opposite directions.

Muscle Focus

- Pectorals
- Abdominals

Objectives

- To improve shoulder horizontal adductor strength and flexibility
- To develop trunk and scapular stabilization

RESISTANCE

Light Medium Heavy

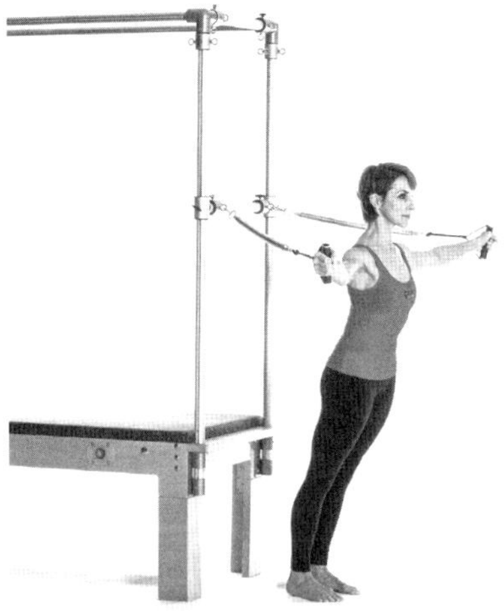

Setup. Stand approximately 12-24 inches (30-60 centimeters) away from the cadillac, with the back to the apparatus and the crossbar at eye level (when facing it). Reach the arms out to the sides in a T position and hold the handles with either an open-hand or a fist. (I prefer the open-hand position as long as it is comfortable and does not induce tension in the hands.) Bend the elbows slightly (micro-bend), with the hands facing forward and some tension in the springs. Lean forward and engage the abdominals.

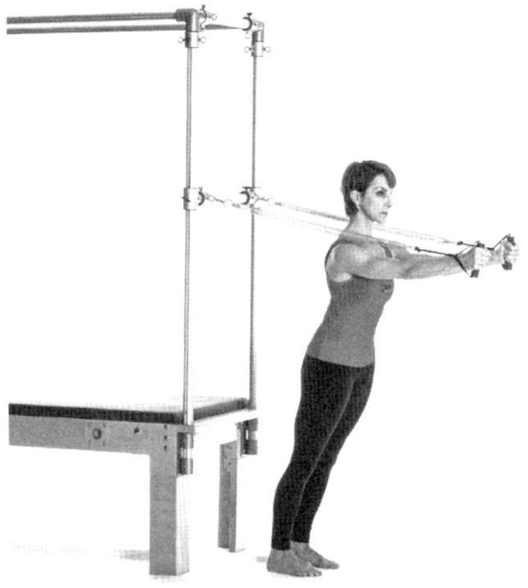

Exhale. Bring the arms together until they are in line with the shoulders, parallel to each other and to the floor.

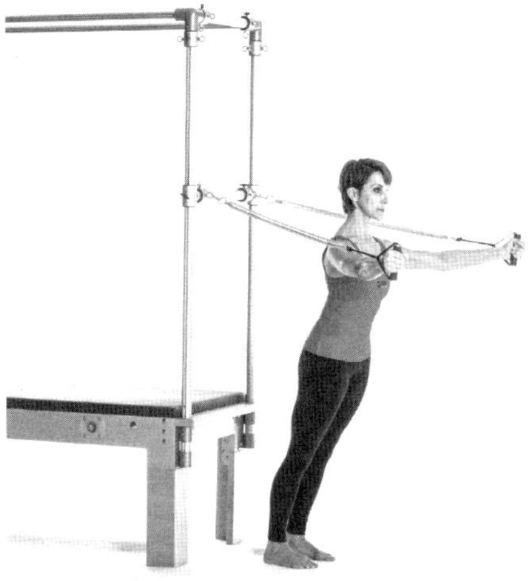

Inhale. Open the arms to the sides, maintaining tension in the springs. Return to the start position. Repeat 10 times.

Arm Circle—Standing

Muscle Focus

- Shoulder extensors
- Shoulder adductors and abductors
- Shoulder horizontal adductors
- Abdominals

Objectives

- To improve shoulder horizontal adductor and shoulder extensor strength
- To improve shoulder adductor and abductor control
- To improve shoulder flexibility
- To develop trunk and scapular stabilization

RESISTANCE

Light — Medium — Heavy

The Cadillac: Arm Circle—Standing highlights control and range of motion of the shoulder complex. It is an extension of the Cadillac: Hug-a-Tree—Standing, but after the horizontal adduction of the shoulders, the arms circle overhead and back around to the T position. The Arm Chair: Circle (chapter 10), which I recommend learning as a preparation to this exercise, is similar. However, this exercise relies on the body's ability to hold itself up without the external support of a chair, making it far more challenging. This is the essence of progression in many Pilates exercises—the movements become more challenging as a higher level of stabilization and internal support is required. Building a solid foundation is the key to later success when performing more advanced exercises. Remember that the level of resistance can be adjusted by stepping farther from, or closer to, the cadillac.

Imagery

Imagine the arms moving through a thick gel—not thick enough to create tension, but sufficient to provide a sense of consistent resistance at every point of the circle.

- ○ Face the palms forward in the first phase of the exercise.
- ○ Rotate the shoulders when the arms are directly forward, hands facing the floor, and prepare to take them overhead.
- ○ Take the arms as far overhead as possible without affecting the alignment of the trunk.
- ○ Avoid elevating the scapulae as the arms are lifted overhead.
- ○ Keep the hands within peripheral vision as the arms circle around.

VARIATION

In order to work the muscles differently and add variety to the movement, you can reverse the direction of the circles. Beginning from the T position, raise the arms overhead, then lower them in front of the body parallel to each other, palms facing down. Rotate the arms when they are directly in front of the shoulders so that the palms face one another, then open them out to the T position.

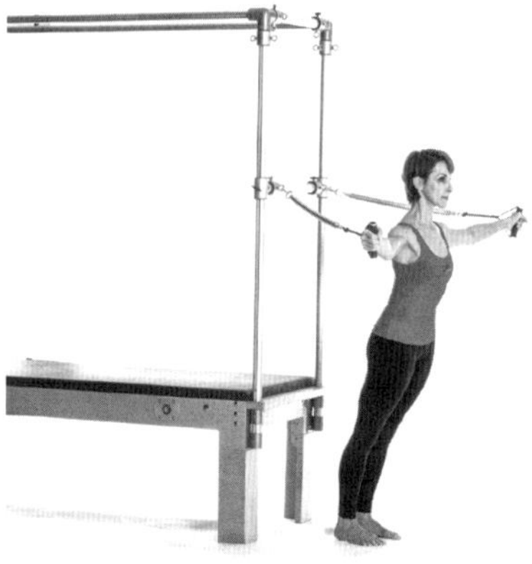

Setup. Stand approximately 12-24 inches (30-60 centimeters) away from the cadillac, with the back to the apparatus and the crossbar at eye level (when facing it). Reach the arms out to the sides and hold the handles with either an open hand or a fist. Bend the elbows slightly (micro-bend), with the hands facing forward and some tension in the springs. Lean forward and engage the abdominals.

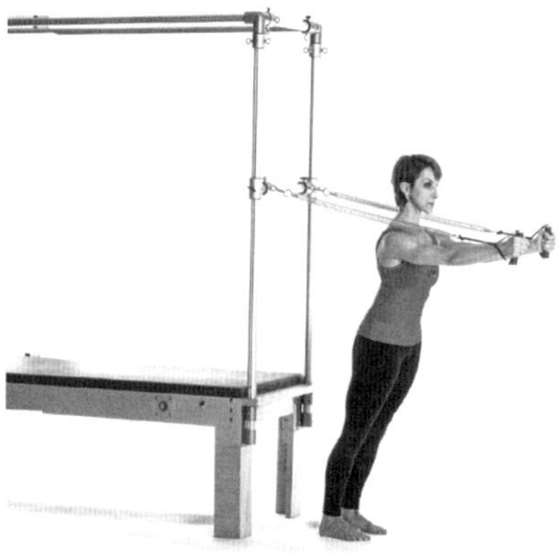

Exhale. Bring the arms together until they are in line with the shoulders, parallel to each other and to the floor, as in the Cadillac: Hug-a-Tree—Standing.

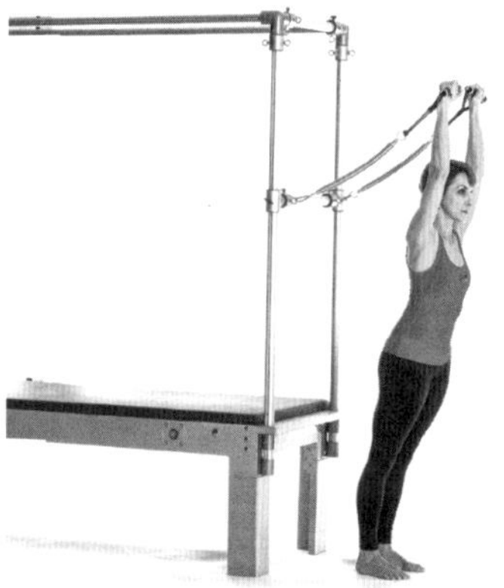

Inhale. Rotate the arms so that the palms face the floor, and lift the arms overhead. Circle the arms out to the sides to the T position, with the palms facing forward. Return to the start position. Repeat 10 times.

Arm Punch—Standing

INTERMEDIATE

Besides the obvious element of developing arm strength, this movement also develops core strength. It demands tremendous trunk stabilization because of the natural tendency to rotate the trunk with each punch.

Imagery

As the name indicates, the movement should feel like a punch. Imagine a precise point in front of you, in line with the shoulder; envision the hand reaching this target with every punch.

- Focus the movement in the arms, while the trunk and shoulder girdle remain stable.
- Face the fingers (fists) toward the direction of the movement throughout and glide the hands along a horizontal plane as if sliding across a table.

PROGRESSION

Once a high degree of stabilization has been achieved, you can add a trunk rotation to the straightening of each arm. This rotation increases the power of the punch significantly because the action emanates from the very powerful rotators of the trunk rather than from the arm. It also now works the muscles of the trunk as movers as well as stabilizers, with significant strength benefit for the abdominal obliques.

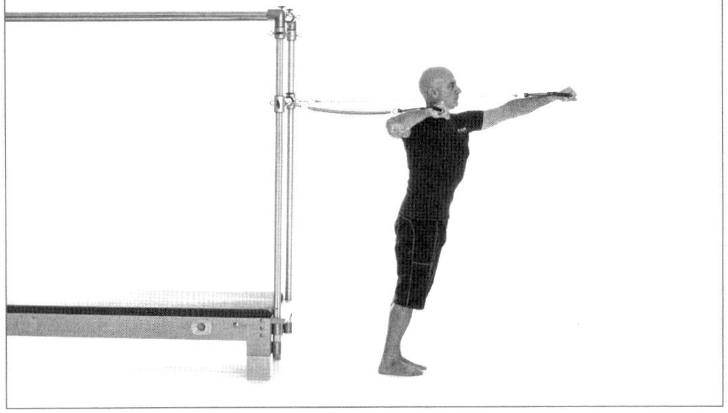

Muscle Focus

- Triceps
- Deltoids
- Pectorals
- Abdominals

Objectives

- To improve elbow extensor strength
- To improve shoulder horizontal adductor strength
- To develop trunk stabilization

RESISTANCE

Light — Medium — Heavy

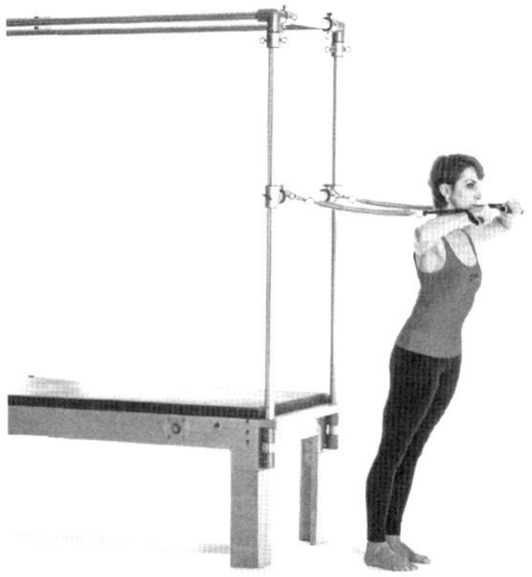

Setup. Stand approximately 12-24 inches (30-60 centimeters) away from the cadillac, with the back to the apparatus and the crossbar at eye level (when facing it). Bend the elbows out to the sides, and hold the handles with the palms facing downward and the fingers forward (the hands will be just above shoulder height). There should be tension in the springs from the outset. Lean forward and engage the abdominals.

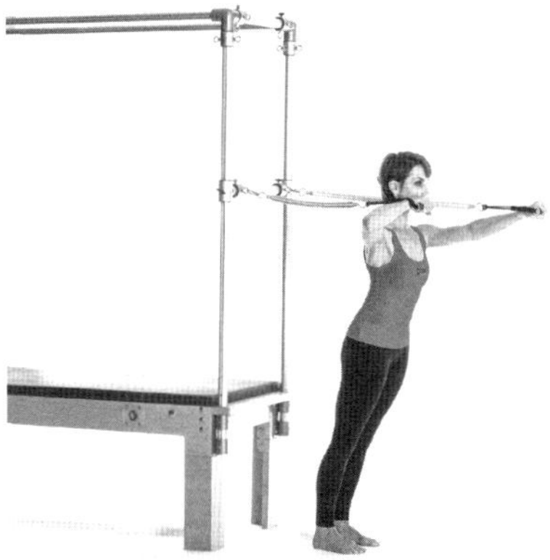

Exhale. Straighten one arm forward, then bend it as you simultaneously straighten the other arm; the hands pass each other midway through the movement on their respective paths.

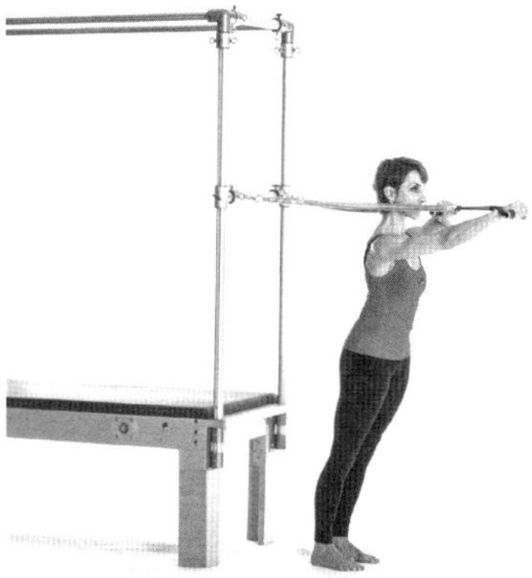

Inhale. Repeat the cycle, performing two punches with each breath. Repeat 10 breath cycles (exhale and inhale).

Biceps—Standing

Muscle Focus

- Biceps
- Abdominals

Objectives

- To improve elbow flexor strength
- To improve shoulder flexor flexibility

RESISTANCE

Light Medium Heavy

Although this movement is essentially a standard biceps curl, the positioning of the arms and trunk offer certain advantages. After working the shoulder horizontal adductors in the Cadillac: Hug-a-Tree—Standing, Arm Circle—Standing, and Arm Punch—Standing, you will feel a significant stretch across the chest when you perform this exercise. The long head of the biceps is held in a fully stretched position, which enhances flexibility and provides a unique angle for developing strength of the biceps.

Imagery

The position of the body can be likened to the figurehead of an old ship. With each bend of the arms, the chest should open more. The feeling should be one of reaching the chest forward (without thrusting the ribs and hyperextending the back).

- Maintain maximum shoulder extension.
- Keep the upper arms stable throughout the movement.
- Keep the elbows parallel to each other (or as close as possible).
- Maintain scapular stabilization, with a feeling of the scapulae opening to prevent them coming together.

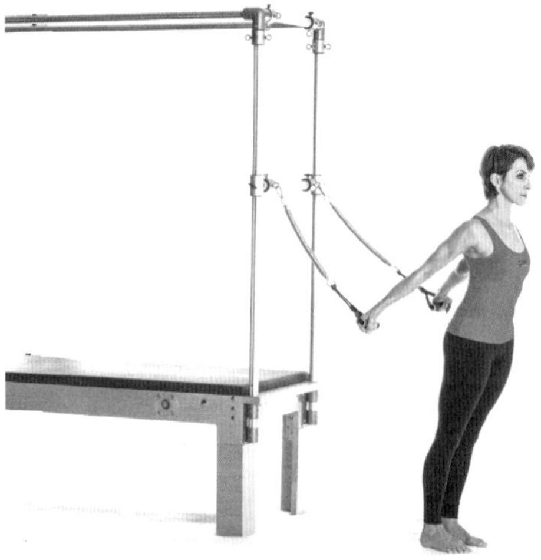

Setup. Stand approximately 48 inches (120 centimeters) away from the cadillac, with the back to the apparatus and the crossbar at eye level (when facing it). Reach the arms behind the body, parallel to each other and straight. Hold a single handle firmly in each hand with a fist, and place the scapulae in a neutral position. Lean forward and engage the abdominals.

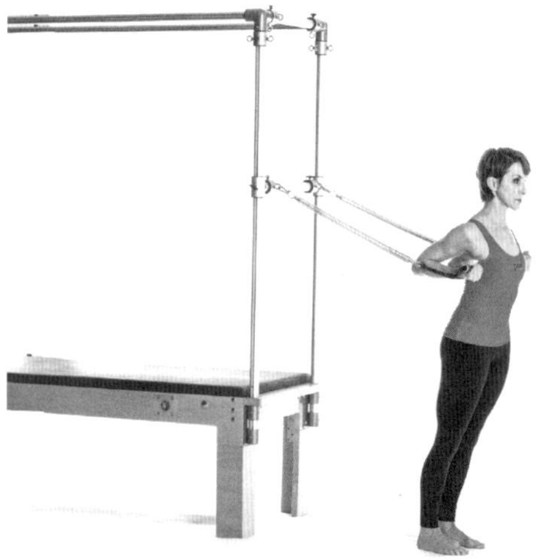

Exhale. Bend the elbows, keeping the upper arms stable and the elbows at the same height, pointing backward.

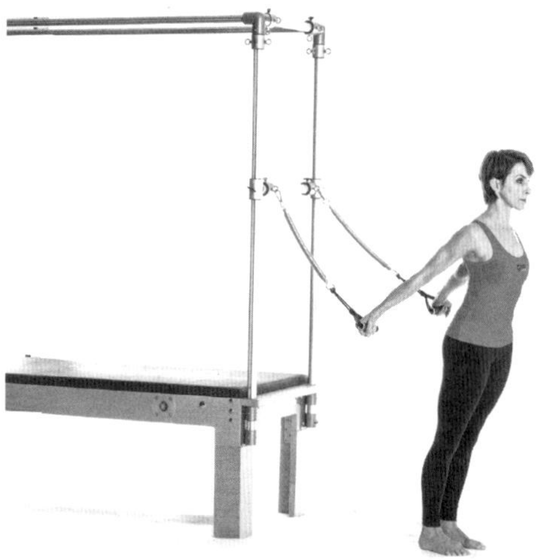

Inhale. Straighten the arms. Return to the start position. Repeat 10 times.

Squat

The Cadillac: Squat is unique in several ways. First, in addition to the obvious challenge for the legs, it presents an even greater challenge for the upper body. Furthermore, the trunk is held in an upright position throughout the movement, rather than the typical forward tilt found in a conventional squat. The upright position encourages neutral alignment and makes the exercise arguably more functional and less risky; the conventional squat position can place excessive load on the lower back.

Because of the benefits for the lower limbs, this exercise appears in the leg work block; however, the Cadillac: Squat addresses many areas of the body and could comfortably fit into the arm work or full body integration blocks as well. The isometric contraction of the biceps, along with the squat action of the legs, develops biceps strength, leg strength, and core strength, particularly the back extensors. Wherever it fits into a session, and whichever block it falls into, it is a valuable addition to any conditioning program.

Imagery

Maintain good alignment of the trunk by imagining that you are leaning backward against a slippery wall as your body slides up and down the smooth surface. To make sure the legs are properly aligned to accommodate the smooth gliding movement of the trunk, picture each leg gliding between two vertical panes of glass.

- ○ Keep the trunk upright in a neutral spine position.
- ○ Hold the upper arms stable and parallel to each other and to the floor.
- ○ Maintain correct tracking of the legs, with the knees aligned over (but not in front of) the feet as they bend and straighten.

Muscle Focus

- Quadriceps
- Biceps
- Back extensors

Objectives

- To improve knee extensor, back extensor, and elbow flexor strength
- To develop trunk stabilization

RESISTANCE

Light — **Medium** — Heavy

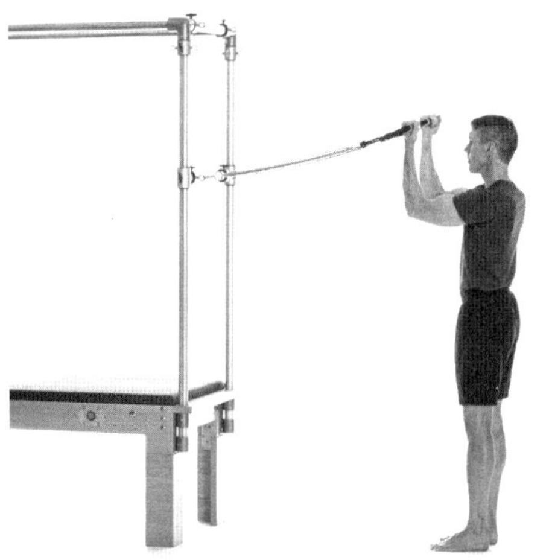

Setup. Stand approximately 36 inches (90 centimeters) away from the cadillac, facing the apparatus, with the crossbar at eye level. Extend the arms in front of the body at shoulder height, hold the handles with slight tension in the springs, and bend the elbows to a 90-degree angle (if the tension is excessive, start with no tension in the springs by moving closer to the cadillac).

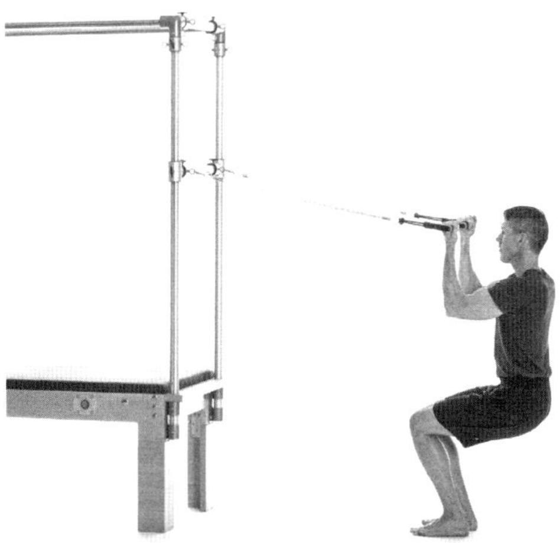

Inhale. Bend the knees into a squat, keeping the heels on the floor. Hold the arms stable and the trunk upright.

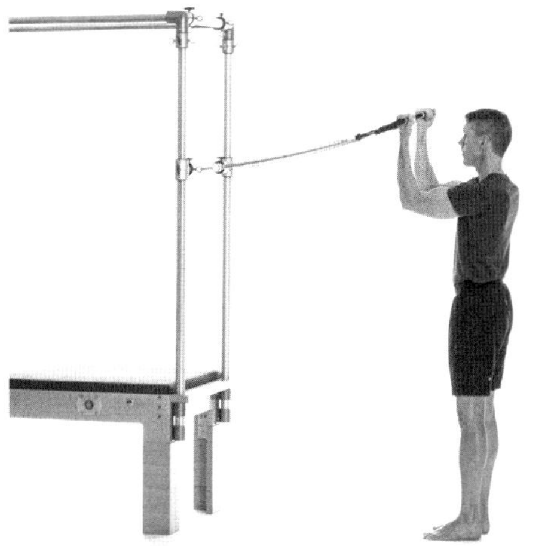

Exhale. Straighten the knees, continuing to maintain the stable arm position. Return to the start position. Repeat 5-10 times. Straighten the arms only after the final repetition.

CADILLAC
Lateral Flexion and Rotation
INTERMEDIATE

Muscle Focus

- Abdominal obliques

Objectives

- To improve abdominal oblique flexibility and control
- To improve lower and mid-back extensor flexibility
- To improve shoulder adductor and extensor control

RESISTANCE

Light — Medium — Heavy

Butterfly

This complex movement with a beautiful name demands significant upper body control, core control, flexibility, and coordination. The movement pattern has two distinct phases: lateral flexion, followed by rotation. This pattern can be found in several advanced Pilates exercises—for instance, the Mat: Twist—as well as in many athletic activities, including golf, volleyball, tennis, and baseball.

In the first phase, the movement is pure lateral flexion with the arms acting as an extension of the trunk. The arms maintain a T position resisting the backward pull of the springs, adding challenge to this simple action. This is followed by the rotation of the trunk; only at the point of maximum rotation do the arms circle around (one overhead and one in front of the body) to reach the "backward" T position (more like a wide inverted V), with the head and upper girdle facing the cadillac. The movement pattern is then reversed to return to the start position.

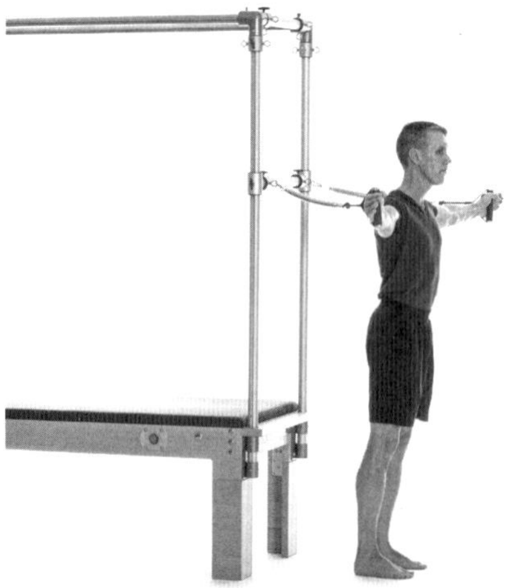

Setup. Stand approximately 12 inches (30 centimeters) away from the cadillac, with the back to the apparatus and the crossbar at eye level (when facing it). Reach the arms out to the sides and hold the handles with either an open hand or a fist. (I prefer the open-hand position as long as it is comfortable and does not induce tension in the hands.) Bend the elbows slightly (micro-bend), with the hands facing forward and some tension in the springs. Lean forward and engage the abdominals.

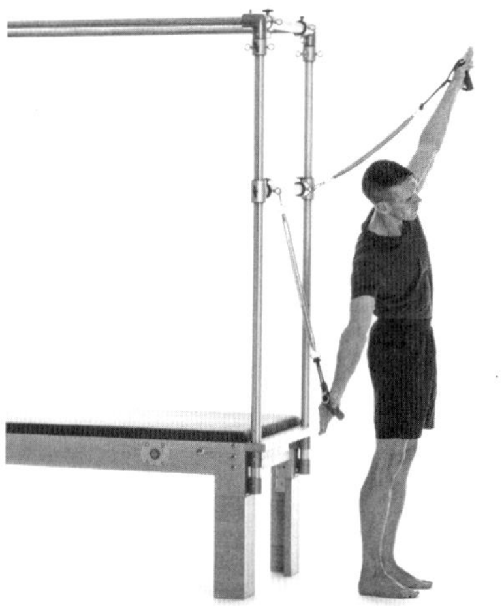

Inhale. Reach over to one side, laterally flexing the trunk.

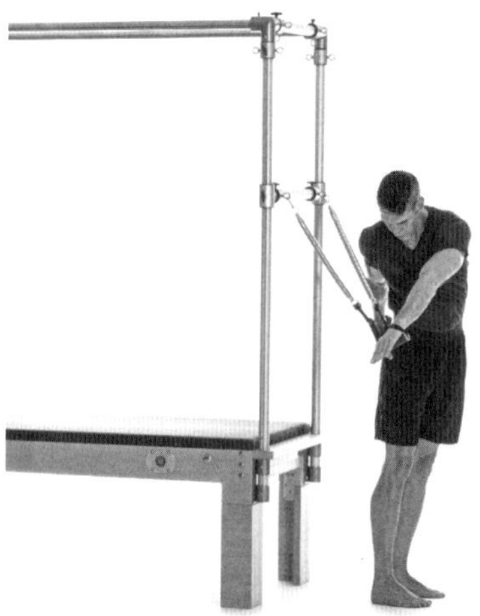

Exhale. Rotate and round the upper body to face the cadillac, bringing the top arm up and over (with the spring going over the head) and the other arm down and across to create a backward T position (wide inverted V position), arms pulled backward, head and shoulder girdle facing toward the cadillac. The arms continue pulling the springs out to the sides and back.

Imagery

The feeling of this movement is like a spring being wound up and then carefully unwound, similar to the dynamic of the Reformer: Mermaid. These two challenging exercises are closely related; finding the connection between them will prove valuable in mastering both. Another image I like to use is simply the name of the exercise: a butterfly. As the arms reach out to the sides throughout the exercise, they should feel like wings.

- Keep the pelvis facing forward as much as possible, while allowing it to adapt to the rotation of the trunk as necessary.
- Maintain constant tension in the springs.
- Keep the arms as wide as possible.

MODIFICATION

Although this exercise is not very physically demanding in terms of strength, it is very demanding in terms of coordination, flexibility, and control. Breaking it up into parts will undoubtedly help lay down a good foundation for success. Start by standing upright with the arms in a T position. Laterally flex to one side, then return to the start position. Repeat to the opposite side. This movement pattern repeats itself in many similar versions on the different apparatus.

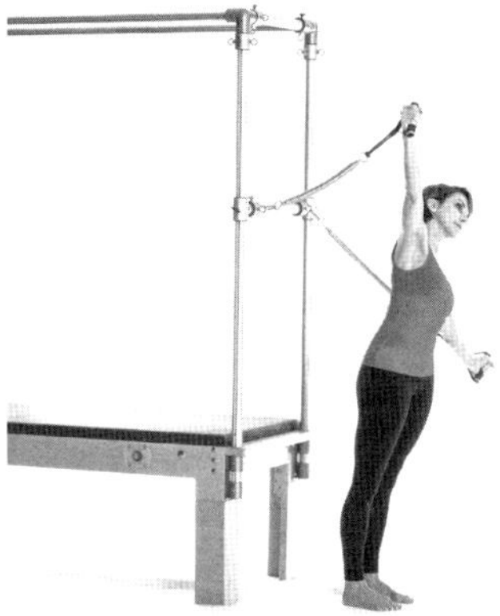

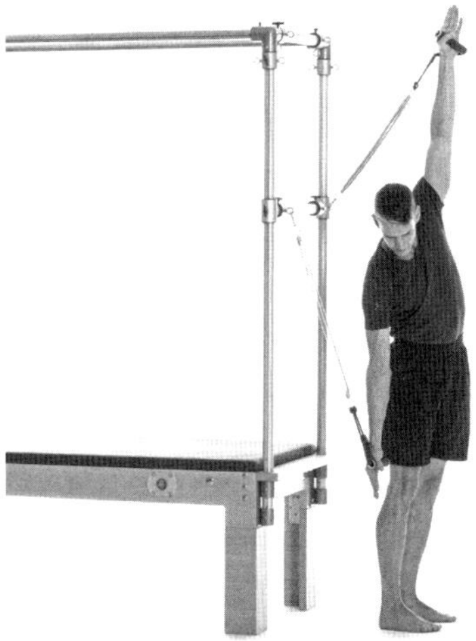

Inhale. Unwind, retracing the movements in reverse, first by taking the top arm over the head and the other arm across the front of the body. Establish the original T position of the arms, returning to lateral flexion.

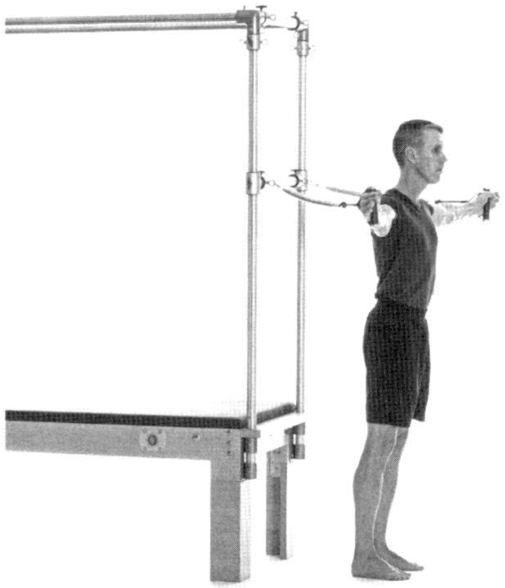

Exhale. Lift the trunk to upright, arms out to the sides. Return to the start position. Repeat 5 times to each side, alternating sides.

Side Lift

Muscle Focus

- Abdominal obliques

Objective

- To improve lateral flexor strength and flexibility

RESISTANCE

Light Medium Heavy

This exercise is not from the classic Pilates repertoire, but I was certainly inspired by the traditional work when creating it. Besides being a valuable exercise for developing the lateral flexors of the trunk, it has a wonderful flow and is exhilarating to perform.

Although the body is ideally in a straight line, it may be necessary to place the legs slightly forward of the center-line, which in turn emphasizes activation of the abdominal obliques. This is helpful when the back extensors, particularly the quadratus lumborum, tend to overpower the abdominals. The same result can be achieved by tipping the upper side of the pelvis slightly back.

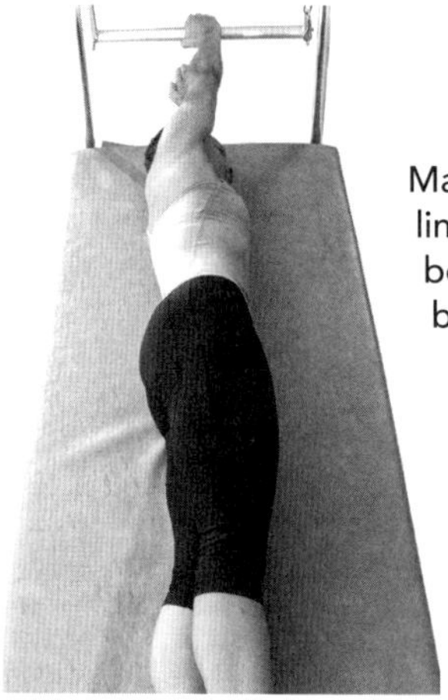

Maintain as close to a straight line as possible with the body, without compromising balanced muscle activation.

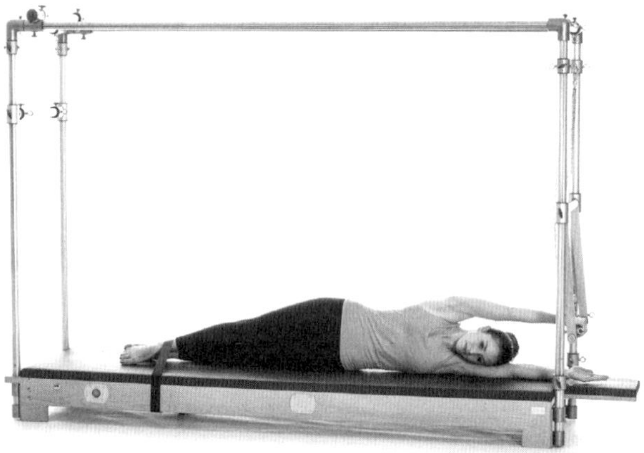

Setup. Lie on one side. Place the feet under the foot strap with the legs straight and the top leg in front of the bottom leg. Rest the head on the shoulder of the bottom arm, which is straight. Hold the push through bar straight overhead with the top arm. Make sure the body is in a long line from the tips of the toes to the tips of the fingers. Align the push through bar with the upright poles, offering a universal starting point for everyone, irrespective of height.

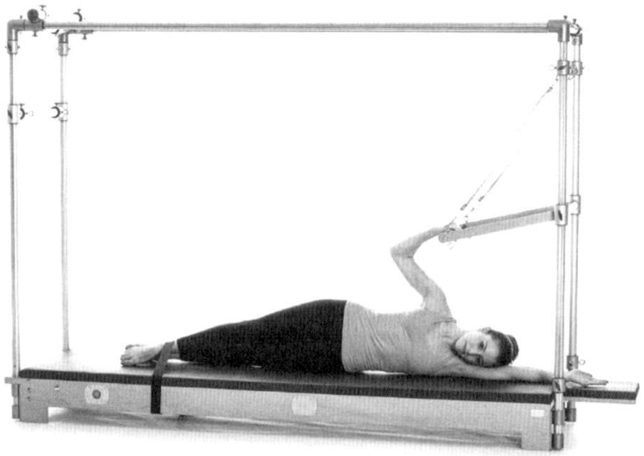

Inhale. Bend the top arm, elbow reaching up toward the ceiling, and bring the push through bar to the inside of the cadillac frame.

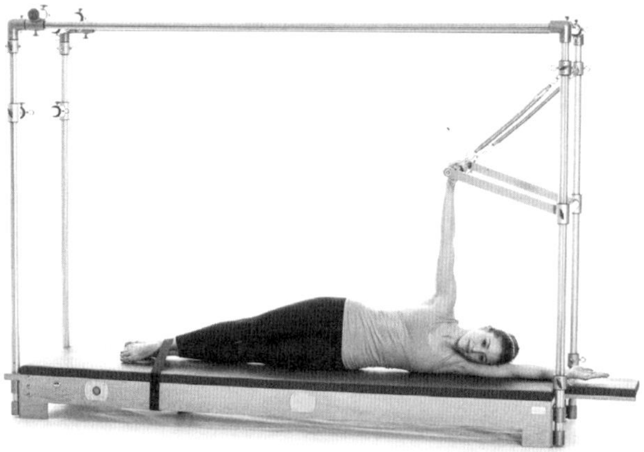

Continuing to inhale, straighten the top arm, lifting the push through bar toward the ceiling.

There is a strong temptation to try to lift the body by bending the elbow and pulling up with the arm holding the push through bar. Avoid this by keeping the top arm straight and focusing on lifting from the waist. Complete the movement by lifting the bottom arm to the push through bar and touching it (or as close as possible). This provides a significant stretch to the underside of the body and works the lateral flexors on the upper side intensely. When lifting, the lateral flexors on the underside should be engaged to help provide a girdle of support and stability around the midsection of the trunk and create an elongated arc shape.

Imagery

This movement always reminds me of flying through the air in a dance leap, using large arcing motions.

- Keep the arm holding the push through bar straight when lifting into lateral flexion.
- Engage the abdominals and back extensors to keep the body aligned.
- Move up and down in the coronal plane, as if between two panes of glass.

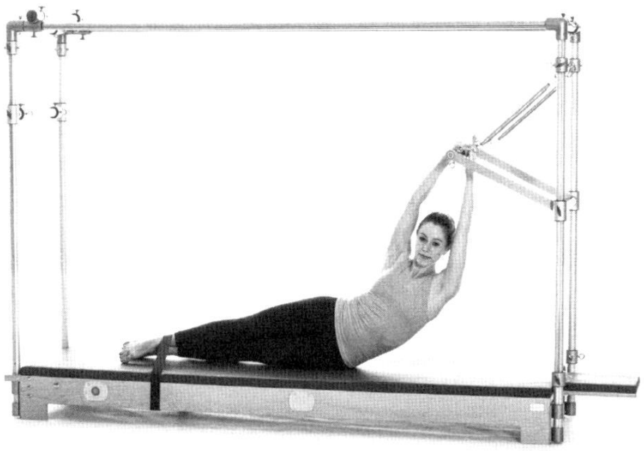

Exhale. Lift the trunk into lateral flexion, then lift the bottom arm to touch the push through bar (or as close as possible).

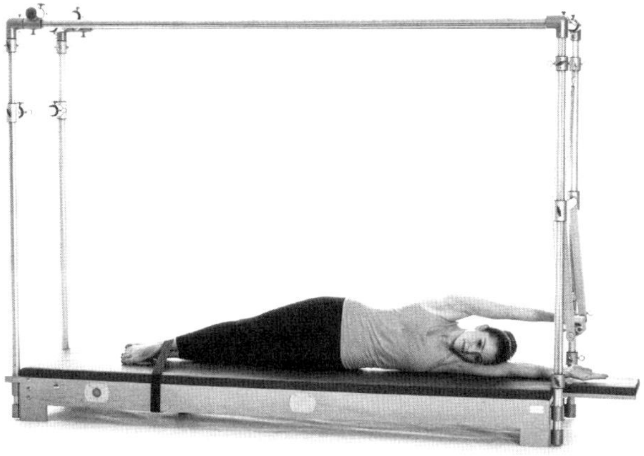

Inhale. Lower the body.

Exhale. Bend the upper arm and straighten it overhead. Return to the start position. Repeat 5 times before switching sides.

CADILLAC

Lateral Flexion and Rotation

INTERMEDIATE

Muscle Focus

- Abdominal obliques
- Intercostals
- Shoulder adductors

Objectives

- To improve abdominal oblique control
- To improve thoracic, shoulder adductor, and abdominal oblique flexibility

RESISTANCE

Light — Medium — Heavy

Side Reach

Few exercises feel as good as this one, providing a focused stretch to the side of the trunk and the underarm. The lumbopelvic region remains in flexion to reinforce the anchoring of the pelvis while the upper trunk flexes laterally on one side and extends laterally on the other, displaying the control we strive for in each segment of the spine, and in the body as a whole. Maintaining a good anchor with the legs and pelvis in order to maximize the stretch is vital.

Imagery

The movement should be a sweeping action of the arm out to the side and back, like a large handheld fan opening and closing. I also like to think of the side of the body and the arm as a rubber band being stretched by an external force attached to the arm; when the force is removed, the body and arm recoil back to the center.

- ○ Maintain lumbopelvic stabilization, particularly when reaching the arm back.
- ○ Press both feet against the upright poles, emphasizing the one on the reaching side.
- ○ Turn the palm of the free hand toward the ceiling while reaching back.
- ○ Allow the head to relax and follow the line of the shoulder and arm, with the gaze directed beyond the hand.
- ○ Allow the ribcage to expand on the stretching side.

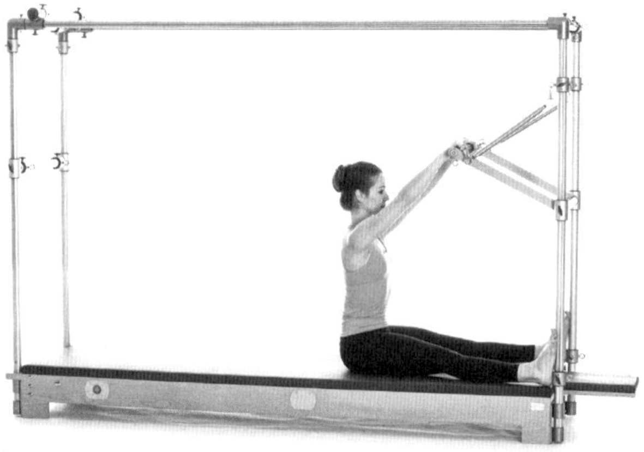

Setup. Sit upright, facing the push through bar. Place the feet against the upright poles and the hands on the push through bar, shoulder width apart. Keep the arms straight.

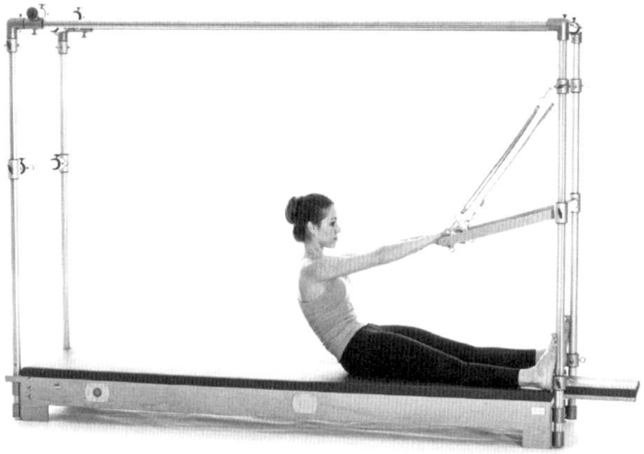

Exhale. Round the trunk and glide the pelvis under in a posterior tilt. Hang back on the push through bar and continue pressing the feet into the upright poles.

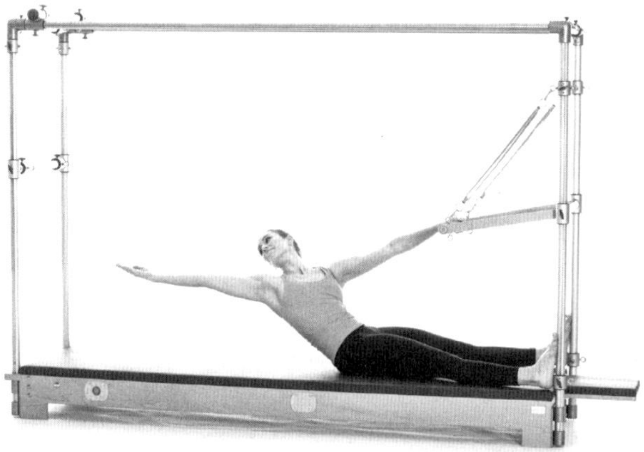

Inhale. While maintaining lumbar flexion, release one hand and sweep it out to the side and back, parallel to the mat with the palm up, to maximize the stretch. Allow the head to relax toward the shoulder and direct the gaze beyond the hand.

Exhale. Return to the previous position, placing the hand back on the push through bar and deepening the spinal flexion.

Inhale. Extend the spine to the upright sitting position. Return to the start position. Repeat 10 times, alternating sides.

Prone 1

Prone 1 is the foundation movement of a wonderful series of back extension exercises on the cadillac. It teaches the fundamental principle of distributing the extension throughout the spine, with specific focus on the mid- and upper back. This is achieved by recruiting the abdominals in concert with the spinal extensors, which assists in protecting the lower back from excessive pressure. It also reinforces coordination of scapular stabilization with spinal extension. Note that the supporting musculature should remain engaged throughout, including between repetitions.

Imagery

The image of an archer's bow being stretched and then released works well to create the powerful, arching shape of the body. The energy is never completely released; the power is held within the musculature at all times, available on demand.

- ○ Articulate the spine, beginning with the crown of the head.
- ○ Keep the abdominals engaged.
- ○ Lift only as high as the lower ribs and reach the sternum forward during the extension.
- ○ Press down on the push through bar continuously, with the arms straight.
- ○ Wrap the fingers and thumb around the push through bar for safety.

Muscle Focus

- Back extensors
- Abdominals
- Shoulder extensors

Objectives

- To improve back extensor strength
- To develop shoulder extensor and abdominal control

RESISTANCE

Light Medium Heavy

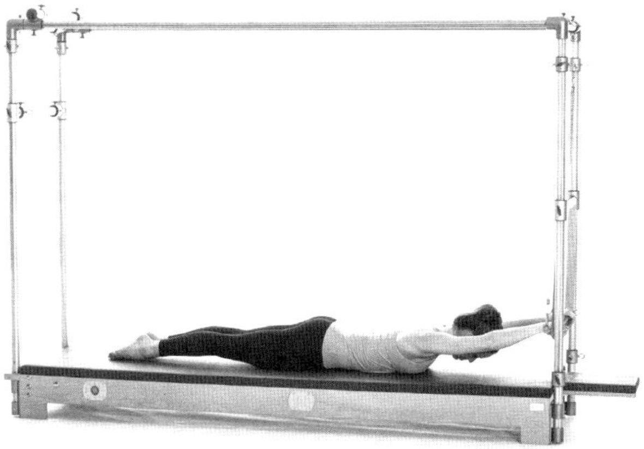

Setup. Lie prone, holding the push through bar with the arms straight overhead (forward), shoulder width apart. Align the push through bar with the upright poles, offering a universal starting point for everyone, irrespective of height.

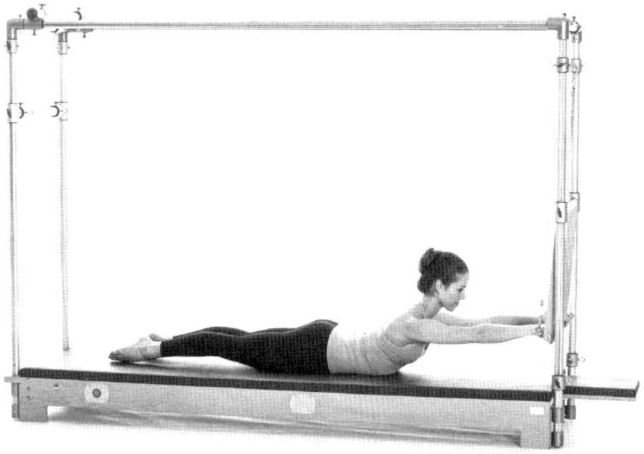

Inhale. Lift the trunk into spinal extension, pressing the arms down gently on the push through bar, pausing at the point where the lower ribs are lightly touching the mat.

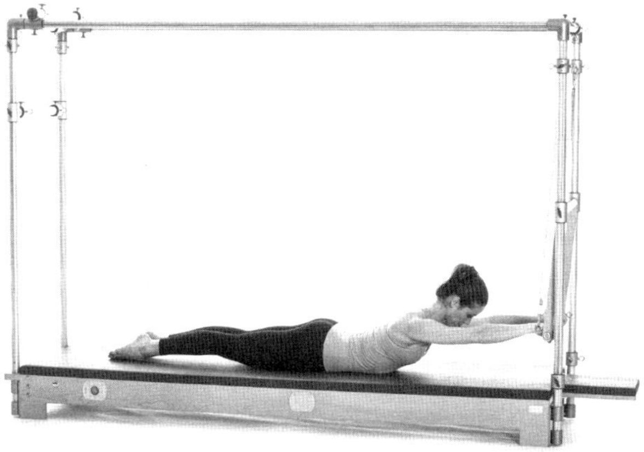

Exhale. Lower the trunk. Return to the start position. Repeat 5-10 times.

Prone 2

Muscle Focus

- Back extensors
- Abdominals
- Shoulder extensors

Objectives

- To improve back extensor strength
- To improve shoulder extensor and abdominal control
- To improve shoulder flexibility

RESISTANCE

Light Medium Heavy

Few exercises integrate spinal extension with the strength and flexibility of the shoulder girdle as beautifully and intricately as the Cadillac: Prone 2. Although the shoulder stretch and the back extension are linked, they should be regarded as two separate movements. It is important to stretch the shoulders as far as possible, allowing the push through bar to start lifting upward before extending the back. The shoulders should feel free and unrestricted, as if the springs are doing the lifting. Then, when the trunk reaches full extension, the effort is transferred largely to the back extensors, without relying on the arms or the push through bar to maintain the elevation of the trunk.

When you reverse the movement, again maximize the stretch of the shoulders before bringing the push through bar down and forward and lowering the trunk.

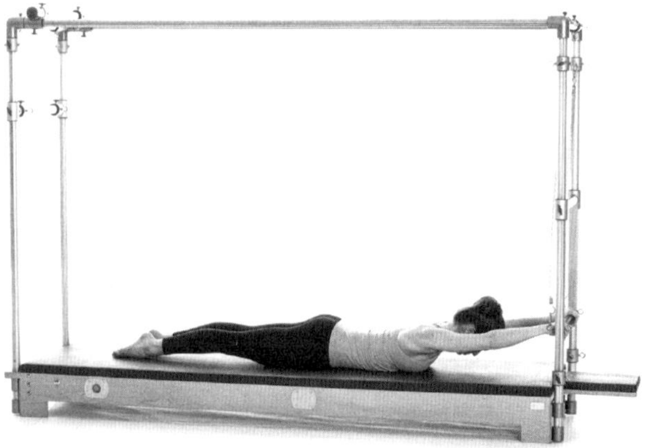

Setup. Lie prone, holding the push through bar with the arms straight overhead (forward). Align the push through bar with the upright poles, offering a universal starting point for everyone, irrespective of height.

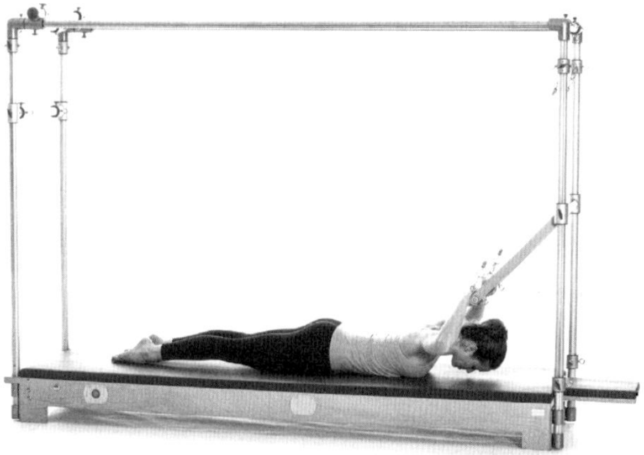

Inhale. Bend the elbows out to the sides, bringing the arms back and behind the head. Begin straightening the arms upward.

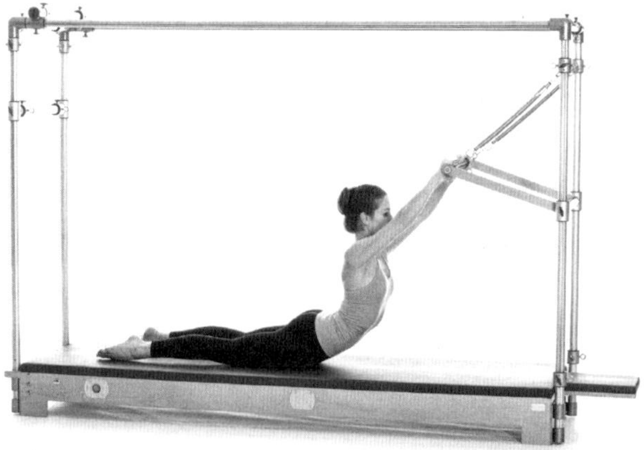

Exhale. When the arms can move no farther, lift the trunk and continue straightening the arms until the elbows and back are fully extended.

Imagery

The image of stretching and releasing an archer's bow used in Cadillac: Prone 1 works well in this exercise, although here it is taken even further as the body reaches a higher, more extreme bow shape. As you begin to lower the trunk after the full back extension, you should feel like you are hanging from the shoulders.

- Achieve maximum stretch of the shoulders before lifting the trunk into extension.
- Allow the push through bar to lift upward before extending the spine.
- In the second part of the exercise, lower the trunk as far as possible and stretch the shoulders before bringing the arms through to complete the movement.
- Keep the abdominals engaged.
- Wrap the fingers and thumb around the push through bar for safety.

PROGRESSION

The following progression takes advantage of the exceptional stretch for the shoulders in the first phase and challenges the stability and strength of the back extension in the second phase. Begin the exercise exactly as described in Cadillac: Prone 2. Following the back extension, rather than reversing the pattern, maintain the maximum back extension while lowering the push through bar in front of the chest, followed by pushing the push through bar forward. Lower the body to the start position.

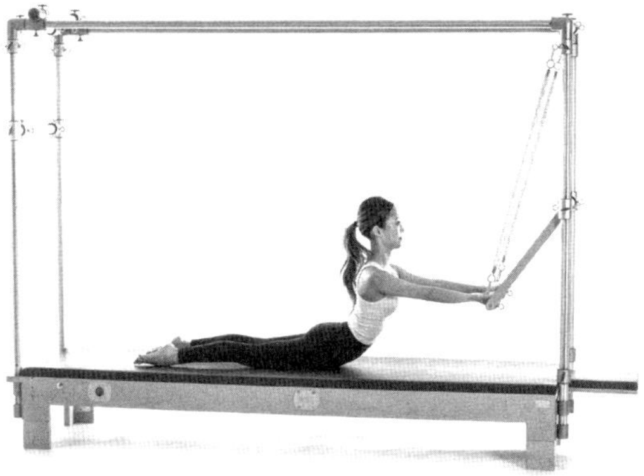

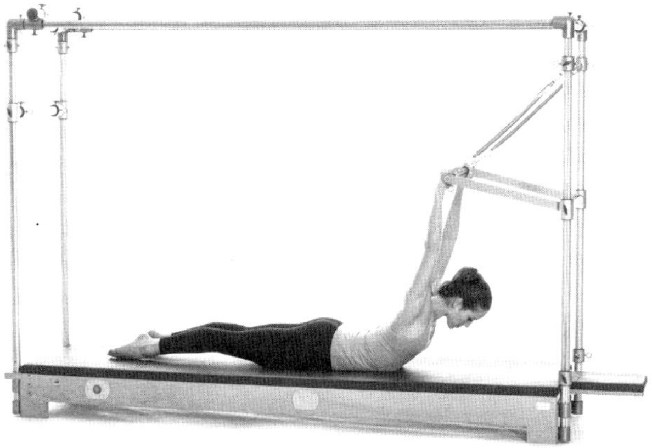

Inhale. Lower the trunk, keeping the arms straight and reaching up.

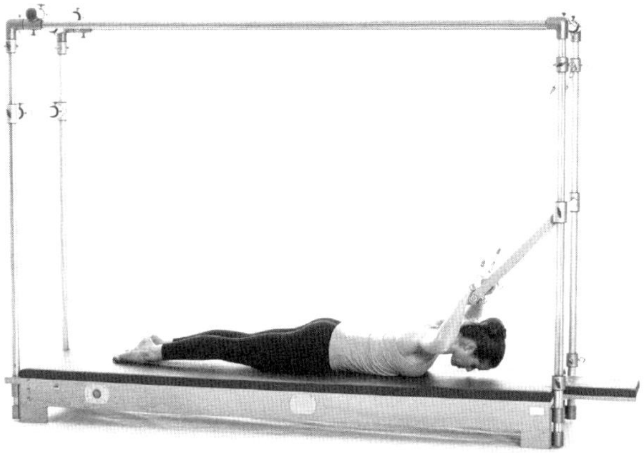

Exhale. Bend the elbows and lower the trunk, bringing the push through bar down, then straighten the arms directly overhead (forward). Return to the start position. Repeat 5 times.

Hanging Back

Muscle Focus

- Back extensors
- Hip extensors
- Scapular stabilizers

Objectives

- To improve back extensor strength
- To improve thoracic flexibility
- To improve hip extensor control
- To develop scapular stabilization

RESISTANCE

Light Medium Heavy

This exercise is impressive to watch and even more fun to do. Although categorized as an advanced exercise, it is within reach of many people, even those who may not believe they can perform such a challenging movement. It encapsulates several fundamental concepts, such as spinal articulation, distribution of forces in back extension, scapular stabilization, abdominal support, and the relationship between back extension and hip extension.

I like to focus this movement in the mid-back, between and just below the scapulae. When you reach the plank position with the body straight and parallel to the floor, maintain lumbopelvic stabilization. Begin articulating the spine into extension starting from the crown of the head. Once the crown of the head is facing directly down, continue through the thoracic spine. Once the thoracic spine is fully extended, add lumbar extension and finally hip extension to provide the finishing touch to the movement.

The arms serve simply as rods or levers connecting the body to the crossbars. The shoulders, however, fulfill an important role; good shoulder function is critical to successful execution of this exercise. The head follows the line of the spine. Avoid the tendency to throw the head back too far when in the hanging back position, hyperextending the cervical spine (eyes gazing down at the mat). This will inevitably result in neck tension. Instead, you should feel like the crown of the head is reaching down toward the mat, completing the gentle, arcing shape.

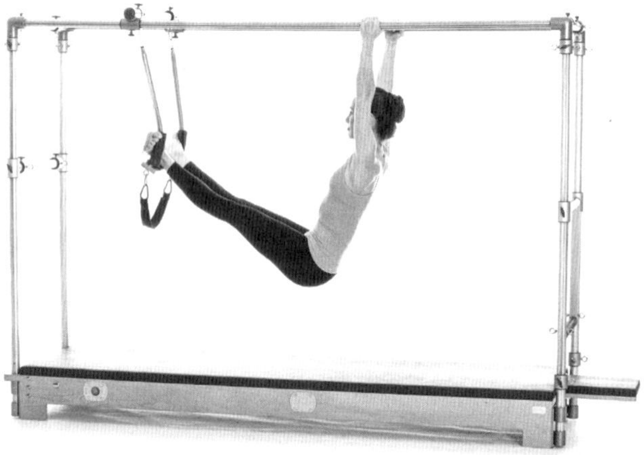

Setup. Hold on to the crossbars of the cadillac with straight arms. Place the feet on the trapeze swing, dorsiflexed, so they wrap around the springs, with the hips externally rotated. Establish a neutral spine position (or as close as possible) when hanging, creating a V position with the body.

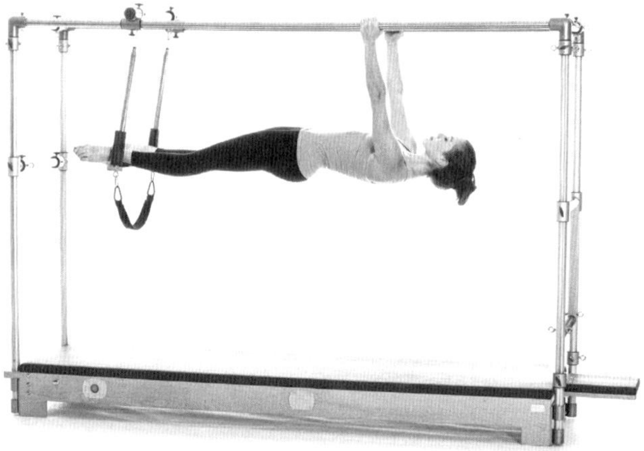

Exhale. Roll up, beginning with the pelvis, articulating through the spine into a plank position so that the body hangs parallel to the mat in neutral alignment. (Plantarflexing the feet is optional at this point.)

Imagery

Visualizing energy lines works well for this exercise. In the start position there is one energy line running through the legs and another running through the trunk, which meet at the pelvis to create a V shape. The pelvis is then lifted, and a straight line is established prior to arching into the hanging back position. In the hanging back position, one long energy line runs from the feet to the pelvis, then gently bends through the trunk and head, tracing the arch shape of the body.

- Reach the tailbone toward the mat when hanging in the start position.
- Establish scapular stabilization in the hanging position before starting the movement.
- Draw in the abdominals, creating deep spinal flexion, to initiate the movement.
- Achieve maximum extension in the mid- and upper back before proceeding to lumbar extension, followed by hip extension, which completes the movement.
- Reach the crown of the head toward the mat in the extended position, avoiding neck tension.

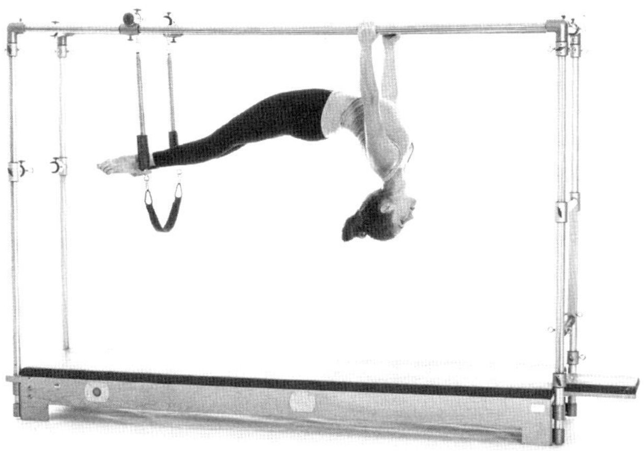

Inhale. Extend further, articulating through the spine starting from the crown of the head. Maximize thoracic extension, keeping the crown of the head directed toward the mat, before adding lumbar extension followed by hip extension. Pivot around the shoulders, keeping the arms straight.

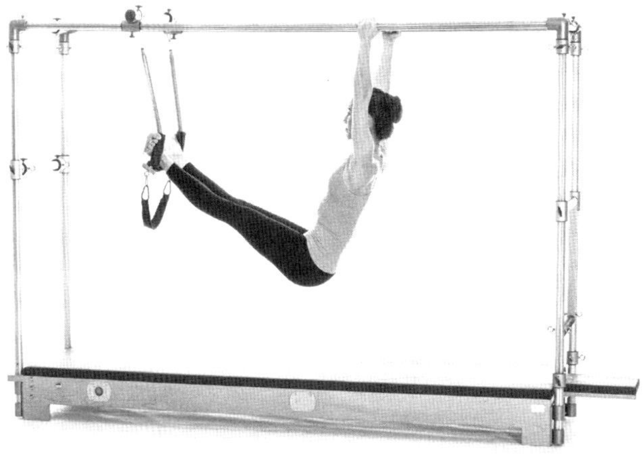

Exhale. Return to the plank position, then articulate through the spine down to the V position. Return to the start position. Repeat 5 times.

Wunda Chair

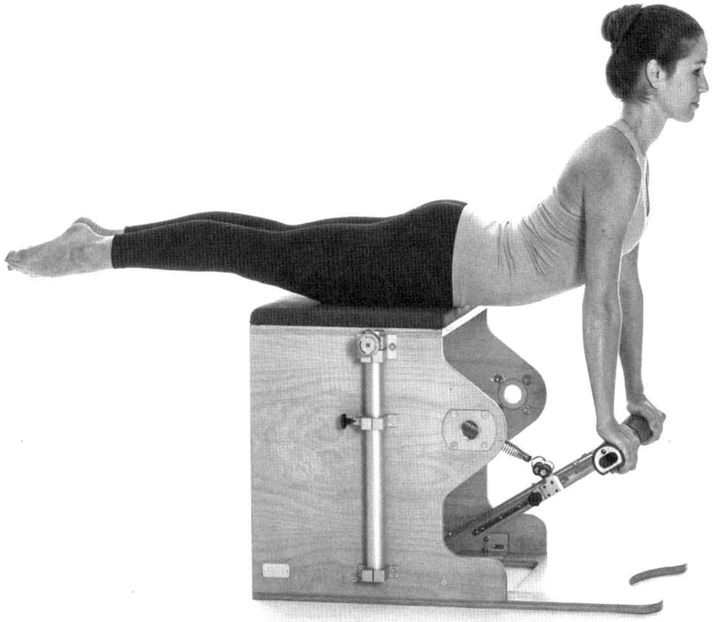

I have a special sentiment for the wunda chair. The genius of this unassuming box never ceases to amaze me. Its versatility is not only in the vast repertoire, but in the fact that the original version could flip over and double as a piece of furniture, a comfortable armchair! Even today there are few, if any, pieces of equipment that can rival the wunda chair's capability: hundreds of exercises for every part of the body and every fitness level in a very small package.

The chair is not easy to use and it often proves quite unforgiving, readily highlighting imbalances and weaknesses. However, it also provides tremendous possibilities and is well suited for improving general fitness and enhancing athletic performance. In many ways, the wunda chair is more functional than other exercise equipment, even other Pilates apparatus, because many exercises are performed upright, which more closely simulates everyday movements. This position demands greater activation of the trunk stabilizers than the reformer or cadillac when performing foot work.

However, because of its design, the wunda chair does not readily accommodate full ranges of motion in many of the exercises. Also, the chair offers fewer possibilities for developing flexion of the joints than for developing extension. As long as you are aware of these possible shortcomings, the wunda chair is simply a must-have apparatus.

I had the privilege of being introduced to the wonders of this apparatus by one of the greatest Pilates teachers to grace our community, Kathy Stanford Grant. Although I had worked on the wunda chair prior to meeting Kathy, it was this insightful teacher who truly opened my eyes to its possibilities and taught me much of its classical repertoire. Kathy was among Mr. Pilates' early students, and one of only two people to receive a teacher's certification from him. (The other is Lolita San Miguel, also a teacher of great distinction and one I am honored to call a friend.) Kathy and I often discussed strategies to make its use more widespread. In fact, Kathy may have been singularly responsible for the rebirth of the wunda chair, bringing it from relative obscurity to center stage in the early 1990s. Today it is possibly one of the most popular pieces of apparatus, both in Pilates studios and in gym environments, where it is frequently used for large group classes. Kathy loved the wunda chair as I do and shared my fascination with its complex simplicity.

I recall as if it were yesterday meeting Kathy and naively volunteering to perform several moves on the chair. I had limited experience on this apparatus even though I had been doing Pilates for about 12 or 13 years. Kathy, who was small in stature and large in presence, quickly homed in on every compensation and imbalance in my body. This was an epiphany for me. I recognized a depth of work that I had previously ignored. I had relied on a strong body and athletic skill to perform choreography well—but that was clearly superficial. My movement was lacking depth. This humbling experience on the chair taught me the meaning of moving from within and set my teaching on a new and exciting path. I had to go back to square one, learning and exploring every movement anew. The experience also taught me to use what I call "MRI vision" (beyond X-ray vision!) to see deeply into other people's bodies and to detect where a movement is coming from even before it happens. This heightened awareness taught me to move differently, to cue differently, to teach differently, and to anticipate more profound results. I often think of my dear friend and mentor, Kathy, and the gift of insightfulness that she gave me.

In early 2021 I was teaching Master I, the second part of my four-part Legacy Program. I was talking about seeing movement and identifying the recruitment of muscles and not only looking at the outside form. At times the alignment may not be ideal due to certain limitations, yet the goal is being achieved. I thought of Kathy when I said: "*Strive for perfection, recognize intention.*" This is vital when cueing people. It is not only a matter of the form being perfect, although of course, that is what we aim for. It is important that the targeted muscles are being activated in the correct way as we strive for that illusive ideal.

Parallel Heels and Toes

The foot work on the wunda chair duplicates the foot positions used on the reformer and the cadillac. However, the positions of the trunk and legs are quite different—on the wunda chair, the trunk is upright and the legs push down toward the floor. Interestingly, each of these apparatus requires that the legs move in a different direction when doing the foot work—horizontal (reformer), upward (cadillac), and downward (wunda chair). Each movement and its accordingly diverse muscle actions have unique benefits.

The dynamic of the leg movement on the wunda chair is like a pumping action, with a relatively short range of motion compared to the full-range knee extension on the reformer and cadillac. It may prove advantageous to sit on pads or a small box during the foot work, particularly if tall, to elevate the body and increase the range of motion of the legs. Feeling the quadriceps more prominently is common on the wunda chair; I refer to this as having "wunda chair legs," a delightful, wobbly sensation often experienced after completing the foot work.

The arm position is unique in that it offers support for the trunk and at the same time provides an excellent stretch for the front of the shoulders and chest. Try not to rely on the arms too much; rather, think of them as a frame for the body.

Imagery

On the cadillac the feeling is like supporting the ceiling, with the legs as pillars. On the reformer the feeling is like propelling yourself on a horizontal plane by pushing against a wall. On the wunda chair the feeling is like pressing against the floor, becoming taller with each leg extension, to the point of feeling levitated above the chair.

- Maintain a stable, upright trunk.
- Push down through the heels when in the heels position.
- Maintain plantarflexion when in the toes position.
- Keep the elbows slightly bent and facing back.

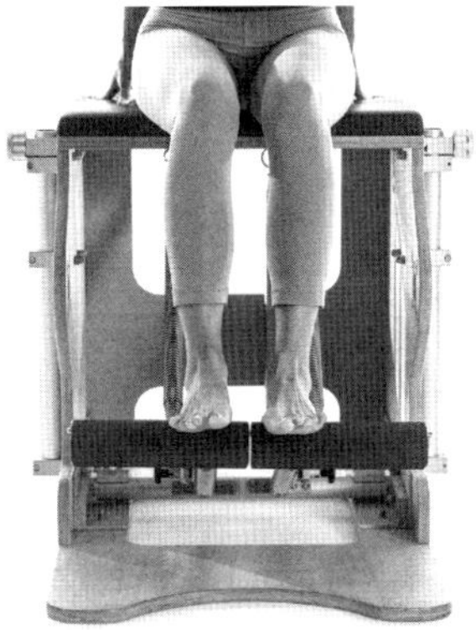

Parallel heels position.

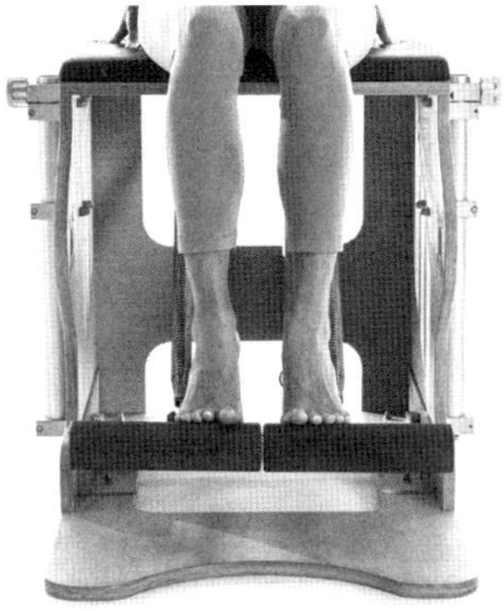

Parallel toes position.

PROGRESSION

Once you have established good stability of the trunk and pelvis, you can try different arm positions, such as down by the sides (not touching the chair), in a T position, reaching to the ceiling, or hands behind the head.

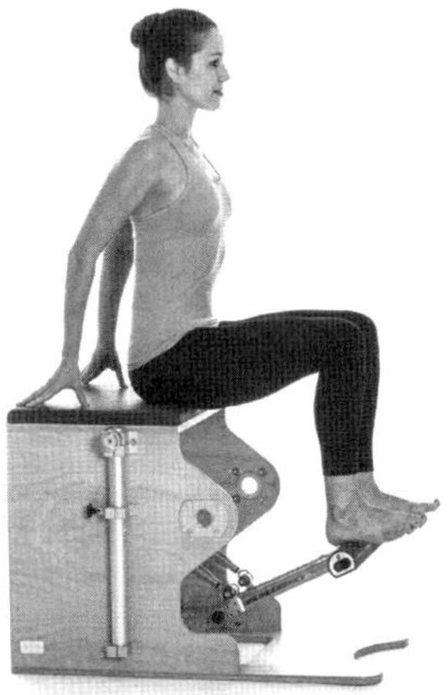

Setup. Sit upright on the front part of the chair, hands resting on the fingertips near the rear of the platform, elbows bent and facing back, scapulae open. Place the feet on the pedal (on the wunda chair the footbar is referred to as the pedal), legs parallel, either on the heels or toes. Start the movement with the thighs slightly higher than horizontal (approximately 5 degrees).

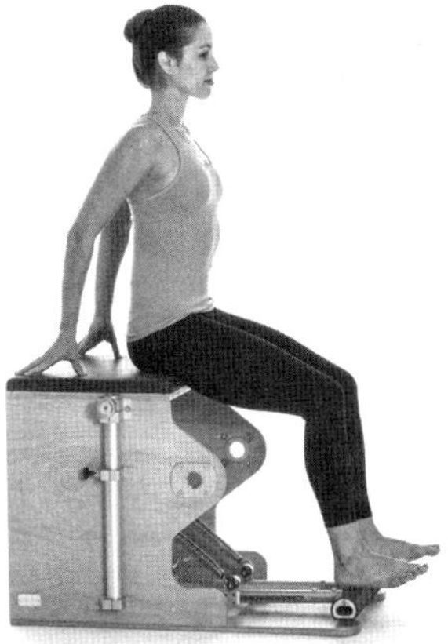

Exhale. Press down with the legs, lowering the pedal until it is about to touch the base (or until the pelvis is no longer stable).

Inhale. Lift the legs, raising the pedal. Return to the start position. Repeat 10 times.

Muscle Focus

- Quadriceps
- Hamstrings
- Abdominals
- Back extensors

Objectives

- To improve knee extensor strength
- To improve hip extensor control
- To develop trunk and lumbopelvic stabilization

RESISTANCE

Light — Medium — Heavy

V Position Toes

Muscle Focus

- Quadriceps
- Hamstrings
- Abdominals
- Back extensors

Objectives

- To improve knee extensor strength
- To improve hip extensor control
- To develop trunk and lumbopelvic stabilization

RESISTANCE

Light Medium Heavy

As with the other apparatus, create the small V position by simply bringing the heels together from the Wunda Chair: Parallel Toes position. It is important to keep the heels actively pressing together throughout. This will in turn engage the hip external rotators and hip adductors. Maintain plantarflexion and feel like you are pressing through the feet in order to keep the resistance constant. Avoid the tendency to drop the heels, which releases the tension in the springs.

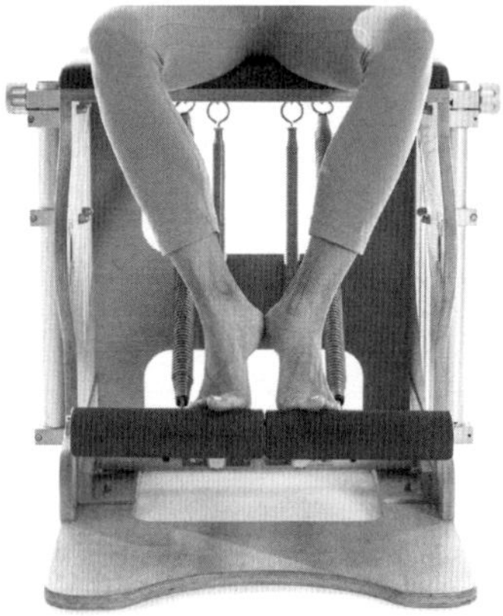

V position toes.

Imagery

The image of a frog leaping is an excellent one for this position. The fact that the body is upright makes the image feel all the more real.

- Maintain a stable, upright trunk.
- Maintain plantarflexion.
- Keep the elbows slightly bent and facing back.

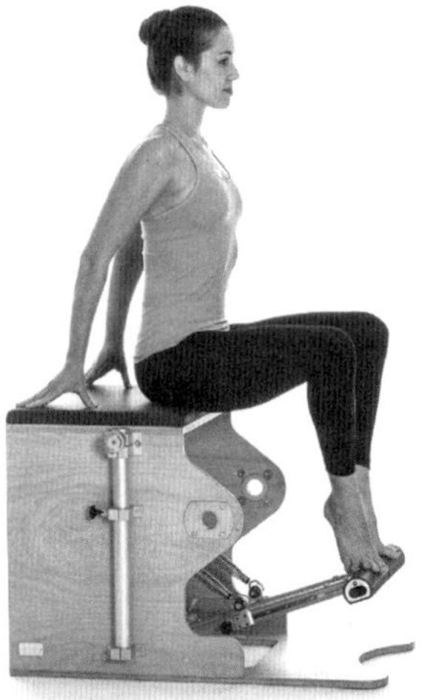

Setup. Sit upright on the front part of the chair, hands resting on the fingertips near the rear of the platform, elbows bent and facing back, scapulae open. Place the toes on the pedal, heels pressing together, creating a V position. Start the movement with the thighs slightly higher than horizontal (approximately 5 degrees).

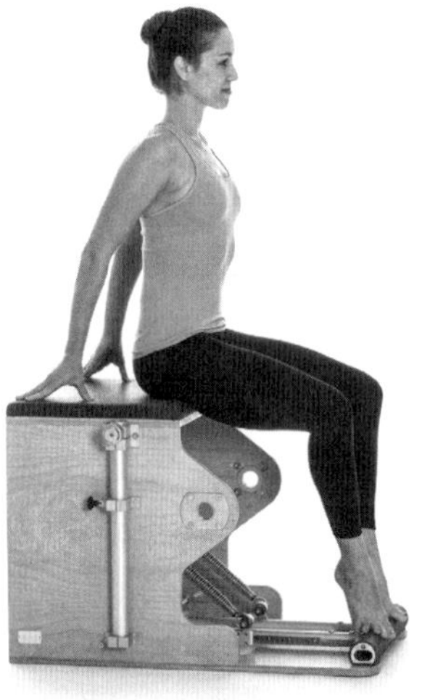

Exhale. Press down with the legs, lowering the pedal until it is about to touch the base (or until the pelvis is no longer stable).

Inhale. Lift the legs, raising the pedal. Return to the start position. Repeat 10 times.

Open V Position Heels and Toes

The open V positions on the wunda chair will not be as wide as those on the reformer or cadillac because the pedal is narrower. However, the same benefits of working the hip external rotators and the hip adductors, plus the knee extensors, hip extensors, and trunk stabilizers, will apply.

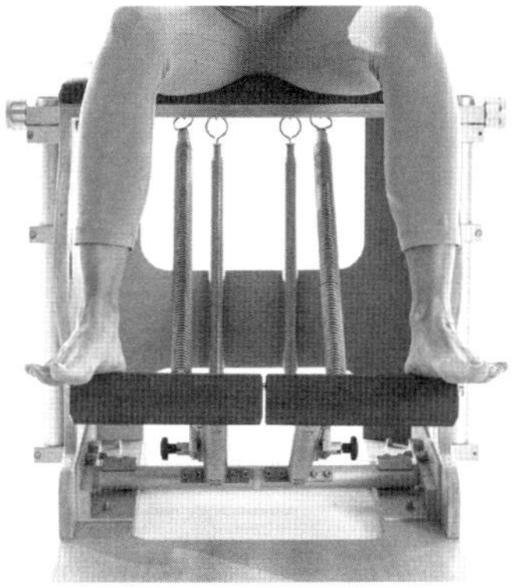

Open V position heels.

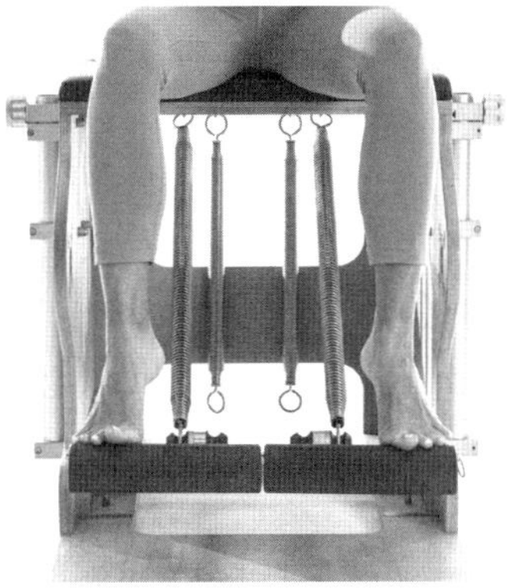

Open V position toes.

Imagery

Imagine the feeling of pressing down into the ground with the legs and at the same time reaching up with the trunk through the top of the head. I sometimes reach the arms overhead, which furthers the feeling of the arms and upper body being lifted.

- Maintain a stable, upright trunk.
- Maintain plantarflexion (toes position).
- Keep the elbows slightly bent and facing back.
- Push down through the heels when in the heels position.

Muscle Focus

- Quadriceps
- Hamstrings
- Abdominals
- Back extensors

Objectives

- To improve knee extensor strength
- To improve hip extensor control
- To develop trunk and lumbopelvic stabilization

RESISTANCE

Light Medium Heavy

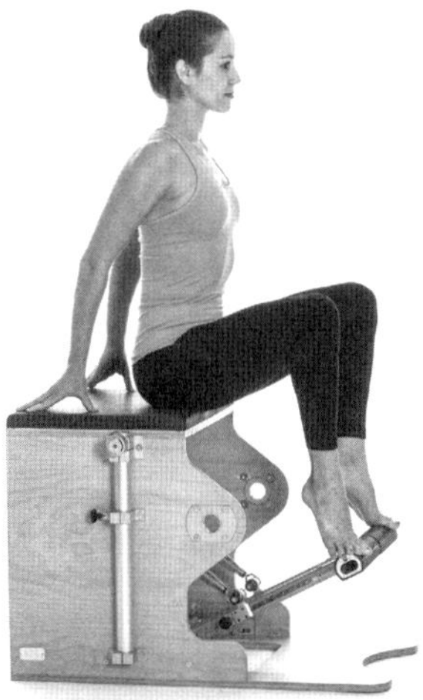

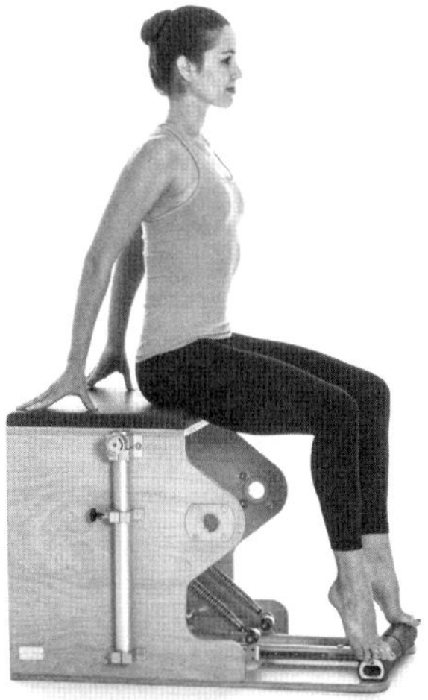

Setup. Sit upright on the front part of the chair, hands resting on the fingertips near the rear of the platform, elbows bent and facing back, scapulae open. Place the heels or toes on each end of the pedal, hips externally rotated the same degree as the Wunda Chair: V Position Toes, but now with the feet apart. Start the movement with the thighs slightly higher than horizontal (approximately 5 degrees).

Exhale. Press down with the legs, lowering the pedal until it is about to touch the base (or until the pelvis is no longer stable).

Inhale. Lift the legs, raising the pedal. Return to the start position. Repeat 10 times.

WUNDA CHAIR
Foot Work
FUNDAMENTAL

Calf Raises

Muscle Focus

- Ankle–foot plantarflexors
- Abdominals
- Back extensors
- Hip flexors

Objectives

- To improve ankle–foot plantarflexor strength
- To improve ankle–foot plantarflexor and hip flexor flexibility
- To develop foot alignment

RESISTANCE
Light Medium Heavy

This position exemplifies the concept of multidimensional, full body integration. Although the calf of the moving leg is the focus of the exercise, trunk stability is being challenged, the hip flexors and calf of the opposite leg are being stretched, and even the shoulder stabilizers are being activated. This exercise is exceptional for highlighting correct foot and trunk alignment as well as lumbopelvic stabilization.

Imagery

The diagonal position of the body in this exercise reminds me of a ski jumper flying down the ramp. Add to this powerful image the completely isolated movement of the foot, as if pressing down on an accelerator pedal of a car.

- ○ Maintain a level pelvis, as close to neutral position as possible.
- ○ Keep the legs parallel rather than externally rotated.
- ○ Keep the back heel pressing into the floor (or as close as possible).
- ○ Utilize the full range of motion of the ankle, moving from full plantarflexion to full dorsiflexion.

PROGRESSION

To add challenge in terms of balance and increased stretch for the hip flexors of the back leg, hold the arms in a T position or place the hands behind the head. At the same time, raise the trunk from the diagonal line to an upright position so that it is in vertical alignment.

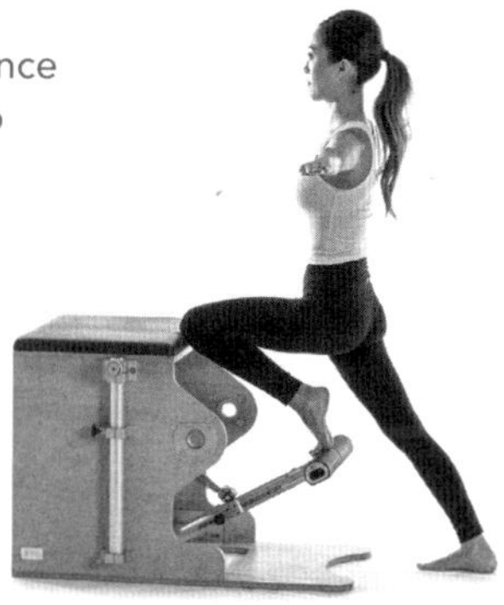

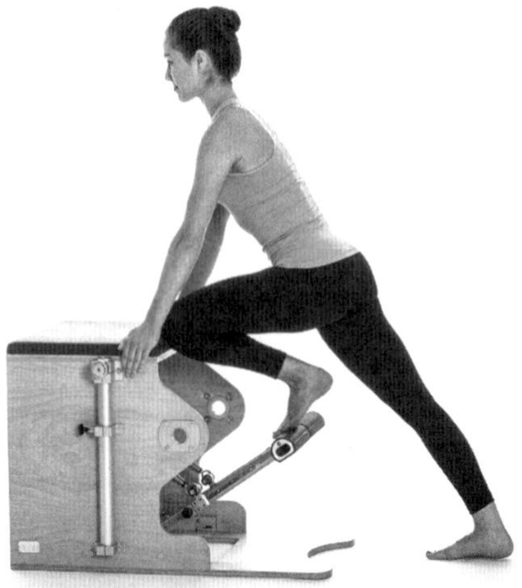

Setup. Stand facing the chair, with the trunk stable on a diagonal line, and place the hands firmly on the front section of the wunda chair, holding on to the sides. Place the toes of one foot on the pedal and press the pedal partway down. Set the leg, just below the knee, firmly onto the front edge of the wunda chair. Hold the back leg straight and place it quite far back from the chair, with the heel pressing into the floor, creating a long diagonal line running from the heel up the trunk and out through the head.

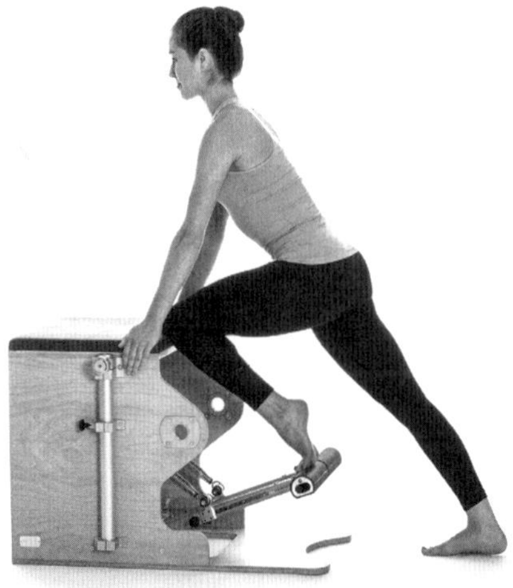

Exhale. Plantarflex the foot, lowering the pedal.

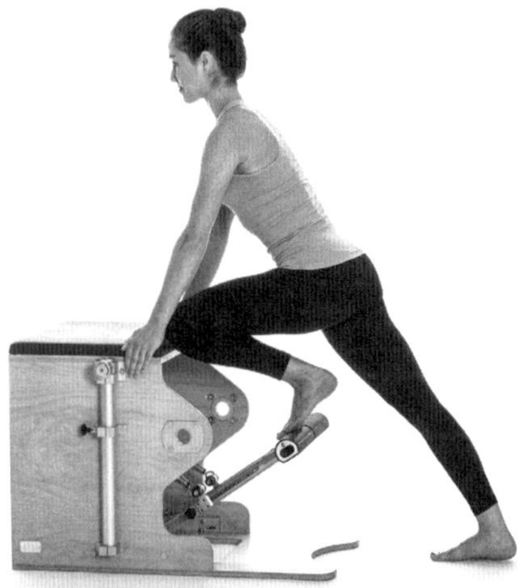

Inhale. Dorsiflex the foot, raising the pedal. Return to the start position. Repeat 10-20 times on the same leg before switching to the other side.

Single-Leg Heel and Toes

All of the advantages and benefits of doing single-leg work on the other apparatus are magnified on the wunda chair. Stabilization is challenging in the sitting position and every possible weakness, imbalance, and compensation is brought to the fore. Few pieces of apparatus, if any, are as valuable as the wunda chair for developing and improving leg function while stabilizing the pelvis and trunk.

Imagery

I find the movement similar to kick-starting an older-style motorcycle while keeping the rest of the body stable. (This image may only make sense to those of you old enough to remember motorcycles with a kick start!)

- Maintain equal weight on both sit bones.
- Keep the pelvis and trunk stable, avoiding rotation as the leg presses down.
- Stabilize the supporting leg.

MODIFICATION

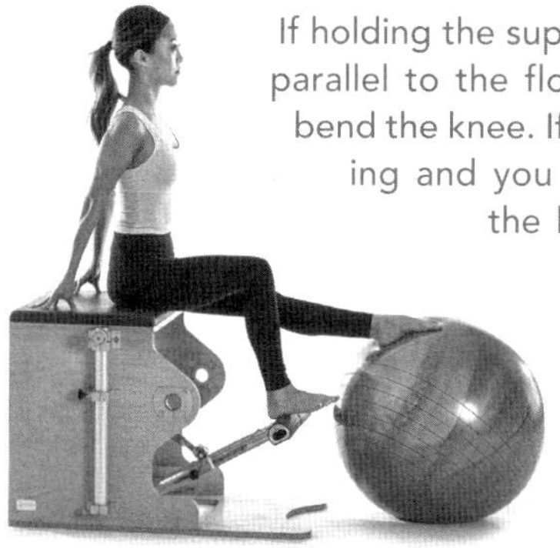

If holding the supporting leg straight and parallel to the floor proves too difficult, bend the knee. If this is still too challenging and you are unable to stabilize the body or hold the leg in the air, rest the leg on a large ball or on the reformer box.

Muscle Focus

- Quadriceps
- Hamstrings
- Abdominals
- Back extensors

Objectives

- To improve knee extensor strength
- To improve hip extensor control
- To develop trunk and lumbopelvic stabilization

RESISTANCE

Light — Medium — Heavy

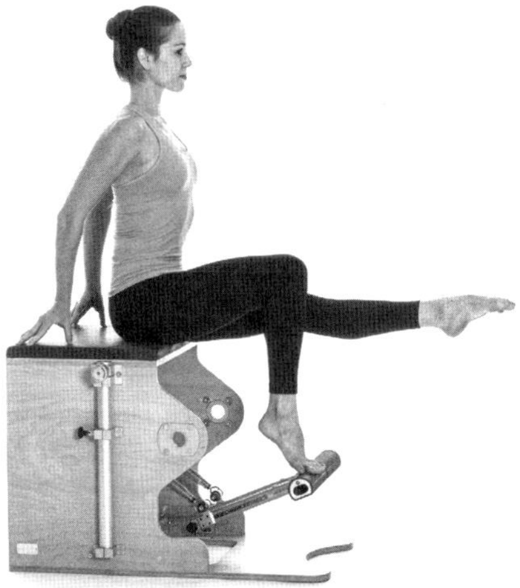

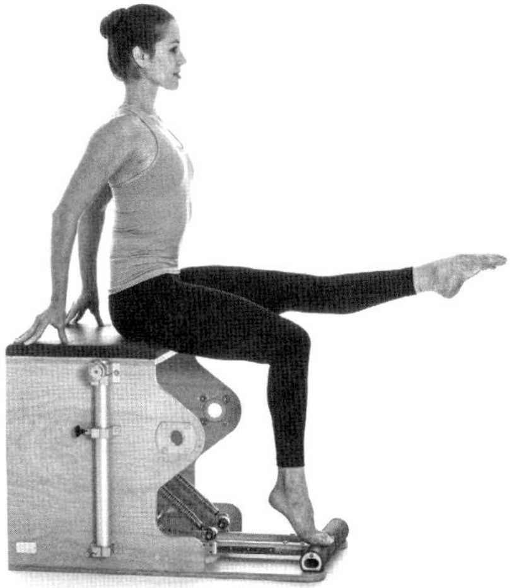

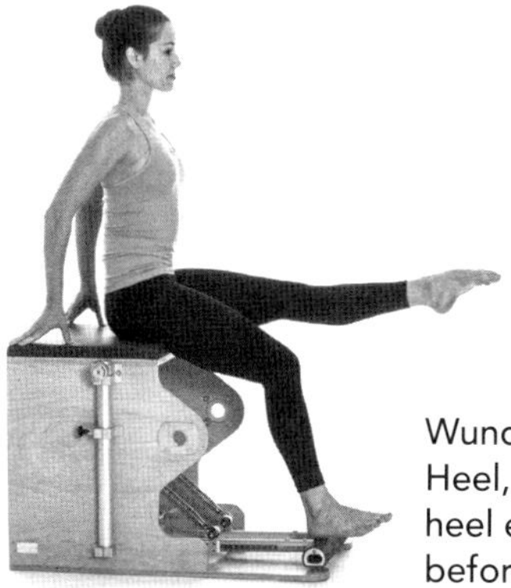

Wunda Chair: Single-Leg Heel, down position. The heel exercise is done before the toes.

Setup. Sit upright on the front part of the chair, hands resting on the fingertips near the rear of the platform, elbows bent and facing back, scapulae open. Place one foot on the pedal in either the single-leg heel or the single-leg toes position. Hold the opposite leg straight and directly forward, parallel to the floor (or as close as possible). Start the movement with the thigh slightly higher than horizontal (approximately 5 degrees).

Exhale. Press down with the leg, lowering the pedal until it is about to touch the base.

Inhale. Lift the leg, raising the pedal. Return to the start position. Repeat 10 times on the same leg before switching to the other side.

Pike—Standing

Muscle Focus

- Abdominals

Objectives

- To improve abdominal control
- To improve lower back flexibility
- To develop scapular stabilization

RESISTANCE

Light — Medium — Heavy

The movement of this exercise is similar to the Mat: Roll-Down described in chapter 2, but it has the advantage of support provided by the spring. This alleviates potential strain on the spine, particularly when it is done with straight legs. This exercise lays the foundation for many abdominal exercises on the various apparatus. The pike position relies on deep flexion of the trunk and excellent scapular stabilization. Note that, in this context, "pike position" simply refers to the body being folded at the waist with the trunk over the thighs. Although some pike positions require the trunk be as straight and flat as possible with the chest held close to the legs, in this pike and others, the trunk is rounded and not held close to the legs.

Imagery

All the pike exercises in Pilates conjure up the feeling and image of a diver in mid-flight, body folded in two, the trunk close to the thighs. This is despite the fact that most versions of the pike position in Pilates demand spinal flexion and are much rounder with space between the trunk and the legs.

- ○ Strive for maximum lumbar flexion.
- ○ Maintain scapular stabilization.
- ○ Keep the knees straight and the legs vertical.

VARIATION

There is tremendous value in combining spinal flexion and spinal extension; this variation takes advantage of this movement pattern. Rather than maintaining spinal flexion throughout the exercise, extend the back when the pedal is lowered during the inhale, followed by the exhale, rounding the trunk, and lifting until the shoulders and hip joints are aligned horizontally.

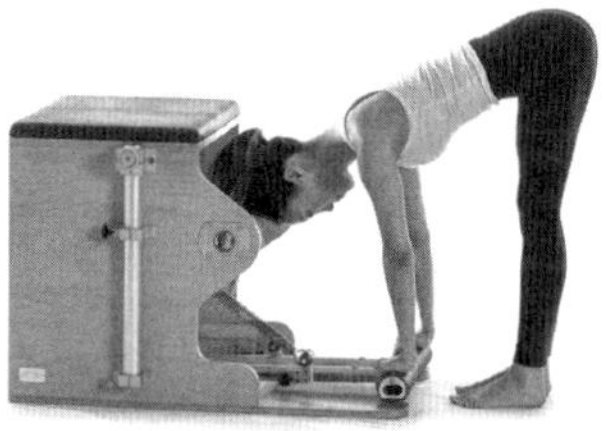

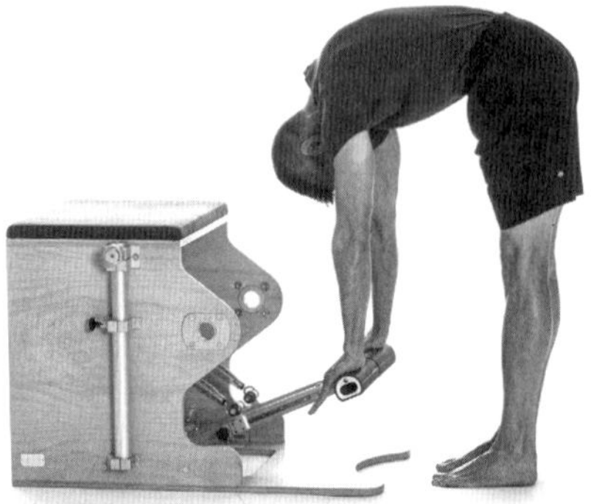

Setup. Stand facing the chair, close to the front, with the legs parallel. Roll down, placing the hands on the pedal, with the shoulders aligned over the wrists.

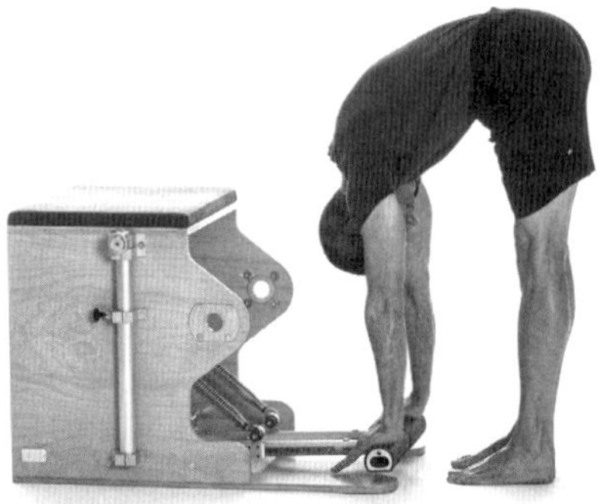

Inhale. Roll down, pressing the pedal toward the floor.

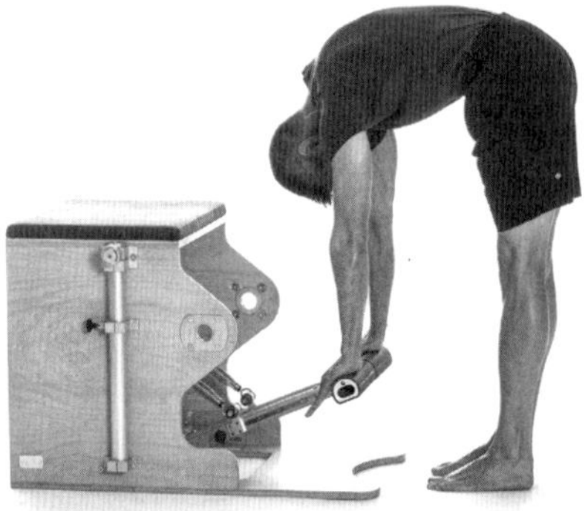

Exhale. Roll up, increasing the spinal flexion and raising the pedal until the shoulders and hips are aligned horizontally. Repeat 5-10 times.

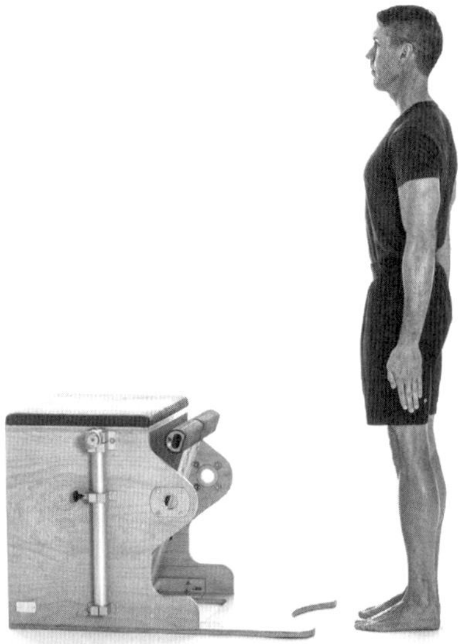

After the final exhale, roll up all the way. Return to the start position.

Pike—Forward

Few exercises exemplify masterful muscle coordination and full body integration better than the Wunda Chair: Pike—Forward. And few exercises can be as humbling for even the fittest and strongest among us. The abdominal and shoulder work is profound and produces a degree of muscle activation few other exercises can match. It must be performed on a medium spring (or lighter); otherwise, there is a tendency to rely on the lift of the spring rather than the work of the abdominals and shoulders. It is important to note that the abdominal work emanates from maximizing the round pike position, not from directly overloading the abdominals such as in the Mat: Double-Leg Stretch or Criss-Cross. It is more about control than pure strength. Layered on top of the abdominal work is the intense shoulder work, which can be likened to performing a handstand from a standstill. The clear influence gymnastics had on the development of the Pilates repertoire is evident in this movement. It is a personal favorite!

Imagery

In this exercise, the sensation should be of floating upward—a feeling of levitation that can be achieved only when all physical and mental components are aligned and working symbiotically.

- ○ Maximize lumbar flexion.
- ○ Keep the shoulders over the wrists and the head aligned with the spine, the crown of the head reaching down toward the chair.
- ○ Maintain plantarflexion of the feet.

Muscle Focus

- Abdominals
- Scapular stabilizers
- Deltoids

Objectives

- To improve abdominal control
- To improve shoulder flexor strength
- To develop scapular stabilization

RESISTANCE

Light Medium Heavy

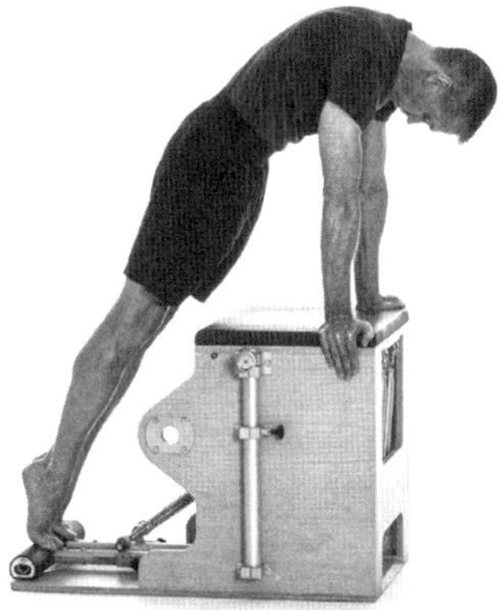

Setup. Stand on the pedal, facing the chair. Place the hands on the back of the chair, holding it from the sides. Align the shoulders directly over the wrists. Keep the scapulae stable and round the trunk, establishing a solid pike position.

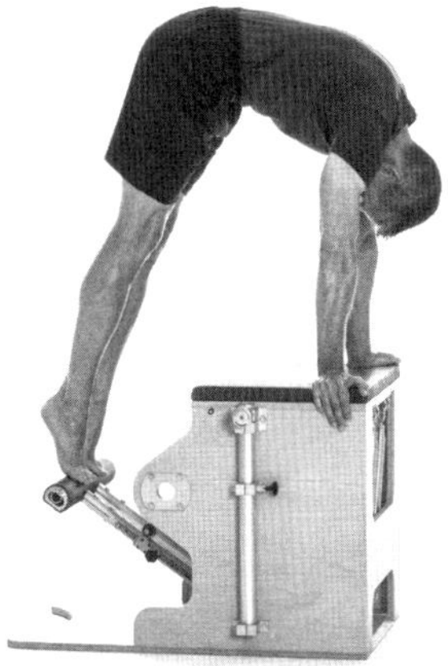

Exhale. Draw deeper into spinal flexion and engage the shoulder flexors, raising the pedal as high as possible.

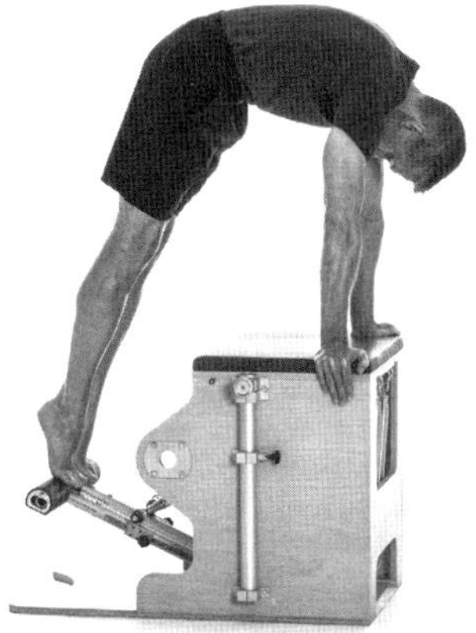

Inhale. Lower the pedal (hovering above the base), maintaining the pike position. Repeat 5 times.

Cat Stretch—Kneeling

Muscle Focus

- Abdominals
- Back extensors

Objectives

- To improve abdominal and back extensor control
- To improve lower back flexibility
- To develop scapular stabilization

RESISTANCE

Light — Medium — Heavy

In some respects, the Wunda Chair: Cat Stretch—Kneeling can be regarded as part of the group of abdominal exercises that focuses on deep spinal flexion, along with the Wunda Chair: Pike—Standing and Pike—Forward. At the same time, this exercise incorporates the all-important spinal extension and a high degree of scapular stabilization. For this reason, it fits comfortably into both the abdominal and the full body integration categories. Based on its all-encompassing nature, I chose the latter.

During the spinal extension, reach the head toward the floor, keeping it between the arms. Aim for 180-degree flexion of the shoulders, creating a straight line (or as close as possible) from the hips, through the trunk and arms to the wrists. Try to keep the hips over the knees so that the thighs remain vertical (or as close as possible). This helps ensure that the movement occurs in the spine, as opposed to the whole body rocking back and forth. Encourage a deep, hollow, round shape of the trunk as the pedal is lifted. There will inevitably be slight movement of the thighs backward as the body lifts; the degree of the movement will depend on the flexibility of the spine and the proportions of the body. This is a normal adaptation of the body to the movement. It is important to discern the difference between adaptation and compensation: Compensation would be rocking the body back in order to lift the pedal and rocking forward to push the pedal down.

Imagery

The name says it all—the shape, the intricate articulation of the spine, the flexibility, and the control—there is no better image to strive for than a cat stretching.

- ○ Align the hips over the knees (or as close as possible).
- ○ Keep the head aligned with the spine, both when the spine is rounded and straight.
- ○ Reach the head down between the arms during the spinal extension.

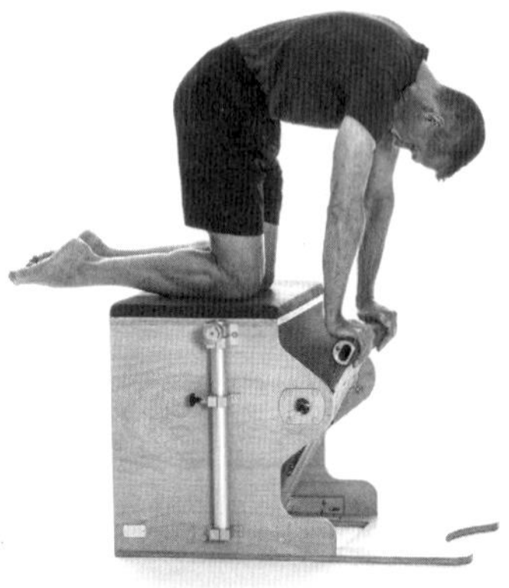

Setup. Kneel on the chair, close to the front edge and facing the pedal, with the body upright and the hips over the knees. Roll down, placing the hands on the pedal, with the shoulders aligned over the wrists.

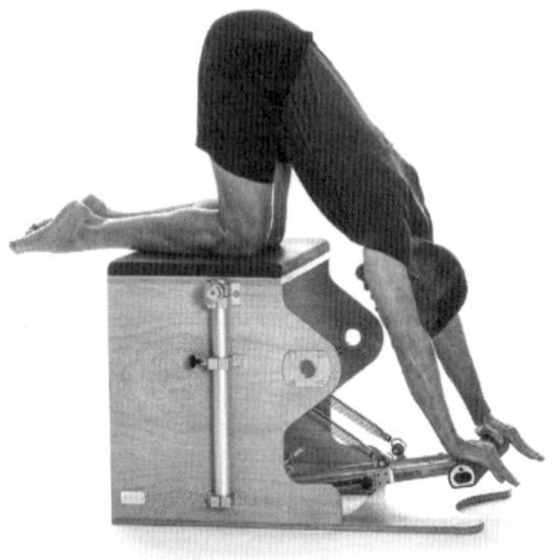

Inhale. Roll down, pressing the pedal toward the floor, extending the spine, and keeping the head between the arms.

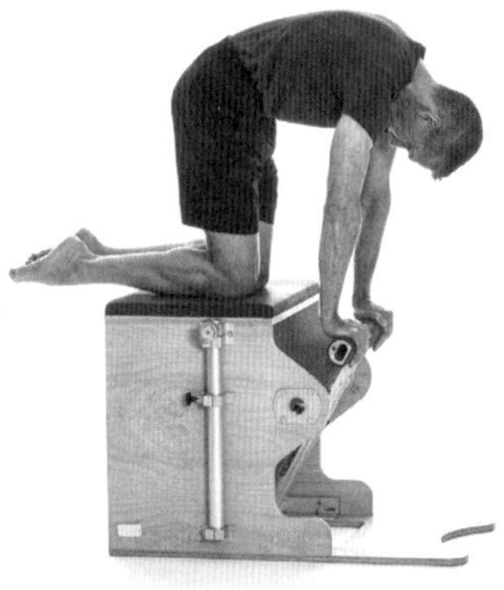

Exhale. Roll up, rounding the trunk into deep spinal flexion until the shoulders and hips are aligned horizontally. Keep the hips above the knees when raising the pedal (or as close as possible). Repeat 5-10 times.

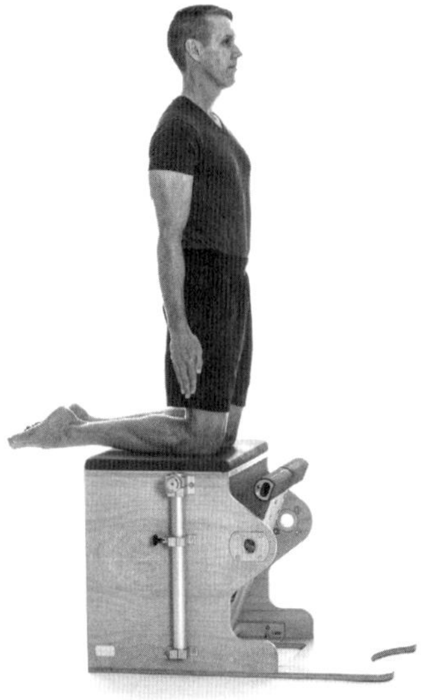

After the final exhale, roll up all the way to an upright kneeling position. Return to the start position.

Torso Press Sit

With the legs stable and parallel to the floor and the trunk acting as one solid, integrated unit, the movement in this exercise occurs at the hip and shoulder joints. Control of the hip flexors is important, but the focus should be on the abdominals and back extensors working in co-contraction to keep the trunk stable. This exercise demands a high level of precision and coordination. It serves as a good preparation for advanced abdominal exercises, such as the many versions of the teaser; however, rather than articulating the spine when lowering and lifting the trunk, the focus in the Wunda Chair: Torso Press Sit is a hinging action, keeping the spine stable. Because of the arm position, this exercise offers a significant stretch for the shoulders and the chest, which many people will benefit from.

Imagery

I liken this position to a drawbridge: Initially lying flat, then hinging in the center, one segment lifts as a solid unit (the trunk), with the remainder of the bridge (the legs) remaining still.

- ○ Keep the legs stable and parallel to the floor.
- ○ Maintain co-contraction of the abdominals and back extensors.
- ○ Align the head with the spine.
- ○ Maintain shoulder stability, with the shoulders externally rotated and fingers facing away from the body.

MODIFICATION

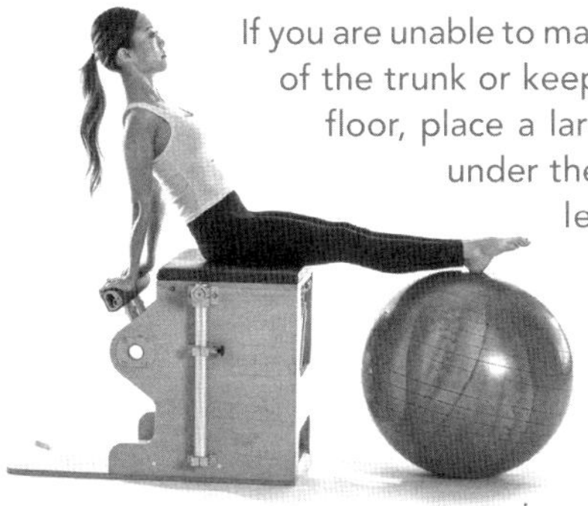

If you are unable to maintain the stable position of the trunk or keep the legs parallel to the floor, place a large ball or reformer box under the feet. This supports the legs and decreases the load on the hip flexors, making it easier for the abdominals and back extensors to maintain trunk alignment.

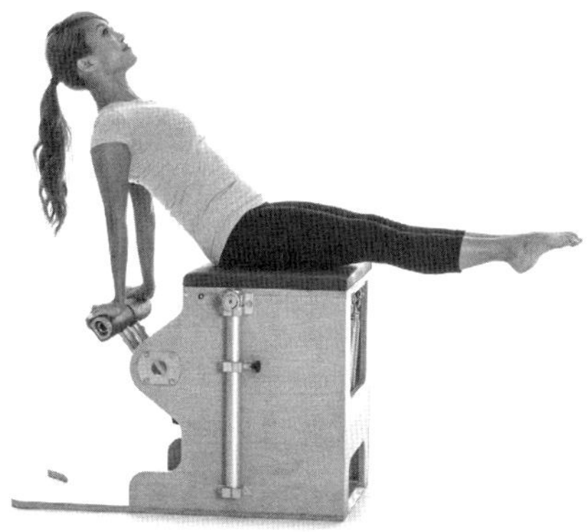

Setup. Sit on the platform facing the back of the chair. Place the hands on the pedal with the fingers facing backward and the shoulders aligned over the wrists. Hold the legs directly forward, parallel to the floor, with the trunk in a neutral spine position on a diagonal line.

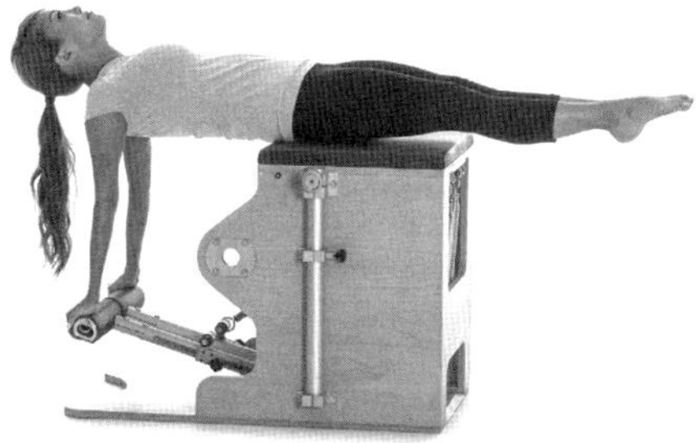

Inhale. Lower the trunk to a flat, supine position parallel to the floor, pressing the pedal down.

Exhale. Lift the trunk, raising the pedal. Return to the start position. Repeat 5-10 times.

Muscle Focus

- Abdominals
- Back extensors
- Hip flexors

Objectives

- To improve abdominal and back extensor strength
- To improve hip flexor control
- To improve shoulder and thoracic flexibility

RESISTANCE

Light — Medium — Heavy

Triceps—Seated

Muscle Focus

- Triceps
- Shoulder flexors
- Abdominals
- Back extensors

Objectives

- To improve elbow extensor and shoulder flexor strength
- To develop trunk and scapular stabilization

RESISTANCE
Light Medium Heavy

This exercise teaches the fundamentals of what are commonly called *dips*. I cannot overemphasize the importance of good trunk alignment and stability, in addition to excellent scapular stabilization. The movement is a combination of shoulder flexion, highlighting the long head of the biceps and the anterior deltoid, along with elbow extension, with a focus on the triceps.

I like to lead into this exercise with shoulder shrugs, allowing the shoulders to lift toward the ears and then pressing them down to engage the scapular depressors, particularly the lower trapezius. This is done with arms straight. (Note that in terms of muscle action this is the opposite of a typical shrug, in which the shoulders are actively lifted, engaging the upper trapezius. Here the shoulders are actively lowered with a focus on the lower trapezius.) Once trunk and scapular stabilization in a neutral position has been established, the triceps exercise can commence.

Imagery

Visualize lifting the body off the ground rather than merely straightening the arms. The involvement of the back extensors and the image of the scapulae gliding down the back are vital to the success of this movement.

- Keep the elbows parallel to each other and facing back.
- Maintain scapular stabilization.
- Maintain an upright and stable trunk.

PROGRESSION

As we know, one side of the body is often stronger than the other. For this reason, I recommend working each side independently whenever possible. When the arms are bent, *cautiously* remove one hand from the pedal and place the arm by your side or behind your head. Straighten and bend the working arm. After 10 repetitions, switch to the other side—again, being extremely cautious when changing.

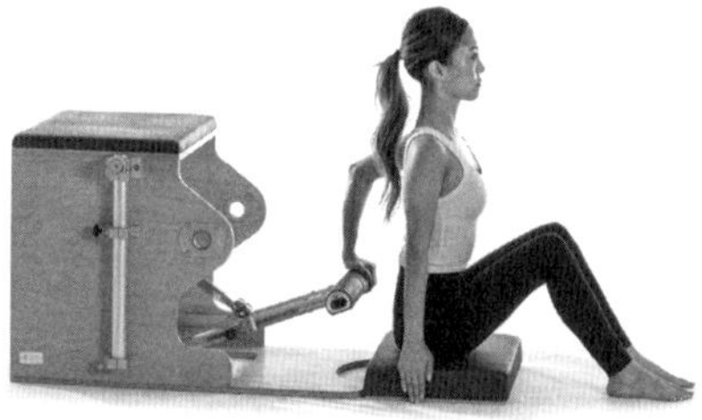

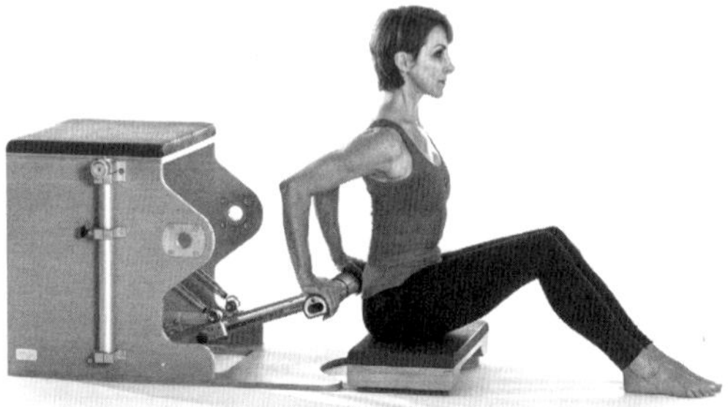

Setup. Sit upright on a box approximately 6-12 inches (15-30 centimeters) high, facing away from the front of the chair. Legs should be parallel, knees bent, and feet placed firmly on the floor hip width apart. Place the hands on the pedal with the fingers facing the body, the elbows bent and facing back.

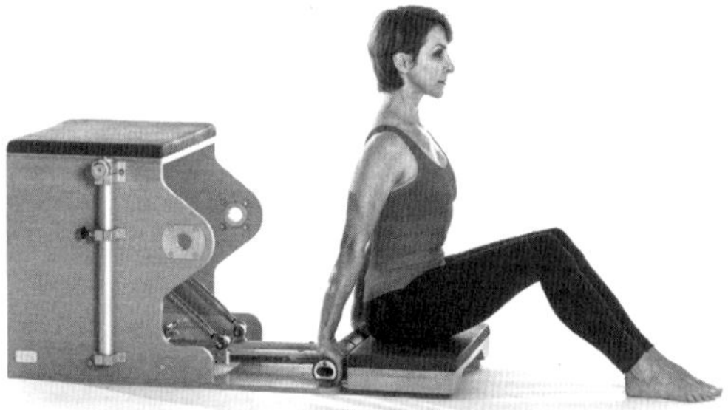

Exhale. Straighten the elbows, pushing the pedal down.

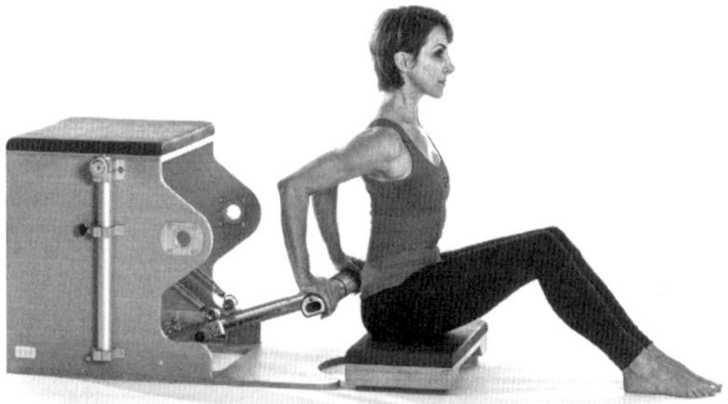

Inhale. Bend the elbows, raising the pedal. Return to the start position. Repeat 10 times.

Triceps—Prone

WUNDA CHAIR
Arm Work
INTERMEDIATE

Muscle Focus
- Triceps
- Back extensors

Objectives
- To improve elbow extensor strength
- To develop trunk and scapular stabilization

RESISTANCE
Light — Medium — Heavy

This exercise resembles the classic push-up with relatively low load (certainly less than the weight of the body) and can teach correct and precise technique. Two areas should be highlighted: The first is the lumbopelvic region, which is partially supported by the platform of the chair and is therefore less likely to collapse. The other is the scapulae, which tend to adduct and elevate. The trunk and scapulae must remain stable in a neutral position so that the movement occurs in the arms alone.

I recommend initially doing this exercise with the arms parallel and bringing the elbows close to the sides of the body when raising the pedal. This is equivalent to a triceps-driven push-up.

Imagery

Although it is the pedal that is being lowered and lifted, the sense should be that the entire body is being lowered and lifted as one integrated and stable unit.

- ○ Keep the body stable and parallel to the floor.
- ○ Maintain scapular stabilization.
- ○ Keep the elbows close to the sides of the body and traveling directly back when bending.

VARIATION

The exercise can also be performed with the elbows reaching out to the sides and fingers facing inward, in which case it more closely resembles a pectorals-driven push-up.

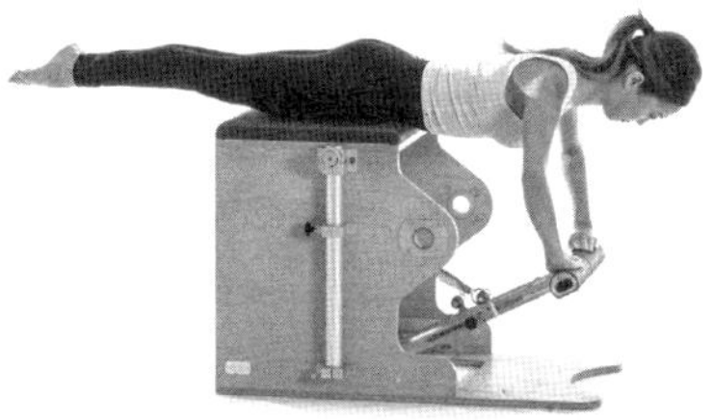

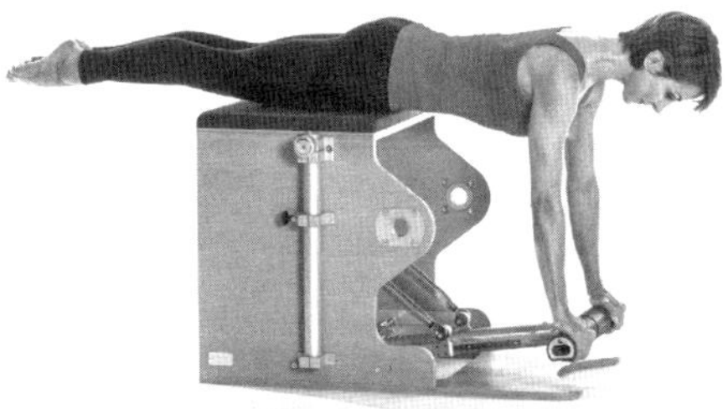

Setup. Lie prone on the chair, with the entire body parallel to the floor, legs straight and together, feet plantarflexed, and hands on the pedal with fingers facing forward. Align the wrists directly under the shoulders and straighten the arms.

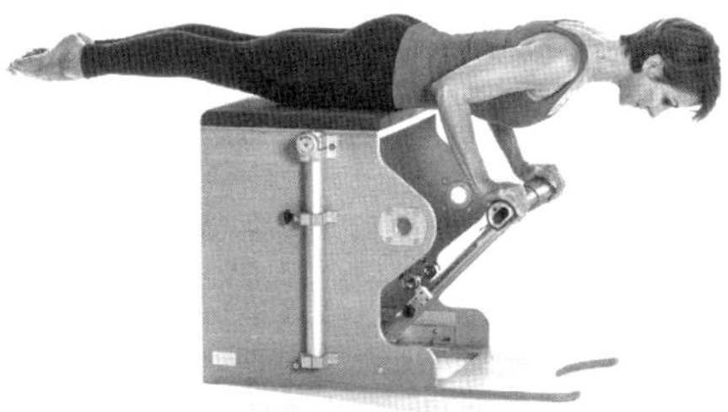

Inhale. Bend the elbows, bringing them to the sides of the body and raising the pedal.

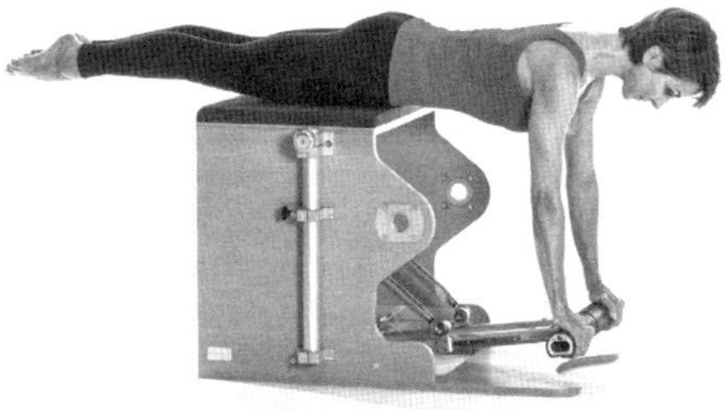

Exhale. Straighten the elbows, pressing the pedal down. Return to the start position. Repeat 10 times.

Dip—Back

Muscle Focus

- Triceps
- Shoulder flexors
- Abdominals
- Back extensors

Objectives

- To improve elbow extensor and shoulder flexor strength
- To improve back extensor control
- To develop trunk and scapular stabilization

RESISTANCE

Light — Medium — Heavy

The similarity of the Wunda Chair: Dip—Back to the dip commonly seen in a gym ends with the name. The placement of the body amplifies the intensity of the exercise, requiring tremendous strength as well as body control, awareness, and muscle integration. As in the Wunda Chair: Triceps—Seated (an excellent preparation for this exercise), the movement combines shoulder flexion with elbow extension. Scapular stabilization should precede the actual movement to counter scapular elevation, which commonly occurs. As always, good trunk alignment and stability are essential.

The body must maintain vertical alignment and be in line with the pedal, holding true to the plumb line (or as close as possible—due to varying body types and chair designs, absolute vertical alignment may not be possible). The most common tendency when executing this exercise is to lean back, bring the shoulders over the handles, and rely almost entirely on the triceps, which sacrifices some of the key benefits of the exercise. Height of the handles should ideally be set so that the upper arms are parallel to the floor (elbows at approximately a 90-degree angle) when starting—however, this will depend on the flexibility of the shoulders. Some wunda chairs do not have side handles, in which case this particular exercise is not possible.

Imagery

This exercise should feel effortless, as if the body is levitating. It should feel as if the force is being generated from under the pedal, as opposed to the arms.

- ○ Keep the elbows facing back and parallel to each other (or as close as possible).
- ○ Maintain scapular stabilization.
- ○ Maintain an upright, stable trunk.

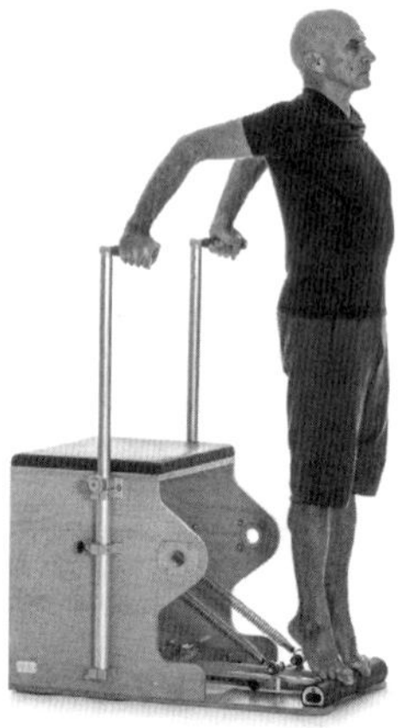

Setup. Stand upright on the pedal, facing away from the chair, and place the hands on the handles with the elbows reaching back.

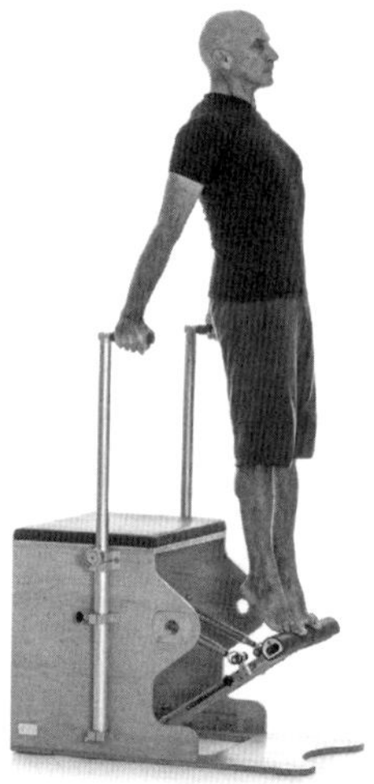

Exhale. Flex the shoulders and straighten the arms completely, pushing down into the handles and elevating the body and the pedal.

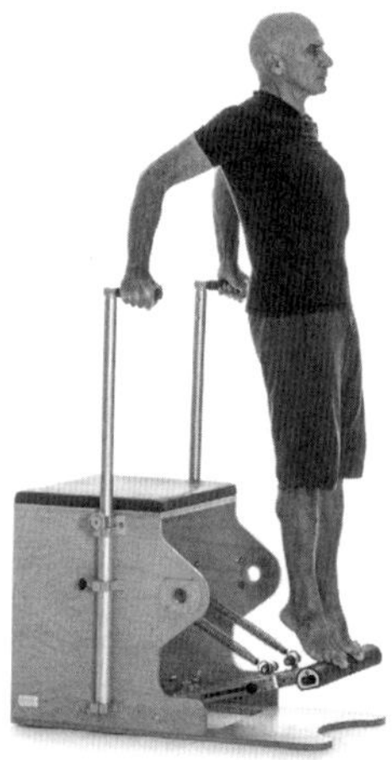

Inhale. Bend the arms, lowering the body and the pedal (not touching the floor). Repeat 5 times. On the final repetition, lower all the way. Return to the start position.

Hamstring Curl

WUNDA CHAIR

Leg Work

FUNDAMENTAL

Muscle Focus

- Hamstrings
- Abdominals
- Back extensors

Objectives

- To improve knee flexor strength
- To develop lumbopelvic stabilization

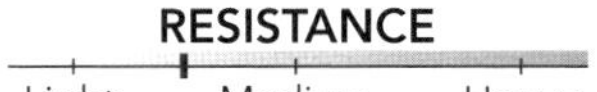

The Wunda Chair: Hamstring Curl is very focused and effective, with the body in a stable and comfortable position. The back is not in danger of being pulled into hyperextension, as is the case with some other hamstring curl exercises performed in a prone position. Another advantage is the ability to perform this hamstring curl with each leg independently—a particular benefit when a significant imbalance is present.

The range of motion of this curl is somewhat limited on most wunda chairs: from approximately 120 degrees at the knee joint to 70 degrees of knee flexion. However, on the BASI Systems wunda chair, the range is relatively large, with the resistance starting at 180 degrees (knees straight) to 70 degrees of knee flexion. (Only the top part of the pedal's arc, which entails pure knee flexion, is used in this exercise—the bottom part requires hip extension together with knee flexion, which is not the objective of this exercise.)

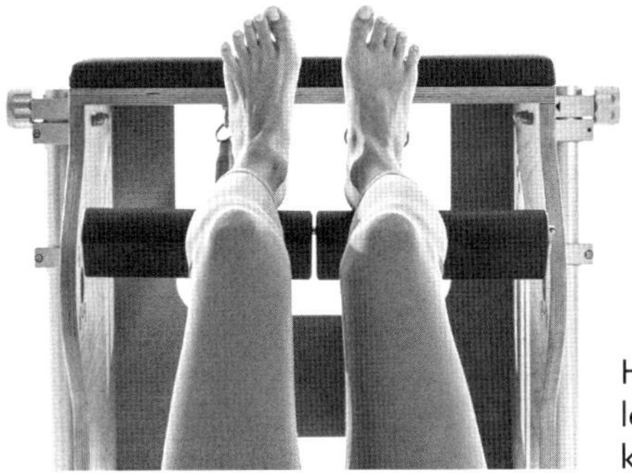

Heels on the pedal, legs parallel, and knees bent.

Imagery

When pulling the heels toward the sit bones, visualize a rubber band connecting each heel to the opposite sit bone to ensure the precise direction of pull. When you have maximized the knee flexion (before starting to extend the hips), straighten the knees and lift the pedal slowly, resisting the pull of the imaginary rubber band as you return to the start position. Never fully release the tension. The feet should feel like there is a floor beneath them, remaining stable throughout.

- ○ Maintain a neutral pelvis.
- ○ Isolate the knee flexion.
- ○ Keep the feet stable.

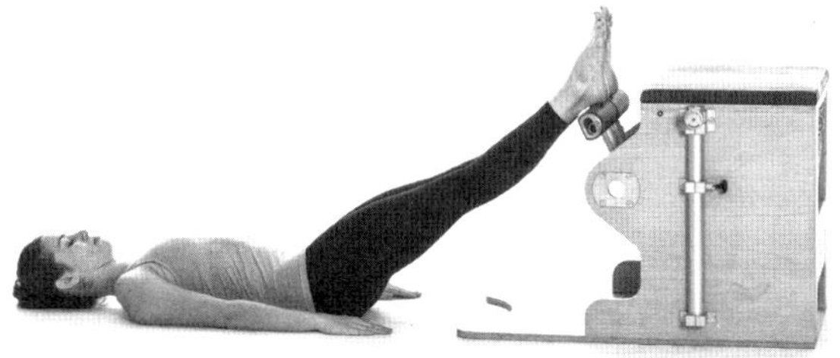

Setup. Lie supine on the floor. Place the heels on the pedal hip width apart, legs parallel and straight (on some chairs the knees will start at approximately 120 degrees of flexion), feet in a neutral position. Place the arms by the sides of the body, straight and palms facing down.

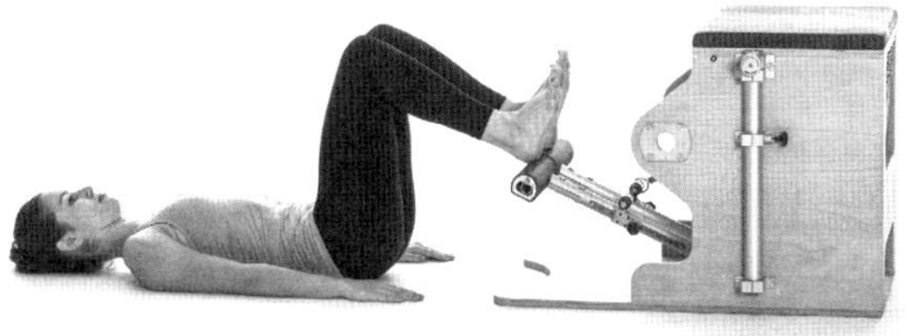

Exhale. Bend the knees, lowering the pedal halfway down. (The feet will be in maximum dorsiflexion when the knees are bent and then they maintain the same angle relative to the pedal when the knees straighten.)

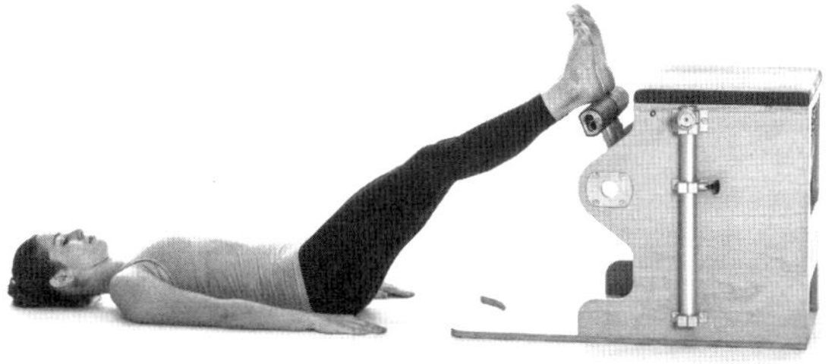

Inhale. Straighten the knees, lifting the pedal. Return to the start position. Repeat 10 times.

Leg Press—Standing

Muscle Focus

- Hamstrings
- Quadriceps
- Hip abductors

Objectives

- To improve hip extensor, knee extensor, and hip abductor control
- To develop lumbopelvic stabilization
- To develop alignment and balance

RESISTANCE

Light | Medium | Heavy

This exercise is important in teaching functional movement of the leg, improving alignment and balance, and perfecting muscle recruitment patterns pertaining to knee and hip extension. The combination of a stable standing leg and keeping the pelvis and trunk in optimum neutral alignment facilitates disassociation of the leg from the rest of the body. The moving leg presses down without disturbing the alignment of the body. Maintaining stability and balance in this exercise highlights the meaning and value of functional movement.

The alignment of the body is key to activating the correct muscles and ensuring a successful outcome. In order to challenge the hip extensors, the standing leg must be sufficiently far back from the chair and the initiation must occur in the hip extensors. Avoid the tendency to stand too close to the chair and lean forward; this transforms the movement, placing the focus on the quadriceps, and eliminates much of the challenge.

Imagery

Visualize climbing a vertical staircase while keeping the body perfectly upright. Another visual that helps is dragging the foot backward like a dog digging in the sand, or an agitated horse digging its hooves in the dirt.

- ○ Initiate the movement with the hamstrings.
- ○ Maintain plantarflexion with the pressing foot.
- ○ Maintain upright posture; avoid leaning forward.

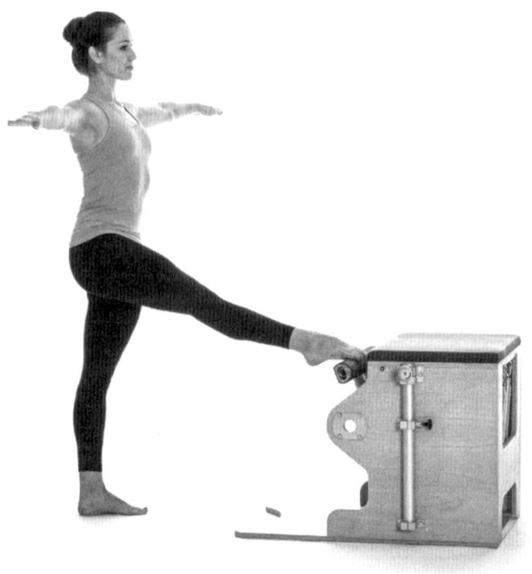

Setup. Stand upright, placing one foot on the pedal in a plantarflexed position with the leg straight and the pedal in its top position. Hold the arms out to the sides in a T position.

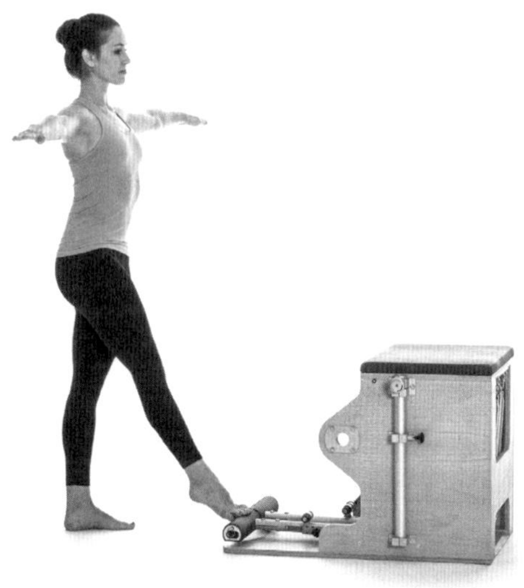

Exhale. Bend the knee and extend the hip. Continue extending the hip and straighten the knee, pressing the pedal down.

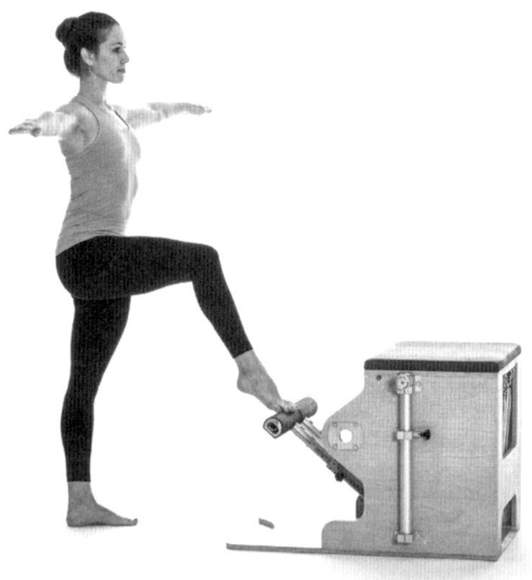

Inhale. Bend the knee and flex the hip. Continue flexing the hip followed by straightening the knee, controlling the pedal as it lifts. Return to the start position. Repeat 5-10 times on the same leg before switching to the other side.

Forward Lunge

The forward lunge is another favorite of mine. I have helped many athletes improve their running, leaping, jumping, and overall performance with this exercise. It is a great equalizer—no matter how strong the legs are, the exercise will not be successful without good body awareness, correct muscle activation patterns, lumbopelvic stabilization, good balance, full body integration, and an optimal strength ratio between the hip extensors, hip abductors, and knee extensors.

Sequencing the muscle activation is key, starting with the hip extensors as the body moves upward and the pedal rises, followed by the hip abductors (particularly the gluteus medius) as the back foot begins to lift off the pedal, and finally the knee extensors as the knee straightens completely. It is of paramount importance to maintain ideal vertical alignment. The tendency to lean forward, using the strength of the quadriceps from the outset, should be avoided. There are many possible modifications, variations, and progressions for select populations and specific activities; however, the basic movement should first be mastered.

Imagery

This exercise is all about feeling as if you are levitating. There should be a sensation of rising from the start position, as if a force under the pedal is propelling you upward or a string from the sky is lifting you up.

- ○ Activate the muscles sequentially: hip extensors, hip abductors, then knee extensors.
- ○ Maintain a stable, neutral pelvis (particularly challenging as the foot lifts off the pedal).
- ○ Move on a vertical line, avoiding leaning forward.

Muscle Focus

- Hamstrings
- Hip abductors
- Quadriceps

Objectives

- To improve hip extensor, hip abductor, and knee extensor strength
- To develop lumbopelvic stabilization
- To develop alignment and balance

RESISTANCE

Light — Medium — Heavy

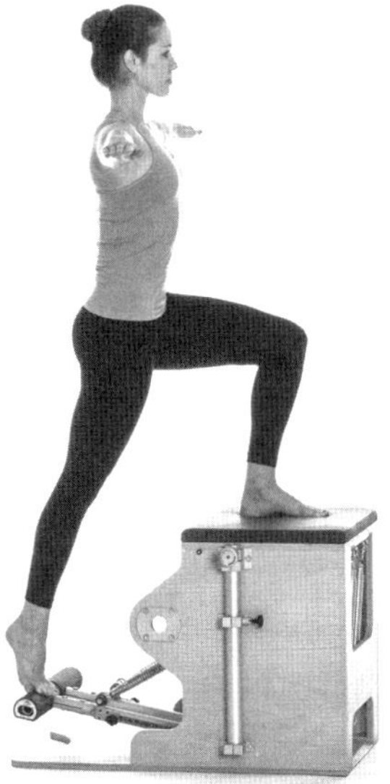

Setup. Stand facing the chair, holding the sides of the platform for support. Place one foot on the pedal, plantarflexed, and press the pedal down. Step onto the platform with the other foot and place it in the middle of the platform. Make sure the knee is at approximately a 90-degree angle, with the thigh parallel to the floor (this may require that shorter people place a pad or a small block under the pedal). Align the knee above the ankle. Stand upright with the hip joints over the pedal and holding true to the plumb line (or as close as possible—due to varying body types and chair designs, it may not be possible to align the hips over the pedal). Place the hands behind the head or out to the sides in a T position.

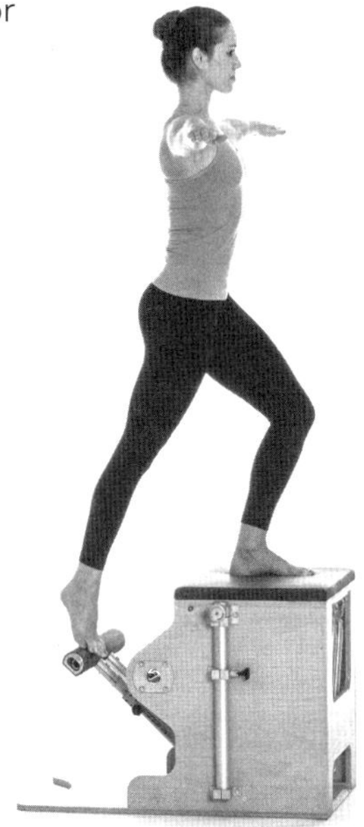

Exhale. Extend the hip, pressing down onto the platform of the chair, and begin to straighten the leg as the pedal rises.

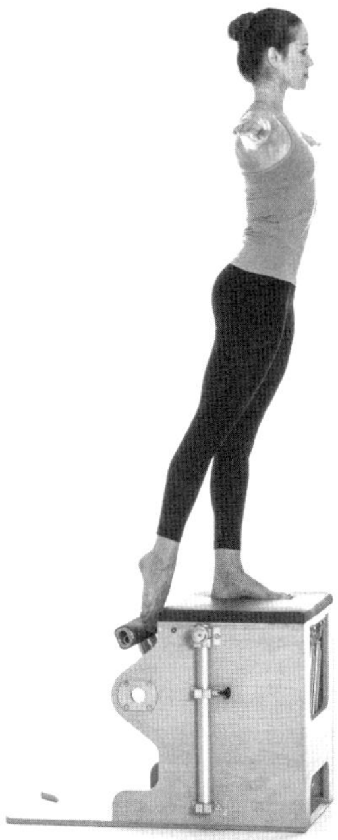

Continuing to exhale, straighten the leg and lift the back foot off the pedal, completing the knee extension.

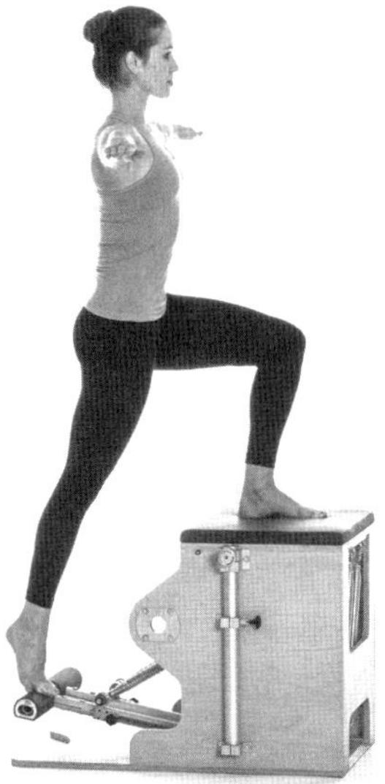

Inhale. Bend the knee, place the foot back on the pedal, and lower the pedal down to the start position. Repeat 5 times on the same leg before switching to the other side.

FUNDAMENTAL

Muscle Focus

- Abdominal obliques

Objectives

- To improve lateral flexor control
- To improve lateral flexor flexibility

RESISTANCE

Light Medium Heavy

Side Over

This is an excellent exercise for teaching precise lateral flexion and correct alignment, thereby laying a foundation to perform this movement in more challenging positions on other pieces of apparatus. The exercise can also be made more or less challenging by incrementally adjusting the spring tension (lighter is more difficult and heavier is less difficult). From a teacher's perspective, the student's body is in an ideal position for cueing and offering input and corrections.

Imagery

Imagine the movement as two-dimensional, occurring between two panes of glass.

- Lift no higher than the diagonal line created by the straight leg and trunk.
- Keep the legs and pelvis stable, with the big toe of the straight leg anchored on the floor (add a block if the toe doesn't reach the floor).
- Move from the waist area.

PROGRESSION

To increase both the intensity and the stretch of the lateral muscles of the trunk and underarm, reach the top arm overhead, with the shoulder internally rotated and the palm facing up toward the ceiling.

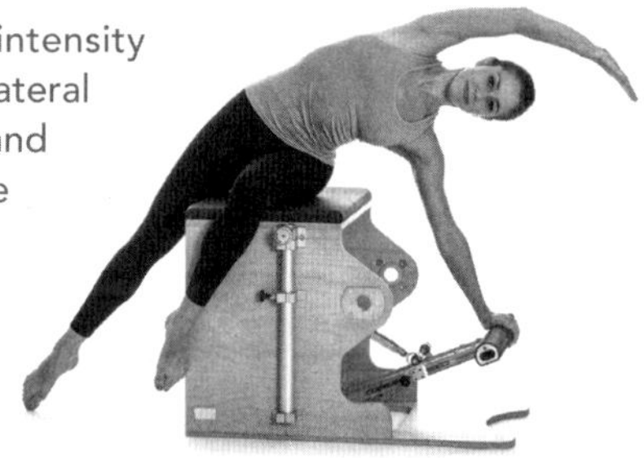

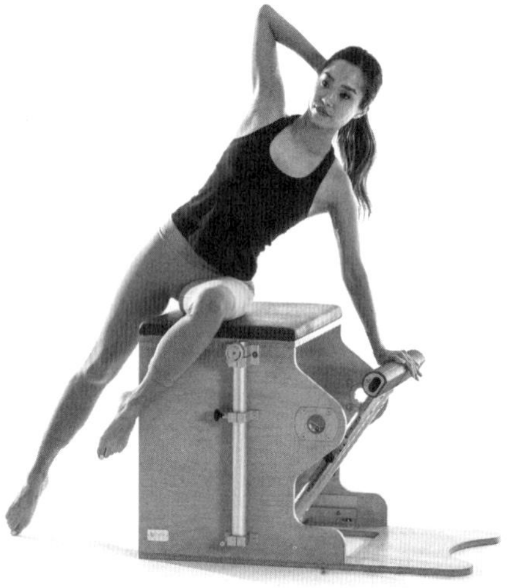

Setup. Sit sideways on the chair, hooking the lower leg on the side of the chair and keeping the other leg straight and in line with the body. Establish a long diagonal line with the trunk, leg, and foot, with the foot touching the floor. Place the lower hand on the pedal and the other hand behind the head.

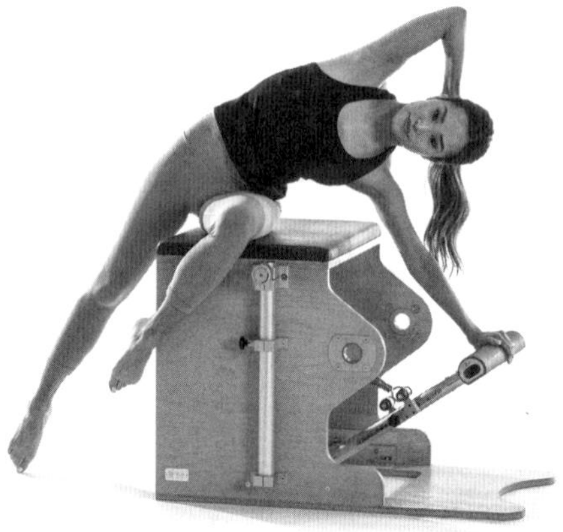

Inhale. Laterally extend the trunk, lowering the pedal.

Exhale. Laterally flex the trunk, lifting the pedal. Return to the start position. Repeat 5-10 times before switching to the other side.

Swan

As with the Wunda Chair: Side Over, this exercise can be made easier or more challenging by incrementally adjusting the spring tension (lighter is more difficult and heavier is less difficult). This adjustability is invaluable when dealing with back problems: The springs can move the body through a predetermined range of motion, using almost-passive movement as neuromuscular patterns are reeducated, and then the muscles can be progressively challenged as improvement takes place.

This exercise is also valuable for teaching the skill of load distribution through the spine when executing back extension exercises. Often, there is a tendency to draw the trunk into flexion as soon as the abdominals are activated. As a result, when the trunk is then lifted, the majority of the extension occurs in the lumbar spine, placing excessive load on this region. This is completely counterproductive to the effect we are striving for. Correct abdominal activation should provide support for the spine and, together with the back extensors, assist in creating a long, evenly distributed arc through the trunk.

Imagery

Visualize a reverse articulation of the spine, starting with the head and moving down the spine, lifting the trunk into extension. This tends to distribute the work throughout the back and establishes a gentle arc shape, rather than excessive hyperextension in the lumbar region.

- ○ Maintain abdominal engagement.
- ○ Keep the legs parallel to the floor.
- ○ Press the hands into the pedal, extending the shoulders, as the body lifts.

MODIFICATION

To reduce the challenge, place the feet on a box or ball so that the body is still parallel to the floor, but the feet are supported. If this still proves too challenging, the feet can be placed on the floor with the knees bent and the thighs pressing against the back of the chair.

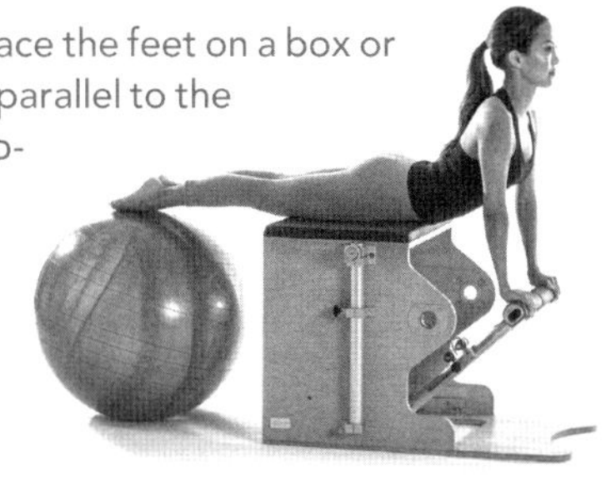

Muscle Focus

- Back extensors

Objectives

- To improve back extensor strength
- To improve abdominal control
- To develop scapular stabilization

RESISTANCE

Light — Medium — Heavy

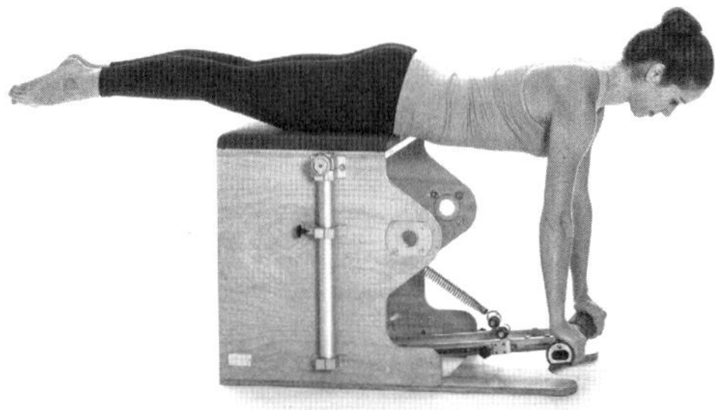

Setup. Lie prone on the chair, parallel to the floor, with the legs straight and together. Place the hands on the pedal, aligning the wrists directly under the shoulders (or as close as possible), and straighten the arms. The pedal may not be all the way down on the base of the chair; this will depend on the length of the arms.

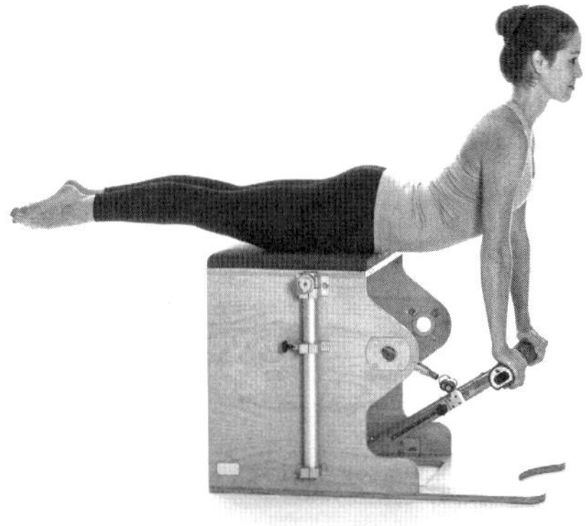

Inhale. Extend the back, lifting the pedal.

Exhale. Lower the back and pedal. Return to the start position. Repeat 5-10 times.

8

Barrels

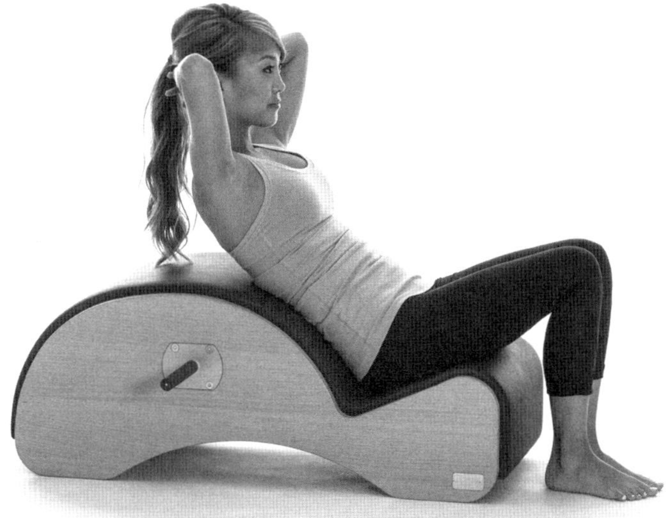

The barrels are as unique in their offerings as they are in appearance, providing exceptional opportunities for both active and passive back extension at all ability levels. But they are not limited to back extension—like the entire lineup of Pilates apparatus, the barrels have endless potential to work the body in every range of motion.

There are two main categories of barrels: The ladder barrel (also known as the high barrel) stands several feet off the ground and is attached to a ladder of the same height. The step barrel (also known as the spine corrector) sits on the floor.

Lighter and more portable versions of the step barrel, such as the half-barrel (also known as the arc), are available. There are many applications for the half-barrel, including using it in conjunction with other apparatus, such as the cadillac or reformer. This opens up a world of opportunity for creative and varied repertoire.

The step barrel I prefer using is called the F2 spine corrector. In addition to the modifications that have been made to the shape of the barrel itself to accommodate a wider range of body types than the original, it offers the option of using an adjustable handle in order to more easily adapt exercises to different body types. The handles also double as a highly adjustable resistance mechanism, which facilitates new and unique repertoire while expanding the scope of the existing repertoire. This chapter includes instructions for exercises on the traditional step barrel and, where appropriate, instructions for F2 spine corrector variations.

As I have emphasized throughout this book, spinal extension is crucial to developing back strength and good posture. The barrels are exceptional tools for strengthening the back extensors and for passively relaxing in a position of spinal extension, thereby stretching the trunk flexors. When doing forward flexion abdominal exercises on the step barrel, the barrel supports the lower back in a neutral position; this is very important in conditions where flexion of the lumbar spine is contraindicated. The barrels also support the trunk during lateral flexion exercises at all levels, facilitating improvement of both strength and flexibility. Unique hip and arm work, full body integration exercises, and stretches can be performed on the barrels, many of which cannot be easily duplicated on other apparatus.

The traditional barrels utilize gravity for resistance, an important consideration when making exercises less or more difficult. I often add ankle or hand weights to the work on the barrels to increase the challenge when developing strength or to facilitate a deeper stretch when doing flexibility exercises. The F2 System integrates springs to facilitate resistance while doing the exercises on the barrels.

I highly recommend ending a session by spending a few minutes in relaxation, lying supine over the step barrel, with the option of a cushion supporting the head if need be. It will leave you stretched out, with a delightful open feeling.

The ladder barrel used for the purposes of demonstration in this book is called the F2 chair. A unique apparatus that I designed over many years, it is essentially a combination of a ladder barrel and an arm chair that facilitates all the original exercises performed on both individual pieces, plus many more. For the purposes of the ladder barrel exercises in this book, there is no difference between the F2 chair and the ladder barrel. The F2 chair will be used for the arm chair exercises presented in chapter 10.

The order in which the following exercises are presented is not necessarily the sequence in which they would be taught or performed. Typically, we would not do an entire session on the barrels (although this is becoming more common with the addition of springs), but would rather include exercises from the rich and diverse repertoire performed on the barrels to fulfill various blocks in a comprehensive session.

Students often wonder whether they should learn the ladder barrel before the step barrel or vice versa. In my opinion, either is fine; both have much to offer at every level of the work.

Hamstring Stretch

This is a comfortable and relatively easy way to stretch the hamstrings. Although this exercise can be performed on a variety of apparatus (as can the Ladder Barrel: Gluteal Stretch), the ladder barrel helps keep the body in optimal alignment to achieve an effective stretch of the hamstrings.

Muscle Focus

- Hamstrings

Objective

- To improve hamstring flexibility

Imagery

Visualize the body functioning like a hinge, with the trunk and pelvis being the top part of the hinge and the lower limb the bottom part. The hip joint is where the actual hinging takes place. The standing leg maintains contact with the ladder and remains stable throughout. The other leg is placed on the barrel and is also part of the stable structure. The upper section of the hinge (trunk and pelvis) moves as one piece, closing over the stretching leg and then opening up again.

- Keep the back extensors engaged and the pelvis tilted in an anterior direction during the stretch.
- Dorsiflex the foot of the leg being stretched to intensify the stretch.
- Maintain contact between the ladder and the back of the standing leg and pelvis.
- Use the arms to support and intensify the stretch.

PROGRESSION

In order to intensify the stretch further, bring the arms around and place them on the barrel on each side of the leg, palms facing down. Press the arms down to help extend the back and lower the trunk closer to the leg.

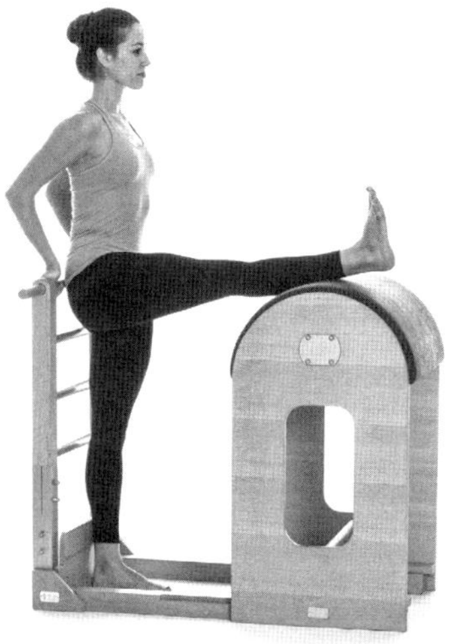

Setup. Stand on one leg facing the barrel, with the leg straight and the back of the leg and pelvis positioned against the ladder. Place the other leg on top of the barrel, keeping it as straight as possible (without hyperextending the knee). Hold the ladder with the hands, arms parallel, elbows facing backward, scapulae stable, and the chest open.

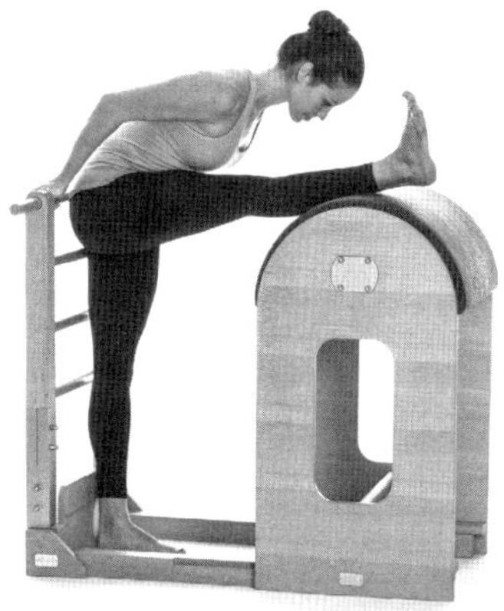

Exhale. Lean forward over the stretching leg, keeping the back as flat as possible. Straighten the arms, pressing them against the ladder while reaching the trunk further over the stretching leg. Dorsiflex the foot to intensify the stretch. Hold this position for 3-5 breath cycles.

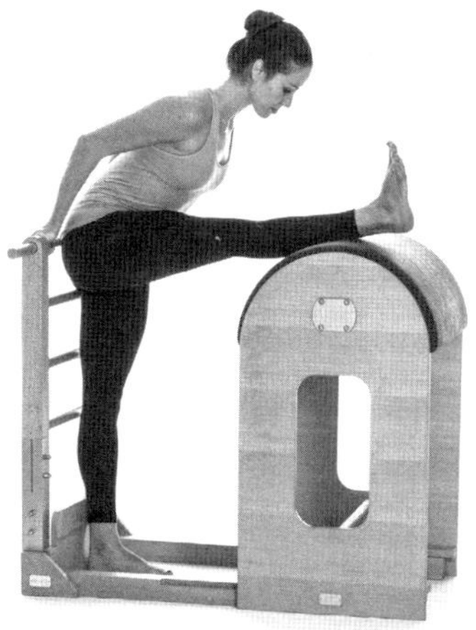

Inhale. Lift the trunk. Return to the start position. Repeat the cycle 1-2 times before switching to the other side.

Gluteal Stretch

Muscle Focus

- Gluteals

Objective

- To improve gluteal flexibility

The gluteals tend to get very tight and are often imbalanced, with the gluteus medius tending to be weak and the gluteus maximus strong. Any imbalances should be addressed in a comprehensive program. Besides strength, a good stretch is often needed, and the ladder barrel, which places the body in excellent alignment to maximize the stretch, is a comfortable location to perform it. Note that this position potentially places stress on the knee of the stretching leg, particularly when the hip joint is tight. Move into the position with caution, and do not exceed your own limits. This stretch can be very intense, so remember to breathe!

Imagery

As with all stretches, focus on the stability of the areas above and below the region that is to be stretched, and then visualize the stretched region becoming soft like rubber and elongating with each breath.

- ○ Keep the back extensors engaged and the pelvis tilted in an anterior direction during the stretch.
- ○ Bring the barrel closer to intensify the stretch.
- ○ Use the arms to support and intensify the stretch.

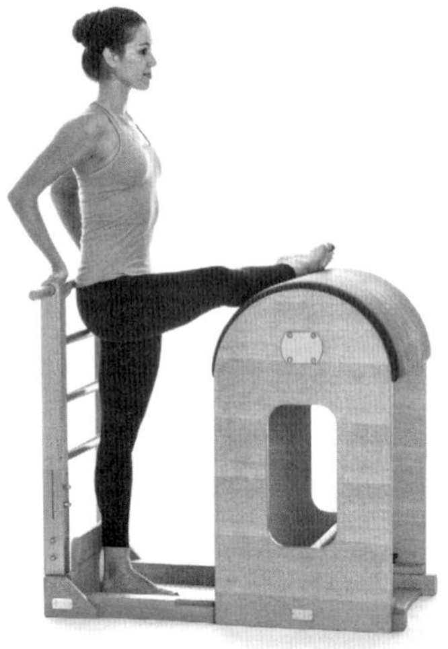

Setup. Stand on one leg facing the barrel, with the leg straight and the back of the leg and pelvis positioned against the ladder. Place the lateral aspect of the other leg on the barrel, bend the knee, and externally rotate the hip. Hold the ladder with the hands, arms parallel, elbows facing backward, scapulae stable, and the chest open.

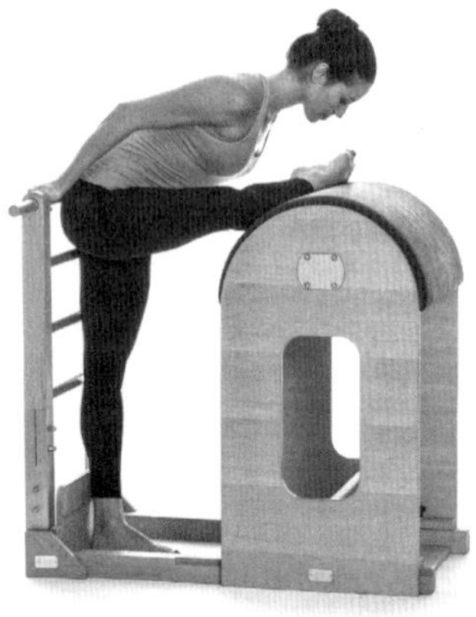

Exhale. Lean forward over the stretching leg and keep the back as flat as possible. Straighten the arms, pushing against the ladder while reaching the trunk further over the leg to intensify the stretch. Hold the position for 3-5 breath cycles.

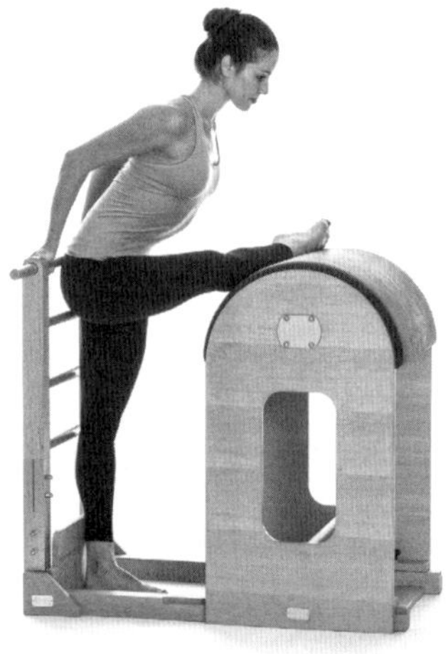

Inhale. Lift the trunk. Return to the start position. Repeat the cycle 1-2 times before switching to the other side.

Adductor Stretch

This stretch is similar to a ballet stretch at the barre. It is most effective when you turn out (externally rotate) the hip of the stretching leg, a position familiar to dancers. The rotation of the hip joint helps keep the pelvis level, so that it doesn't hike up on the stretching side. If this position is not familiar to you, take particular care to achieve correct alignment of the pelvis so that undue stress is not placed on the joints, particularly the hip and knee joints. This exercise also stretches the lateral flexors of the trunk and the shoulder adductors on the upper side of the trunk.

Imagery

I like to imagine the stretching leg and the trunk creating the two sides of a wishbone. The foot of the stretching leg and the hand of the stretching arm should reach as far as possible in the same direction, with the leg and arm almost parallel when in maximum stretch. Visualize the area between the pelvic crest and the lower ribs on the upper side of the trunk opening and expanding. At the same time, the region under the armpit of the stretching arm also opens, allowing the arm to reach further overhead. Breathing correctly is important in any stretch, but particularly so when stretching the muscles of the trunk. Visualize directing the breath into the upper lung, feeling the trunk expand and the ribs open in moderation and with control.

- Keep the pelvis level.
- Dorsiflex the foot of the stretching leg to intensify the stretch.
- Prevent the ribs from flaring excessively on the upper side of the trunk.
- Accentuate elongation of the trunk, particularly as it is initially lowered and then lifted in the final phase.

Muscle Focus

- Adductors
- Hamstrings
- Lateral flexors
- Shoulder adductors

Objective

- To improve hip adductor, lateral flexor, shoulder adductor, and hamstring flexibility

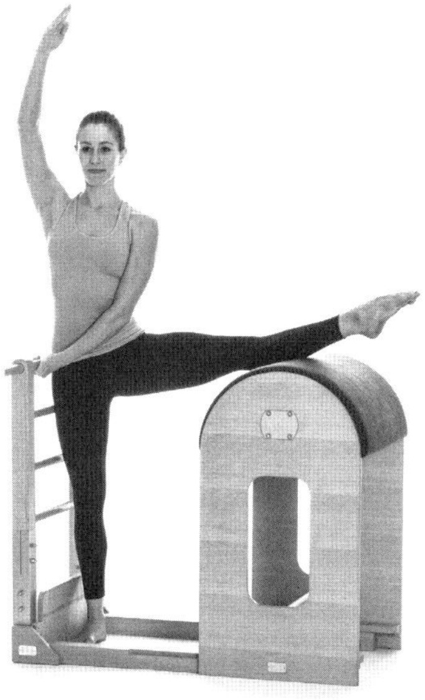

Setup. Stand on one leg with your side to the barrel and the lateral aspect of the leg and pelvis pressing against the ladder. The standing leg is straight and the hip parallel, and the arm on that side is lifted overhead. Place the stretching leg up on the barrel with the hip externally rotated, keeping the leg as straight as possible (without hyperextending the knee). The stretching leg will be forward of the pelvis; the angle of the leg to the body will depend on the flexibility of the hip joint. Place the other arm in front of the body and, using an underhand grip, hold on to one of the steps of the ladder (which one will depend on height and arm length).

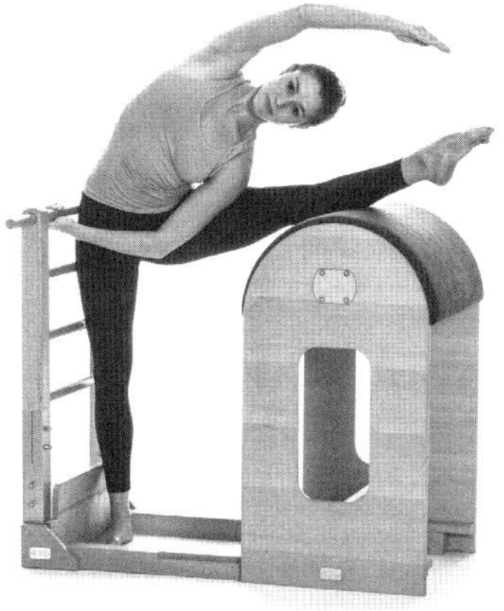

Exhale. Laterally flex the trunk over the stretching leg, reaching the overhead arm as far to the side as possible. Pull toward the ladder with the bottom arm. Hold this position for 3-5 breath cycles.

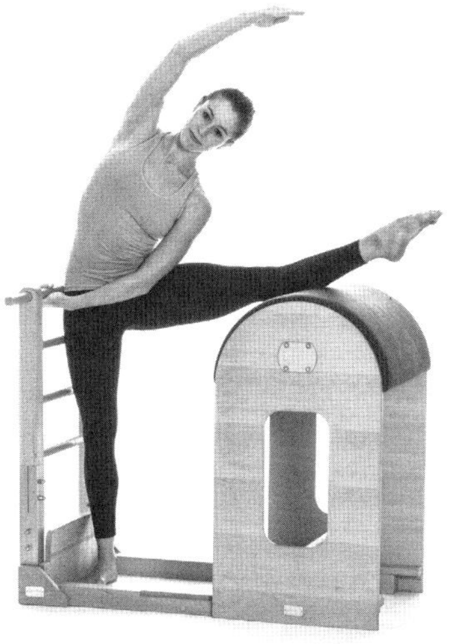

Inhale. Lift the trunk together with the overhead arm. Return to the start position. Repeat the cycle 1-2 times before switching to the other side.

Side Over

Muscle Focus

- Abdominal obliques
- Back extensors

Objectives

- To improve lateral flexor strength and flexibility
- To develop trunk stabilization

This exercise closely resembles the Reformer: Side Over and incorporates many of the same principles. An excellent preparation to both is the Wunda Chair: Side Over. However, performing the exercise on the ladder barrel offers two additional benefits: It requires more balance, which demands deep activation of the core muscles for stabilization, and the shape of the barrel supports the body in perfect lateral alignment, facilitating a wonderful stretch for the upper side.

Imagery

At the start of the exercise, a straight energy line runs through the length of the body, highlighting the elongated diagonal line. The next phase in the exercise, lateral flexion, is all about curve and elasticity—think of soft, cascading fabric as the body is draped over the barrel. Another helpful image is that of a young, flexible tree being bent over and then slowly released. A good visual to help maintain correct alignment of the trunk is to imagine the movement occurring in the coronal plane between two panes of glass.

- ○ Keep the elbows wide and the fingers loosely interlaced behind the head.
- ○ Engage the internal support system (ISS) prior to the movement to stabilize the trunk.
- ○ Keep the upper leg stable, pressing the heel into the rung of the ladder as if trying to straighten the leg.
- ○ Avoid pulling up with the foot that is hooked under the ladder.
- ○ Elongate the trunk, creating a large arc, as the body is lowered and lifted.

MODIFICATION

This modification is essentially the same exercise as the Ladder Barrel: Side Over, but the trunk has far more support and is more stable. In addition, the lever arm created by the trunk and its distance from the fulcrum is shorter, making the exercise less challenging in terms of load on the lateral flexors of the trunk. Create a more stable base by placing the feet on the lowest rung near the base of the ladder, or even on the floor in front of the base. Place the top leg behind the bottom leg, and establish the same straight diagonal line with the trunk. Lower the trunk over the barrel and then lift the trunk. This is an extremely effective exercise for all fitness levels.

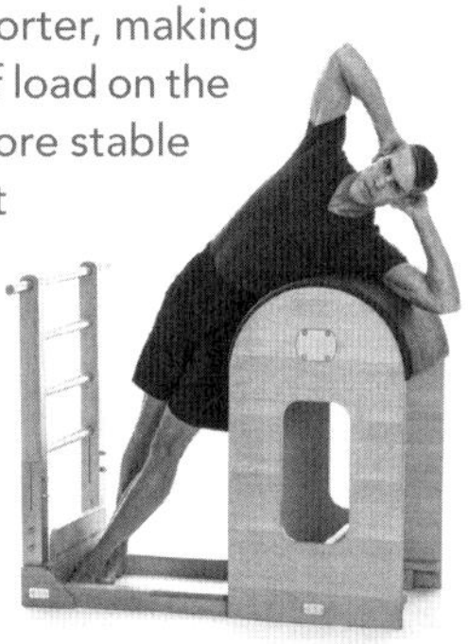

Setup. Rest one side of the pelvis on the barrel. Place the bottom foot on the first rung of the ladder, with the leg straight and the hip parallel. Externally rotate the upper hip, bend the knee, and press the heel onto the second rung, with the foot under the top rung (it should not actually touch the top rung). Establish a straight diagonal line from the lower foot through the entire body, and place the hands behind the head, fingers loosely interlaced.

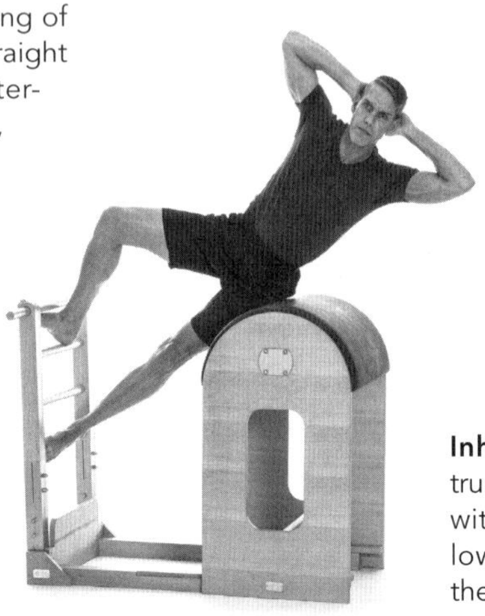

Inhale. Lower the trunk over the barrel with the head following the line of the spine.

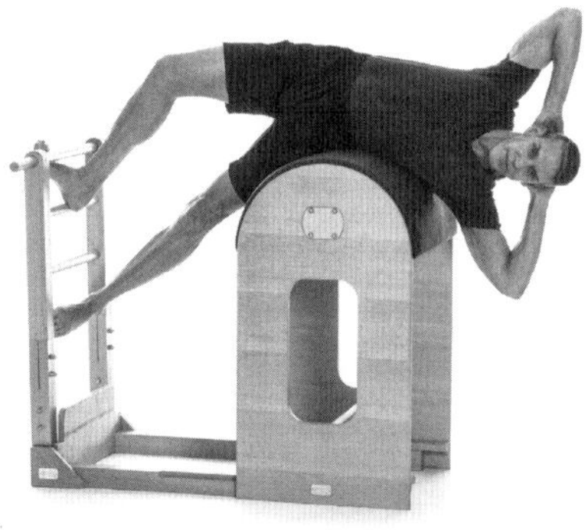

Exhale. Lift the trunk to the diagonal line. Return to the start position. Repeat 5-10 times before switching to the other side.

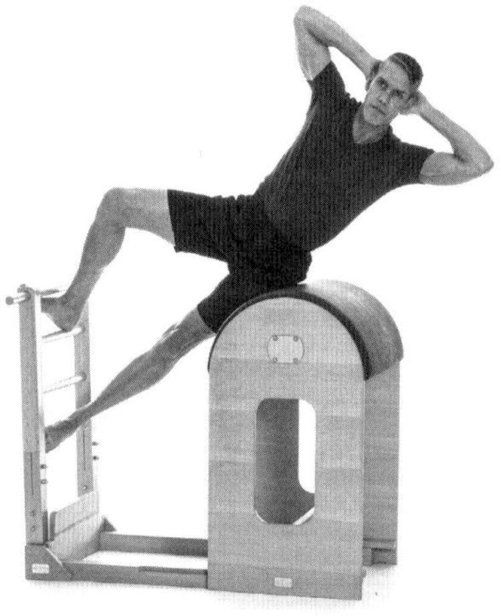

Back Extension

In all back extension exercises, it is vital to keep the abdominals engaged throughout the movement. This protects the back, facilitates correct muscle recruitment and body alignment, and distributes the load throughout the spine. When setting up the ladder barrel, be aware that the distance between the barrel and the ladder dictates where the work is focused and how much load is placed on the musculature. The closer the barrel is to the ladder, the greater the load on the back extensors—the fulcrum is lower in the body, the lever arm is longer, and the work is focused lower in the back. If the intention is to work the mid- or upper back, set the barrel farther from the ladder and place the feet lower down on the ladder.

Imagery

I encourage visualizing a reverse spinal articulation, beginning from the crown of the head, and then moving sequentially down through the spine, through the mid-back, and finally through the lumbar spine and sacrum. Emphasize elongation as opposed to height, reaching out from the top of the head.

- ○ Keep the abdominals engaged.
- ○ Bias toward a posterior tilt of the pelvis, pressing the pubic symphysis gently forward.
- ○ Align the head with the spine.
- ○ Create a straight diagonal line with the legs and the trunk when lifted in extension.

VARIATION

As an alternative, this exercise can be performed facing the opposite direction and utilizing springs for stability rather than the ladder. When using the ladder, the legs are on a stable, fixed base, which allows the legs to (potentially) do more of the work than desired, and compensations may appear. On the F2 chair the legs are supported by springs, which makes the stabilization dynamic. This challenges the balance and encourages trunk and lumbopelvic stabilization. The ISS will be recruited and the back extensors will work to their full potential. The exercise is felt deeply and intensely, not only in the back extensors but also the hip extensors. The breath and movement pattern remain the same as the original; however, the body position and the effect are clearly different.

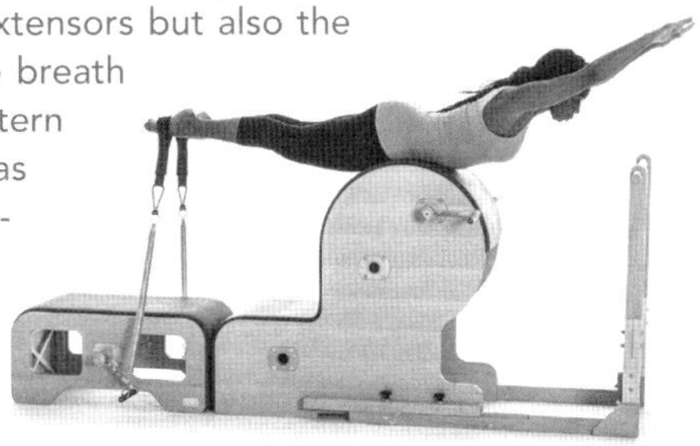

Muscle Focus

- Back extensors
- Abdominals

Objectives

- To improve back extensor strength
- To develop trunk stabilization

Setup. Lie prone, with the trunk draped over the barrel. Place the toes on the first rung of the ladder, with the feet in a V position. Anchor the heels under the second rung. Place the hands behind the head, fingers loosely interlaced.

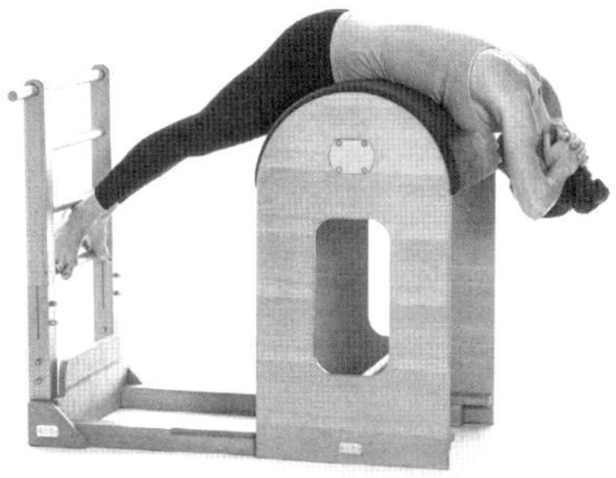

Inhale. Lift the trunk, extending the back.

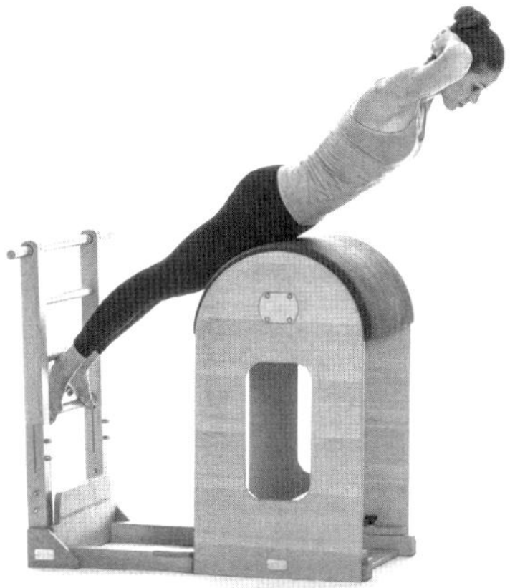

Exhale. Lower the trunk. Return to the start position. Repeat 5-10 times.

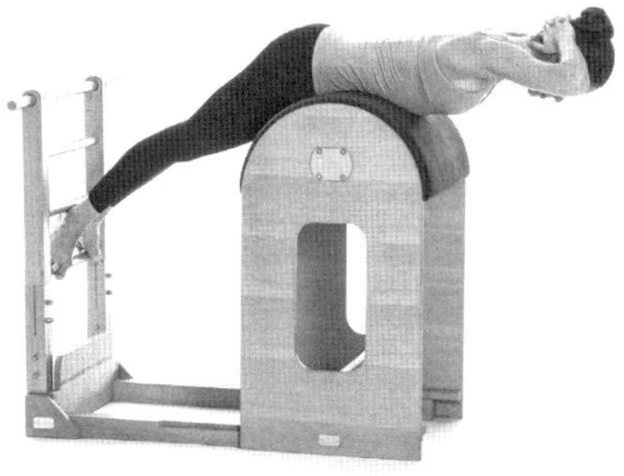

Swan

Muscle Focus

- Back extensors
- Abdominals
- Hip extensors

Objectives

- To improve back extensor strength
- To improve hip flexor flexibility
- To develop hip extensor and abdominal control

The swan is one of the most aesthetically beautiful movements in the repertoire and very gratifying to perform. It is an advanced back extension exercise that builds strength, flexibility, and tremendous control, and is particularly helpful for those gymnasts and dancers who tend to rely almost entirely on flexibility and the extension emanating from the lumbar spine. The key is integrated and organic movement through the knees, hips, shoulders, and every vertebral joint in the spine to create the desired shape. Many people focus only on the back, specifically the lower back. This results in shearing forces on the lower back and the body folding over, rather than arcing from the knees through the thighs and trunk all the way through to the fingertips. The combination of moderate knee flexion together with hip extension will help prevent the body from sinking as the knees bend. In fact, it should feel like the body is lifting even higher as the knees bend and the thighs press into the barrel.

Engaging the abdominals is critical to protecting the back and achieving the desired form. Note that the barrel should be set relatively close to the ladder so that the thighs are pressing against the barrel. In the final phase of the extension, gravity is actually pulling you further into extension, making this exercise not only advanced but also potentially dangerous. It is vital to maintain abdominal support throughout.

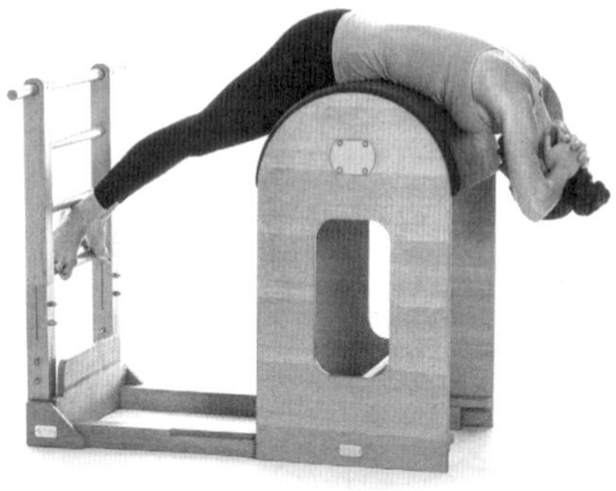

Setup. Lie prone, with the trunk draped over the barrel and the thighs pressing against it. Place the toes on the first rung of the ladder, with the feet in a V position. Anchor the heels under the second rung. Place the hands behind the head, fingers loosely interlaced.

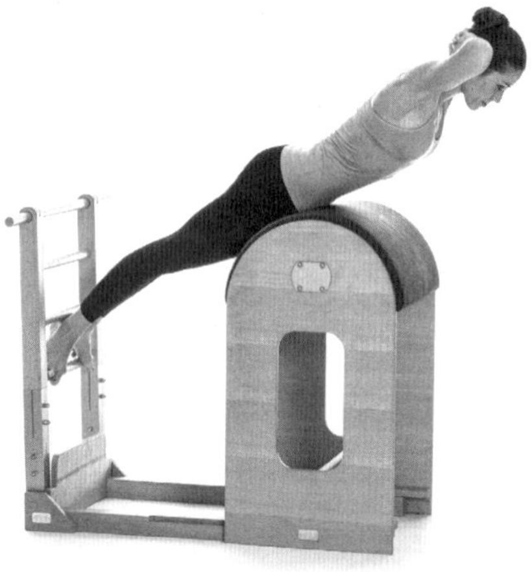

Inhale. Lift the trunk and extend the back, creating a diagonal line with the trunk and the legs.

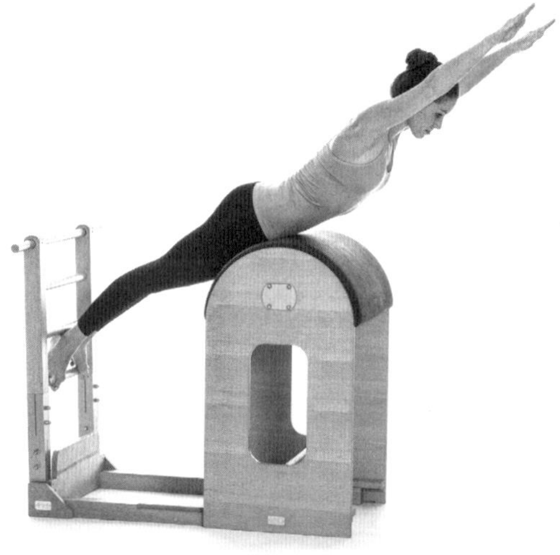

Exhale. Straighten the arms overhead in a wide V position in line with the ears, establishing a long line from the fingers to the toes.

Imagery

The image of an arc is important to create the correct movement pattern and muscle recruitment sequence when in full extension. As with many of the other back extension exercises, I also like to imagine an archer's bow being pulled taut, poised to unleash tremendous power.

- Keep the abdominals engaged, particularly in the final phase.
- Bend the knees (without sinking) as the trunk arches back and the hips extend, pushing the thighs further into the barrel.
- Distribute the extension through the entire spine and the hips, adding shoulder flexion to complete the shape.
- Keep the head aligned with the spine.

VARIATION

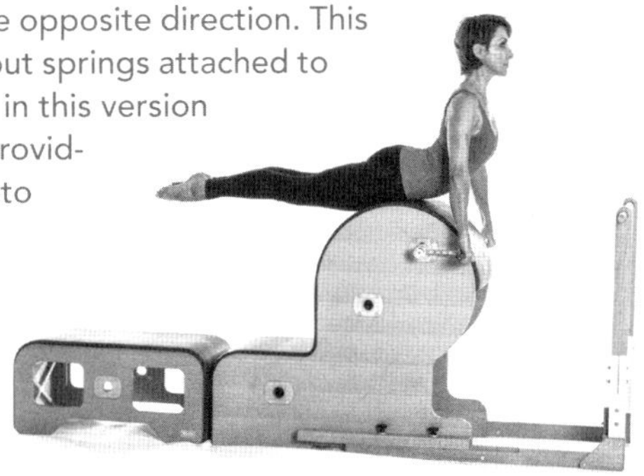

This variation is similar to the Ladder Barrel: Back Extension variation, with the body facing the opposite direction. This version can be done with or without springs attached to the legs, feet in straps. However, in this version the hands are on the F2 handles, providing support as the body is lifted into maximum extension. Performing this variation of the Ladder Barrel: Swan offers distinct advantages. First, using springs requires dynamic stabilization, as opposed to the static support provided by the ladder (using no springs provides even less support, making it more challenging). Second, the handles can be used to ease the back into its full range of motion as much as needed without placing excessive strain on the spine and the supporting musculature.

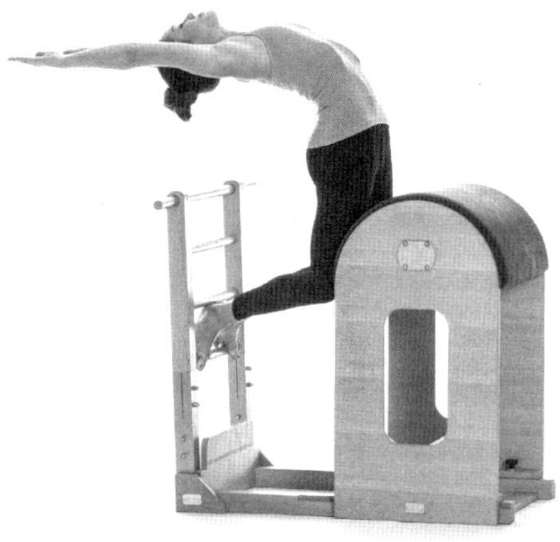

Inhale. Reach up toward the ceiling with the arms, drawing a large arc with the body, while simultaneously bending the knees and pressing the thighs into the barrel.

Continue to inhale as you press the thighs further against the barrel and extend the hips to the point of maximum extension. Take the trunk and the arms back until they are parallel to the floor (or as close as possible).

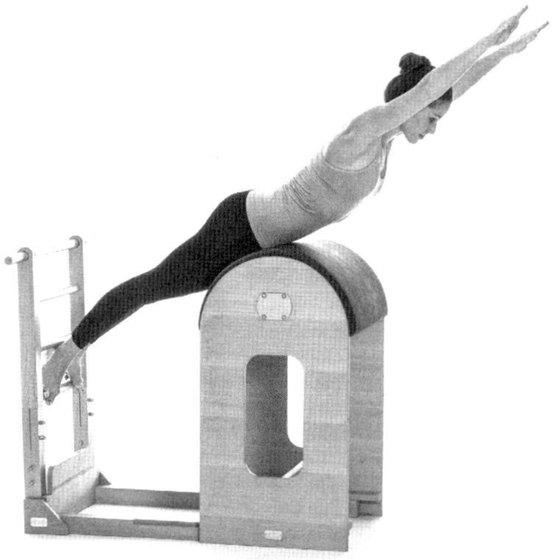

Exhale. Lift the body, reaching the arms toward the ceiling, and continue lowering the trunk to the long diagonal line.

Inhale. Place the hands behind the head.

Exhale. Lower the body. Return to the start position. Repeat 3-5 times.

Reach

Muscle Focus

- Abdominals
- Shoulder extensors and flexors

Objectives

- To improve abdominal control
- To improve abdominal, shoulder extensor, and thoracic flexibility

This exercise offers a wonderful interplay between spinal flexion and spinal extension, with the added bonus of a valuable shoulder stretch. The stretch for the back, particularly the lower back, should be maximized when in the C curve position, as should the stretch for the abdominals, chest, and shoulders when in the supine position.

This exercise focuses on the lower back and the shoulders, two areas that tend to become tight. In the supine position, the spine should be neutral, the legs straight, and the arms reaching overhead in a straight diagonal line, supported by the barrel. This is an ideal position in which to stretch the shoulders. However, be aware of the tendency to thrust the ribs forward in an endeavor to achieve more range in the shoulders. Doing so can result in hyperlordosis and possible stress on the lower back. In addition, this will actually *release* the stretch in the shoulders, making the stretch completely ineffective. The ISS must be activated to help maintain a stable, elongated position when supine and to assist when transitioning from supine to sitting, and vice versa.

Imagery

The visual of a green branch being pulled into an arc with twine tied to each side (like a bow) and then opening out to the straight position conjures up the perfect dynamic for this exercise.

- ○ Maximize the C curve when in the sitting position.
- ○ Maintain a straight line with the body when in the supine position.
- ○ Keep the head aligned with the spine at all times, placing it between the arms when in the supine position.

PROGRESSION

Once good form and control have been established, take the body from the straight line into further extension. Rest the back of the head on the barrel to avoid straining the neck, and continue reaching back with the arms. To reverse it, lift the head and arms, reestablishing a distinct straight line with the body, before returning to the start position. The F2 spine corrector has a gentler curve than the traditional step barrel, enabling the upper back and head to be supported when in hyperextension. In addition, the F2 spine corrector offers springs to better activate the muscles and develop strength, as well as provide increased stretch for the shoulders.

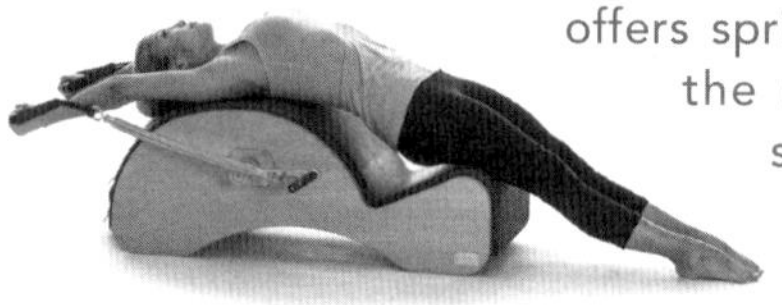

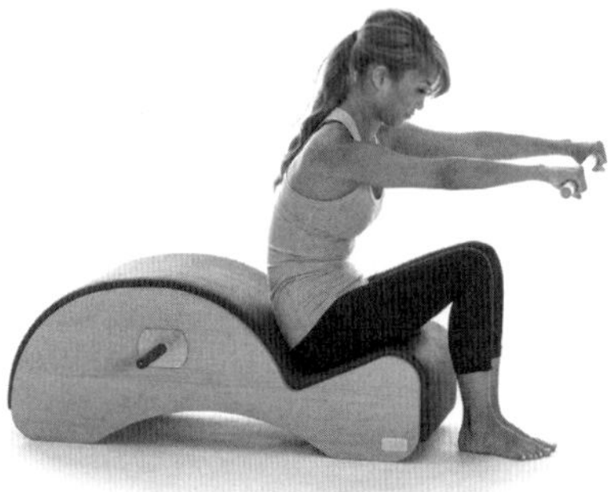

Setup. Sit in the dip between the step and the barrel, with the trunk in a C curve, holding a roll-up bar approximately 36 inches (90 centimeters) in length. Arms are reaching forward, shoulder width apart at shoulder height. Bend the knees, keeping the legs together, shins perpendicular to the floor, and place the feet firmly on the floor.

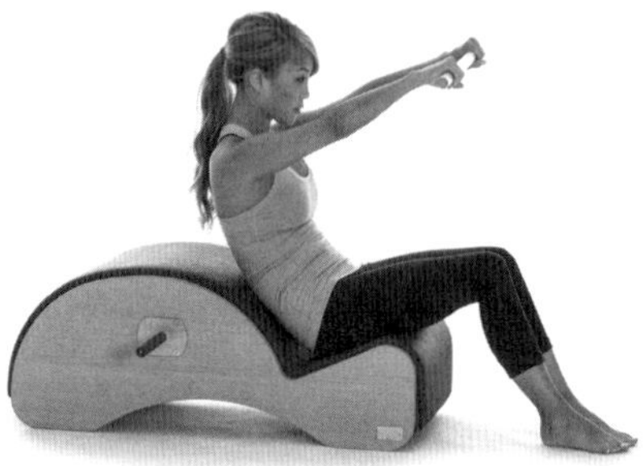

Exhale. Roll down onto the barrel, straightening the legs.

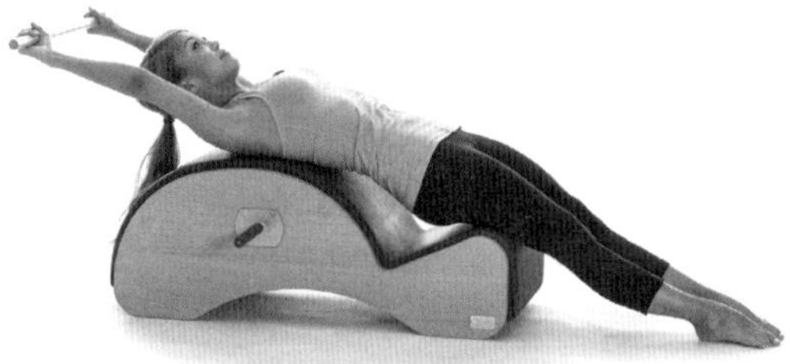

Continuing to exhale, extend the trunk, straighten the legs, and reach the arms overhead to form a straight line with the legs, trunk, and arms.

Inhale. Stretch the shoulders further while maintaining the straight line.

Exhale. Draw the trunk back into the C curve, bending the legs and bringing the arms forward. Return to the start position. Repeat 5 times.

Overhead Stretch

This exercise resembles the Step Barrel: Reach but offers a more intense stretch for the shoulders and chest, taking the trunk into hyperextension. The abdominals must be activated throughout to avoid excessive stress on the lower back. The apparatus itself also offers valuable support, as it does with many of the exercises.

An important element of this exercise is the sequential movement that progresses through the body—starting at the core, the movement proceeds through the spine as you roll down, and then continues to the arms. The arms then circle around and "pick up" the spine again to initiate the roll-up into a sitting C curve. The completion of the exercise is another sequential movement through the spine, transitioning from trunk flexion to sitting upright. Note that this exercise challenges the mobility of the shoulder, so anyone with shoulder restrictions should approach it with caution.

Imagery

The dynamic of this exercise should be of a perpetual rolling wave moving through the body as it goes through the full spectrum of movement: extension, hyperextension, and flexion.

- Lower the trunk onto the barrel before circling the arms.
- Keep the head aligned with the spine and the neck relaxed.
- Lift the head and spine sequentially as the arms circle around.

PROGRESSION

Once good form and control have been established, you can enhance the work of both the shoulder flexors and back extensors with this progression. Rather than completing the movement with the arms reaching forward at shoulder height, lift the arms overhead, reaching up to the ceiling. Once proficiency has been achieved, you can hold small hand weights to amplify both the strength and flexibility gains of the exercise.

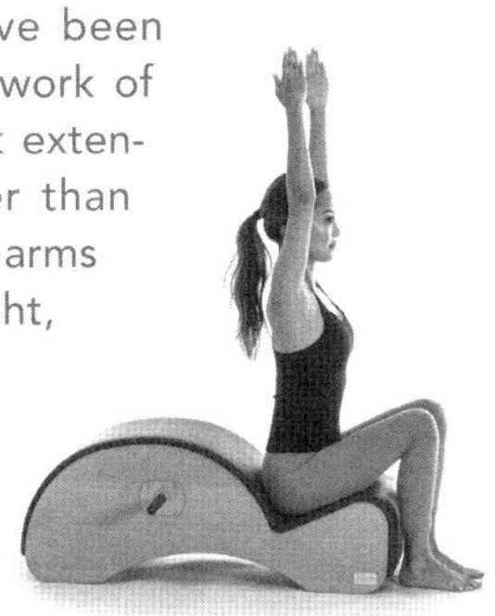

Muscle Focus

- Abdominals
- Shoulder extensors and flexors

Objectives

- To improve abdominal control
- To improve abdominal, shoulder extensor, and thoracic flexibility

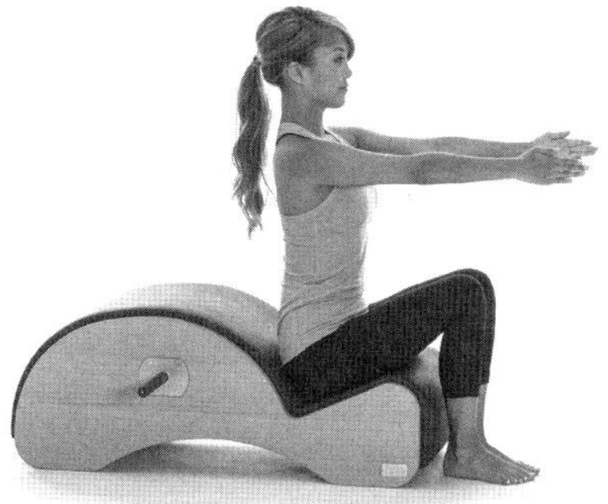

Setup. Sit in the dip between the step and the barrel, with the trunk in an upright position. Arms are reaching forward, shoulder width apart at shoulder height, palms facing each other. Bend the knees, shins perpendicular to the floor, and place the feet firmly on the floor hip width apart.

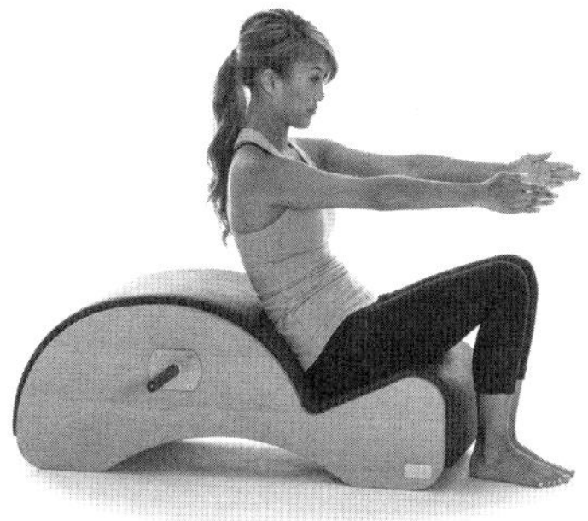

Exhale. Roll down onto the barrel.

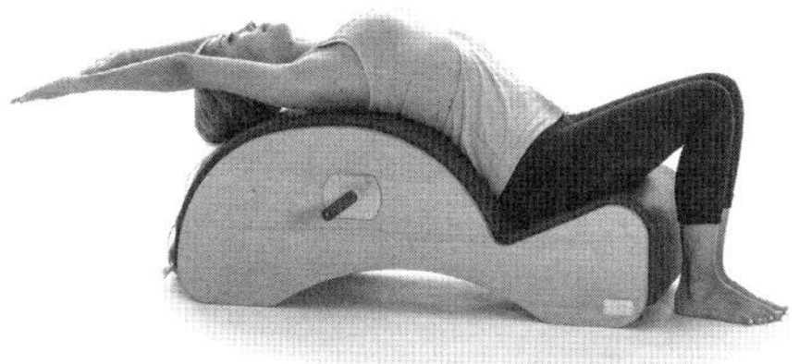

Inhale. Reach the arms overhead and circle them around.

Exhale. Roll up to the sitting C curve position, with the shoulders over the hips and the spine in flexion. Extend the spine to an upright position. Return to the start position. Repeat 5 times.

Chest Lift

Muscle Focus

- Abdominals

Objectives

- To improve abdominal strength and flexibility
- To improve thoracic flexibility

This exercise on the step barrel is similar to the Mat: Chest Lift, with two fundamental differences. First, the range of motion achieved on the step barrel is greater, spanning from spinal hyperextension to spinal flexion, which is valuable because the abdominals are seldom strengthened or stretched beyond a neutral spine position. Second, the lower back remains in either a neutral position (when the trunk is lifted) or in hyperextension (when the trunk is lowered) while it is supported by the barrel throughout, which protects the spine in these ranges and minimizes the risk of pressure on the discs. This could be particularly important in certain circumstances—for example, if a medical practitioner recommends that a patient with a disc problem in the lower back improve abdominal strength but advises against flexion of the lumbar spine. This exercise also has the added benefit of a significant stretch for the chest, which most people desperately need.

Imagery

Imagine the lumbar region remaining absolutely stable, as if part of a statue, and the movement occurring from a hinge or pivot point directly below the sternum. In addition, imagine a rubber band connecting the pubic symphysis to the sternum. As the body goes into extension the rubber band is stretched, but is never released. As the body lifts forward into flexion, the band shortens and assists the abdominals. Visualize the lift beginning from deep within the pelvic bowl.

- ○ Support the head with the hands (rest the head on a cushion when in spinal extension if necessary).
- ○ Keep the elbows wide.
- ○ Maintain contact between the lumbar spine and the barrel.

VARIATION

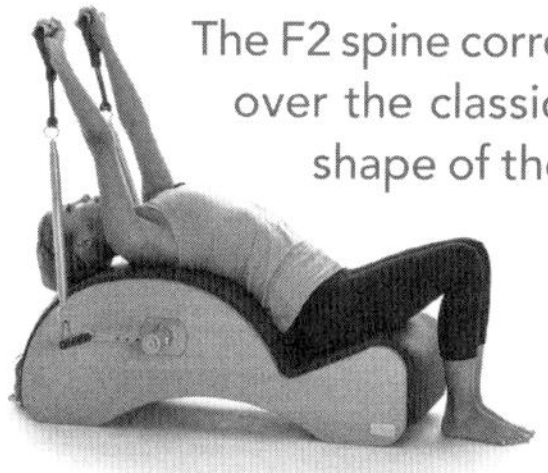

The F2 spine corrector has several additional benefits over the classic step barrel for this exercise. The shape of the barrel provides excellent support for the trunk in extension, and the springs offer the added component of resistance, facilitating greater strength gains for the abdominals.

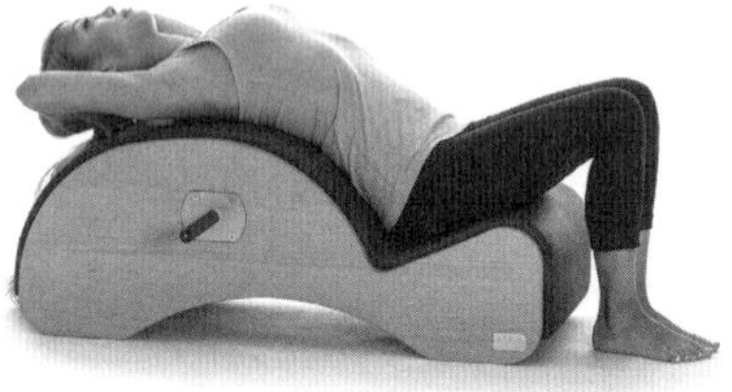

Setup. Lie supine on the barrel with the pelvis anchored in the dip of the step barrel. Interlace the fingers behind the head and stretch the thoracic spine over the barrel. Bend the knees, shins perpendicular to the floor, and place the feet firmly on the floor hip width apart.

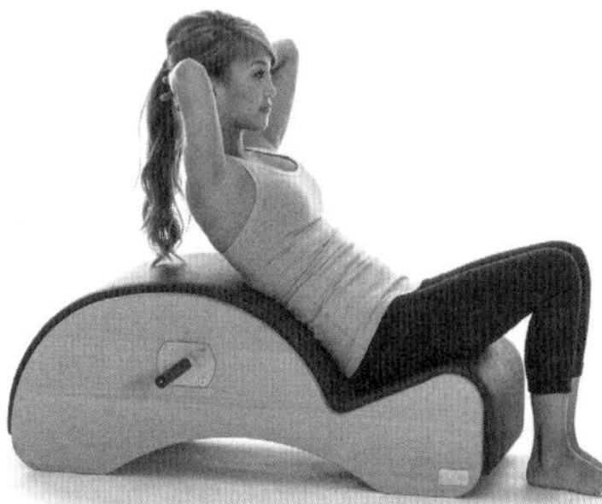

Exhale. Lift the head and chest into spinal flexion.

Inhale. Pause in this position.

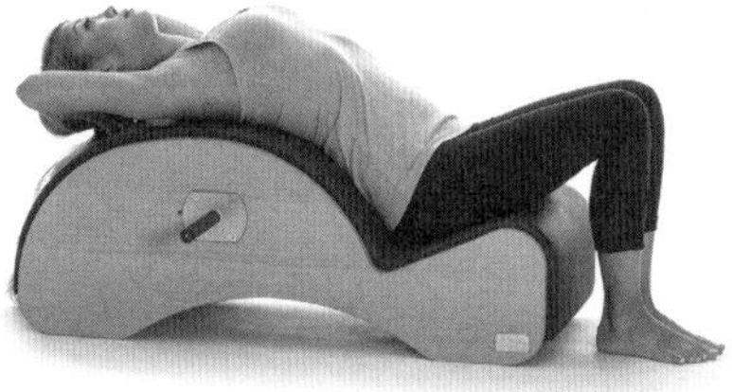

Exhale. Lower the head and chest. Return to the start position. Repeat 5-10 times.

Teaser Prep

The Step Barrel: Teaser Prep assists in building a foundation for the many versions of the teaser performed on almost all the Pilates apparatus, including the step barrel. It also prepares the body well for the pike movements, particularly those performed on the wunda chair and reformer. Observing the intricate connections among the many exercises on all the different apparatus in the Pilates method is fascinating. These connections can be viewed as branches of a large family tree. Understanding these relationships helps immensely in preparing the body for the next level, whatever it may be.

There are three areas of particular focus in most of the teasers: abdominals, back extensors, and hip flexors. This Step Barrel: Teaser Prep focuses on the abdominals and hip flexors but does not emphasize the back extensors. The barrel provides unique and welcome support for the body: When the body is straight on a diagonal line it supports the legs and upper back, and when the body is in the pike position it supports the mid-back, allowing the pelvis and lower back to sink into the dip between the step and the barrel. As with all the teasers, although often categorized as abdominal work, they in fact involve the entire body. I have elected to place the Step Barrel: Teaser Prep in the abdominal work block due to the focus on flexion of the trunk and the profound abdominal engagement during this phase of the exercise.

Imagery

Imagine the body opening out and then closing like a switchblade; the action is sharp, precise, and controlled.

- ○ Keep the head aligned with the spine.
- ○ Activate the abdominals prior to lifting the legs.
- ○ Focus the eyes directly forward when in the pike position.

VARIATION

The movement pattern of the Step Barrel: Teaser Prep on the F2 spine corrector is the same as on the classic step barrel; however, springs are used to provide resistance. This challenges the abdominals more and offers the potential for increased strength gains.

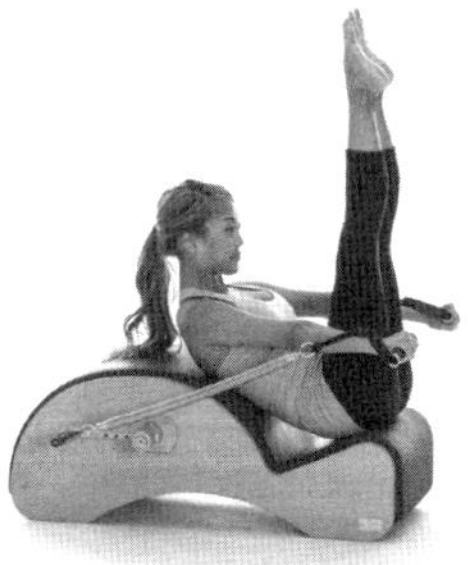

Muscle Focus

- Abdominals
- Hip flexors

Objectives

- To improve abdominal and hip flexor strength
- To improve hamstring and shoulder flexibility

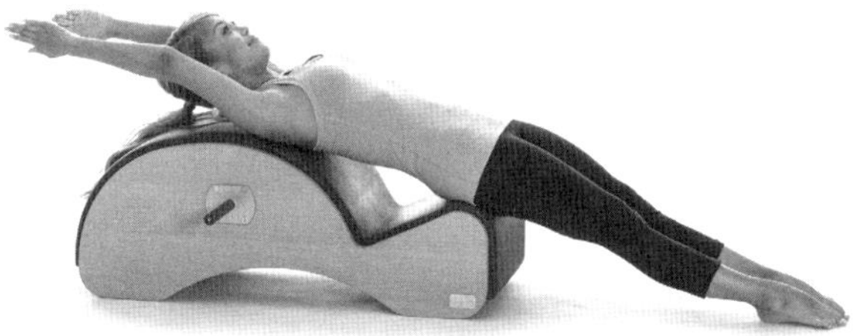

Setup. Lie supine on the barrel with the tailbone on the edge of the step and the upper back resting on the barrel. Reach the arms overhead, creating a straight line from the tips of the toes to the tips of the fingers.

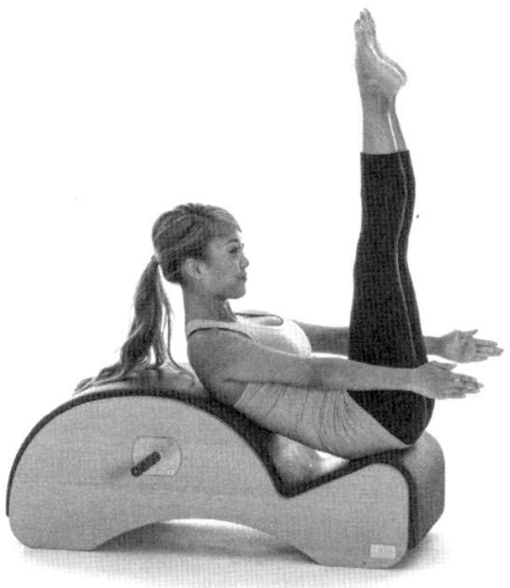

Exhale. Lift the arms and trunk forward and simultaneously lift the legs toward the ceiling, creating a deep pike position, with the legs perpendicular to the floor and the arms parallel to the floor.

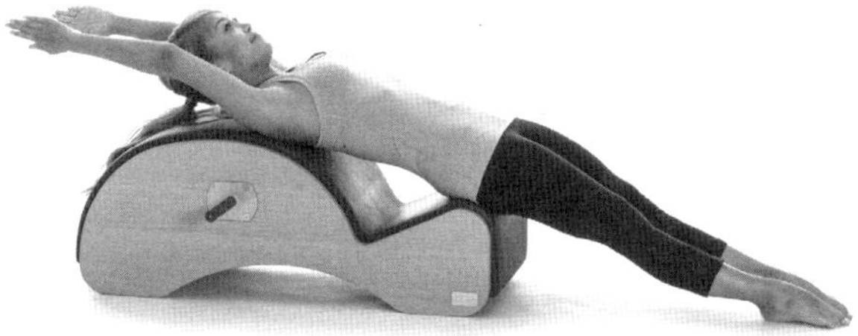

Inhale. Lower the trunk and legs. Return to the start position. Repeat 5 times.

Muscle Focus

- Hip adductors
- Abdominals

Objectives

- To improve hip adductor flexibility and control
- To develop lumbopelvic stabilization

Opening

The step barrel is an excellent piece of apparatus to work the hip adductors, particularly for those with tight hamstrings. The elevated position of the pelvis on the barrel places less stretch on the hamstrings than a supine position on the floor does, therefore requiring less hip flexor activation to keep the legs lifted and allowing maximum focus on the hip adductors and on maintaining a stable pelvis and trunk.

Imagery

Whether using resistance or not, imagine pressing against a huge spring or moving through heavy gel, creating internal resistance as the legs open and close.

- Open the legs as wide as possible without forgoing control or pelvic alignment.
- Pause with the legs perpendicular to the floor after each opening.
- Keep the hips externally rotated.

PROGRESSION

Once excellent control has been achieved, you can add ankle weights to this exercise to facilitate a deeper stretch and develop strength. Alternatively, you may use the F2 spine corrector, which offers convenient handles to hold on to and provides resistance through the full range of motion via the spring mechanism (keep tension in the springs throughout). However, employ extreme caution when using resistance, because it increases the potential danger of pressure on the lower back and excessive load on the hip adductors.

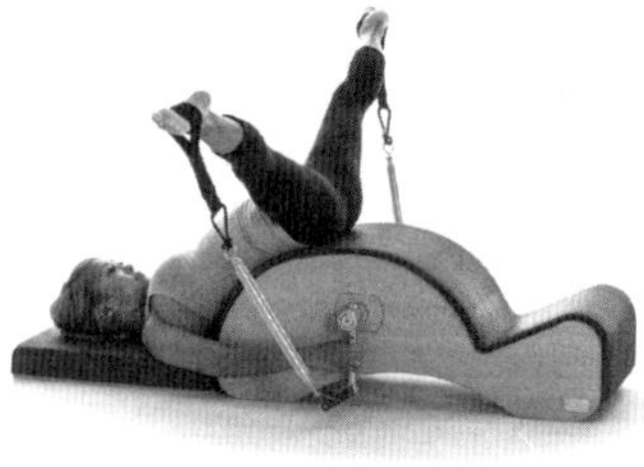

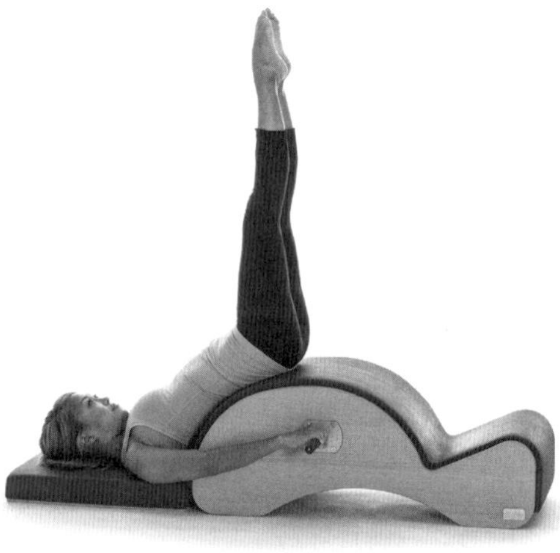

Setup. Lie with the back and pelvis on the barrel, the legs perpendicular to the floor, the hips externally rotated, and the shoulder girdle on the floor. Hold the barrel firmly with the hands. (Place a mat under the shoulder girdle and head to elevate the body in relation to the barrel, if necessary.)

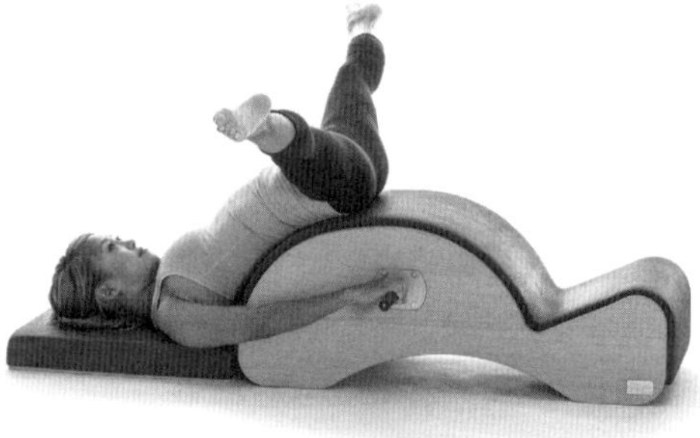

Inhale. Abduct the legs, opening them to a wide V position.

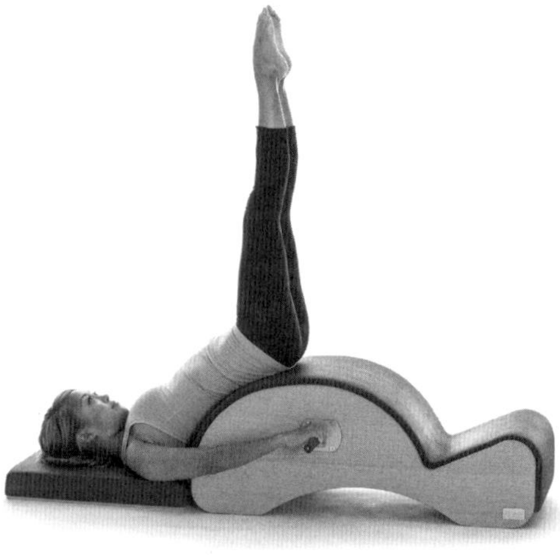

Exhale. Adduct the legs, closing them to the perpendicular position. Return to the start position. Repeat 10 times.

Helicopter

Coordination plays a key role in this exercise. As the legs travel in opposite directions, each leg must move at the same pace and achieve the same range of motion. This exercise combines the Step Barrel: Opening with the Step Barrel: Scissors (both prerequisites).

Imagery

The name of this exercise serves the image well—visualize the blades of a helicopter circling around, preparing for takeoff. (Stay grounded!)

- Touch each point of a large circle with the legs.
- Pass the legs through the perpendicular position after each circle.
- Keep the feet at a consistent height from the floor.
- Maintain lumbopelvic stabilization.

VARIATION

Once excellent control has been achieved, you can add ankle weights to this exercise to facilitate a deeper stretch and develop strength. Alternatively, you may use the F2 spine corrector, which offers convenient handles to hold on to and provides resistance through the full range of motion via the spring mechanism (keep tension in the springs throughout).

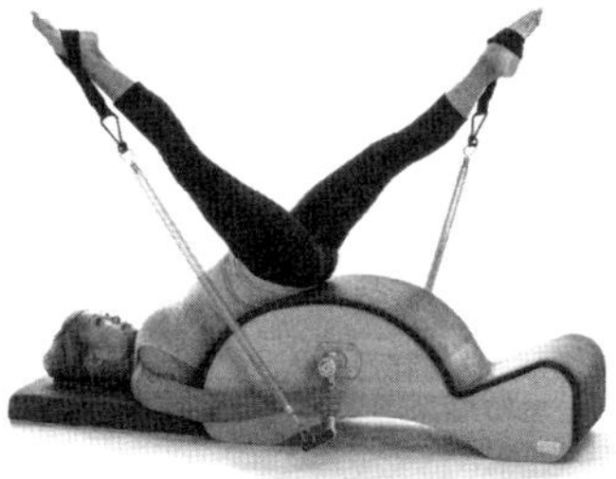

Muscle Focus

- Hip flexors
- Hamstrings
- Hip adductors
- Abdominals

Objectives

- To improve hip adductor strength and flexibility
- To improve hamstring and hip flexor control and flexibility
- To develop hip joint mobility
- To develop lumbopelvic stabilization

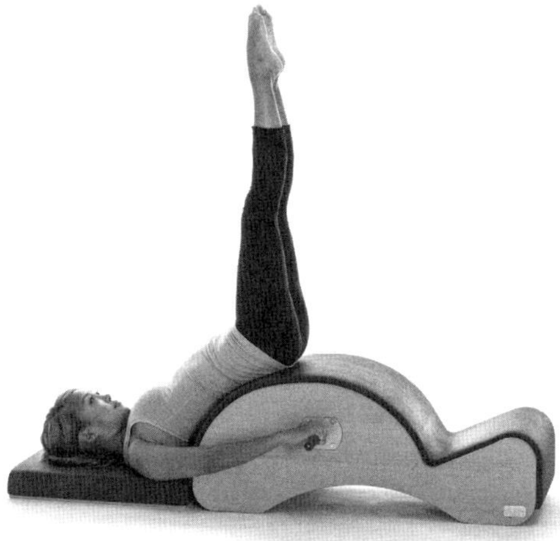

Setup. Lie with the back and pelvis on the barrel, the legs perpendicular to the floor, the hips externally rotated, and the shoulder girdle on the floor. Hold the barrel firmly with the hands. (Place a mat under the shoulder girdle and head to elevate the body in relation to the barrel, if necessary.) Hold the legs perpendicular to the floor, hips externally rotated (turned out).

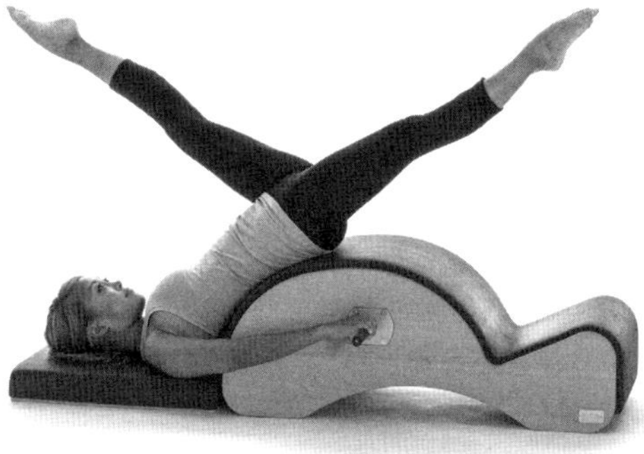

Inhale. Open the legs as wide as possible to the back and front in a scissor-like motion.

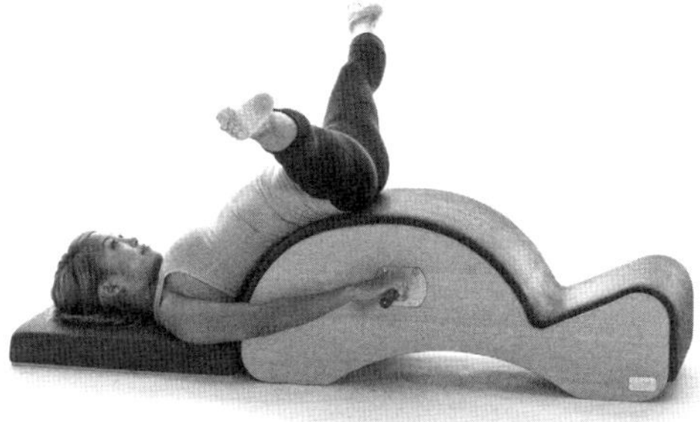

Exhale. Circle the legs in opposite directions. (The front leg circles to the back; the back leg circles to the front.) Return to the start position. Repeat 5 times in the same direction, and then reverse direction.

Scissors

Muscle Focus

- Hamstrings
- Hip flexors
- Abdominals

Objectives

- To improve hamstring and hip flexor flexibility
- To improve hamstring and hip flexor control
- To develop lumbopelvic stabilization

The Step Barrel: Scissors provides a wonderful stretch for the hamstrings and hip flexors and develops control of not only these muscle groups, but of all the muscles surrounding the hip joint. The spine is in a hyperextended position and the hip flexors are pulling on the lower back with a very long lever (the legs). Keeping the pelvis stable and maintaining abdominal activation throughout the movement is of paramount importance. Without abdominal support, you are at risk of placing excessive pressure on the lower back. This exercise is a great preparation for the Mat: Scissors. On the mat, the barrel is replaced by the arms, making it far more challenging.

Imagery

The name says it all—visualize long scissors opening and closing with a sharp, direct, and precise movement.

- Pause momentarily with the legs perpendicular to the floor after each opening.
- Create a V shape with the legs, opening them an equal distance to the back and front.
- Keep the trunk and pelvis connected to the barrel.

VARIATION

Once excellent control has been achieved, you can add ankle weights to this exercise to facilitate a deeper stretch and develop strength. Alternatively, you may use the F2 spine corrector, which offers convenient handles to hold on to and provides resistance through the full range of motion via the spring mechanism (keep tension in the springs throughout). Note that when using springs the hips are externally rotated (turned out), which allows for a greater range of motion of the hip joint. The movement should be smooth and unencumbered, as if being done with no springs.

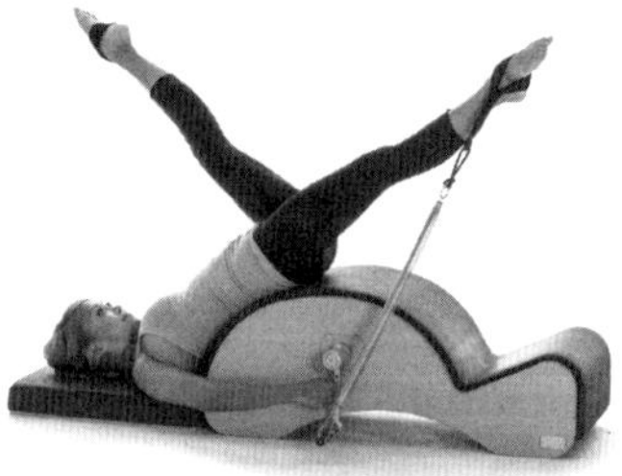

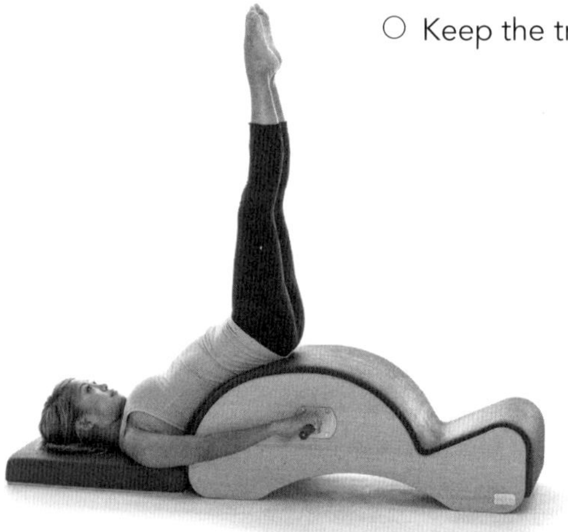

Setup. Lie with the back and pelvis on the barrel, the legs perpendicular to the floor, the hips parallel, and the shoulder girdle on the floor. Hold the barrel firmly with the hands. (Place a mat under the shoulder girdle and head to elevate the body in relation to the barrel, if necessary.)

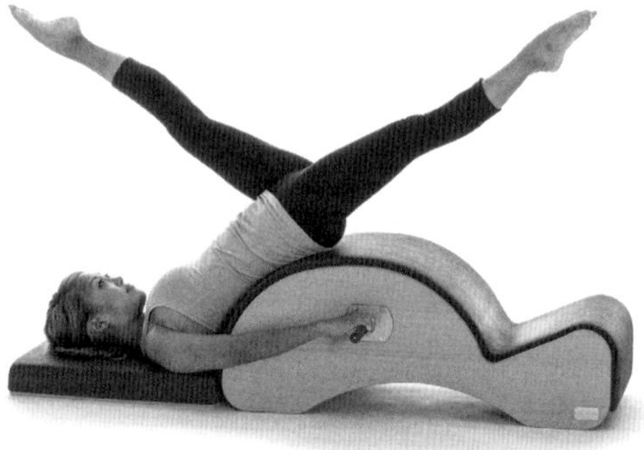

Exhale. Open the legs as wide as possible to the back and front in a scissor-like motion. Do two pulses with the legs when they reach maximum range, attempting to open a little further with the second pulse.

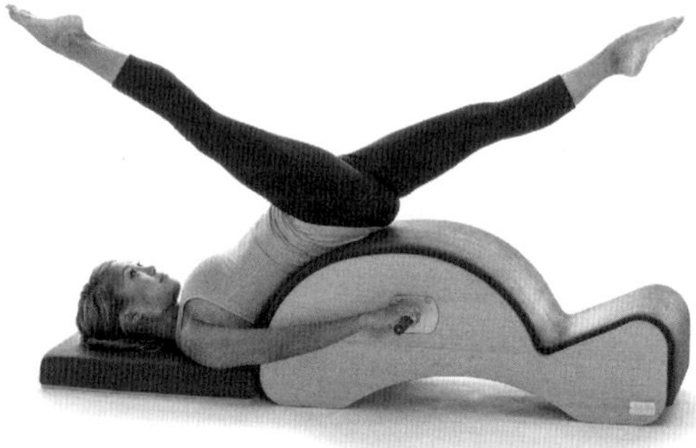

Inhale. Switch the legs, passing through the perpendicular position with each repetition. Return to the start position. Repeat the cycle 10 times, finishing in the perpendicular position.

Bicycle

As with the Step Barrel: Helicopter, coordination is possibly the greatest challenge in this exercise. The legs move simultaneously, with one bending while the other straightens. The cycling movement should be as large and elongated as possible. As with the Step Barrel: Scissors, which is an excellent preparation for this exercise, the legs are parallel (as opposed to externally rotated), and the path they follow should be close to the centerline. Passing through this position is important to ensure that the circular motion remains very large and stretches the hip flexors and hamstrings.

This version of the bicycle serves as an effective preparation for the Mat: Bicycle; here the barrel supports the body, as opposed to the arms holding the pelvis in an elevated position. As with the mat version, the movement pattern in this bicycle can be reversed.

Imagery

Imagine cycling a bicycle with very large wheels and pedals. The movement should be circular, not linear, with each leg drawing a large circle.

- ○ Touch the step of the step barrel with the toes as the back leg bends to come in.
- ○ Keep the legs parallel to each other; avoid splaying the knees, particularly as the back leg bends.
- ○ Maintain lumbopelvic stabilization.

VARIATION

Once excellent control has been achieved, you can add ankle weights to this exercise to facilitate a deeper stretch and develop strength. This particular exercise is not well suited to springs because they hamper the smooth, flowing motion. Note that when reversing the movement the toes will also touch the step (this adds more challenge).

Muscle Focus

- Hip flexors
- Hamstrings
- Abdominals

Objectives

- To improve hamstring and hip flexor flexibility
- To improve hamstring and hip flexor control
- To develop lumbopelvic stabilization

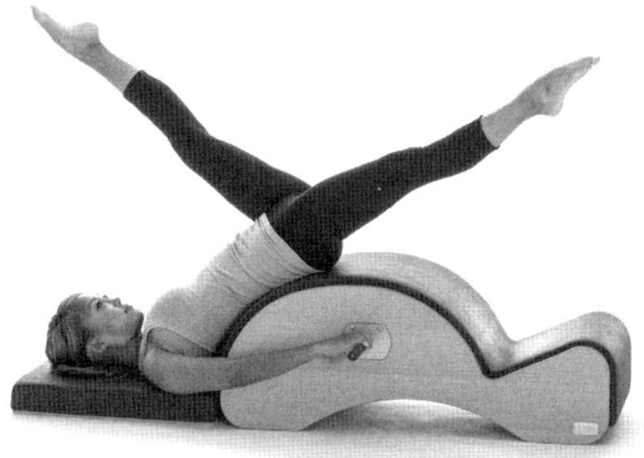

Setup. Lie with the back and pelvis on the barrel, the legs perpendicular to the floor, the hips parallel, and the shoulder girdle on the floor. Hold the barrel firmly with the hands. (Place a mat under the shoulder girdle and head to elevate the body in relation to the barrel, if necessary.)

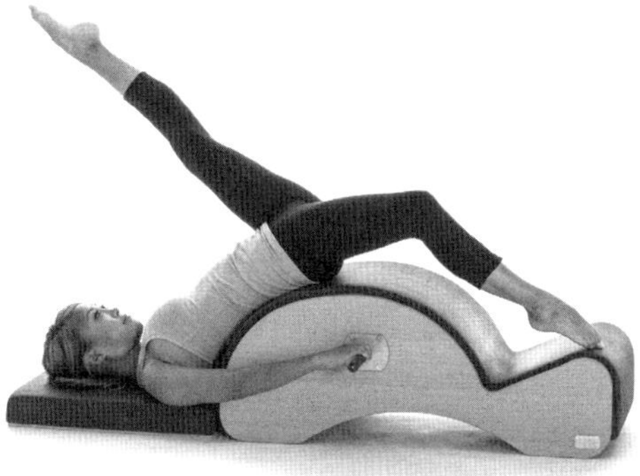

Exhale. Bend the back leg, touching the step with the toes. Simultaneously, begin to extend the front leg, reaching it up to the ceiling.

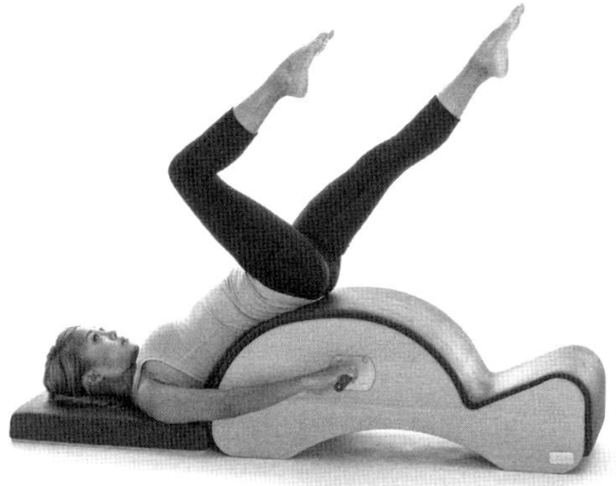

Continuing to exhale, draw the bent back leg toward the chest, crossing the other leg, which is now passing through the perpendicular position on its way to the back.

Inhale. Open to the scissors position, straightening what is now the front leg opposite the face. Return to the start position. Repeat 5 times on each leg, then reverse direction.

Roll-Over

Muscle Focus

- Abdominals
- Hip flexors

Objectives

- To improve abdominal and hip flexor control
- To improve hip flexor, hamstring, and back extensor flexibility
- To develop spinal articulation

Those who find the Mat: Roll-Over difficult may have success with the Step Barrel: Roll-Over. The barrel elevates the pelvis, placing it in a position that alleviates the pull on the hamstrings and lower back. It also allows gravity to assist the abdominals in the roll-over phase of the exercise, which can be very challenging.

Once you have mastered this exercise on the step barrel, it will likely be easier to perform it on the mat. Be cautious when lowering the legs, which function as a long lever arm, back to the start position. The lower back can easily be overloaded or pulled into hyperextension; the abdominals must be firmly engaged throughout to counteract this danger. However, once excellent lumbopelvic stabilization has been achieved, lowering the legs until the pelvis and legs create one straight line provides an excellent stretch for the hip flexors.

Note that this exercise demands deep spinal flexion and can also place pressure on the cervical spine. Both these aspects of the exercise may be contraindicated in certain circumstances. If in doubt, consult with a medical professional. Ideally, very little pressure should be placed on the cervical spine. Along with the shoulders, the barrel helps support the weight of the body and alleviates pressure from the cervical spine. It also assists in controlling the degree of spinal flexion.

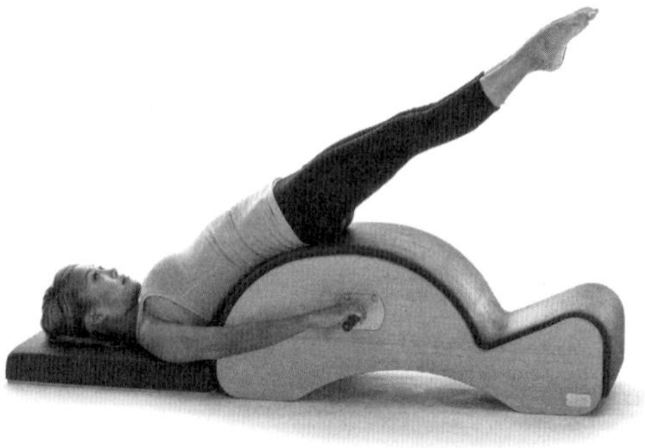

Setup. Lie with the back and pelvis on the barrel, the shoulder girdle on the floor, and the legs perpendicular to the floor. Lower the legs to form a straight diagonal line with the pelvis (0 degrees of hip flexion). This position demands exceptional lumbopelvic stabilization. Start with the legs lifted higher if there is any pressure on the lower back. Hold the barrel firmly with the hands. (Place a mat under the shoulder girdle and head to elevate the body in relation to the barrel, if necessary.)

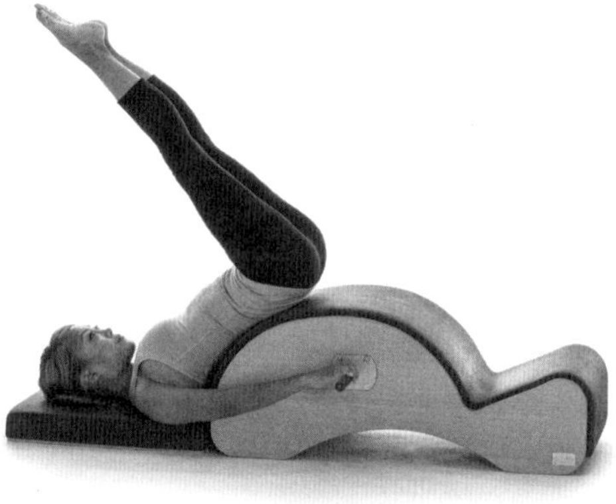

Inhale. Lift the legs to a 90-degree angle in the hip joint (note that this will be beyond the perpendicular position).

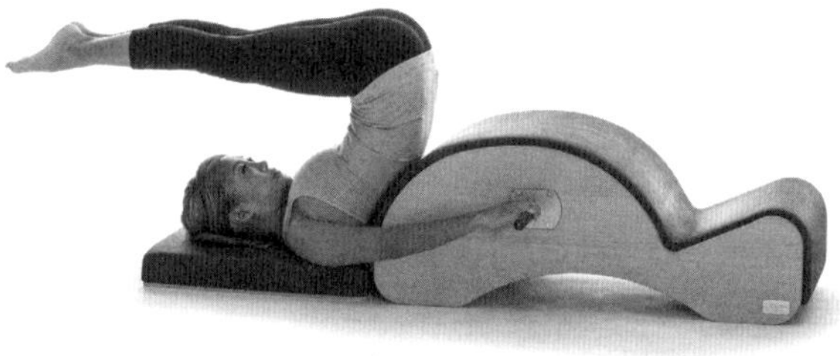

Exhale. Roll over, transferring the legs overhead. Pause with the legs parallel to the floor.

Imagery

The visual of the vertebrae being gently lifted off the barrel and then placed back on like a necklace of pearls helps achieve the desired spinal articulation.

- Maintain abdominal support.
- Keep the barrel connected to the back, even when in spinal flexion and the legs are overhead.
- Establish a 90-degree angle in the hip joint prior to rolling over.
- Bring the legs to perpendicular and plantarflex the feet when returning to the start position.

PROGRESSION

Once excellent control has been achieved, you can add ankle weights to this exercise to facilitate gains in strength and flexibility. Alternatively, you may use the F2 spine corrector, which offers convenient handles to hold on to and provides resistance via the spring mechanism. As always, employ extreme caution when using any type of resistance, because it increases the potential for excessive pressure on the neck and lower back. Note that the beginning position of this exercise demands tremendous abdominal and hip flexor control, which is magnified when resistance is added, whether via weights or springs.

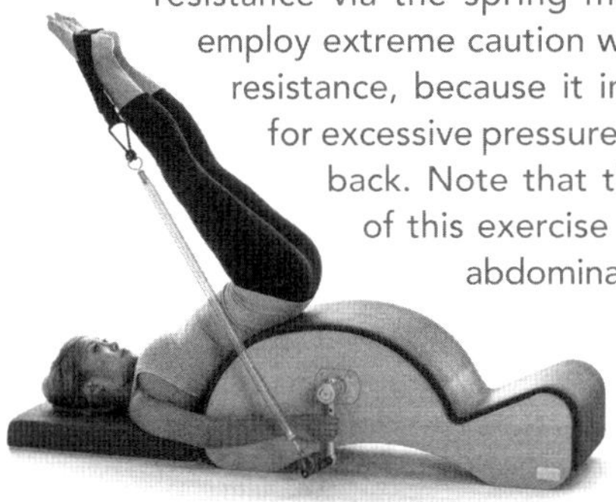

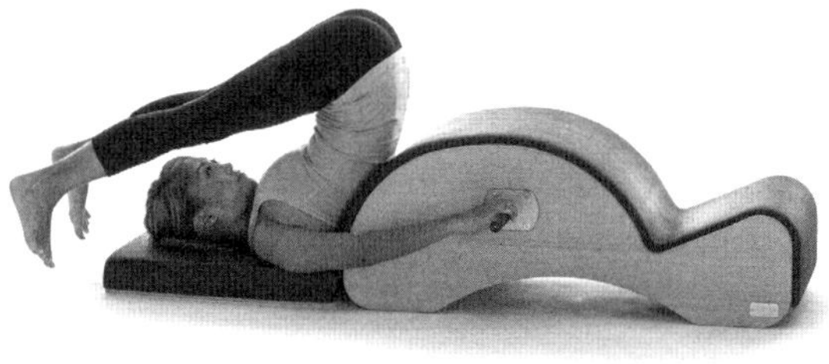

Inhale. Dorsiflex the feet, separate the legs to shoulder width, and lower the feet toward the floor (or as close as possible).

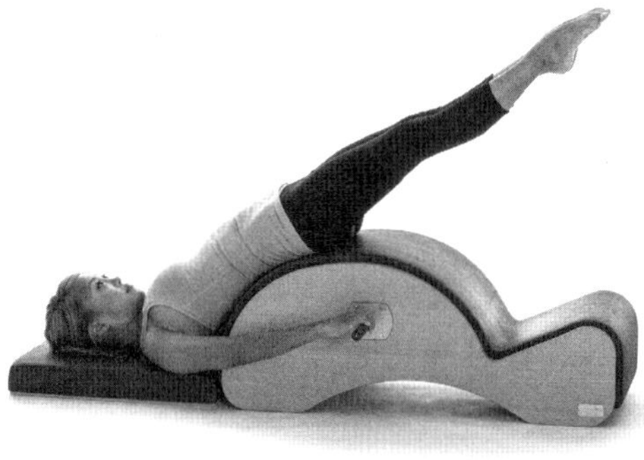

Exhale. Roll down through the spine, placing each vertebra on the barrel until the pelvis is anchored. Continue lifting the legs. When they are perpendicular to the floor, plantarflex the feet, lower the legs, and bring them back together. Return to the start position. Repeat 5 times.

Muscle Focus

- Abdominal obliques
- Back extensors

Objective

- To improve lateral flexor strength and flexibility

Side Over

The step barrel is exceptionally helpful in achieving correct alignment and muscle recruitment for lateral flexion. It supports the body and virtually guides it in the desired direction. This exercise addresses both strength and flexibility of the lateral flexors and lays a solid foundation for many other lateral flexion exercises in the Pilates repertoire, including the Reformer: Side Over and the Ladder Barrel: Side Over.

There is a strong tendency to try to lift with the head, tilting it sideways, a common compensation in this movement. Keeping the head aligned with the spine and the neck uninvolved is extremely important. The muscles of the trunk, particularly the abdominals and back extensors, support this integrated movement and help create both the elongated line as well as the arc shape when draped over the barrel.

Imagery

Visualize tall grass being blown sideways in a soft breeze; then the breeze subsides and the grass lifts back up. I encourage you to strive for this effortless, soft quality.

- ○ Lift the trunk only as high as the straight diagonal line created by the trunk and the top leg.
- ○ Stabilize with the muscles of the core.
- ○ When lifting, direct the movement up toward the ceiling, rather than "crunching" sideways.

VARIATION

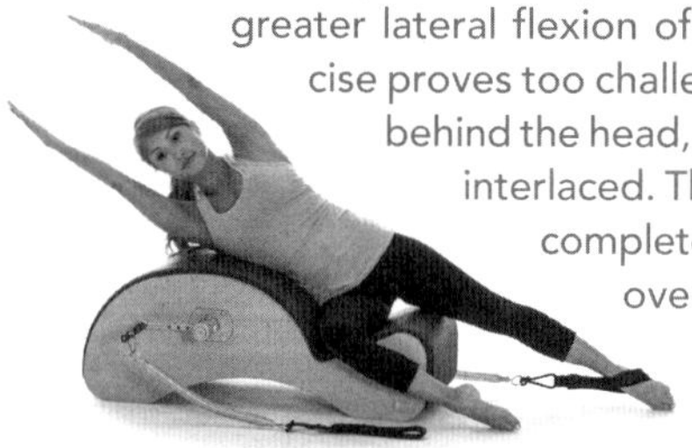

When performing this exercise on the F2 spine corrector, a spring can be placed on the straight leg to assist in dynamically stabilizing the body. This facilitates greater lateral flexion of the trunk. If the exercise proves too challenging, place the hands behind the head, with the fingers loosely interlaced. This exercise may also be completed by relaxing sideways over the barrel, stretching the lateral flexors and underarm.

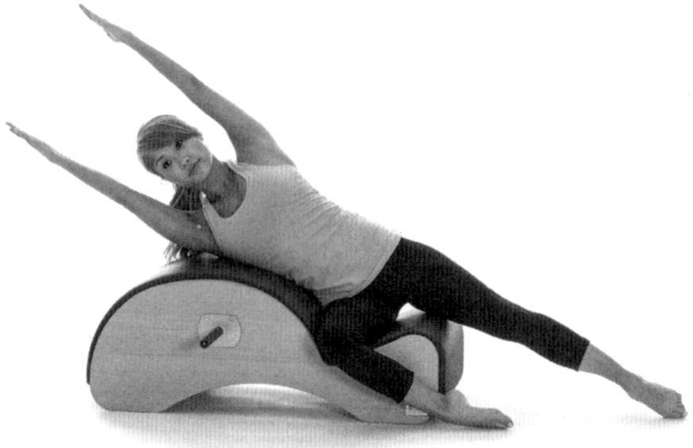

Setup. Lie on the step barrel on one side of the body. Bend the bottom leg to a 90-degree angle in the hip and knee joints and rest it in the step of the barrel. Straighten the top leg (not externally rotated), with the foot plantarflexed and anchored on the floor. Straighten the arms overhead.

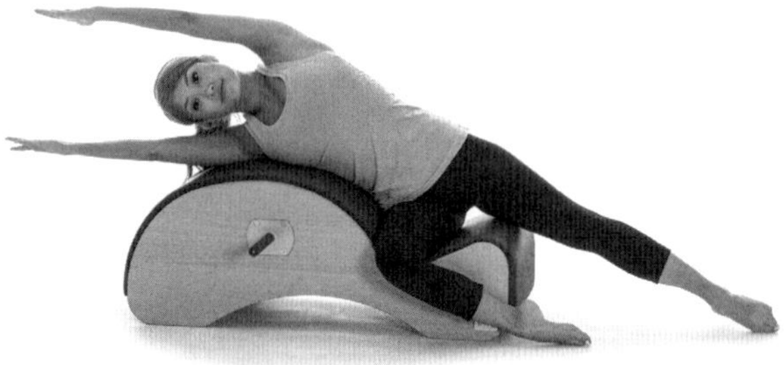

Inhale. Lower the trunk over the barrel.

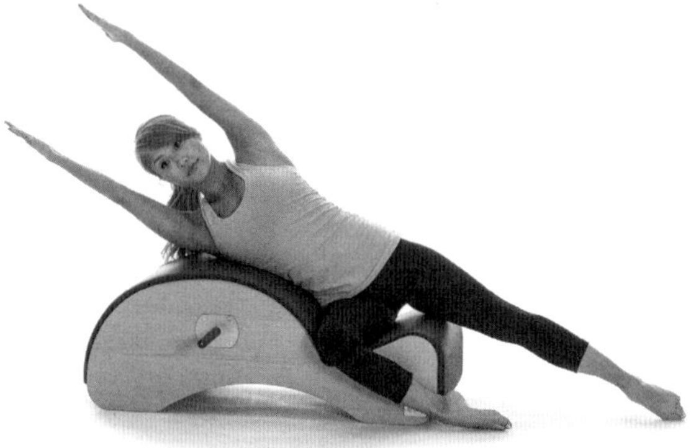

Exhale. Lift the trunk, creating a straight diagonal line with the arms, trunk, and top leg. Return to the start position. Repeat 5-10 times before switching to the other side.

Swan

Muscle Focus

- Back extensors
- Hip extensors
- Abdominals

Objectives

- To improve back extensor strength
- To improve hip extensor control

Versions of this exercise are done on almost every piece of Pilates apparatus. The step barrel is no exception and is an excellent place to teach the positioning, alignment, and muscle recruitment for this popular exercise. The step barrel supports the trunk and the legs, thereby alleviating some of the potential stress on the back and assisting the back extensors and hip extensors to achieve the perfect bow shape. Of course, the abdominals are vital to supporting the movement, achieving the correct form, and protecting the back.

Imagery

The image of an archer's bow being pulled taut helps to visualize the position and the dynamic, as well as to illustrate the important concept of distributing the work evenly through the back.

- ○ Engage the abdominals.
- ○ Continue to adduct the legs as they lift into hip extension.
- ○ Stabilize the scapulae prior to lifting the trunk.

VARIATION

Using the handles of the F2 spine corrector for this exercise offers the benefit of arm support, which allows you to explore the full range of spinal extension without placing excess pressure on the lower back. Activate the back extensors and use the arms only for support. There is a strong tendency to straighten the arms while allowing the shoulders to lift (scapular elevation); however, the arms do not need to straighten completely. It is more important to keep the scapulae in a neutral position than to achieve more height with the back at the expense of scapulae placement.

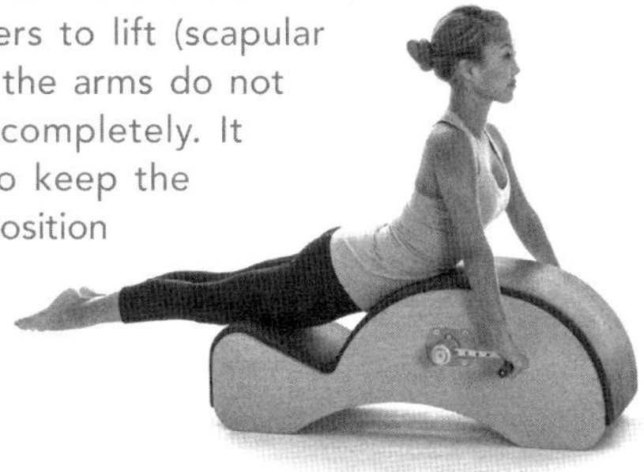

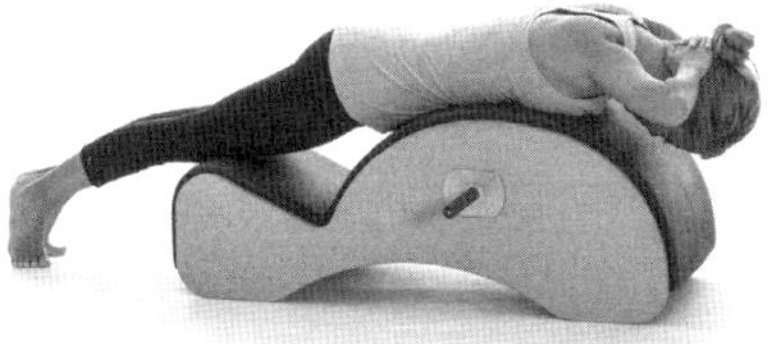

Setup. Lie prone over the barrel with the knees slightly bent, the hips externally rotated, the feet in a small V position with the toes anchored on the floor, and the fingers loosely interlaced behind the head.

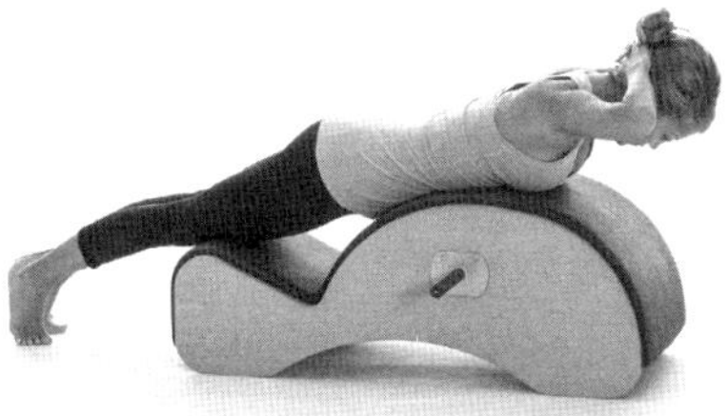

Inhale. Lift the head and trunk, extending the back.

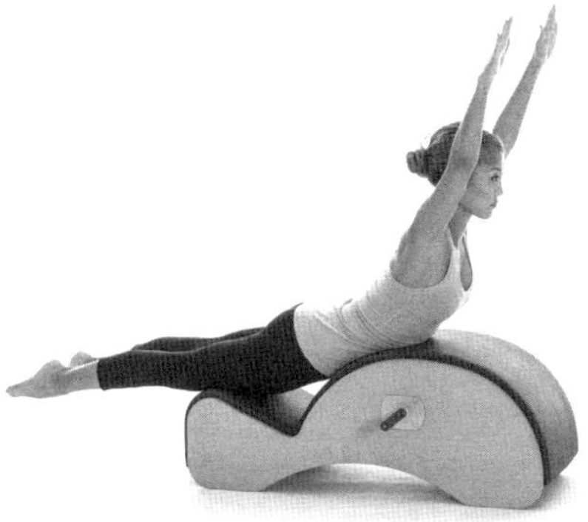

Exhale. Lift the trunk higher as the arms reach forward and up to create a wide V position. Simultaneously straighten and lift the legs, plantarflexing the feet.

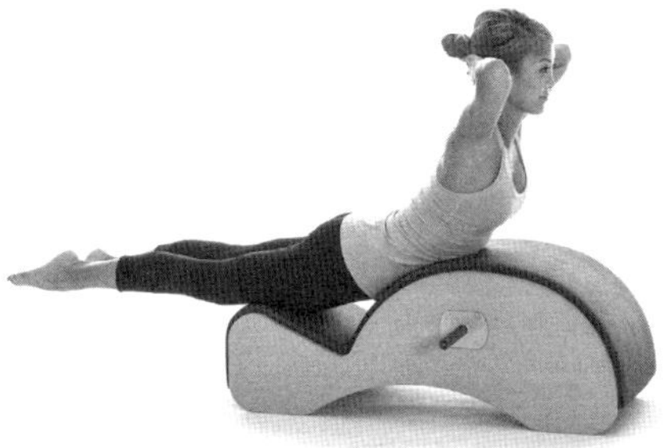

Inhale. Place the hands back behind the head.

Exhale. Lower the trunk and legs. Return to the start position. Repeat 5 times.

Ped-a-Pul

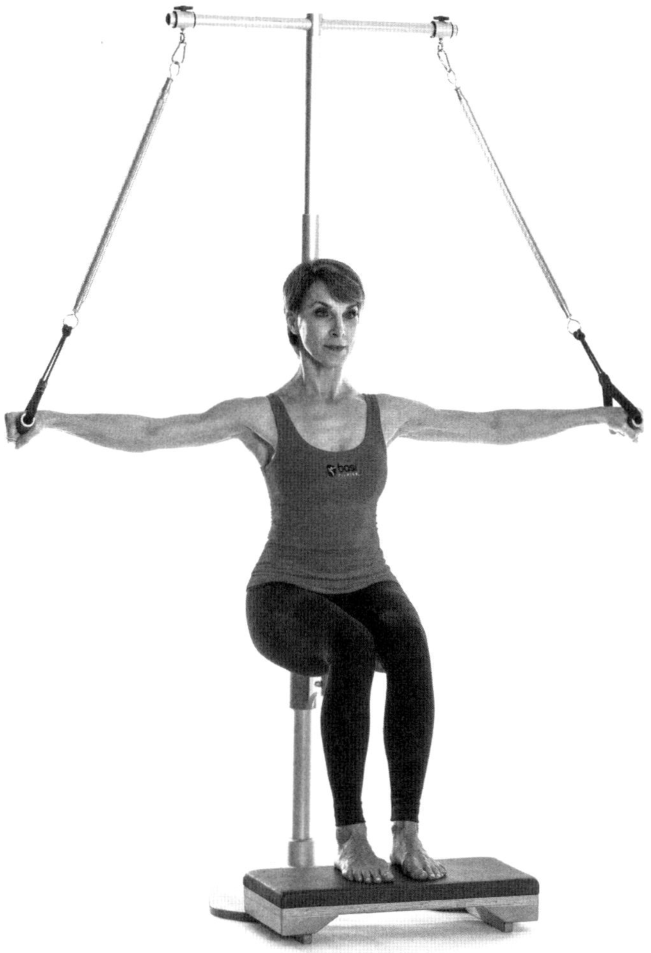

The ped-a-pul is one of Joseph Pilates' original apparatus, but it is not as commonly used as others, such as the cadillac and the reformer. However, it has unique capabilities that cannot be easily duplicated on the other equipment. The ped-a-pul focuses on the arms and shoulder complex, working the body in a standing or sitting position, and is therefore excellent for developing upright alignment and balance.

I have created a series of exercises for the ped-a-pul that works the shoulders below shoulder height. Working at this height is particularly advantageous when teaching scapular stabilization and working with shoulder ailments, such as impingement syndrome. These exercises are the same as in the supine arm work series on the reformer; however, here the body is in an upright position. This position is more functional by nature and further challenges the postural muscles and alignment of the spine. In addition, the arms work independently, which eliminates the possibility of a dominant side doing more of the work. This series has proven to be invaluable when rehabilitating the shoulder and for general conditioning of the upper body.

Although most modern ped-a-puls have adjustable resistance to meet individual needs, the original ped-a-pul did not. When working with one that is not adjustable, you can increase the resistance by squatting lower or sitting on a stool. (The lower the body is in relation to the springs, the more resistance there will be.) Sitting on a stool offers more stability, which may be an advantage in certain situations. For this reason, the BASI Systems ped-a-pul (based on my original designs) includes an integrated seat.

Some ped-a-puls may be attached to the wall, whereas others are self-standing. Although each offers unique benefits, I prefer to attach the ped-a-pul to the wall, unless the base is large and stable. It is safer and presents more possibilities both in terms of repertoire and adding resistance, which in turn offers more potential strength gains.

The handles can be held either with an open hand or a fist, whichever feels more comfortable. The open-hand position with fingers straight accentuates the long line of the arms; however, tension often creeps into the fingers, in which case the fist position is preferred.

Extension

This exercise focuses on shoulder extension from shoulder height and below. It develops shoulder extensor control or strength (if there is adequate resistance) in this specific range of motion, utilizing both concentric and eccentric contractions. It is an excellent preparation for shoulder extension together with trunk flexion, a frequently recurring movement pattern found in much of the Pilates abdominal work, including the Mat: Hundred and the Reformer: Coordination. It also serves as a preparation for shoulder extension together with trunk extension, found in exercises such as the Reformer: Pulling Straps 1.

Imagery

Visualize pressing the hands against a big, inflated balloon. Alternatively, you can imagine that you are deep underwater and must use only your arms to propel yourself upward.

- ○ Maintain scapular stabilization.
- ○ Keep the arms straight and moving parallel to each other.

MODIFICATION

If it is difficult to maintain the standing position, it is possible to sit on a stool, a large ball, or the integrated seat.

PED-A-PUL
Arm Work
FUNDAMENTAL

Muscle Focus

- Shoulder extensors
- Triceps

Objectives

- To improve shoulder extensor and elbow extensor control and strength (depending on the resistance)
- To develop trunk and scapular stabilization
- To develop spinal alignment

RESISTANCE

Light Medium Heavy

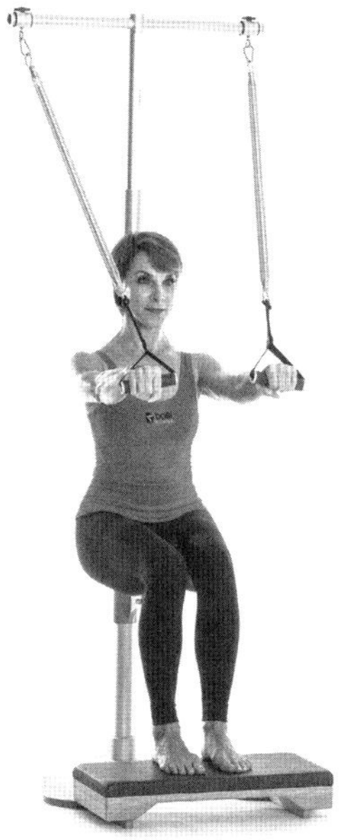

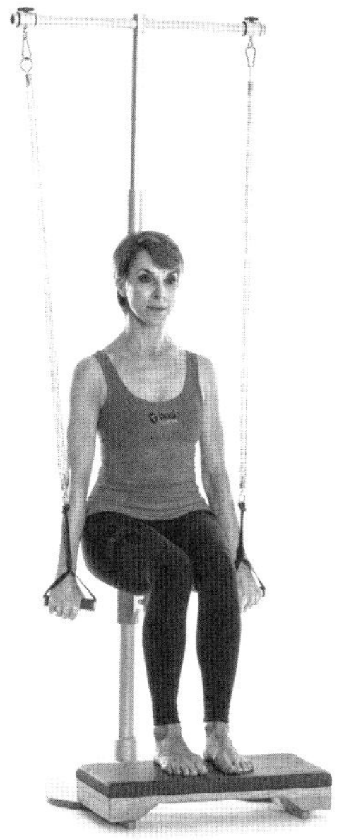

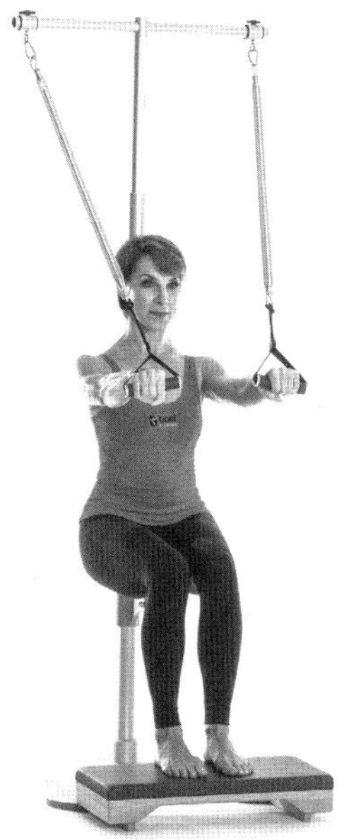

Setup. Stand (sit) with the back against the pole in a neutral spine position and the feet firmly placed on the floor, knees directly above the ankles. Keep the legs hip width apart and parallel to each other. Hold the handles and straighten the arms at shoulder height directly in front of the shoulders, parallel to the floor and to each other, palms facing down.

Exhale. Extend the shoulders, lowering the arms down to the sides of the body in line with the hip joints.

Inhale. Flex the shoulders, lifting the arms to shoulder height. Return to the start position. Repeat 10 times.

PED-A-PUL

Arm Work

FUNDAMENTAL

Muscle Focus

- Shoulder adductors

Objectives

- To improve shoulder adductor control and strength (depending on the resistance)
- To develop trunk and scapular stabilization
- To develop spinal alignment

RESISTANCE

Light — Medium — Heavy

Adduction

This exercise focuses on shoulder adduction from shoulder height and below. Like shoulder extension, shoulder adduction is performed together with the movement of the trunk in many Pilates exercises. It is often accompanied by trunk flexion, as in the case of abdominal work, or back extension, as in the Reformer: Pulling Straps 2.

Imagery

Imagine spreading your arms like the wings of an eagle as they move up and down. This is a powerful image; enjoy the sensation.

- ○ Maintain scapular stabilization.
- ○ Keep the arms straight, with the palms starting out facing the floor and then facing the body.
- ○ Maintain a neutral spine position.

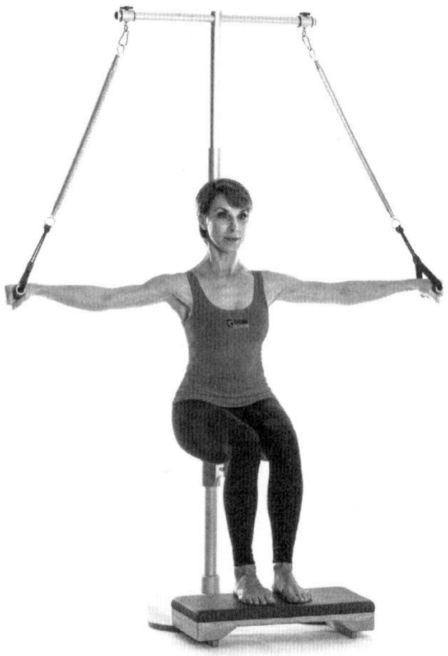

Setup. Stand (sit) with the back against the pole in a neutral spine position and the feet firmly placed on the floor, knees directly above the ankles. Keep the legs hip width apart and parallel to each other. Hold the handles and reach the arms out to the sides in a T position, with the palms facing down and a micro-bend in the elbows.

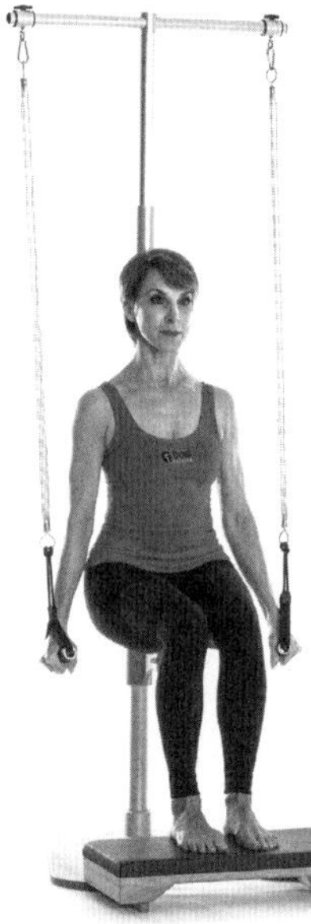

Exhale. Adduct the shoulders, bringing the arms down to the sides of the body in line with the hip joints.

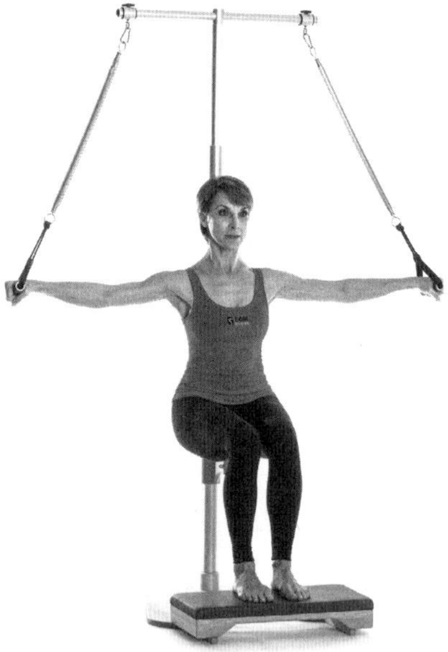

Inhale. Abduct the shoulders, lifting the arms. Return to the start position. Repeat 10 times.

Triceps

This exercise offers extremely focused work for the triceps. Keeping the upper arms stable and close to the sides of the body is key to maximizing the work of the triceps and isolating the movement of the elbow. In addition, keeping the wrist perfectly stable and aligned with the arm is very important. When the wrist bends back, as it tends to do, it places excessive pressure on the joint and releases some of the tension from the springs. The lower arm and wrist should be viewed as one solid unit.

Imagery

Imagine the body levitating with each extension of the elbows. The trunk elongates and the scapulae provide a stable base to push off from. The lower arm should feel like a mechanical lever attached at the elbow, and the joint like a well-lubricated hinge.

- Maintain scapular stabilization.
- Keep the upper arms close to the sides of the body.
- Isolate the movement of the lower arms.
- Maintain a neutral spine position.

Muscle Focus

- Triceps

Objectives

- To improve elbow extensor strength
- To develop trunk and scapular stabilization
- To improve spinal alignment

RESISTANCE

Light — Medium — Heavy

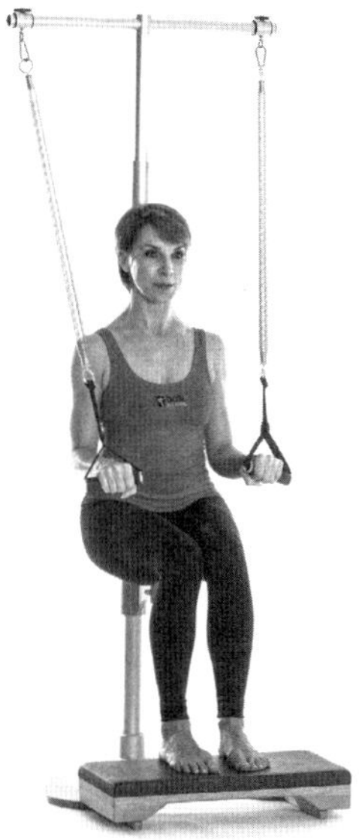

Setup. Stand (sit) with the back against the pole in a neutral spine position and the feet firmly placed on the floor, knees directly above the ankles. Keep the legs hip width apart and parallel to each other. Hold the handles and firmly anchor the arms by the sides of the body with the elbows bent at a 90-degree angle.

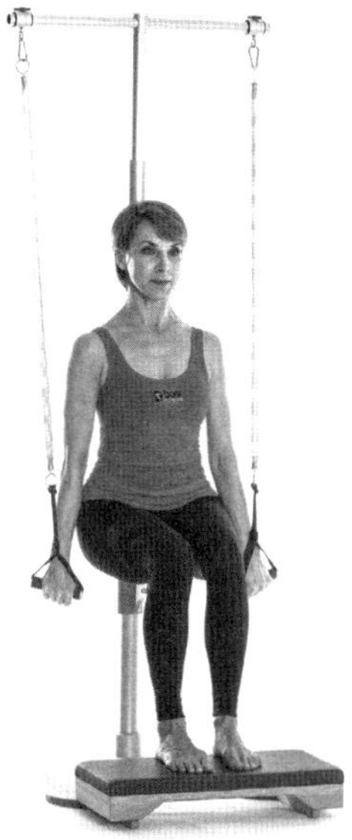

Exhale. Extend the elbows, straightening the arms.

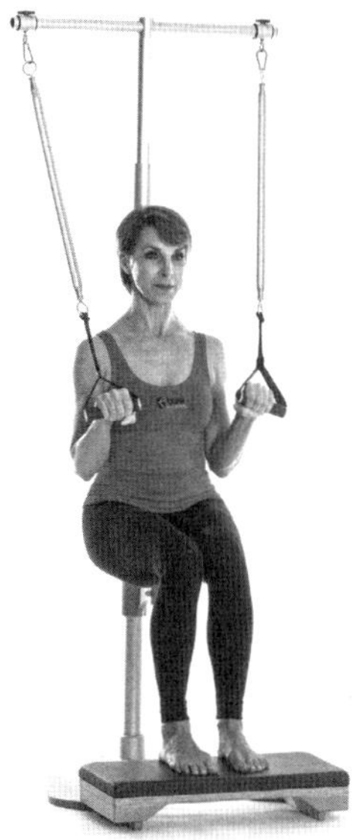

Inhale. Flex the elbows, bending the arms beyond the start position to work a greater range of motion. Repeat 10 times.

Muscle Focus

- Shoulder adductors and extensors

Objectives

- To improve shoulder adductor and extensor control and strength (depending on the resistance)
- To develop shoulder joint mobility
- To develop trunk and scapular stabilization
- To develop spinal alignment

RESISTANCE
Light | Medium | Heavy

Circle

The Ped-a-Pul: Circle combines shoulder adduction and shoulder extension. Starting in a T position, lower the arms to the sides of the body, followed by rotating the shoulders so the hands change from facing the body to facing back. At this point there should be a brief pause before the arms lift up again. Controlling the scapulohumeral rhythm (the relationship between the movement of the humerus and the scapula) is a crucial aspect of this exercise and is very important in establishing healthy shoulder function. The scapulae can rotate slightly to accommodate the movement of the humerus; however, scapular elevation should be avoided. The fact that the movement occurs below shoulder height allows the scapula to remain almost completely still.

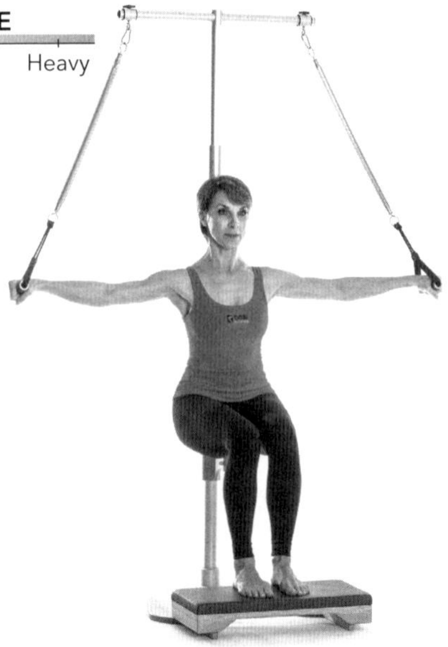

Setup. Stand (sit) with the back against the pole in a neutral spine position and the feet firmly placed on the floor, knees directly above the ankles. Keep the legs hip width apart and parallel to each other. Hold the handles and reach the arms out to the sides in a T position, with the palms facing down and a micro-bend in the elbows.

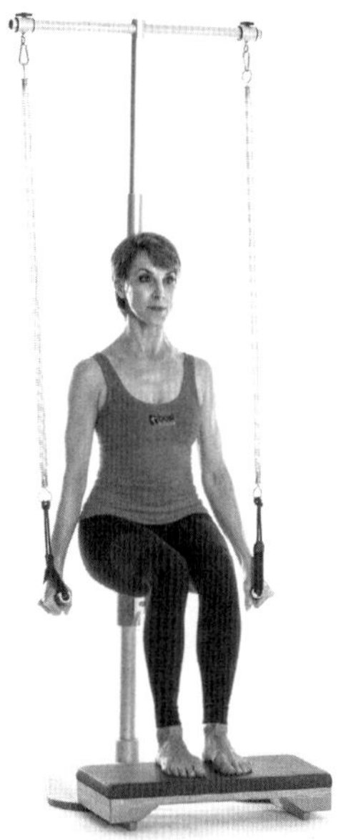

Exhale. Adduct the shoulders, bringing the arms down to the sides of the body.

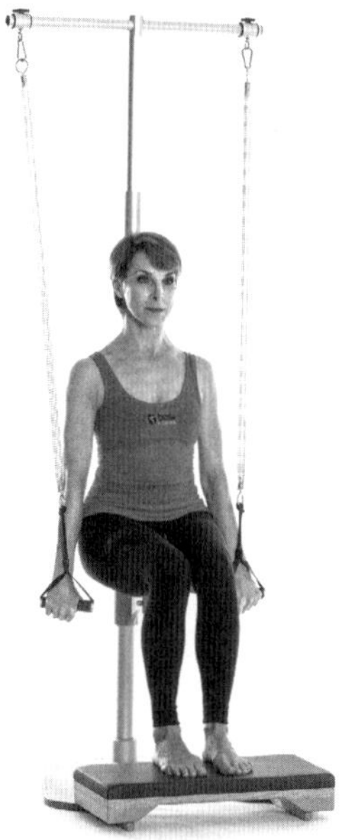

Continuing to exhale, rotate the shoulders so that the palms face back.

Imagery

The feeling should be that of stirring a huge pot of thick porridge. There should be no breaks in the movement, despite the slight pause as the shoulders rotate.

- Maintain scapular stabilization.
- Allow the scapulae to glide and rotate slightly according to the movement of the humerus.
- Maintain a neutral spine position.

VARIATION

Performing the Ped-a-Pul: Circle in both directions is very beneficial in terms of developing coordination and muscular control. To reverse the exercise, begin in the T position, and bring the arms to the front in line with the shoulders. Extend the shoulders, keeping the arms parallel to each other, and bring them straight down to the sides of the body in line with the hip joints. At this point, rotate the shoulders so the hands transition from facing back to facing the body. Lift the arms back to the T position.

In the Ped-a-Pul: Circle, the shoulder extensors work concentrically while the shoulder adductors work eccentrically. In this variation, the reverse applies. In Pilates, we train the muscle in isometric, concentric, and eccentric modes, an approach that is widely supported in the world of exercise science.

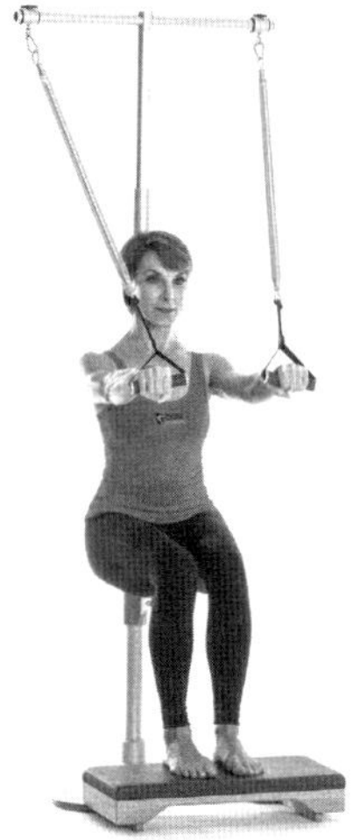

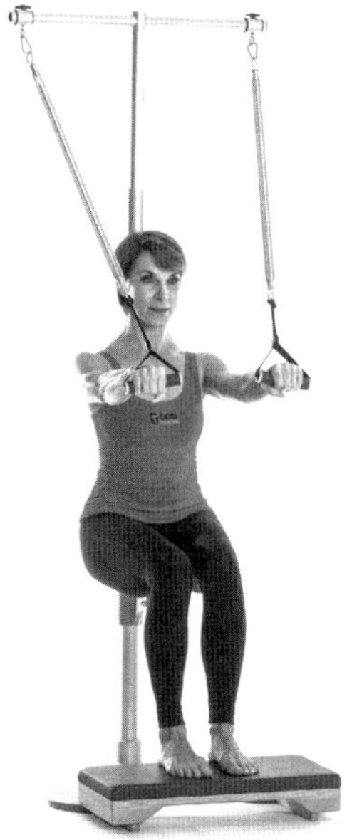

Inhale. Flex the shoulders, lifting the arms in front of the body to shoulder height.

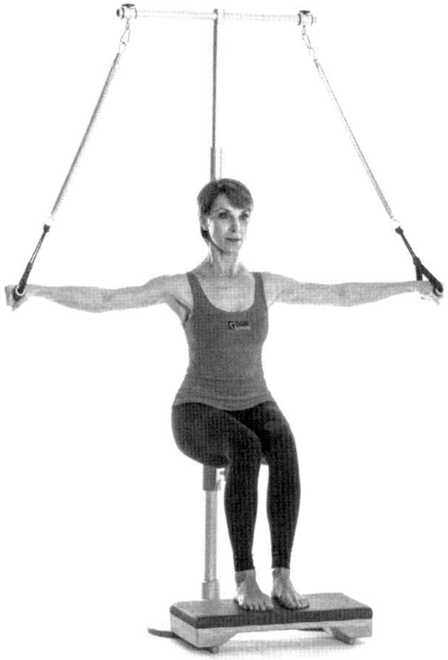

Continuing to inhale, horizontally abduct the shoulders. Return to the start position. Repeat 10 times.

Arm Chair

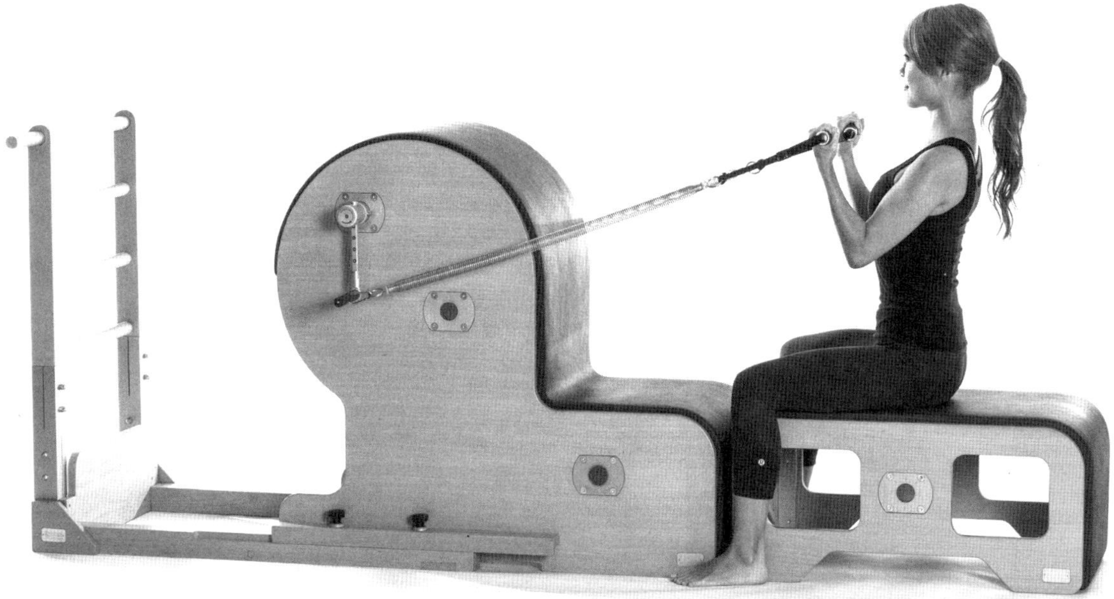

I would find it very difficult to run a Pilates studio without the arm chair. Yet, this piece of equipment is not often used; many Pilates teachers are not even aware of its existence. The arm chair is comfortable, user friendly, convenient, and effective for teaching and cueing arm work. I believe that it has enormous, and largely untapped, potential. As with the wunda chair, it is the simplicity of this apparatus that I find so appealing. The arm chair is relatively small and unassuming, yet it provides an abundance of opportunities for developing the entire body.

As the name implies, the arm chair in its traditional form is used primarily for the arms and shoulder complex. It is an excellent aid for teaching good shoulder mechanics and the concept of scapular stabilization during arm work. It offers support for the trunk, which is invaluable in the early stages of learning Pilates, specifically the upper body exercises.

Several contemporary versions of the arm chair exist, offering a variety of different benefits. In the first and second editions of *Pilates*, the arm chair described was one similar to the classic arm chair designed by Joseph Pilates. Now, in this third edition, I will focus on the F2 chair (introduced in chapter 8), a multifaceted piece of apparatus that addresses the entire body and works it in every conceivable position, range of motion, and plane of motion, which opens up a world of possibilities while offering all of the benefits of the classic arm chair. However, presenting the extensive repertoire of the F2 chair would far exceed the parameters of this book. Here I will focus on the arm work only, and I will continue referring to the apparatus as the arm chair. I encourage those interested to seek out further education and training on the F2 chair, as well as the F2 System in general. An entire universe will open up to you.

Although the resistance mechanism used on the F2 chair is highly adjustable and uses a specialized form of notating the resistance, for the sake of consistency I have simply provided a range of resistance.

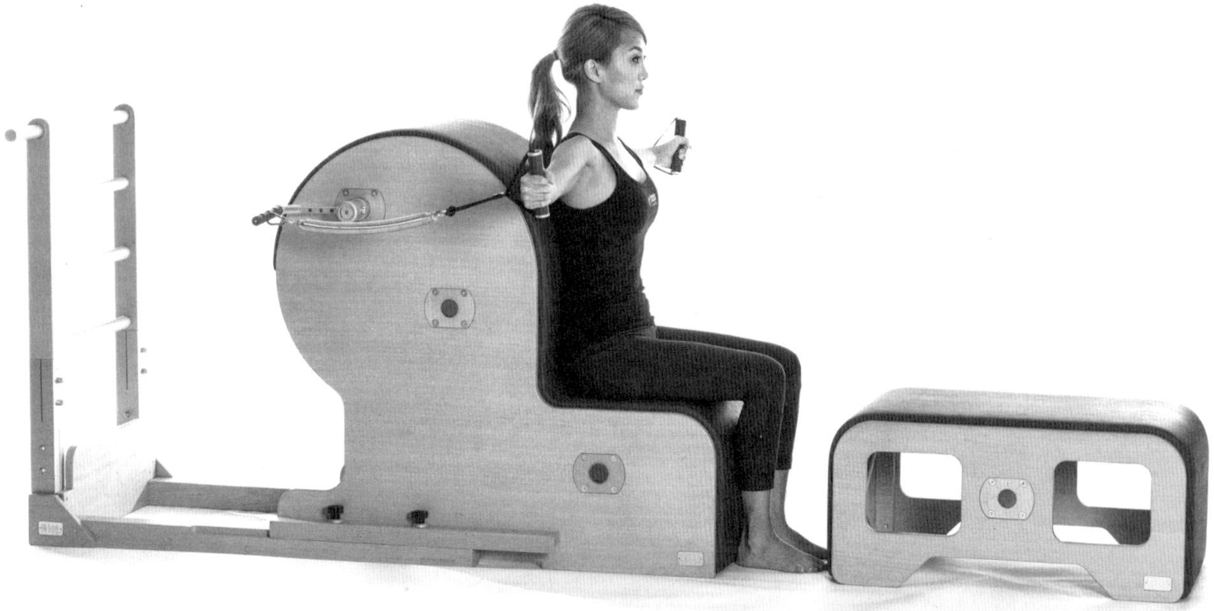

Chest Expansion

The arm chair offers an excellent position for performing this exercise, particularly for those with tight hamstrings who find it difficult to sit upright on the reformer with the legs straight forward (see Reformer: Chest Expansion—Seated). The trunk must be in an optimum position in order to activate the correct muscles and benefit from the exercise. It is surprising how little resistance is required to work the shoulder extensors effectively when the body is aligned correctly.

The most typical compensations or substitution patterns seen in this exercise are shoulder elevation, trunk flexion, and elbow flexion. These compensations occur when the resistance is too high or when strength, body awareness, and control are lacking. The arm chair can assist in overcoming these compensations and in laying the foundation for correct movement of the shoulders and arms.

Imagery

The sitting position on the arm chair promotes the feeling of elongation, of reaching down to the floor with the fingertips (or fists) and up to the ceiling with the crown of the head. I also encourage a slight elevation of the chest, which prompts deeper activation of the mid-back extensors. When I was a young dancer studying the Martha Graham technique, I had a wonderful teacher who spoke about the feeling of having a fishhook placed through my sternum with the fishing line pulling me upward toward the sky. The image, painful though it sounds, has always stuck with me; I think of it whenever I need to achieve a more upright position.

- Keep the range of motion relatively small (approximately 20 degrees forward of the trunk to 10-20 degrees behind the trunk).
- Keep the trunk stable and upright.
- Reach down to the floor with the fingertips (or fists), keeping the elbows straight.

PROGRESSION

Change the resistance and angle of resistance in this progression by moving the F2 lever where the spring attaches. In addition, place the feet on the seat with the legs straight and together, feet dorsiflexed or plantarflexed. This is a more challenging position, particularly for the hamstrings and back extensors, that will prepare you well for the Reformer: Chest Expansion—Seated.

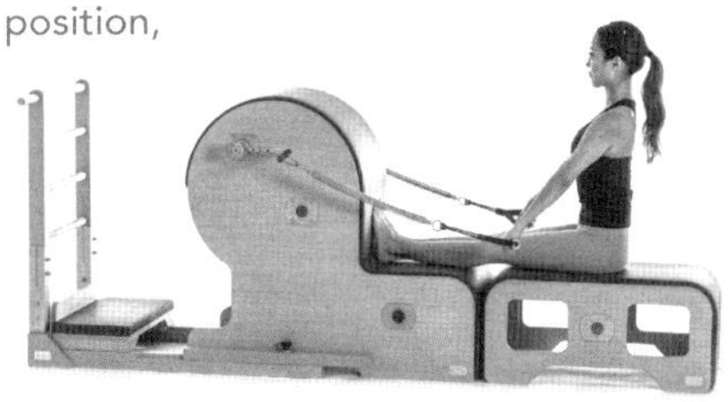

Muscle Focus

- Shoulder extensors
- Triceps
- Abdominals
- Back extensors

Objectives

- To improve shoulder extensor and elbow extensor strength
- To develop scapular and trunk stabilization

RESISTANCE

Light — Medium — Heavy

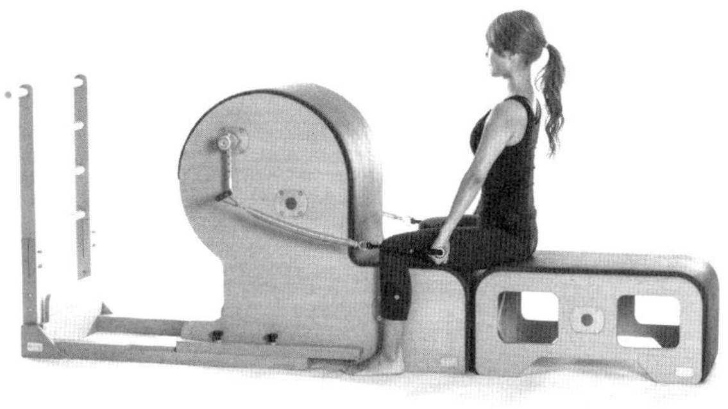

Setup. Facing the backrest, straddle the box in front of the arm chair, feet placed firmly on the floor. Hold the handles, with the arms straight and approximately 20 degrees forward of the trunk, palms facing back. Maintain an open-hand position (or fist) with the fingers reaching toward the floor.

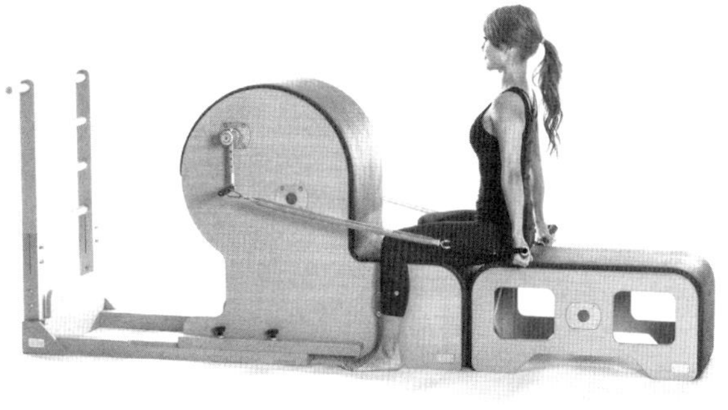

Exhale. Extend the shoulders, moving the arms straight back.

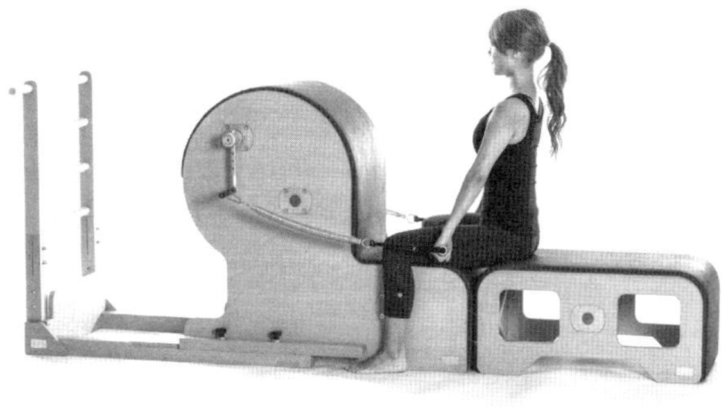

Inhale. Flex the shoulders, bringing the arms forward. Return to the start position (maintaining slight tension in the springs). Repeat 10 times.

Biceps

Muscle Focus

- Biceps
- Deltoids
- Abdominals
- Back extensors

Objectives

- To improve elbow flexor strength
- To improve shoulder flexor control
- To develop trunk stabilization

RESISTANCE

Light — Medium — Heavy

The Arm Chair: Biceps is an addition to the classic Pilates repertoire—one that requires good trunk stabilization with a focus on the back extensors, but is not hampered by tight hamstrings. The position of the body and the nature of the apparatus allow for a more comfortable sitting position and more resistance than the Reformer: Biceps—Seated. This is an advantage when the goal is to develop biceps strength.

Imagery

The arms should feel like they are weightless or resting on a table. This image helps take the stress out of the shoulders. The upper arms remain stable as the lower arms work independently, lifting and lowering like a drawbridge.

- ○ Keep the trunk stable and upright.
- ○ Keep the arms parallel to each other and prevent them from moving up and down.
- ○ Avoid scapular elevation.

PROGRESSION

In this progression the arms are held parallel to each other and to the floor, and the legs are straight forward on the seat. Both of these changes make the exercise more challenging. There is a tendency to flex the shoulders further when bending the elbows, which, although intuitive, is counterproductive. By adjusting the direction of the lever on the F2 chair as in the original version, the resistance originates from a lower angle, reducing the load on the shoulder flexors. This is a good example of the exceptional adjustability of the F2 chair.

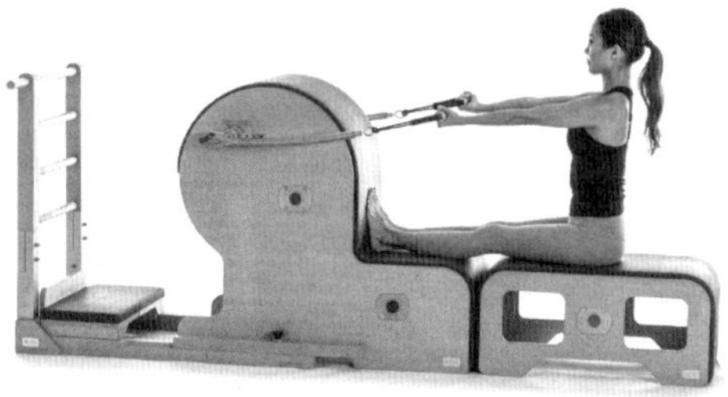

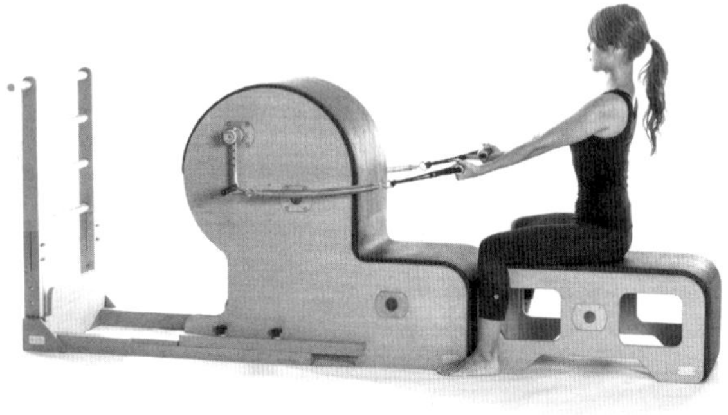

Setup. Facing the backrest, straddle the box in front of the arm chair, feet placed firmly on the floor. Hold the handles with the arms in front of the body, parallel to each other and in line with the spring, palms facing up.

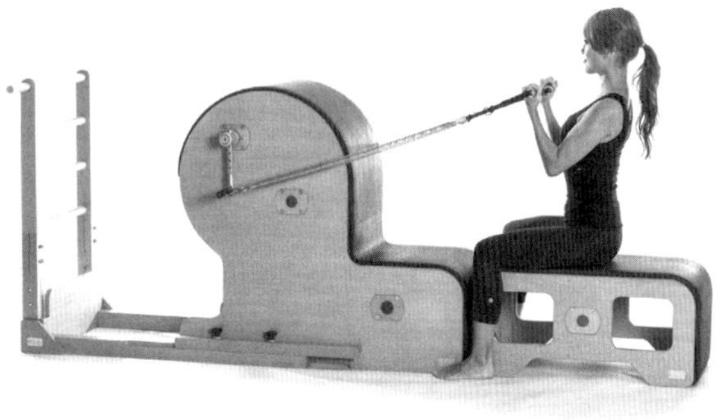

Exhale. Flex the elbows, bending the arms.

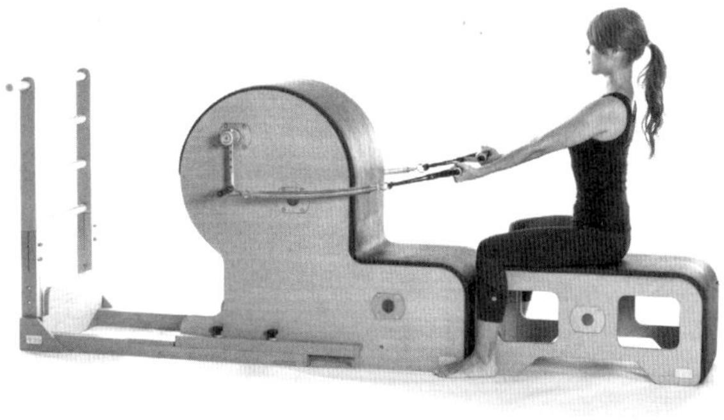

Inhale. Extend the elbows, straightening the arms. Return to the start position. Repeat 10 times.

Rhomboids

This exercise places the body and arms in a different position than the Reformer: Rhomboids—Seated, involving internal rotation of the shoulder as opposed to external rotation. Still, these two exercises have a great deal in common. In both versions the position and stability of the trunk are key to successful execution of the exercise. In both I recommend first isolating the shoulder horizontal abduction and only later adding the scapular adduction. Doing so isolates the glide of the scapula, rather than combining it with the movement of the arm, which invariably results in compensation patterns creeping in.

Imagery

The movement of the arms resembles a rowing action, although the trunk, which provides a stable foundation for the movement, remains still (in actual rowing the trunk would initiate the movement). Despite this difference, the image will assist in achieving the desired action.

- ○ Keep the trunk stable and upright.
- ○ Move the arms on a diagonal line.
- ○ Keep the elbows high, reaching out and back.
- ○ Avoid using the biceps excessively and bending the elbows beyond a 90-degree angle.

PROGRESSION

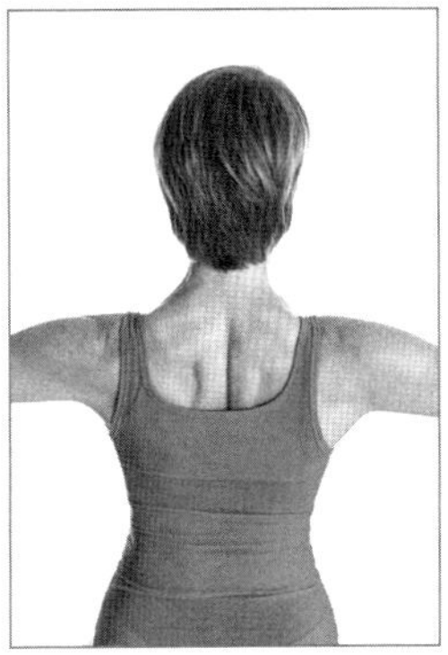

In this progression the arms are held parallel to each other and to the floor, palms facing down. Once the horizontal abduction of the shoulder is complete, add adduction of the scapulae. As you draw the scapulae together, continue pulling the arms back as if the humerus and the scapula are locked together and move as one unit. Reverse the sequence by abducting the scapulae followed by horizontally adducting the shoulders.

Muscle Focus

- Posterior deltoid
- Rhomboids
- Abdominals
- Back extensors

Objectives

- To improve shoulder horizontal abductor and scapular adductor strength
- To develop trunk stabilization

RESISTANCE

Light — Medium — Heavy

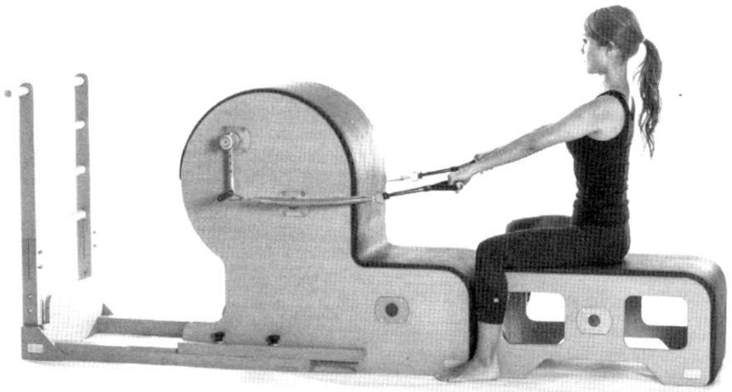

Setup. Facing the backrest, straddle the box in front of the arm chair, feet placed firmly on the floor. Hold the handles with the arms in front of the body, parallel to each other and in line with the spring, palms facing down.

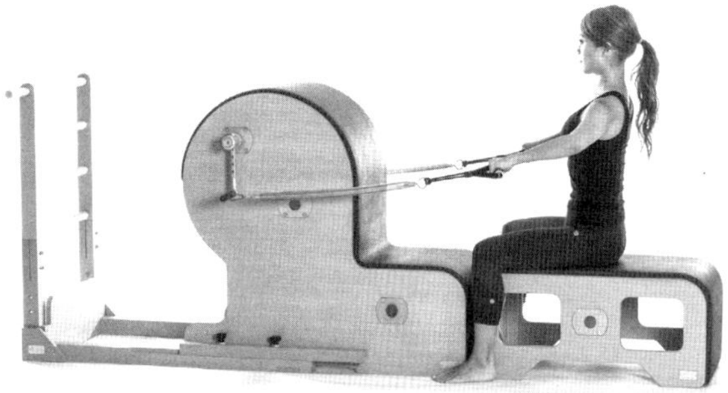

Exhale. Reach the elbows out to the sides and back without moving the scapulae, horizontally abduct the shoulders, and allow the elbows to bend until they are at a 90-degree angle.

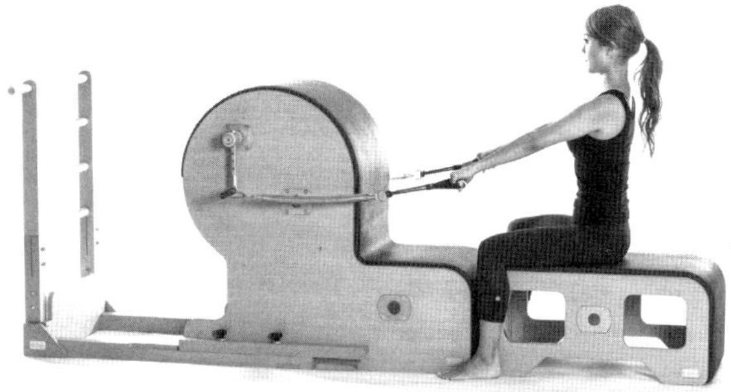

Inhale. Horizontally adduct the shoulders, straightening the elbows. Return to the start position. Repeat 10 times.

Hug-a-Tree

Muscle Focus

- Pectorals
- Abdominals
- Back extensors

Objectives

- To improve shoulder horizontal adductor strength and flexibility
- To develop trunk stabilization

RESISTANCE

Light — Medium — Heavy

Having the back supported while performing this exercise is invaluable. Not only does the arm chair support the trunk in perfect alignment as you develop the strength to hold the body in a good sitting position, but it also assists in maintaining scapular stabilization by providing a solid surface to press the scapulae against. As with the Reformer: Hug-a-Tree—Seated, the feeling of reaching out through the fingertips (or fists) with the arms elongated is important to maximize the work in the shoulder region and maintain the resistance in the springs.

Imagery

I love hugging (trees included!). However, the image of hugging a tree tends to result in the arms being too rounded, decreased range of motion, less load, shoulder internal rotation and possible elevation, and ultimately, diminished return when compared to performing the exercise with the arms straighter and only a micro-bend in the elbows. You should have a sense of being regal, with the arms open as if spreading your wings. As you bring the arms toward each other, imagine pressing against a large balloon. Finally, sitting on the chair should feel like sitting on a throne, upright and proud.

- ○ Keep the back broad and maintain scapular stabilization.
- ○ Avoid rounding the back as the arms close, and thrusting the ribs forward as the arms open.
- ○ Maintain elongation of the arms, without locking the elbows.

VARIATION

An additional variation that can be done with the feet on the floor or on the box is when the arms are parallel and in line with the shoulders, rotate the shoulders so that the palms face the floor. Rotate them back so the palms face each other again before opening the arms and returning to the start position. Besides being an excellent exercise for establishing good scapular stabilization and developing mobility of the shoulder joint, it is a good preparation for the upcoming Arm Chair: Circle.

PROGRESSION

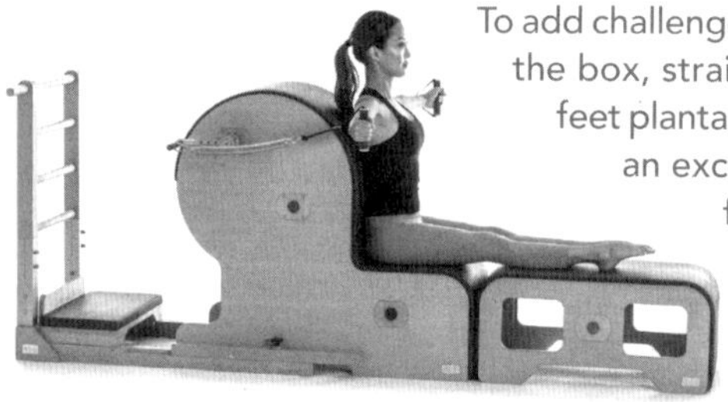

To add challenge place the legs on the box, straight and together, feet plantarflexed. This is also an excellent preparation for the Reformer: Hug-a-Tree—Seated.

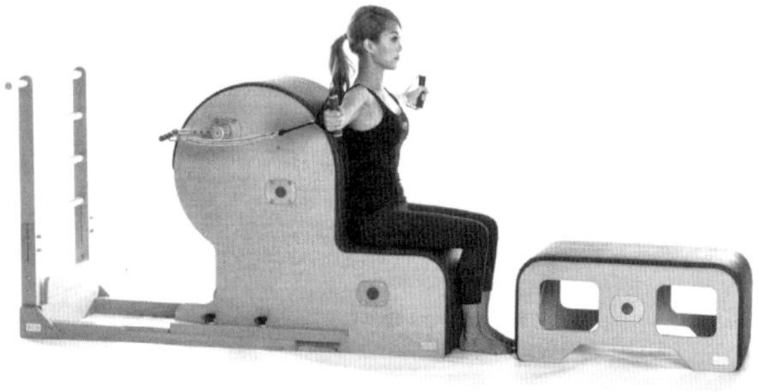

Setup. Sit with the back against the chair, feet placed firmly on the floor hip width apart. Hold the handles with the arms out in a T position, elbows slightly bent (micro-bend) and the palms facing forward. Use a fist or an open-hand position with the fingers reaching out to the sides.

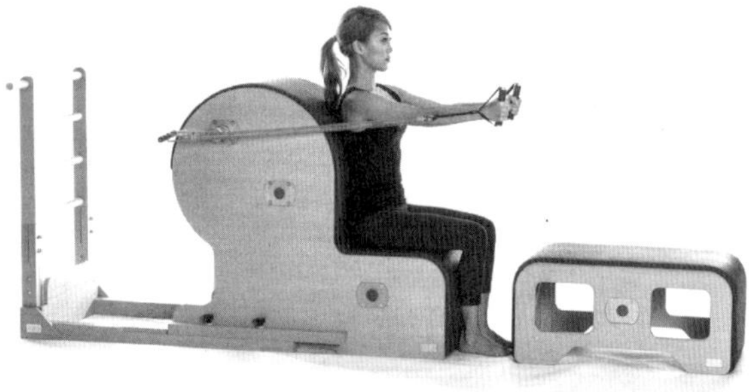

Exhale. Horizontally adduct the shoulders, bringing the arms toward each other until they are parallel and in line with the shoulders.

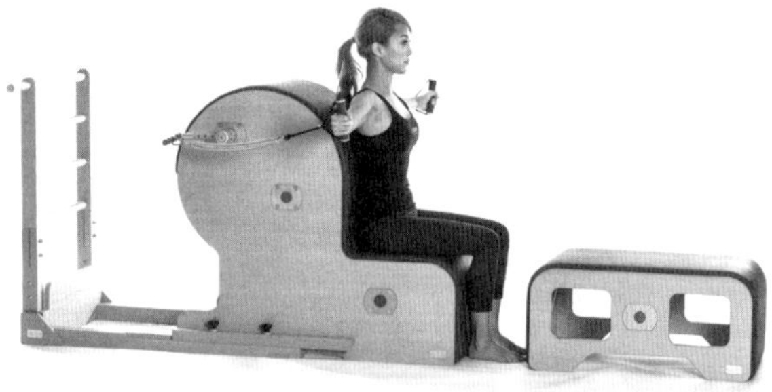

Inhale. Horizontally abduct the shoulders, opening the arms. Return to the start position (maintaining slight tension in the springs). Repeat 10 times.

Circle

ARM CHAIR

Arm Work

FUNDAMENTAL

Muscle Focus

- Shoulder extensors
- Pectorals

Objectives

- To improve shoulder horizontal adductor strength and flexibility
- To improve shoulder extensor control
- To develop shoulder mobility
- To develop trunk and scapular stabilization

RESISTANCE

Light | Medium | Heavy

Shoulder dysfunction is possibly the most common issue that Pilates teachers deal with on a daily basis. We repeatedly give cues regarding correct shoulder placement and shoulder mechanics—to release tension, avoid elevating the shoulders, or maintain scapular stabilization. This exercise is an excellent way to promote shoulder control and mobility. Although the movement may appear to place strain on the shoulders, particularly as the arms lift overhead (which would be contraindicated if any dysfunction, such as shoulder impingement syndrome, were present), this is not the case. Rather than lifting weight overhead, as they would with dumbbells, the arms resist the backward and upward pull of the spring, primarily using the shoulder horizontal adductors and extensors with minimal use of the shoulder adductors, abductors, and flexors. In fact, this exercise and the other arm chair exercises in this series can greatly assist in regaining range of motion after shoulder surgery or injury without loading the muscles excessively or stressing the region.

Imagery

Imagine that the arms are being lifted by a pulley attached to weights. As the weights (the scapulae) are drawn down the back, the arms lift up effortlessly. The weights and the arms are finely balanced; as the arms circle around, the weights move slightly in and out like small pendulums, responding to the movement. However, they always have a downward orientation, providing a feeling of weightlessness in the arms.

- ○ Keep the back broad and maintain scapular stabilization.
- ○ Maintain trunk stabilization.
- ○ Avoid rounding the back as the arms close, and thrusting the ribs forward as the arms open.

VARIATION

Reverse the direction. Starting from the T position, abduct the shoulders and bring the arms overhead. Extend the shoulders, pressing the arms down to shoulder height. Rotate the shoulders so the palms face each other, then horizontally abduct the shoulders, opening the arms.

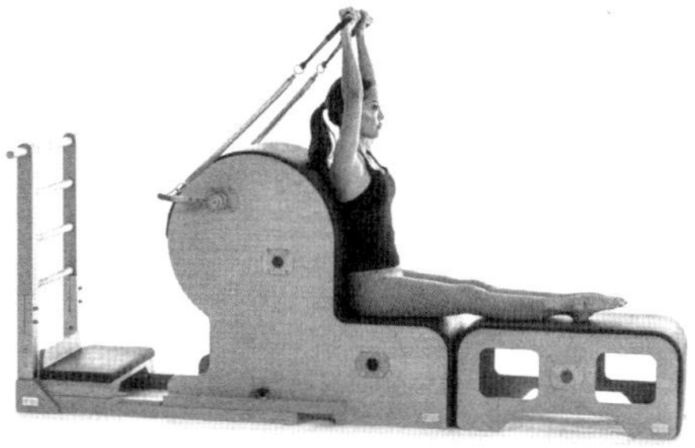

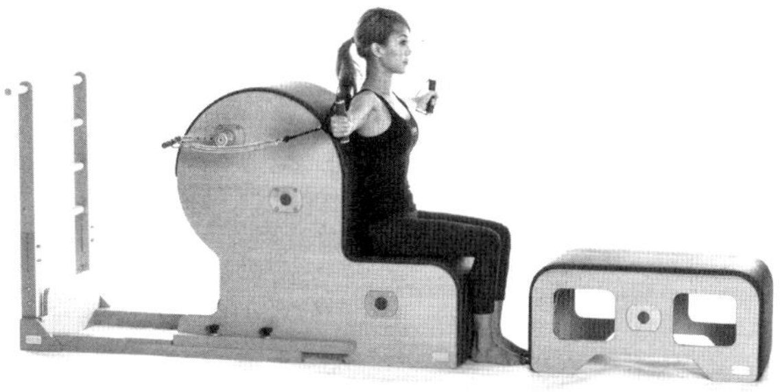

Setup. Sit with the back against the chair, feet placed firmly on the floor hip width apart. Hold the handles with the arms out in a T position, elbows slightly bent (micro-bend) and the palms facing forward. Maintain a fist or an open-hand position with the fingers reaching out to the sides.

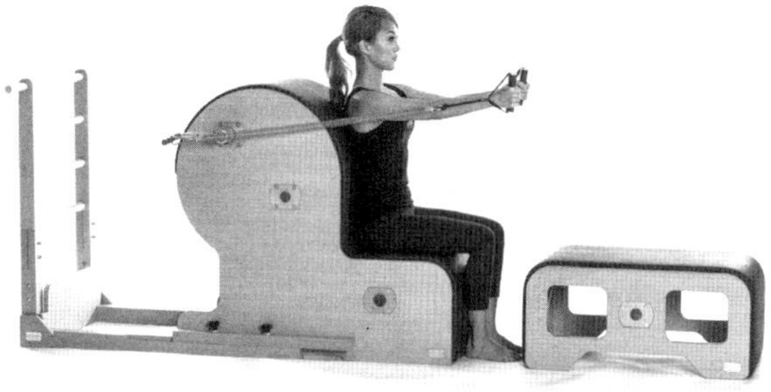

Exhale. Horizontally adduct the shoulders, bringing the arms toward each other until they are parallel and in line with the shoulders.

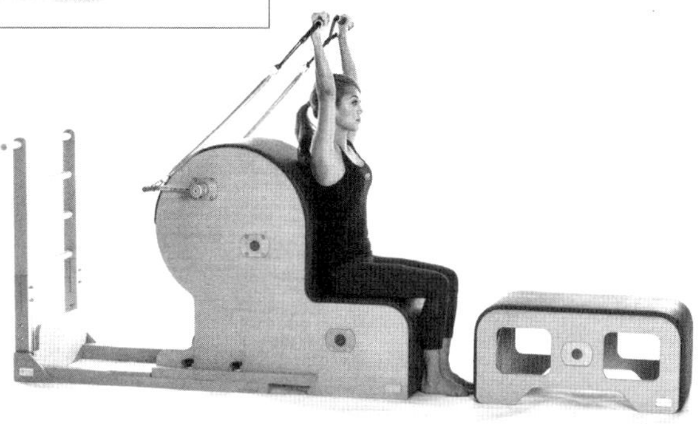

Inhale. Rotate the shoulders so the palms face down. Then lift the arms overhead and circle them around to the T position (maintaining slight tension in the springs). Return to the start position. Repeat 5-10 times.

ARM CHAIR
Arm Work
FUNDAMENTAL

Muscle Focus
- Triceps
- Pectorals

Objectives
- To improve elbow extensor strength
- To develop shoulder horizontal adductor control

RESISTANCE
Light Medium Heavy

Salute

This exercise is very similar to the Reformer: Salute—Seated, and like the other exercises in this series, serves as a good preparation for the more challenging reformer work. Keep tension in the springs throughout the exercise while moving the arms on a slight diagonal line, just above the horizon. Keep the elbows reaching out to the sides while the fingers (or fist) point forward throughout.

Imagery

As with the Reformer: Salute—Seated, imagine the arms gliding along a ramp slightly above the line of the horizon. The angle is no more than approximately 30 degrees, so that shoulder elevation is avoided. Focus on the feeling of an infinite line.

- Keep the back broad and maintain scapular stabilization.
- Direct the fingers (or fist) forward as the arms straighten and bend.
- Focus the work in the arms and avoid rounding the shoulders.

VARIATION

If you wish to focus the work more on the triceps, lower the elbows so that the arms are parallel to each other. This changes the focus from the triceps and pectorals to the triceps alone. As previously stated, the F2 chair allows you to adjust not only the amount of resistance but also the angle of resistance, which is highly beneficial in targeting specific muscles.

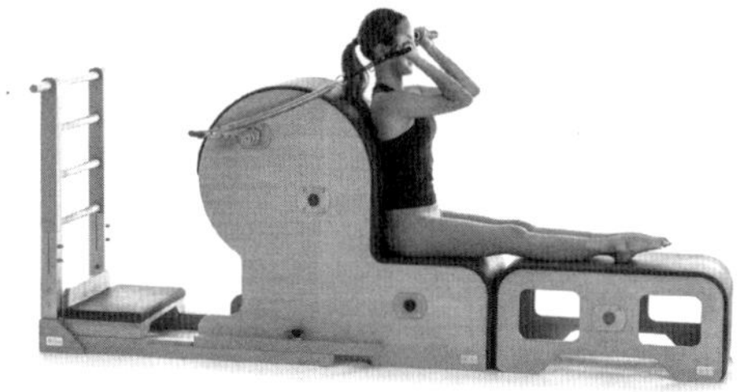

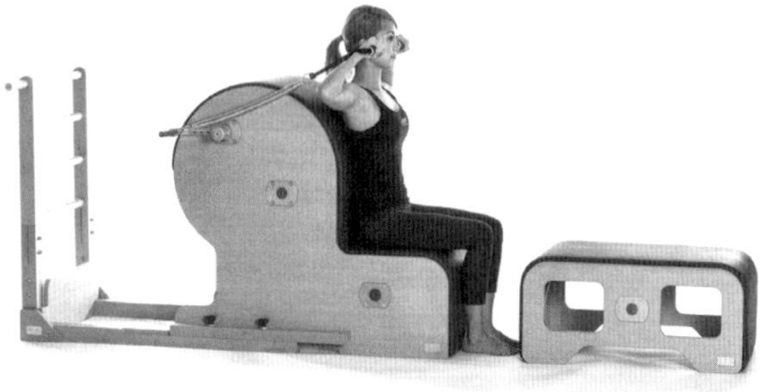

Setup. Sit with the back against the chair, feet placed firmly on the floor hip width apart. Hold the handles with a fist or an open hand. Place the hands opposite the temples at eye level, palms facing down and fingers facing forward.

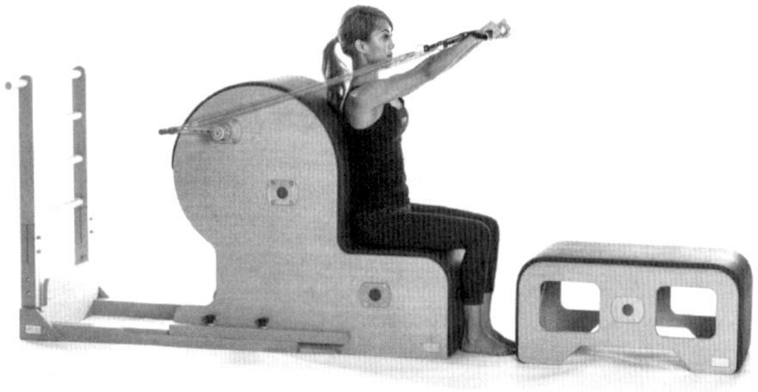

Exhale. Extend the elbows, straightening the arms on a diagonal line.

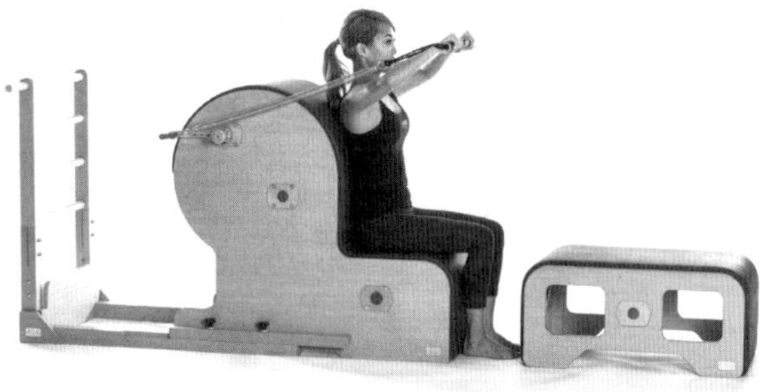

Inhale. Flex the elbows, bending the arms and keeping the fingers pointing in the direction of the movement. Return to the start position (maintaining slight tension in the springs). Repeat 10 times.

Magic Circle

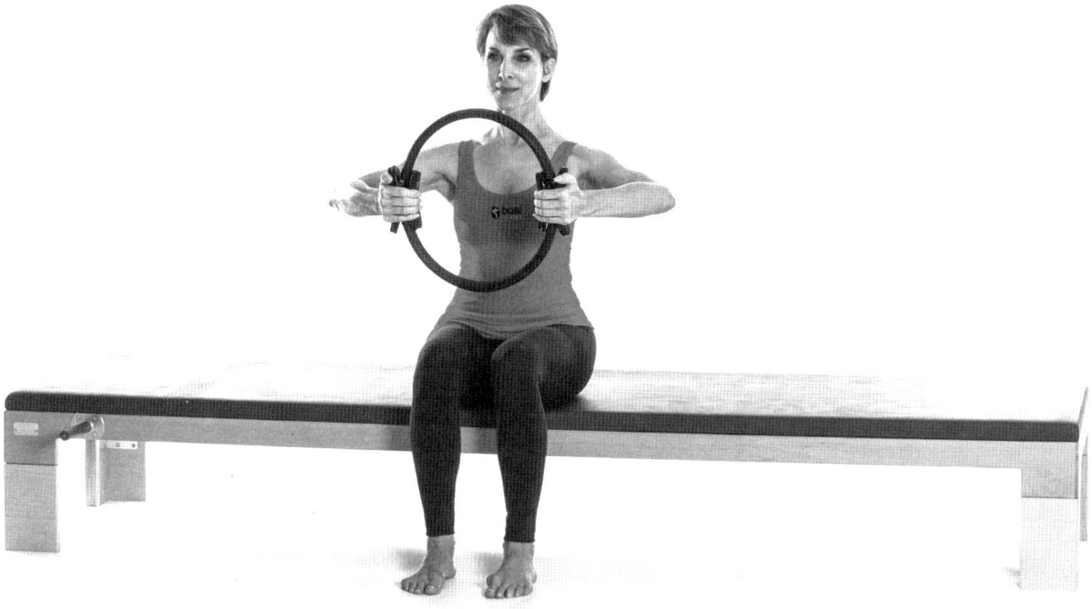

The number of aliases that exist for this simple ring reflects the wide variety of exercises that can be performed with it. It is the perfect travel companion, an ideal complement to a full apparatus session, and an excellent accessory to use in a mat work class to add variety, challenge, and excitement.

The magic circle can be used to keep the body in alignment or the limbs in a desired position—for example, by holding it between the arms opposite the chest or above the head. It can be used to encourage the continuous activation of a certain muscle group—for example, by holding it between the legs to help maintain adductor engagement. It can also be used to add resistance to a movement or heighten the level of coordination.

It often amazes me when I see some similar "new" device that works one or two muscle groups flood the fitness market and sell millions of units; often the magic circle works those same muscle groups, and does so much more. For instance, one popular piece of equipment is an inner-thigh apparatus that works the adductors—and that's it! The magic circle works the adductors just as well, but it also works the abductors, hamstrings, abdominals, back extensors, and arms. The secret is out, and the magic circle is finally receiving its long overdue credit.

Many types of magic circles are now available. Some offer more resistance than others; some are made of a super-light material and others are heavier. Choose one that suits your lifestyle and needs. In terms of resistance, err toward lighter rather than heavier. If you travel frequently and the circle is to become a travel companion, get the ultra-light version. If it is to be used in a studio and will need to stand up to the demands of continuous use, get the one that is the most durable.

The range of motion used in some magic circle exercises is very small (if any at all), requiring a dynamic, pumping action rather than a slow movement. These exercises can be viewed more like isometric exercises than isotonic. However, other exercises—typically those with a larger range of motion or where the muscles are stronger and at a mechanical advantage—demand a slow movement, holding the maximum contraction for several seconds before gradually releasing the tension (never completely), and then repeating.

Arms Bent

This is a fun, effective exercise to develop the chest muscles, and the pumping action involved is well suited to the magic circle. Be aware of recruiting the pectorals with each pump. Keep the round shape created by the arms consistent and the wrists firm as you squeeze the arms together.

Imagery

Although this image may seem a little graphic, try to bounce the pectorals with each pump. (This works for both men and women.)

- ○ Maintain ideal upright alignment.
- ○ Maintain scapular stabilization and avoid rounding the shoulders.
- ○ Perform small pumping movements.

PROGRESSION

This exercise can also be performed with the arms straight, further challenging the horizontal adductors of the shoulder.

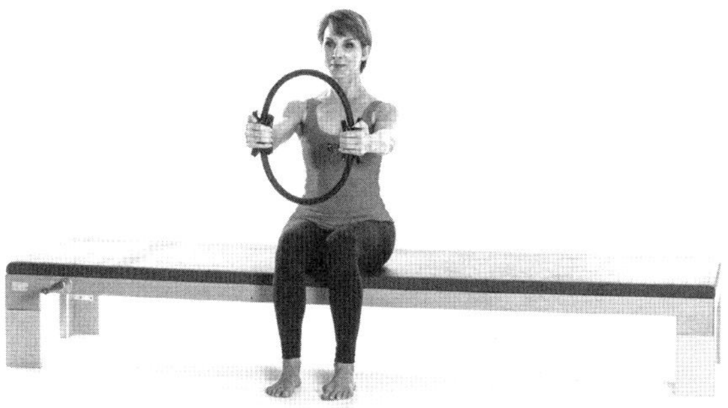

Muscle Focus

- Pectorals

Objective

- To improve shoulder horizontal adductor strength

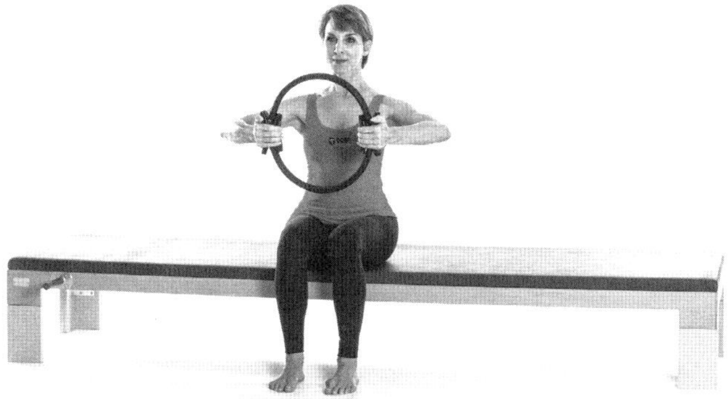

Setup. While sitting or standing upright, hold the circle directly opposite the sternum with the elbows bent.

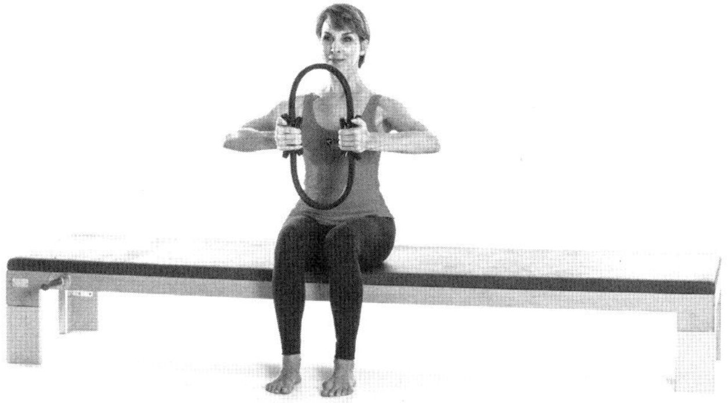

Exhale. Horizontally adduct the shoulders, pressing the arms together with small pumps for 5 counts.

Inhale. Maintain the tension in the circle and continue with small pumps for 5 counts. Return to the start position. Repeat for 5 breath cycles (exhale and inhale).

Arms Overhead

Muscle Focus

- Pectorals
- Deltoids

Objective

- To improve shoulder abductor strength (overhead)

This arm exercise is more difficult than it looks. Maintaining scapular stabilization and avoiding tension in the shoulders and neck are challenging enough, but adding the arm movement makes it even harder. The movement is so challenging that for most people this exercise will be purely isometric—the arms will remain still as they press together.

Imagery

This exercise never fails to evoke the image of a halo!

- ○ Maintain ideal upright alignment.
- ○ Maintain scapular stabilization.
- ○ Perform small pumping movements.
- ○ Lift the arms only as high as shoulder flexibility allows without elevating the scapulae.

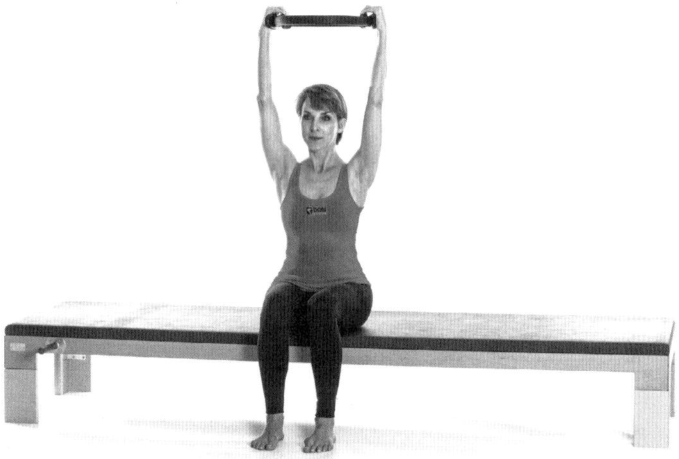

Setup. While sitting or standing upright, hold the circle overhead.

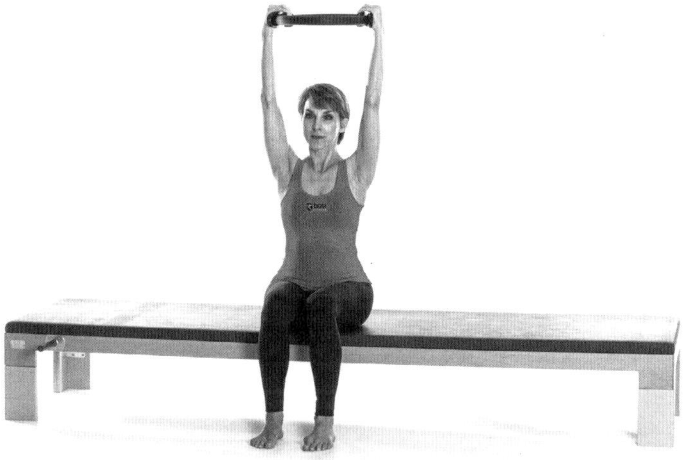

Exhale. Adduct the shoulders overhead, pressing the arms together with small pumps for 5 counts.

Inhale. Maintain the tension in the circle and continue with small pumps for 5 counts. Return to the start position. Repeat for 5 breath cycles (exhale and inhale).

Single-Arm Side Press

Muscle Focus
- Shoulder adductors

Objective
- To improve shoulder adductor strength

This exercise requires that you engage the shoulder adductors, particularly the latissimus dorsi and pectorals, prior to the pumping action and keep them engaged throughout the sequence. Maintaining scapular stabilization with the elbow slightly bent and reaching out to the side is important. The movement occurs in the glenohumeral joint only; the elbow remains stable.

Imagery

Imagine trying to pat the side of your leg, but the air is thick and gel-like and does not allow you to reach it. But you persist!

- Maintain ideal upright alignment.
- Maintain scapular stabilization.
- Perform small pumping movements.
- Avoid neck and shoulder tension.

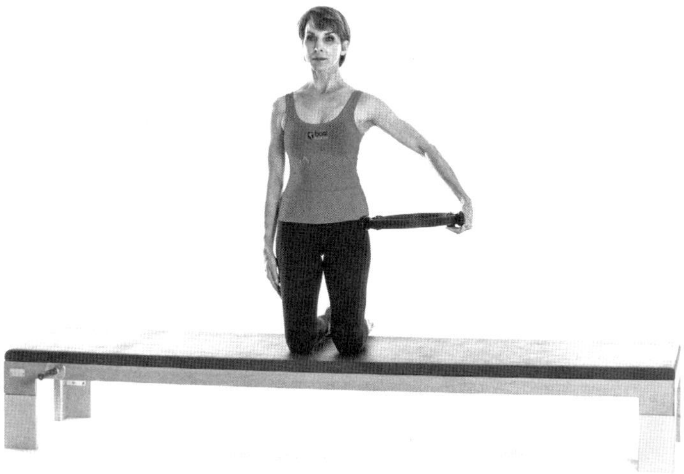

Setup. While kneeling or standing upright, hold the circle in one hand and rest it against the side of the thigh, directly below the hip joint. The elbow should be slightly bent and the shoulder internally rotated.

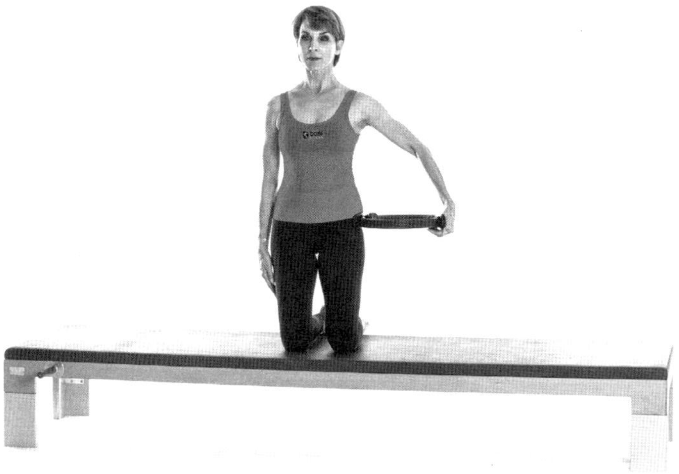

Exhale. Adduct the shoulder, pressing the hand toward the thigh with small pumps for 5 counts.

Inhale. Maintain the tension in the circle and continue with small pumps for 5 counts. Return to the start position. Repeat for 5 breath cycles (exhale and inhale) before switching to the other side.

Single-Arm Biceps

Muscle Focus

- Biceps

Objective

- To improve elbow flexor strength

I added this simple yet effective biceps exercise to the repertoire years ago when I wanted to provide a more comprehensive workout for the arms and upper body using the circle. Contrary to the pumping action of many of the other exercises, this exercise is performed slowly; compress the circle for several seconds before allowing the arm to lift up.

Imagery

This always conjures up an image of Africa, where I grew up. I would see the people, particularly the women, carrying heavy loads on their heads, often balancing them with one hand. Their posture was perfect as they walked gracefully, unencumbered by the enormous weight. This, to me, exemplifies the body in perfect alignment and balance.

- Press the circle straight down.
- Use the palm of the hand, not the fingers.
- Find a comfortable place to rest the circle on the shoulder.

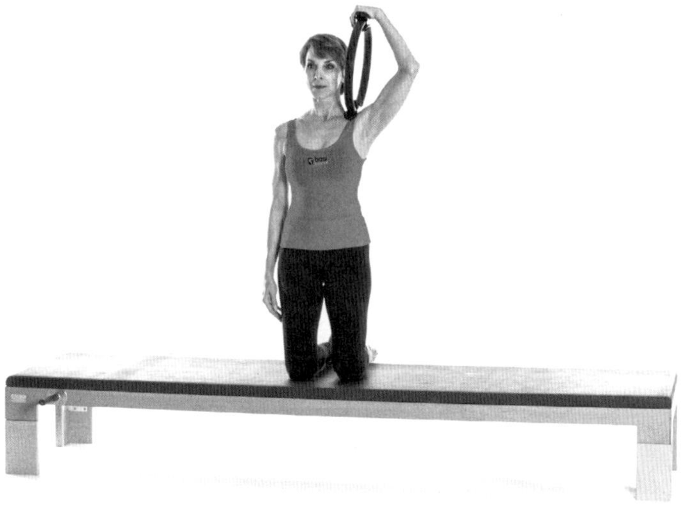

Setup. While kneeling or standing upright, hold the top of the circle in one hand and rest the lower side of the circle on the shoulder, directly above the joint. Bend the elbow and reach it out to the side.

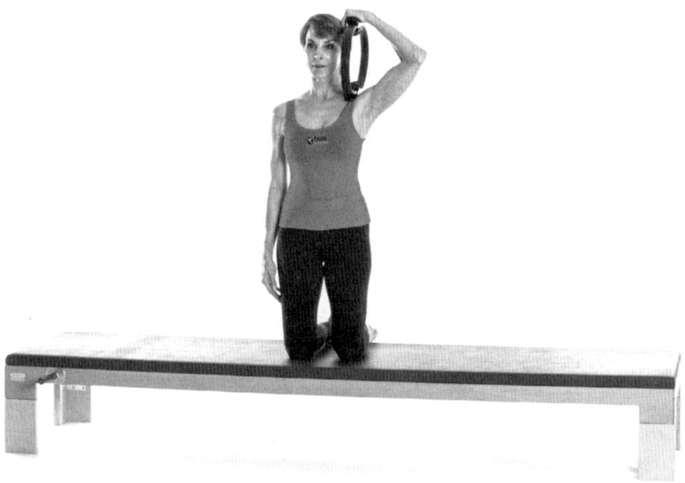

Exhale. Lower the hand down toward the shoulder, bending the elbow further.

Inhale. Lift the hand, maintaining tension in the circle. Return to the start position. Repeat 10 times before switching to the other side.

Above Knees—Seated

Muscle Focus

- Hip adductors

Objective

- To improve hip adductor strength

The hip adductor group is made up of several individual muscles originating and inserting at different points. Changing the position of the magic circle works the hip adductors slightly differently, with each position engaging the muscles in a unique way.

This first movement in this series is a straightforward, effective hip adductor exercise. However, you should also view it as a full body exercise, emphasizing the alignment of the head, trunk, pelvis, and feet.

Imagery

The imagery for the entire series of magic circle hip adductor exercises, whether performed sitting, prone, or supine, is about the hip joints moving freely without affecting the stable alignment of the rest of the body. The feeling should be like the head of the femur is a spoon stirring thick porridge, or moving in a soft gel.

- ○ Find a comfortable location on the inner thighs to place the circle where it will not slip out.
- ○ Press equally with both legs.

VARIATION

Try placing the magic circle directly below the knees and also just above the ankles. Placing the circle just above the ankles works the muscles of the feet as well as the hip adductors. The feeling should be one of gliding the legs toward each other, sliding the feet across the floor.

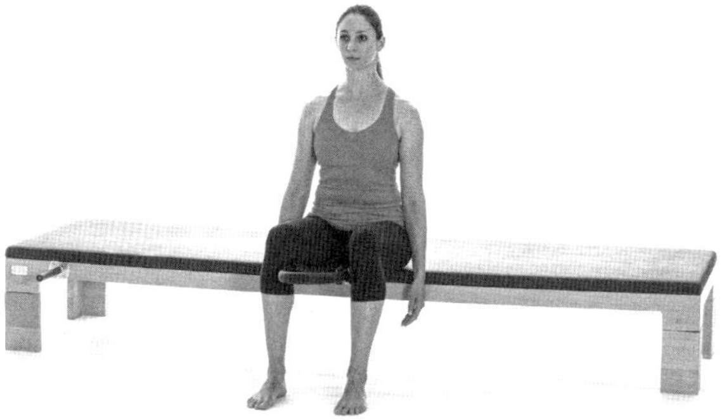

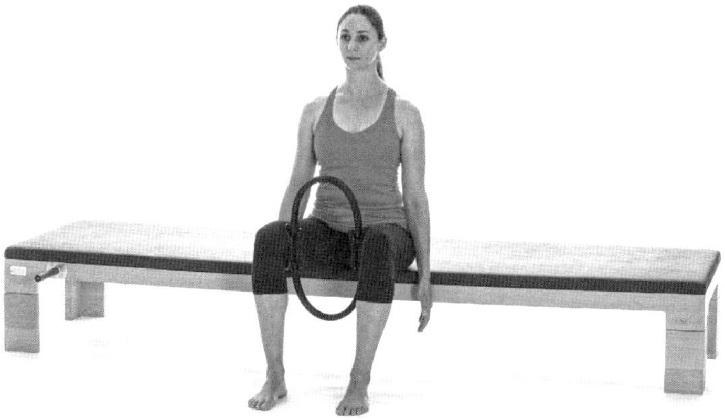

Setup. Sit upright with the hips and knees at a 90-degree angle, feet placed firmly on the floor. Hold the circle between the legs, just above the knees.

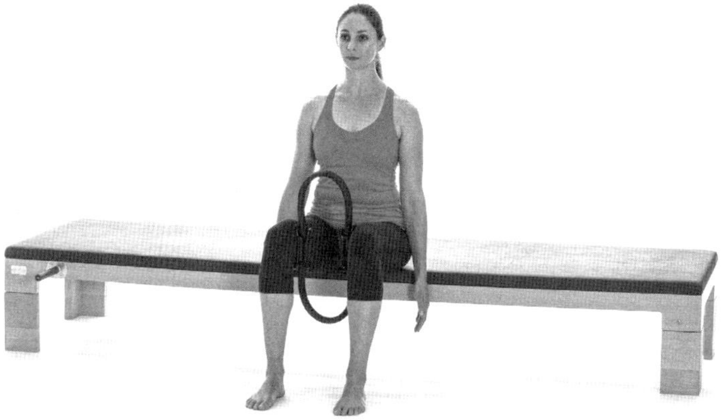

Exhale. Adduct the hips, pressing the legs together.

Inhale. Abduct the hips, opening the legs and maintaining tension in the circle. Return to the start position. Repeat 10 times.

Knees—Supine

Muscle Focus

- Hip adductors

Objectives

- To improve hip adductor strength
- To develop lumbopelvic stabilization

Although this exercise is geared toward strengthening the hip adductors, it requires good abdominal strength and exceptional lumbopelvic stabilization. In addition, it is an optimal position in which to work the pelvic floor muscles.

If you suspect that you lack the abdominal strength needed for this exercise, perform the modification instead.

Imagery

I like to imagine that the tailbone is a tail that lifts up between the legs, drawing the sit bones together. Visualize this image while hollowing the abdominals and squeezing the legs together to help recruit the pelvic floor and abdominal complex and deepen the work of the hip adductors. However, this is only an image and should not cause the pelvis to tuck under into a posterior tilt.

- ○ Maintain a neutral pelvis and neutral spine.
- ○ Keep the hips and knees at a consistent 90-degree angle.

MODIFICATION

If abdominal strength is limited, keep the lower back flat on the floor instead of maintaining a neutral spine position, even if this results in a slight posterior tilt of the pelvis. If the lower back rises off the floor into hyperlordosis or you feel tension in the lower back, place the hands behind the head, interlace the fingers, and lift the upper trunk into forward flexion (such as in the Mat: Chest Lift). If this position continues to place stress on the back, perform the exercise with the feet together on the floor.

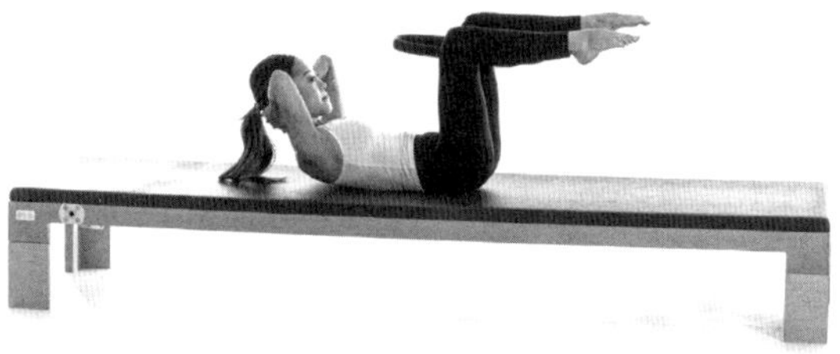

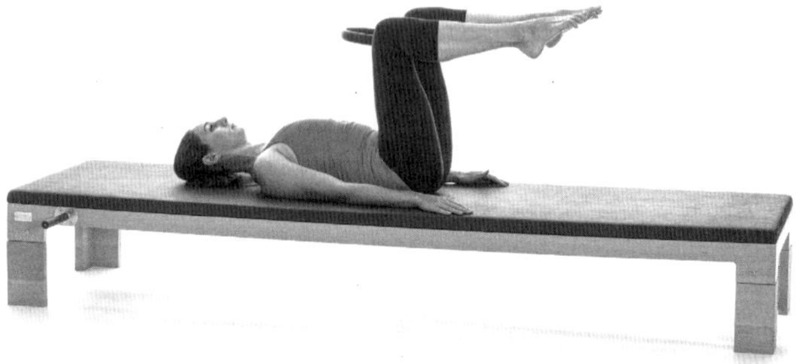

Setup. Lie supine in a neutral spine position, with the hips and knees at a 90-degree angle (tabletop position), legs parallel to each other. Place the circle between the thighs just above the knees.

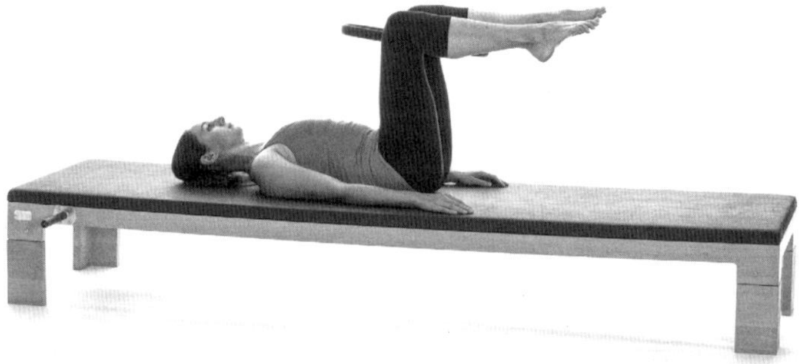

Exhale. Adduct the hips, pressing the legs together. Maintain the tabletop position, with the hips and knees at a 90-degree angle and the shins parallel to each other and to the floor.

Inhale. Abduct the hips, opening the legs and maintaining tension in the circle. Return to the start position. Repeat 10 times.

Ankles—Supine

Like the previous exercise, this one strengthens the hip adductors and requires good abdominal strength and exceptional lumbopelvic stabilization. Again, it has the benefit of providing an optimal position in which to work the pelvic floor muscles. However, because the legs are straight, the lever arm is longer, magnifying the work of the abdominals and hip flexors and demanding a very high level of control.

If you lack the abdominal strength needed for this exercise, perform the modification instead.

Imagery

The image of the tailbone as a tail lifting up while squeezing the legs together also works well here. Recruitment of the pelvic floor muscles and abdominal complex deepens the work of the hip adductors and helps to protect the lower back.

- Maintain lumbopelvic stabilization.
- Keep the legs at a consistent angle to the floor.
- Relax the neck and shoulders.

MODIFICATION

If the lower back rises off the floor into hyperlordosis or you feel tension in the lower back, place the hands behind the head, interlace the fingers, and lift the upper trunk into forward flexion (such as in the Mat: Chest Lift). If it is still too difficult, lift the legs higher, closer to a 90-degree angle. Bend the knees to further decrease the load. I also encourage doing the exercise with hip external rotation (turnout) as opposed to parallel. It works the hip adductors slightly differently and some may find it easier to maintain spinal support in this position.

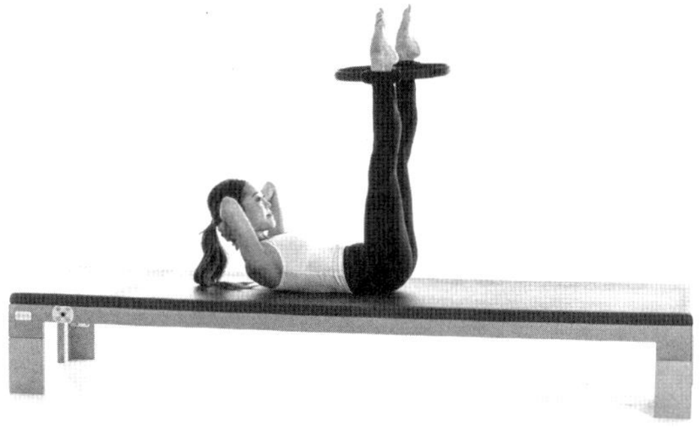

Muscle Focus

- Hip adductors

Objectives

- To improve hip adductor strength
- To develop lumbopelvic stabilization

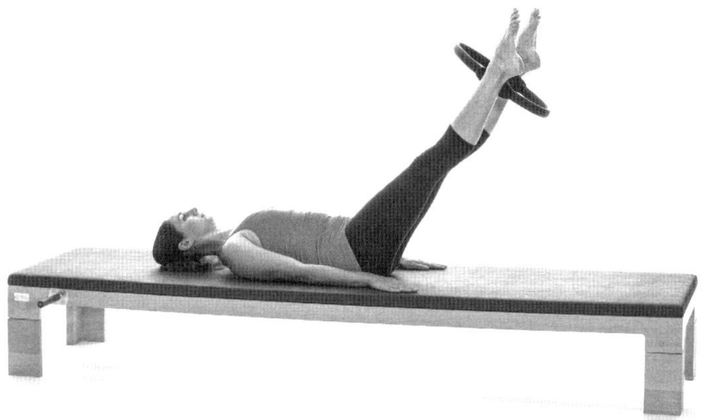

Setup. Lie supine in a neutral spine position with the legs straight, between a 60- and 90-degree angle to the floor (depending on your abdominal strength and lumbopelvic stabilization; the lower the legs, the more difficult the exercise becomes). Place the circle between the legs, just above the ankles.

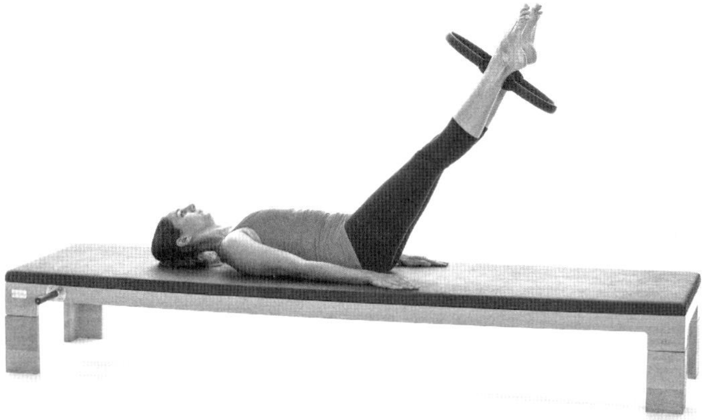

Exhale. Adduct the hips, pressing the legs together.

Inhale. Abduct the hips, opening the legs and maintaining tension in the circle. Return to the start position. Repeat 10 times.

Knees Bent—Prone

Muscle Focus

- Hip adductors
- Hip extensors

Objectives

- To improve hip adductor and hip extensor strength
- To develop lumbopelvic stabilization

This exercise is exceptional for building strength in the hip adductors and hip extensors. Keeping the knees bent and lifting the thighs off the mat throughout the exercise maximizes the work of the hip extensors, using both functions of the hamstrings (knee flexion and hip extension). Avoid the tendency to tilt the pelvis anteriorly and hyperextend the lower back, which places stress on this area. This is particularly pertinent when the hip flexors are tight or when the abdominals are not engaged sufficiently to counteract the anterior pull typically exerted by tight hip flexors. In such cases, draw the abdominals in deeper and push the pubic symphysis forward to emphasize a posterior tilt of the pelvis. If necessary, place a small cushion under the abdominal region to assist in achieving the correct position.

Imagery

The body should feel like an archer's bow that has been pulled taut. As the feet lift higher toward the ceiling with each squeeze, the bow becomes tauter and the arc is accentuated.

- ○ Extend the hips prior to squeezing the legs together and keep them extended.
- ○ Maintain consistent 90-degree flexion in the knees, feet reaching up to the ceiling.
- ○ Keep the hips parallel (as opposed to externally rotated) as the legs squeeze together.

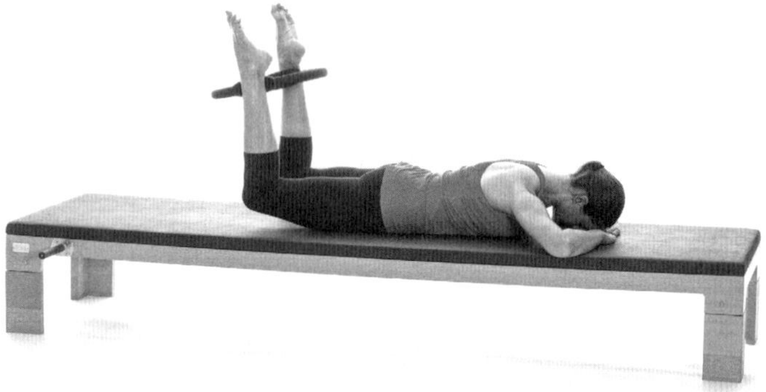

Setup. Lie prone with the knees bent at a 90-degree angle and the thighs lifted off the mat. Place the circle between the legs just above the ankles. Rest the forehead on the hands.

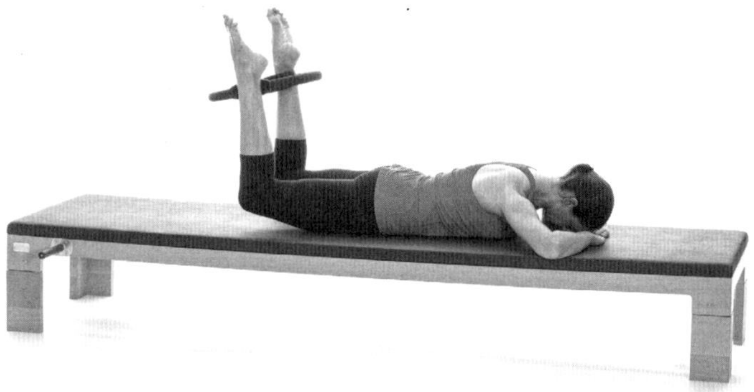

Exhale. Adduct the hips, pressing the legs together.

Inhale. Abduct the hips, opening the legs and maintaining tension in the circle. Return to the start position. Repeat 10 times.

Knees Straight—Prone

Muscle Focus

- Hip adductors
- Hip extensors

Objectives

- To improve hip adductor and hip extensor strength
- To develop lumbopelvic stabilization

Like the previous exercise, this one is exceptional for building strength of the hip adductors and hip extensors. Keeping the thighs lifted off the mat throughout the movement while contracting the adductors promotes profound hip extensor work. Avoid the tendency to tilt the pelvis in an anterior direction. Although the knees are now straight, which releases the taut rectus femoris, the lever arm has been lengthened, challenging the hip extensors and back extensors more and potentially placing stress on the lower back. This position demands a very high level of control.

Imagery

The image of the archer's bow is an excellent one for this exercise as well. In this case, the feeling is one of elongating into the bow shape with each squeeze of the legs, as opposed to lifting high.

- Extend the hips prior to squeezing the legs together and keep them extended.
- Maintain abdominal engagement with a bias toward a posterior pelvic tilt.
- Relax the neck and shoulders.

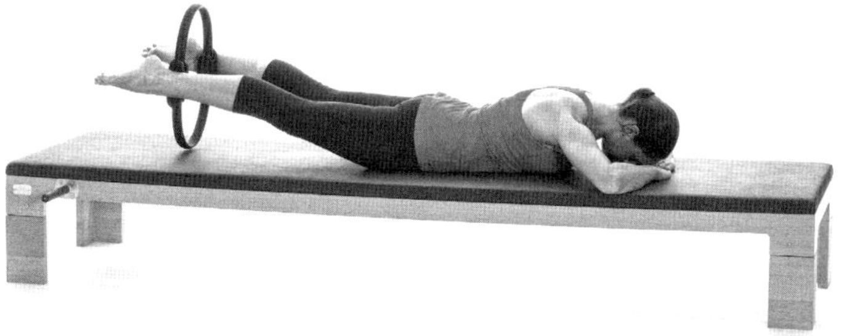

Setup. Lie prone with the legs straight and the thighs lifted off the mat. Place the circle between the legs, just above the ankles. Rest the forehead on the hands.

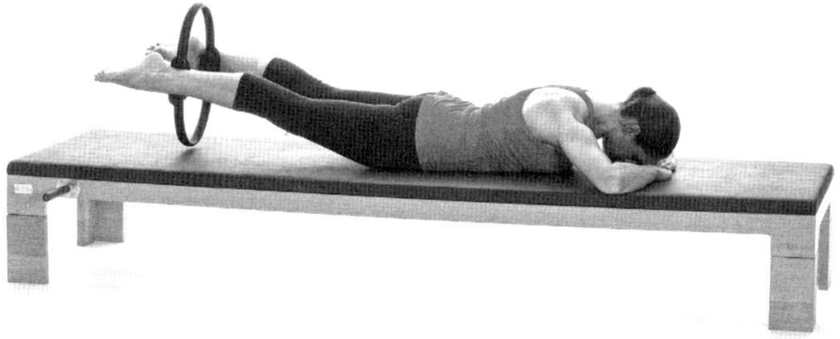

Exhale. Adduct the hips, pressing the legs together.

Inhale. Abduct the hips, opening the legs and maintaining tension in the circle. Return to the start position. Repeat 10 times.

MAGIC CIRCLE

Leg Work

FUNDAMENTAL

Muscle Focus

- Hamstrings

Objectives

- To improve hip extensor and knee flexor strength
- To develop lumbopelvic stabilization

Hamstrings

One of my students came up with this excellent hamstring curl exercise years ago; since then I have added the element of hip extension to it. The knee moves within a very small range of motion, if at all—however, if the goal is a small range of motion or an isometric contraction, then this will prove to be a useful exercise. I suggest orienting the pelvis toward a posterior tilt from the outset, using a cushion under the abdominal region, if necessary. That will counter the tendency to tilt it anteriorly, which often results in hyperextension of the lower back.

Imagery

Visualize the archer's bow position, and add the hamstring curl to further accentuate the arc shape. Maintain the bow shape with the working leg while the straight leg provides an anchor for the movement.

- Extend the hip of the bent leg before pressing the heel down, and keep it extended.
- Avoid externally rotating the working leg and keep the thighs close together.
- Maintain abdominal engagement with a bias toward a posterior pelvic tilt.

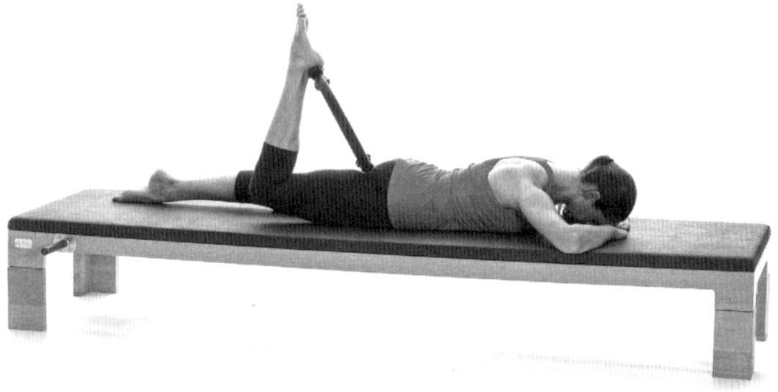

Setup. Lie prone with one leg straight and the other bent at the knee. Lift the bent leg slightly off the mat. Place the circle below the gluteals and above the heel of the bent leg. Rest the forehead on the hands.

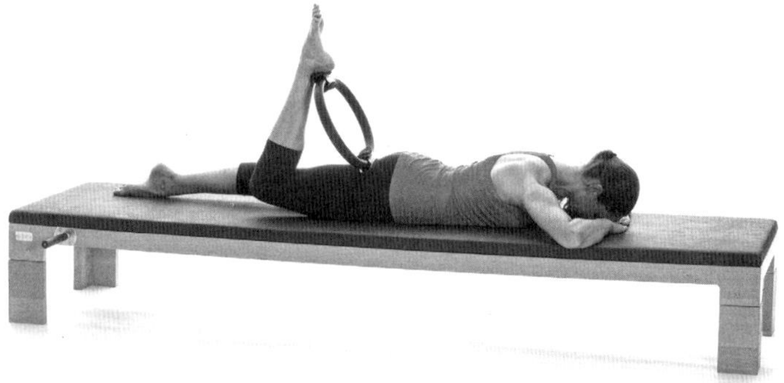

Exhale. Press the heel down toward the pelvis, bending the knee further.

Inhale. Lift the heel, maintaining tension in the circle. Return to the start position. Repeat 10 times before switching to the other side.

Swan

The Magic Circle: Swan is a challenging back extension exercise that is wonderful to integrate into a mat work class. It focuses on the upper and mid-back as opposed to the lower back. The lower back is often hypertonic, which tends to inhibit the recruitment of the mid- and upper back muscles. Extending the hips and lifting the legs immediately activates the lower back, plus it potentially distracts from the focus of the exercise. Therefore, the legs should remain anchored on the mat, as uninvolved as possible in the back movement.

The shoulder flexors feature prominently in keeping the arms aligned with the trunk. Ideally, the arms should line up opposite the ears. Make sure to keep the head aligned with the spine; avoid the tendency to lift it and look straight forward.

Imagery

This position begs the use of the image of a halo above the head (and promotes goodness in the world). This image also keeps the relationship between the head and the arms consistent.

- ○ Adduct the hips.
- ○ Focus on length as opposed to height.
- ○ Move the arms, head, and trunk as one unit.

MODIFICATION

In order to make this exercise a little easier, hold the circle in a horizontal position, parallel to the floor. This way, the back and shoulders start from a less challenging position and are not required to lift as high.

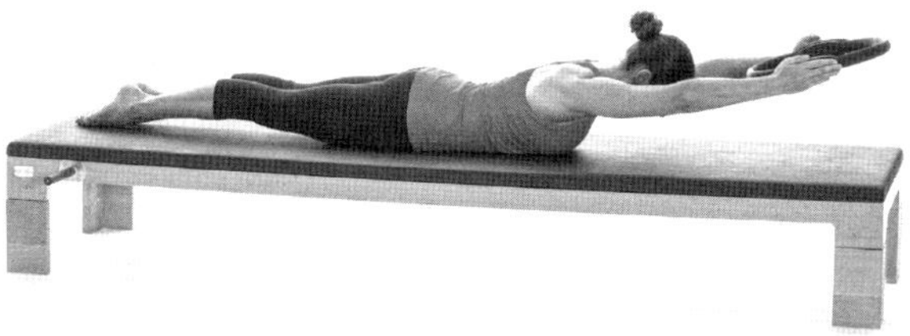

Muscle Focus

- Back extensors
- Shoulder flexors and shoulder abductors

Objectives

- To improve back extensor strength
- To improve shoulder flexor and shoulder abductor control

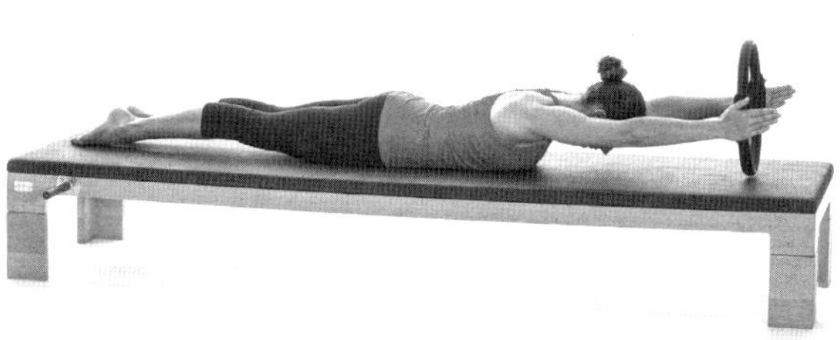

Setup. Lie prone with the arms straight and reaching overhead. Hold the circle in the palms of the hands and keep the legs anchored on the floor. Note that the position of the magic circle, vertical to the floor, will demand that the back is in extension from the outset.

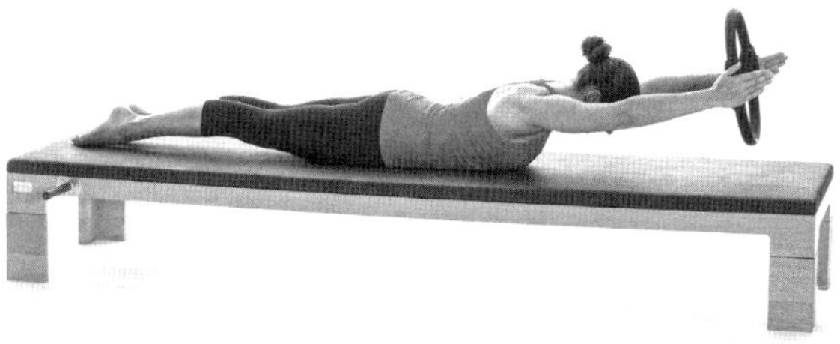

Inhale. Lift the upper body, extending the back and pressing the arms together.

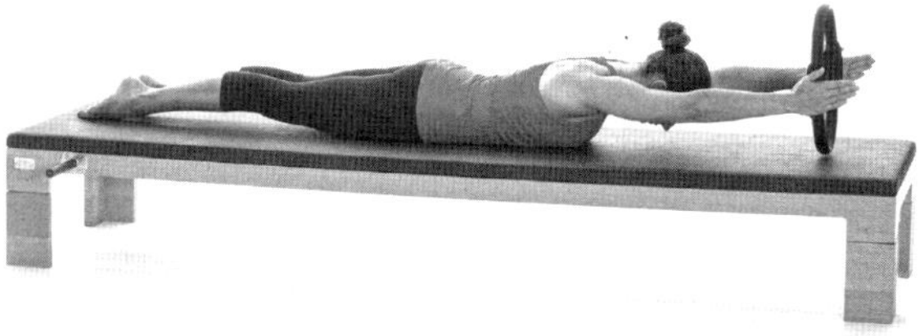

Exhale. Lower the upper body, maintaining the tension in the circle. Return to the start position. Repeat 5-10 times.

12

Sample Exercise Routines

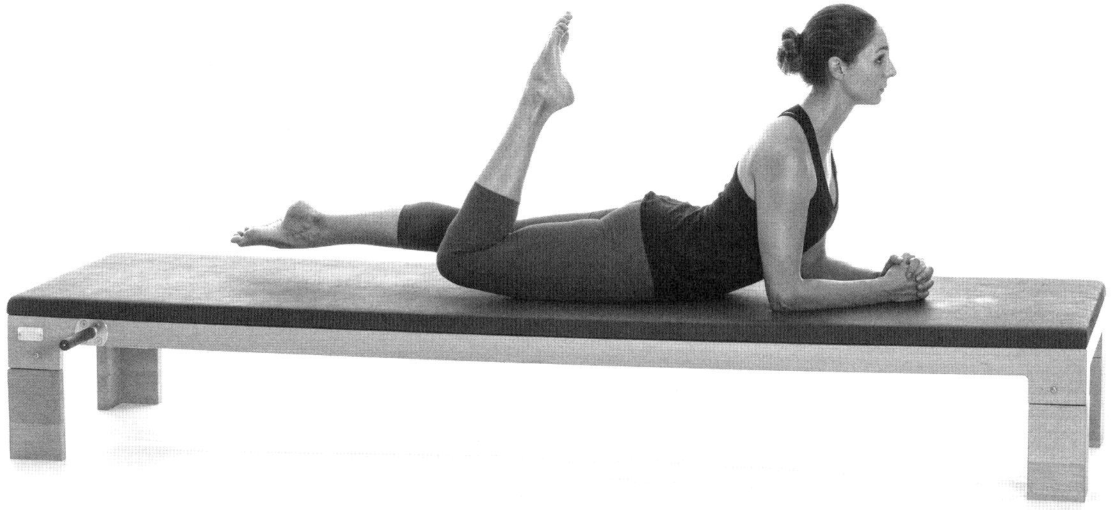

In this chapter, I provide several sample exercise routines for you to use in your Pilates practice. These will help you become acquainted with the exercises and learn how to sequence them effectively within the BASI block system, as described in chapter 3. This in no way implies that the exercises must be practiced in the order I suggest—I believe that keeping things fresh and being able to adapt to different situations is important. The block system merely offers a structure that promotes positive outcomes and opens the door to creativity without sacrificing clarity and direction.

For instance, when choosing arm work exercises, you can select those that best suit your current needs from a large pool of upper body exercises. You may also choose from a selection of *arm series,* a preset compilation of arm exercises that together form a complementary, integrated, and balanced exercise unit. The same goes for each block—you can choose individual exercises or series of exercises (where applicable). Practicing set routines—whether those offered here or those that you create—so that they become second nature will undoubtedly prove advantageous and beneficial. The block system helps you reinforce these routines while keeping the work exciting and fresh.

Sequencing Exercises

Once you have learned the exercises, you should then incorporate them into a comprehensive, flowing routine. The mat work particularly lends itself to seamless transitions and unobstructed flow—one continuous movement from beginning to end. It starts with the first breath of the setup and continues to the final breath of relaxation at the end.

I have been greatly influenced by years of dance and Ashtanga yoga, as well as a familiarity with tai chi and martial arts. These disciplines all share the quality of continuous movement—what I think of as *flow.* As explained in chapter 4, the mat block system incorporates what I call *flow sequences,* and flow is the underlying quality in each exercise and routine. Although maintaining the same degree of flow when working on the apparatus is more difficult, you should always experience a feeling of fluidity and inner focus. Apart from helping you feel good and look beautiful, flow offers physiological benefits: It heightens the cardiovascular effect, elevates the body temperature, and builds muscular endurance. Flow also brings mental benefits, including concentration and release of tension. Together these characteristics culminate in a state I refer to as *meditation in motion.*

Creating transitions from exercise to exercise to make the sequence flow is a stimulating process. Whether on the mat or the apparatus, transitions should be choreographed as an integral part of the routine so that there is no need to stop, reposition, and start again, which wastes energy and breaks concentration. Although they are important, however, the transitions should not dictate the order of the exercises. The order must be determined by physiological principles, addressing the planes of motion, muscle groups, and safe progression. This is the premise of the block system.

The following guidelines will help you in compiling a session. These guidelines apply to every session, whether it lasts 10 minutes or 60 minutes, whether it is done on the mat or on the apparatus, and whether it is fundamental or advanced.

- Progress from less demanding exercises to more demanding ones.
- Perform large muscle group exercises earlier in the session.
- Perform lower risk exercises earlier in the session.
- Keep programs progressive in the use of range of motion, load, complexity, and speed.
- Address as many muscle groups as possible during a session.

- Practice the different functions of the muscles: stabilization and mobilization.
- Incorporate all types of muscle contraction: isometric, concentric, and eccentric.
- Include all ranges of motion (flexion, lateral flexion, rotation, and extension), including in combination.
- Balance the exercises according to the primary joints and their movements (such as hip flexion, hip extension, hip abduction, hip adduction, and hip rotation).
- Emphasize a particular area based on individual needs while maintaining a good overall balance.
- Include more challenging exercises after an adequate warm-up.
- Add exercises that focus on balance and proprioception.
- Work the mind and body together in harmony.

Be cognizant that to make a program effective and to see continued gains, you must gradually and consistently make the exercises more challenging. Effective cueing, using accessories such as rubber bands, modifying the exercises, adjusting the resistance, and introducing variations and more difficult progressions (keeping the muscle focus consistent) can all help achieve this goal.

Individualizing a Sequence

Perhaps the most valuable quality of the Pilates method is its adaptability—it can cater to a broad range of people with differing needs, from those restricted in mobility to elite athletes. It can accommodate the young, older adults, fit, unfit, dancers, athletes, pregnant women, and those rehabilitating from injury or surgery. It is as beneficial for men as for women. I do not believe any other system offers such diversity while still challenging each person's capabilities to the maximum. Best of all is the calm, trusting, nurturing, and noncompetitive environment that is typical of most Pilates studios. It is important to reiterate, however: Although Pilates is suited to *anyone*, not *everyone* will enjoy or relate to this type of work.

The extensive body of exercises, along with the choice of apparatus, allows the compilation of a program to be tailored to each individual. The decision to introduce new exercises should be well thought out. Adding challenging and more advanced exercises is tempting, but new repertoire can be counterproductive if it is not appropriate or you are not adequately prepared for it. You must assess whether an exercise

CHANGING UP YOUR PRACTICE

It is beyond the scope of this chapter to provide exercise sequences to suit every need. However, you can use the routines in this book as a foundation and adapt them to meet your needs or those of your students. In this third edition of *Pilates*, I have provided a modification, variation, or progression for the vast majority of exercises. An excellent way of customizing these routines for different populations or individuals is to maintain the structure and exercises of each program but change out specific exercises with the alternative option offered for that exercise. Your choice can include a modification, progression, or variation based on whether you want the program to be more accessible, more challenging, or just offer more variety. In this way these programs can be refreshed and reused repeatedly, always offering a new perspective.

is of a suitable level, whether it will affect any injured areas adversely, whether it will help achieve a desired goal, and whether you (or your student) have adequate training and skills to perform it.

If you are a teacher designing a program, I encourage you to find out as much as possible about the individual you are working with. More important than what to do is what *not* to do, particularly in cases in which the wrong exercise may result in injury or even irreparable damage. Become intricately familiar with the repertoire, be well educated in the science of human movement, know the body you are working with, and then be creative in developing options—never losing sight of the essence of the exercise. Err on the side of caution and seek further professional advice (medical and otherwise) as needed. Two concepts are ever-present for me, whether practicing the work or teaching it—*when in doubt, find out* and *be safe, not sorry*! When used as it was intended, Pilates can be the answer to anyone's quest for well-being.

Adapting Routines for Select Populations

Select populations is a general term that describes groups with specific needs. There are two main groups: people for whom you may need to *decrease* the intensity of the work and people for whom you may want to *increase* the intensity of the work. The first group, which includes older adults, the injured, and people going through some form of rehabilitation, typically requires modification of the exercises and the use of assists, such as cushions, rubber bands, and springs. The second group, which includes athletes and dancers, consists of those who may need increased intensity or complexity. Both groups need specifically tailored programs, often based on vastly different goals. Some populations may fit both of these categories to varying degrees. Pregnant women, for example, require modification and monitoring to suit their constantly changing bodies, yet at the same time they are often fit, athletic, and not limited in the same sense as those who are going through rehabilitation.

Even within these groupings, the goals may vary greatly. For instance, athletes often need *specificity training*, in which they work on activity-specific skills and develop the neuromuscular system to improve performance. However, they may also need *cross-training* to improve general balance (in the broadest sense of the word) and enhance their overall conditioning program. Pilates is exceptional for both. Making subtle changes in the program—choice of exercises, resistance, and number of repetitions—can all affect the outcome.

FUNDAMENTALS TO TAKE ON THE ROAD

If I told you about the many—and often odd—places I have practiced Pilates, it would surely bring a smile to your face! I do an enormous amount of traveling, and I always take the essentials on the road with me. This usually consists of a mat and some small accessories such as rubber bands and a magic circle (although the circle has become the cause of growing scrutiny at airport security checks). The beauty of Pilates is that you can compile a program for every occasion and any location with the guidelines outlined in this chapter. Remember that consistency is the key, and if you let your Pilates practice lapse while you are traveling, all your hard work is diminished. Regular practice will keep you alert, in shape, and on top of your game at all times, even when sunning yourself on a beach in Hawaii or hiking in the Himalayas!

Considering Safety

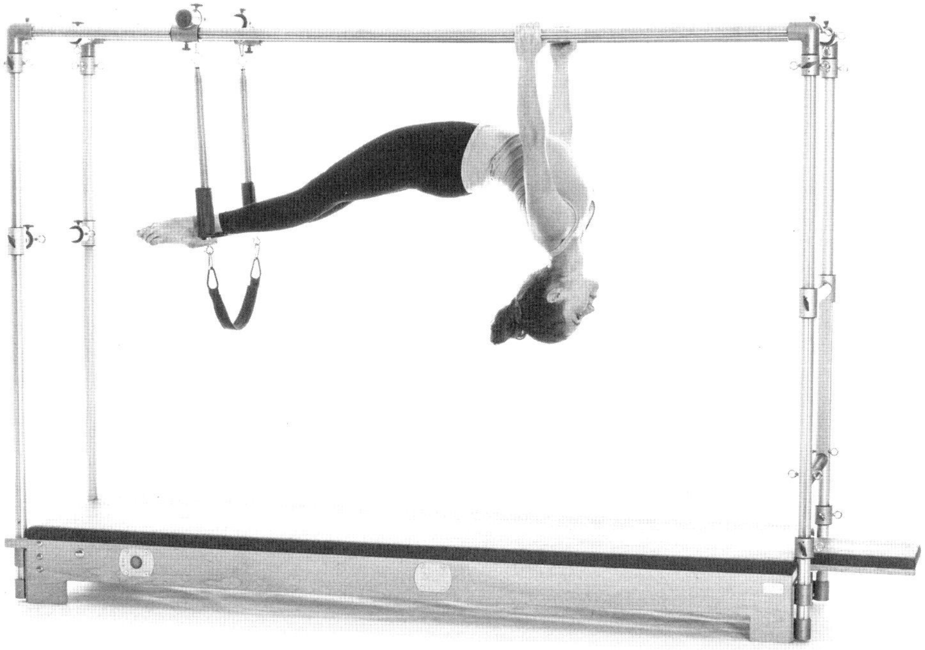

Whether you are doing mat work or working on the Pilates apparatus, safety is of paramount importance. In addition to following the general safety protocols for any exercise class—warming up, preparing the body for action, monitoring heart rate and body temperature, and cooling down at the end of the session—you also need to know how to work safely with the full complement of Pilates apparatus. Although Pilates equipment is generally considered very safe, it is in fact potentially dangerous if not used correctly and with discretion, as the following story illustrates.

In 1989 I was in Australia, teaching and directing the dance department at a performing arts college, where I had also introduced a Pilates program. I had a Pilates studio at the college for my work with the students as well as Pilates enthusiasts, professional dancers, and professional athletes. One morning I was teaching a young dancer, around 12 years old, as she did mini roll-ups on the cadillac. She was a regular student and had done the exercise many times. I was standing in close proximity to her when, intending to explain something to me, she accidentally let go of the push through bar, which was attached to two springs from the top. The bar flew into my mouth, crushing my four front teeth, sending me tumbling into the wall behind me, and knocking me out. I came around with my hand over my mouth, blood dripping out, and pieces of teeth in my hand.

Today, after multiple implants and crowns and more hours spent in dental chairs than I wish to recall, I continue to have oral surgeries and be traumatized by the event. Was it anyone's fault? No—just an unfortunate accident that very clearly speaks to the potential dangers of an apparatus that was never intended for unsupervised mass use. Yet, given the exposure Pilates is now receiving and some of the modern trends in the way it is taught, this fact is often ignored. The features that make the equipment so beneficial for fitness and conditioning and the therapeutic environment also make it potentially harmful. Each exercise requires recruiting the body's stabilizers, which is one reason this work is so functional—the equipment does not support you. If you do not incorporate good stabilization, you risk not doing the movement correctly, and worse, the possibility of an accident and injury. In addition, the equipment has many moving parts including springs, bars, straps, handles, and other attachments, all of which when used as intended are highly effective, yet can also be harmful. Good instruction, proper training, and a need for vigilance are essential.

Starting With Inner Focus

You are now familiar with both the philosophy and the exercises of Pilates and are ready to delve into your practice. I like to begin and conclude each session with a little time for relaxation or inner focus. If you commence the session with tension, that tension will be carried into your exercises and compound as the body is challenged, and the experience will likely be counterproductive, rather than having a calming and rejuvenating effect.

A good warm-up and cool-down exercise to begin and end the session is the Mat: Roll-Down, which draws attention to alignment as well as serving as a path to inner focus. After 3-5 Mat: Roll-Downs, I suggest a short mat work warm-up before moving on to the apparatus. When doing the mat work, a session typically begins and ends by going through a brief inner focus period in a standing, sitting, or supine position.

The following is a suggested outline for achieving inner focus when starting a mat work session.

1. Lie down on the mat in a supine position, with the knees bent and legs parallel to each other, hip width apart. Spread the feet comfortably on the floor. Place the arms by the sides of the body. Allow the spine, which should be in a neutral, natural position, to sink into the mat.
2. Relax the feet, back, and neck.
3. Engage the adductors to prevent the legs from splaying.
4. Imagine the pelvis floating in space with no forces pulling on it.
5. Visualize an elongated spine, relaxing the muscles of the back.
6. Reach the fingers toward the feet, with the scapulae floating in a neutral position.
7. Elongate the neck, sensing the crown of the head reaching away from the body.
8. Relax the muscles of the face.
9. Be present in the moment, focus on the breath, and feel the lateral expansion of the chest on the mat.
10. Become aware of your body down to the last muscle fiber.
11. Engage the internal support system.
12. Take 5 long, deep breaths—you are now ready to move!

Mat Work Sequences

In this section I provide three mat work routines: fundamental, intermediate, and advanced. Each routine builds on the previous one. Practice them while incorporating the principles discussed in this book, and feel free to replace any of the exercises with the suggested modifications, variations, or progressions. Remember, Pilates is about quality, not quantity. Practice the work with integrity and make each movement the best that you possibly can. In the words of Joseph Pilates in his book *Return to Life Through Contrology*, "Make a close study of each exercise and do not attempt any other exercise until you first have mastered the current one and know its routine down to the last detail without any reference to the text" (p. 32).

I have suggested a time frame for each program. This should be used as a guide to help measure whether you are moving too slowly or too quickly.

Fundamental Mat Work Routine

Exercises: 16; approximate time: 25 minutes

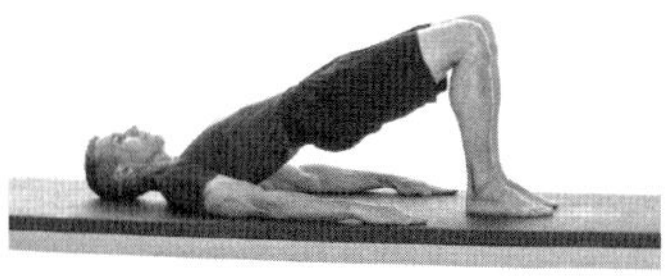

Pelvic Curl, page 49

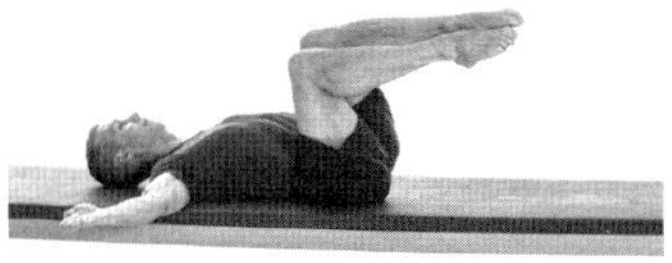

Spine Twist—Supine, page 50

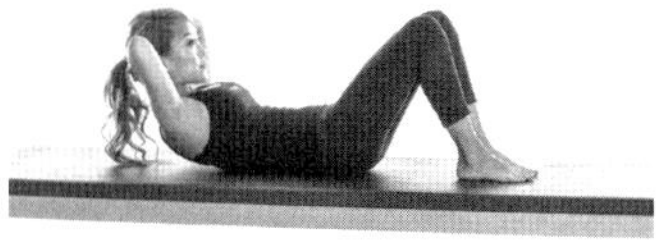

Chest Lift, page 51

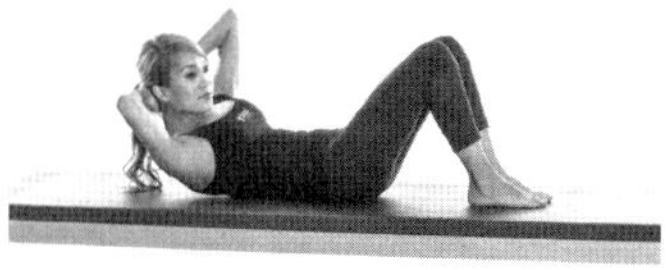

Chest Lift With Rotation, page 52

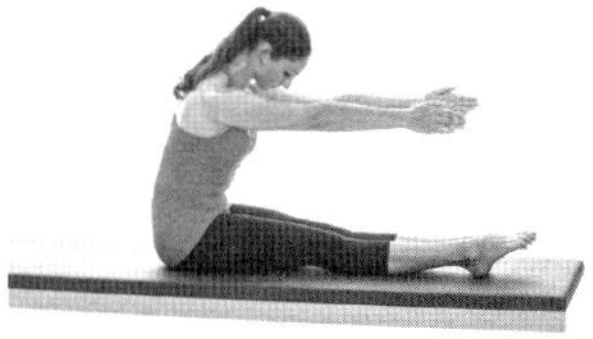

Roll-Up, page 58

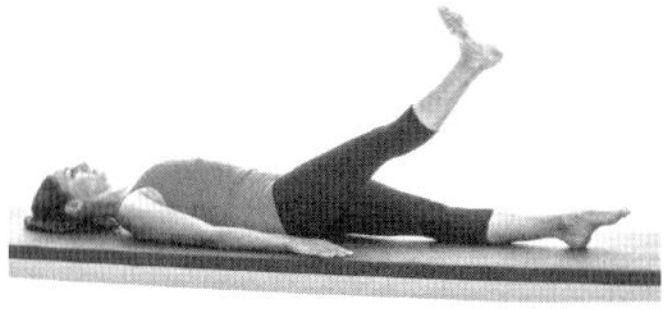

Leg Circle, page 54

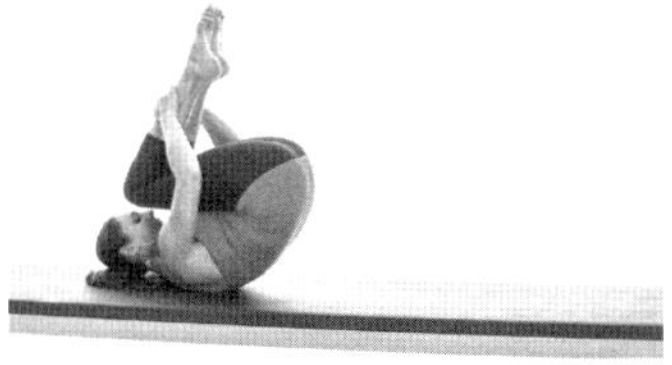

Rolling Like a Ball, page 74

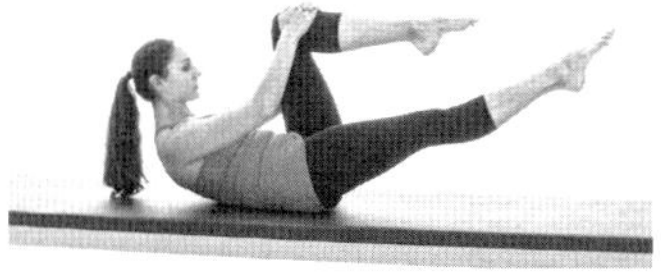

Single-Leg Stretch, page 62

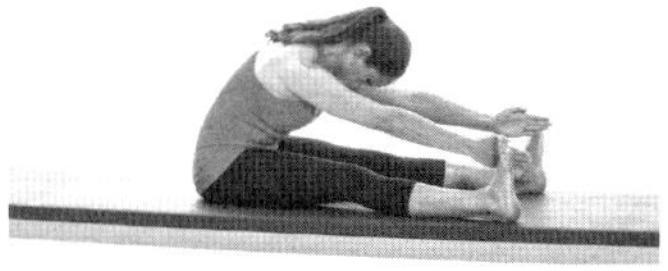

Spine Stretch, page 73

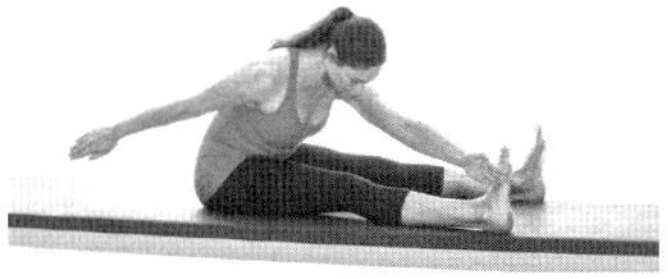

Saw, page 108

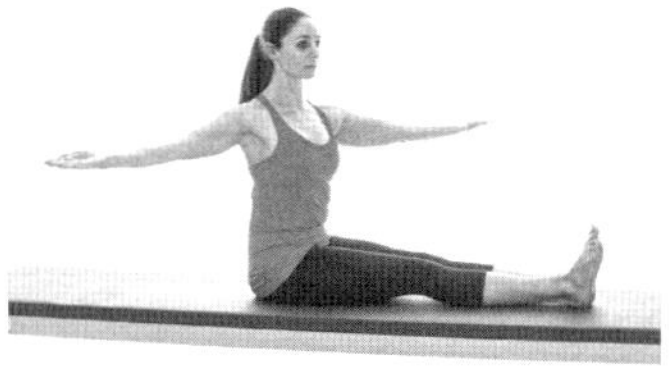

Spine Twist—Sitting, page 106

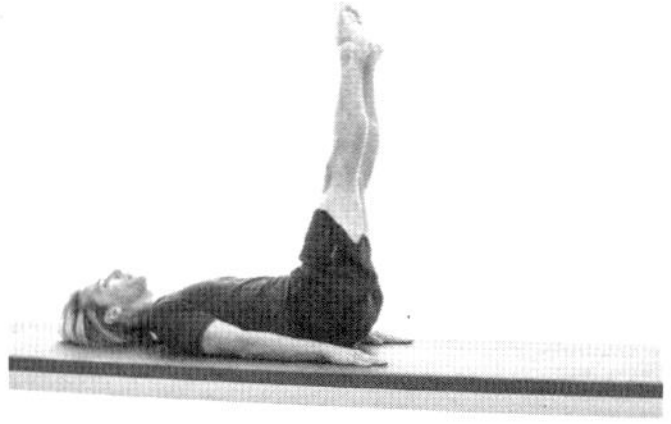

Corkscrew, page 110

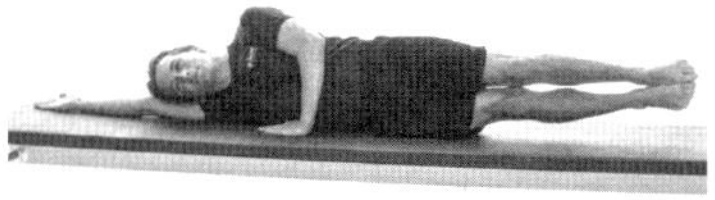

Side Leg Lift, page 101

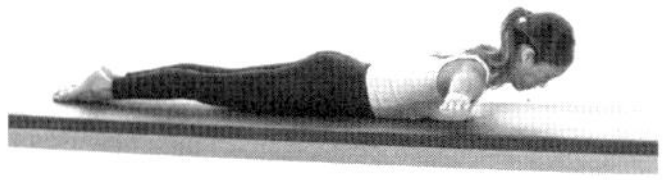

Back Extension, page 115

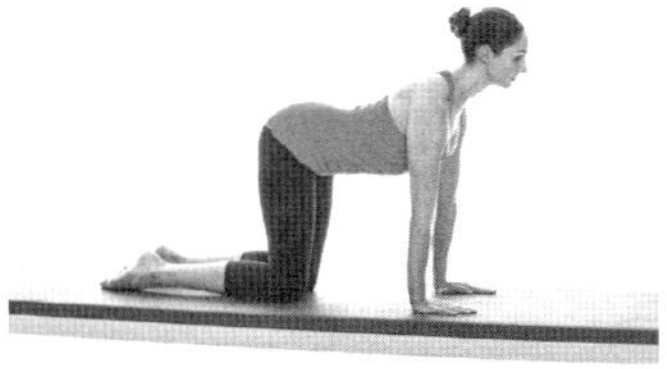

Cat Stretch, page 95

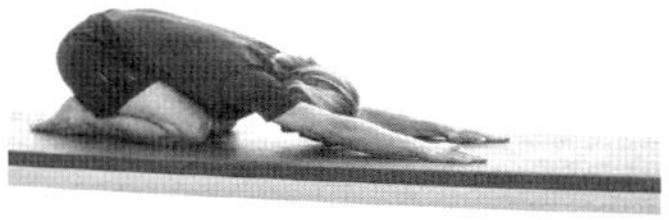

Rest Position, page 121

Intermediate Mat Work Routine

Exercises: 32; approximate time: 45 minutes

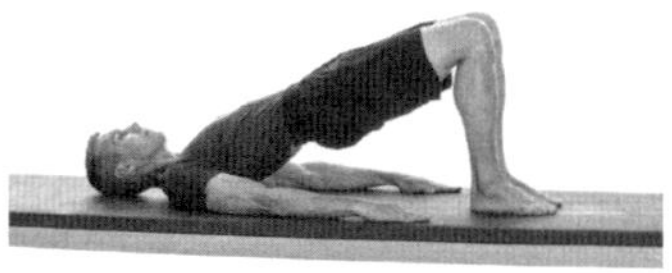

Pelvic Curl, page 49

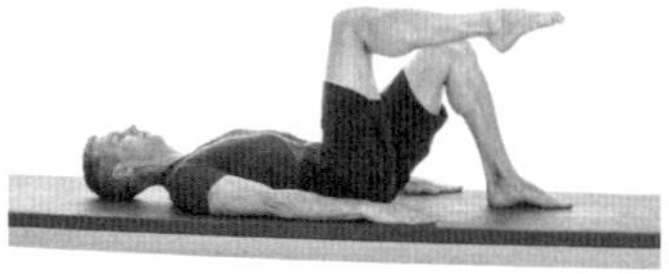

Single-Leg Lift, page 53

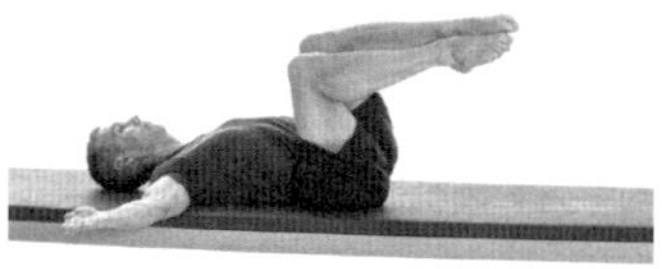

Spine Twist—Supine, page 50

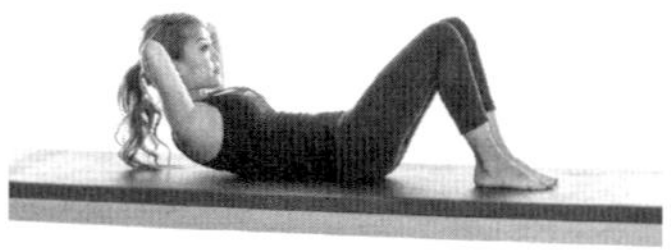

Chest Lift, page 51

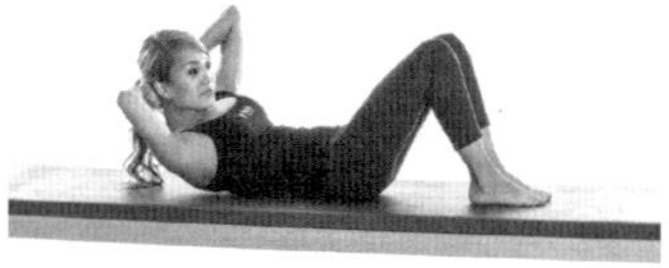

Chest Lift With Rotation, page 52

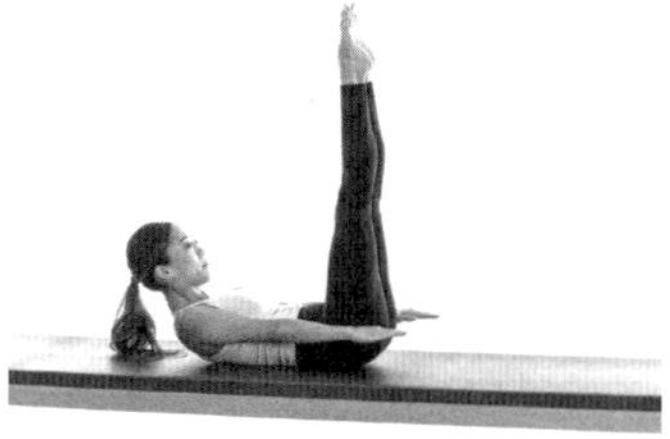

Hundred, page 56

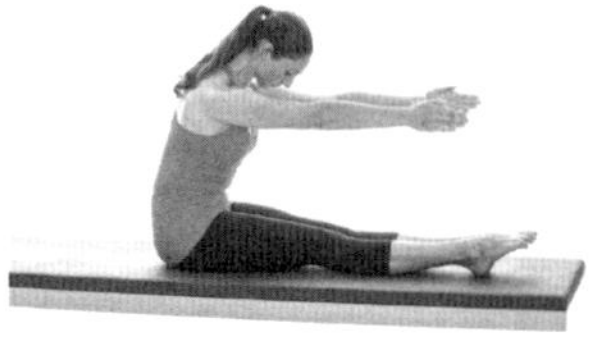

Roll-Up, page 58

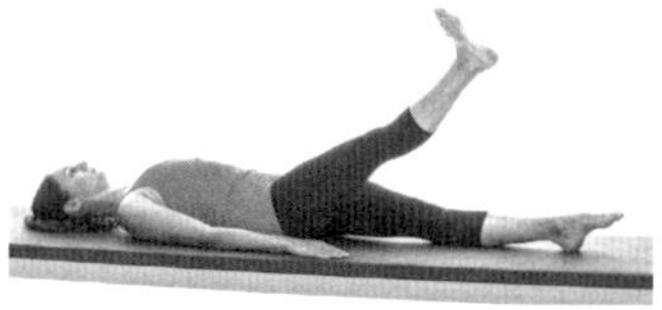

Leg Circle, page 54

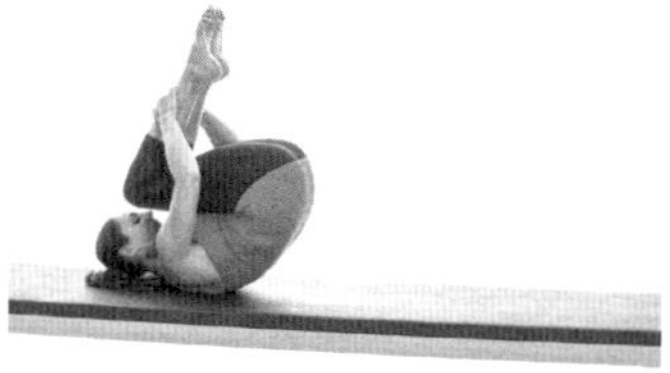

Rolling Like a Ball, page 74

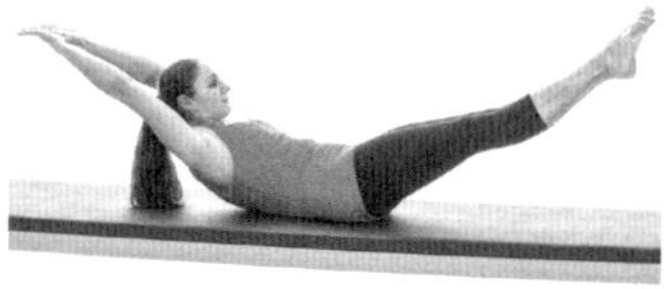

Double-Leg Stretch, page 66

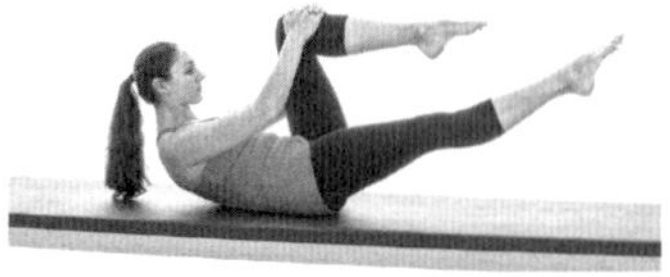

Single-Leg Stretch, page 62

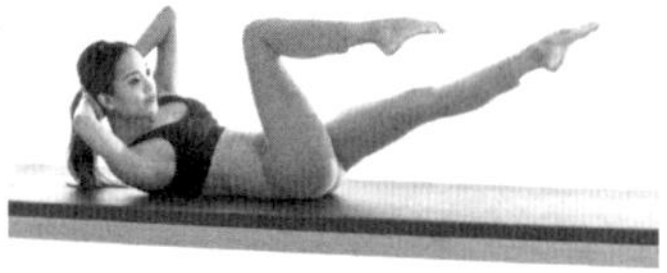

Criss-Cross, page 64

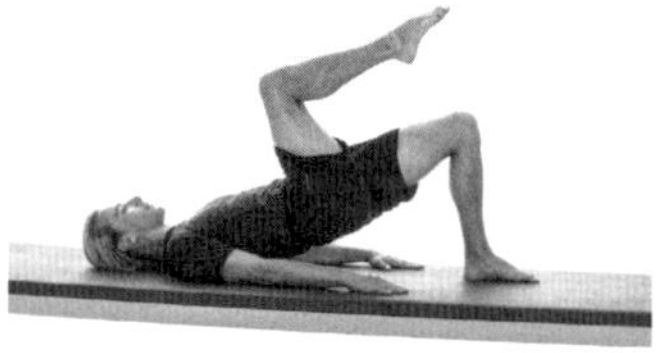

Shoulder Bridge Prep, page 89

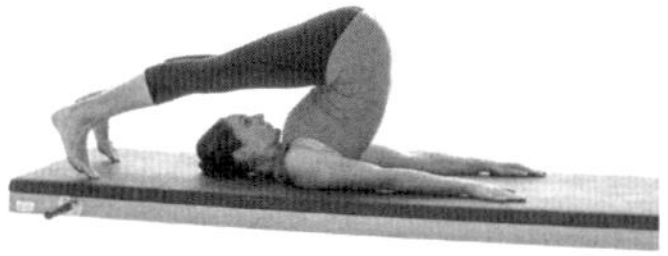

Roll-Over, page 78

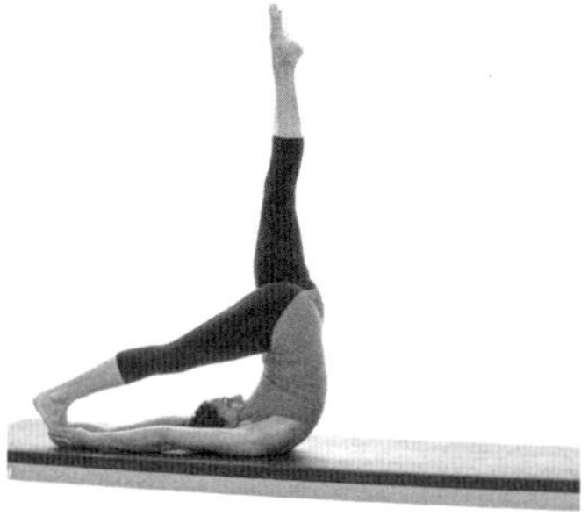

Control Balance, page 80

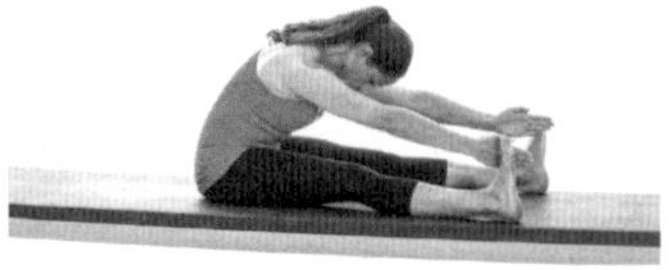

Spine Stretch, page 73

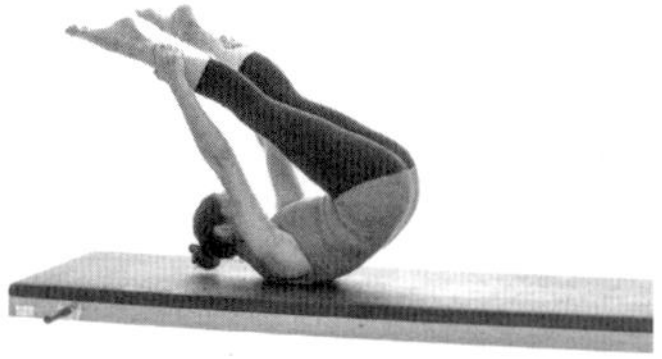

Open-Leg Rocker, page 76

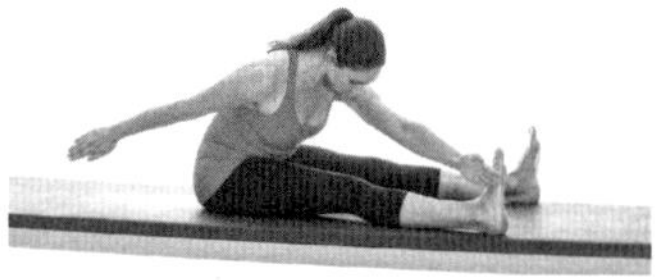

Saw, page 108

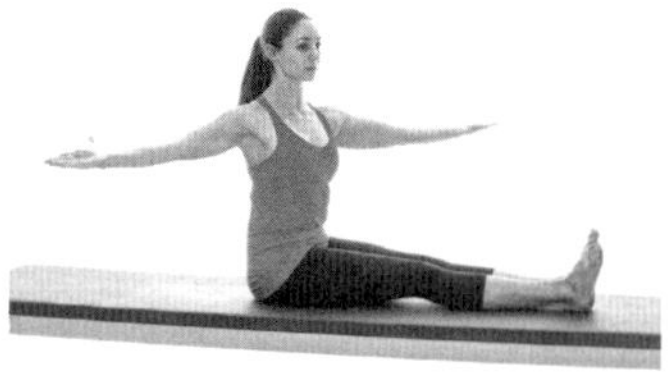

Spine Twist—Sitting, page 106

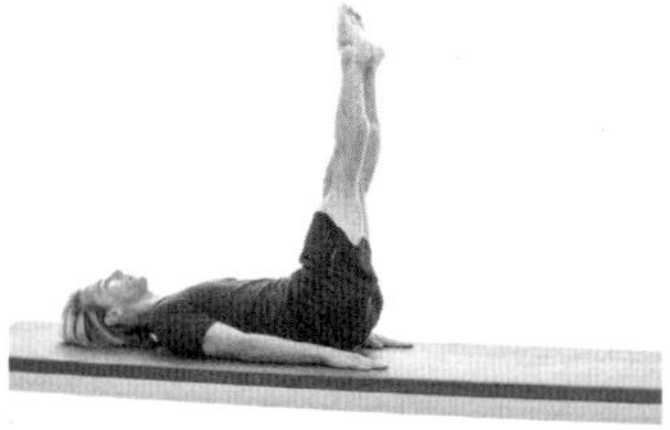

Corkscrew, page 110

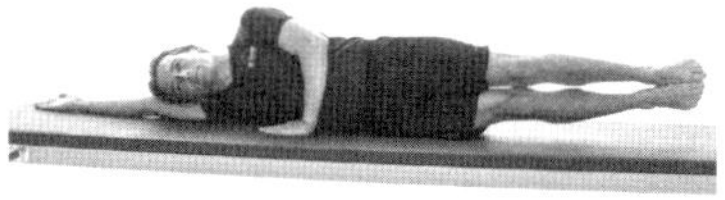

Side Leg Lift, page 101

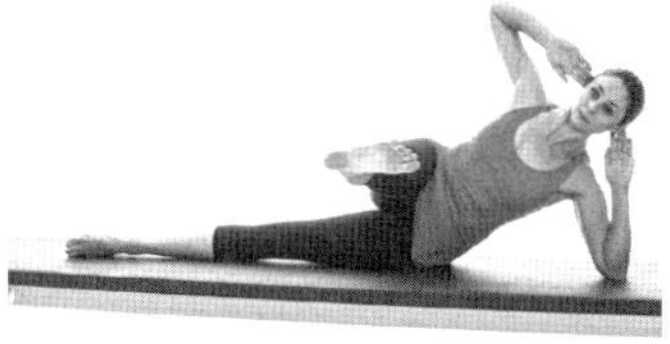

Side Kick, page 102

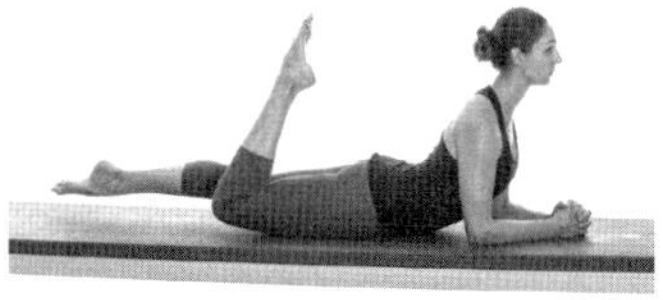

Single-Leg Kick, page 116

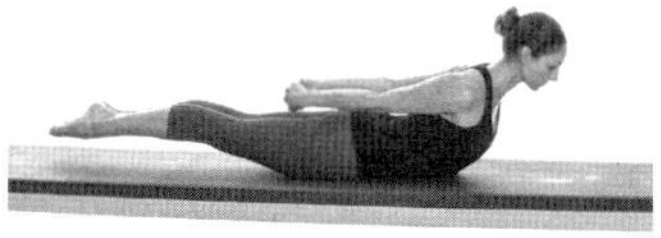

Double-Leg Kick, page 117

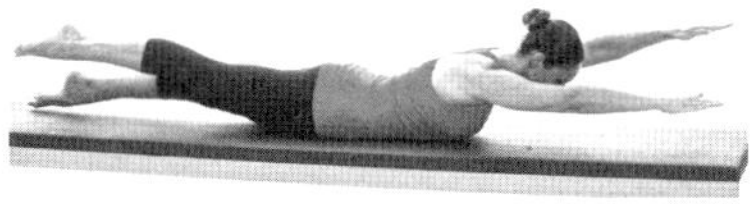

Swimming, page 118

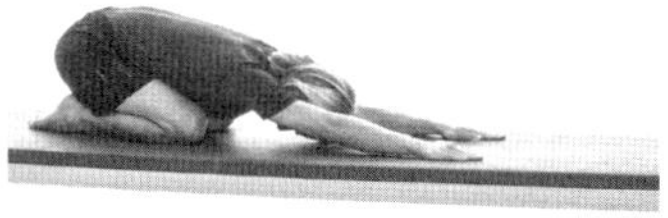

Rest Position, page 121

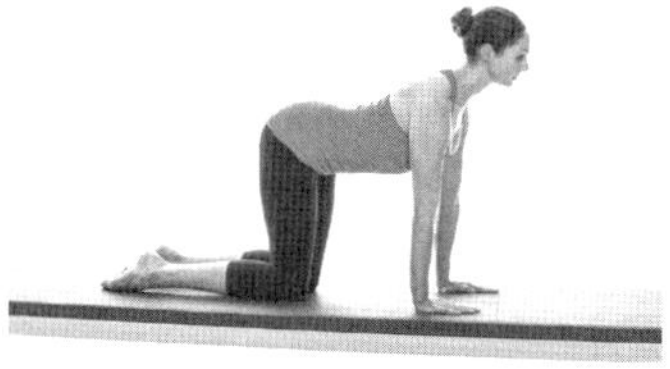

Cat Stretch, page 95

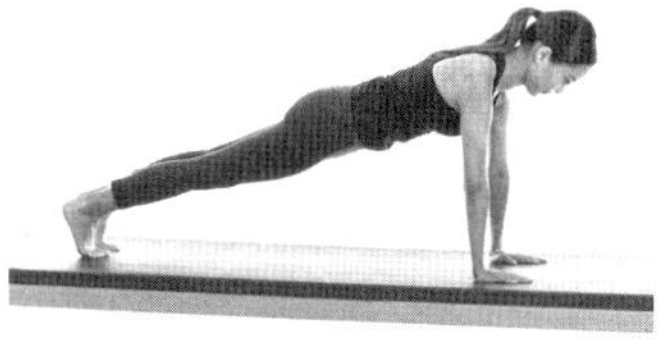

Front Support, page 96

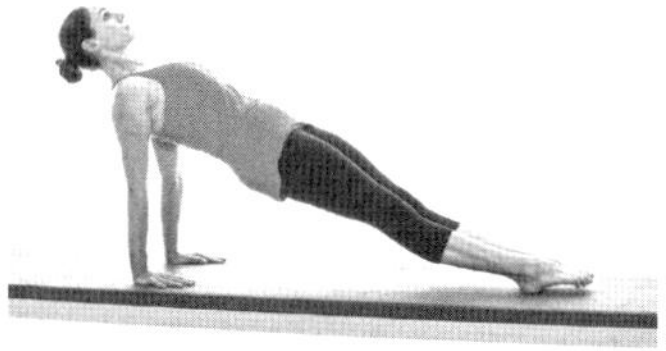

Back Support, page 93

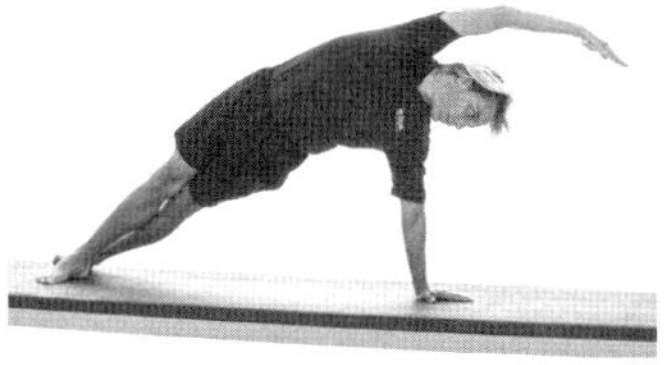

Side Bend, page 104

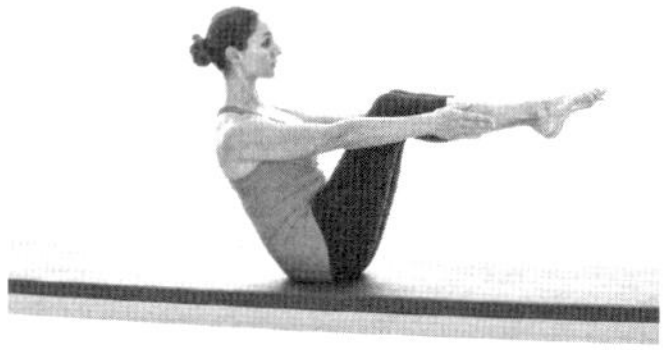

Teaser Prep, page 70

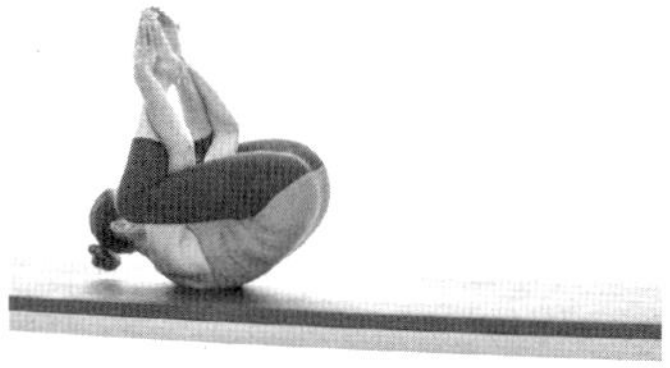

Seal Puppy, page 75

Advanced Mat Work Routine

Exercises: 44; approximate time: 60 minutes

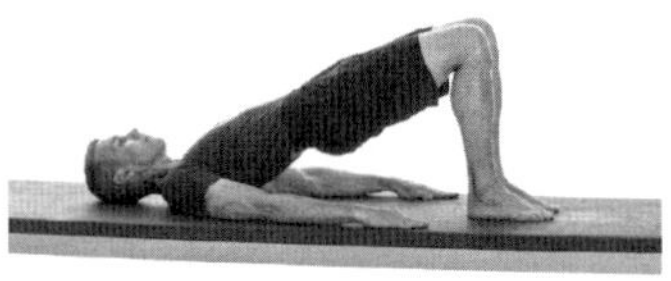

Pelvic Curl, page 49

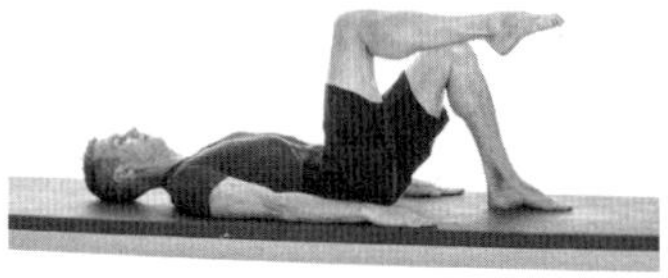

Single-Leg Lift, page 53

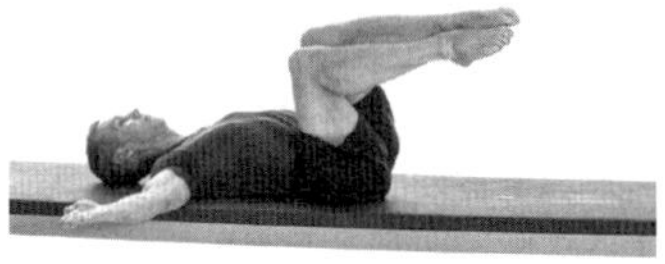

Spine Twist—Supine, page 50

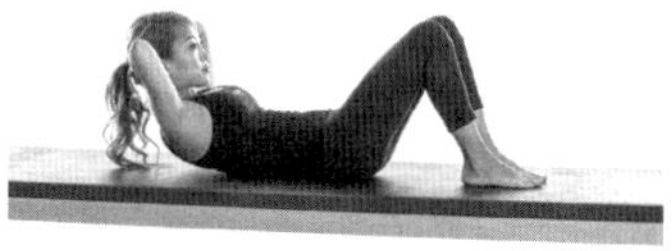

Chest Lift, page 51

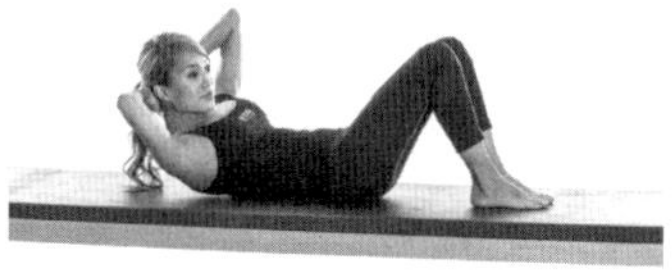

Chest Lift With Rotation, page 52

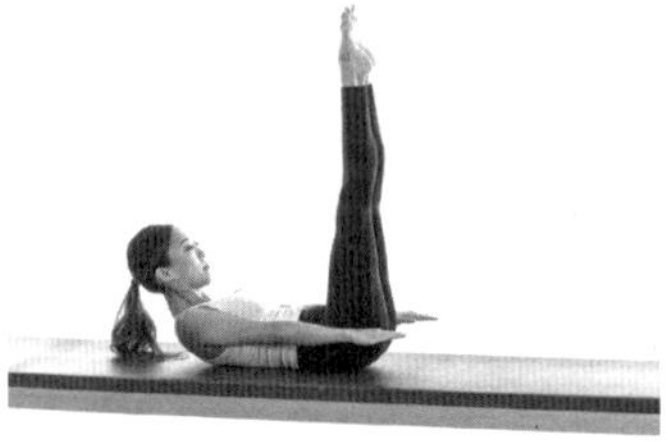

Hundred, page 56

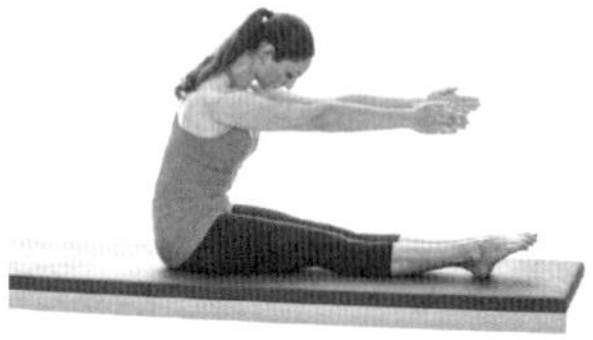

Roll-Up, page 58

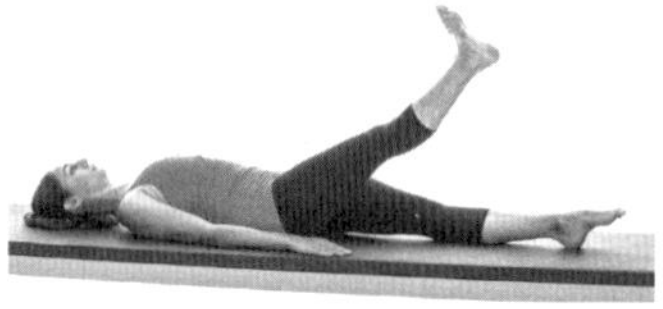

Leg Circle, page 54

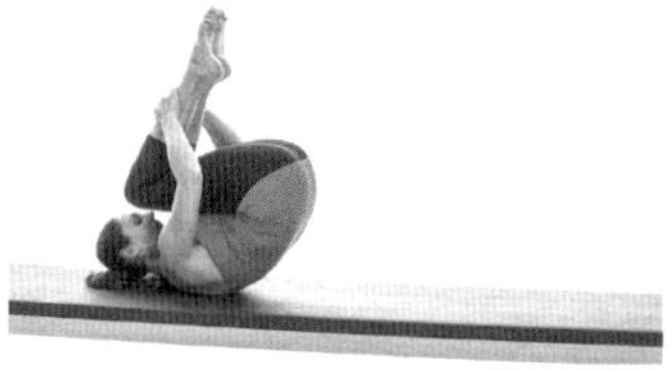

Rolling Like a Ball, page 74

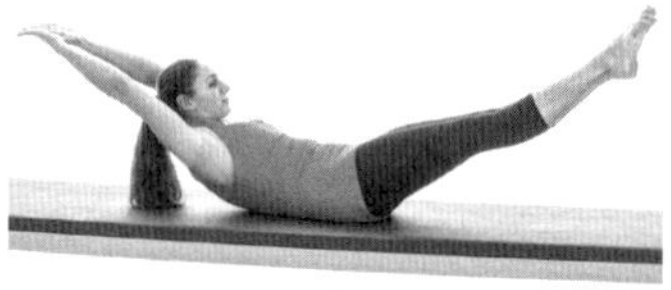

Double-Leg Stretch, page 66

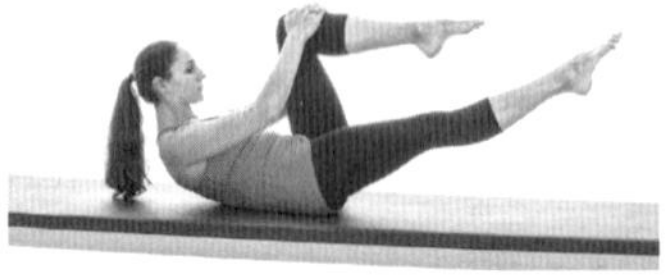

Single-Leg Stretch, page 62

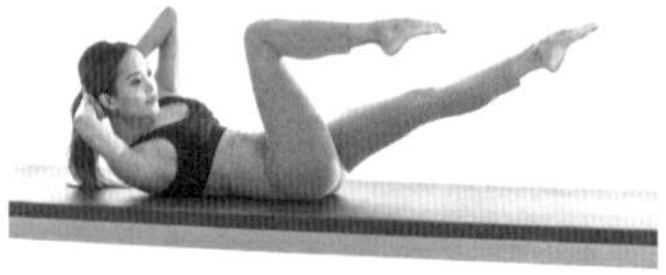

Criss-Cross, page 64

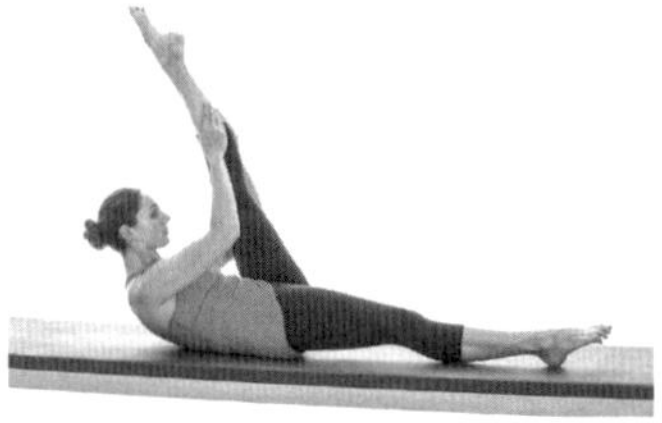

Hamstring Pull, page 68

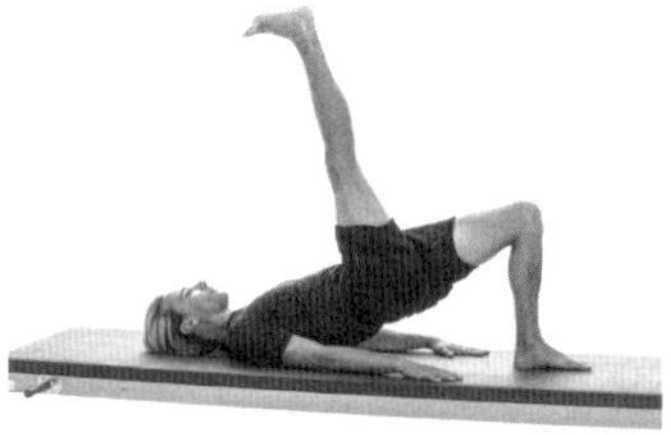

Shoulder Bridge, page 90

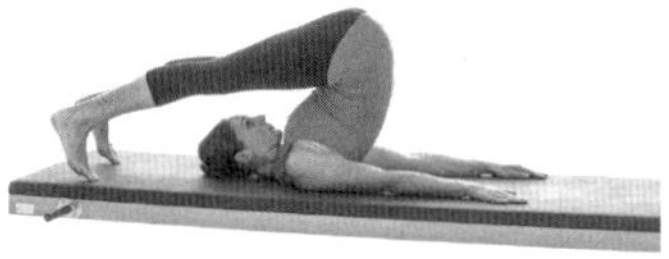

Roll-Over, page 78

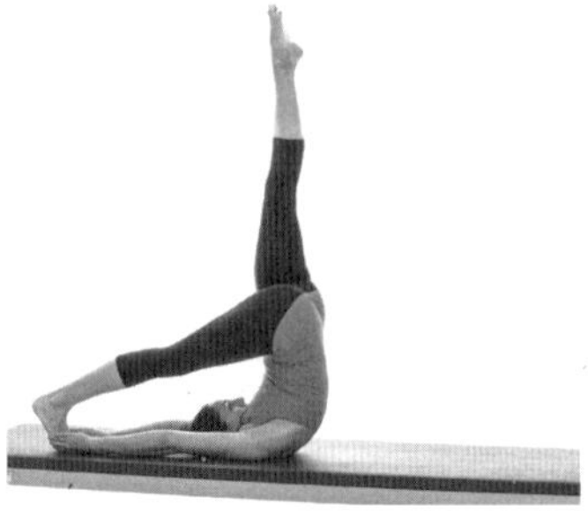

Control Balance, page 80

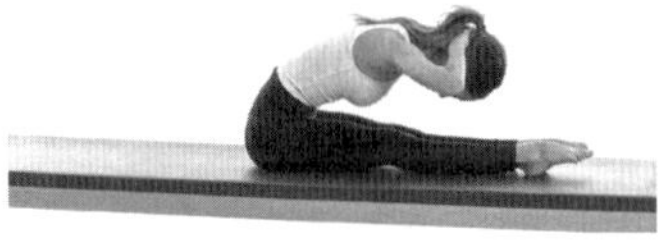

Neck Pull, page 60

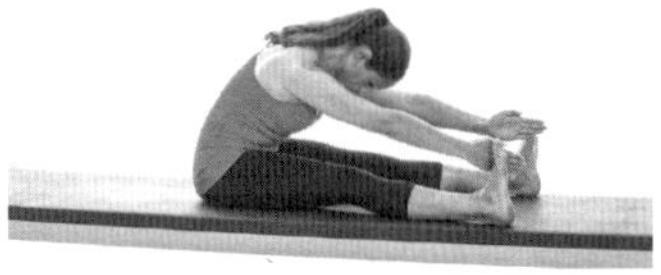

Spine Stretch, page 73

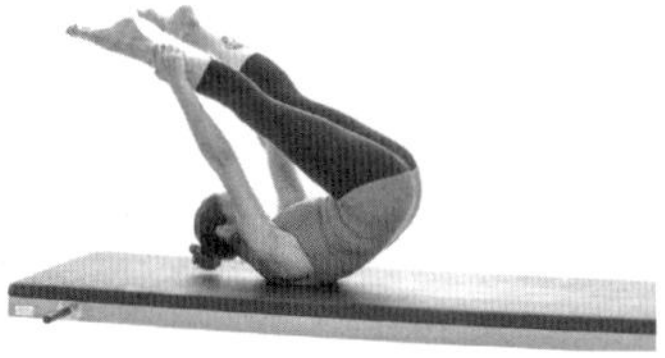

Open-Leg Rocker, page 76

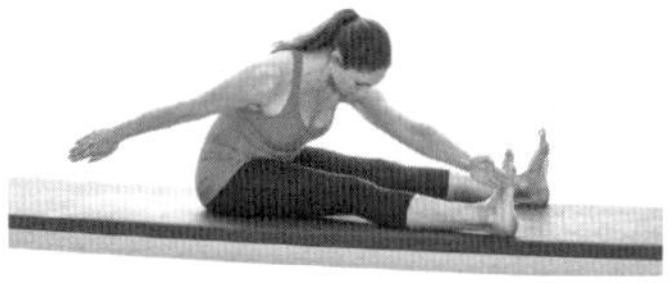

Saw, page 108

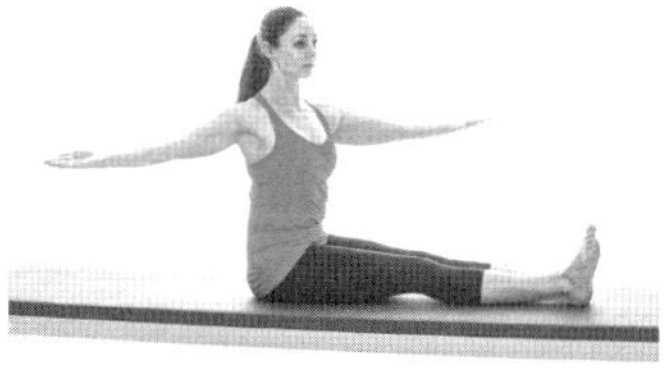
Spine Twist—Sitting, page 106

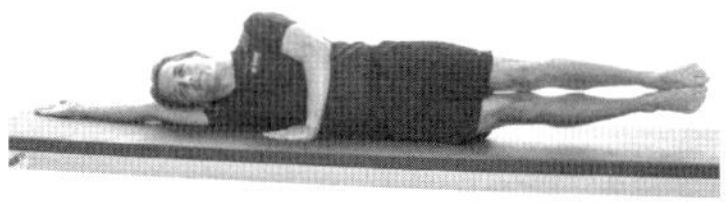
Side Leg Lift, page 101

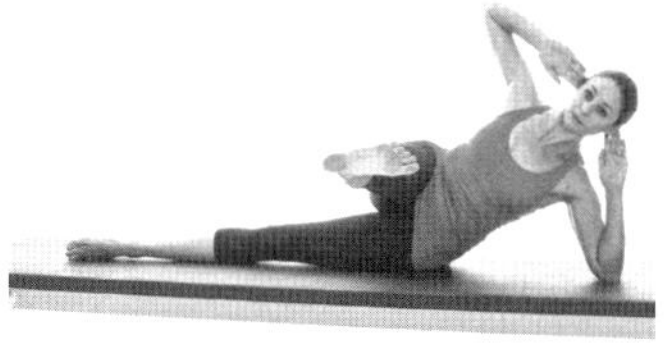
Side Kick, page 102

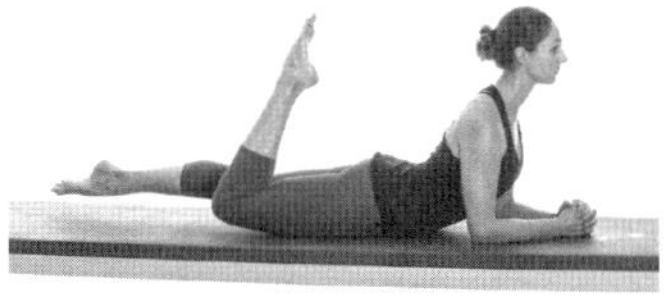
Single-Leg Kick, page 116

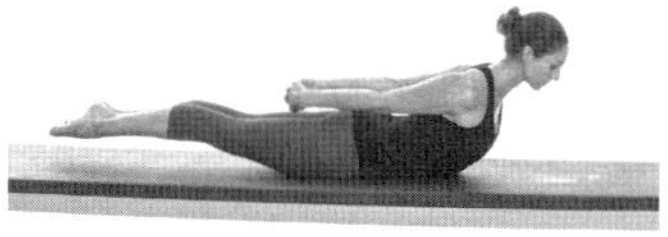
Double-Leg Kick, page 117

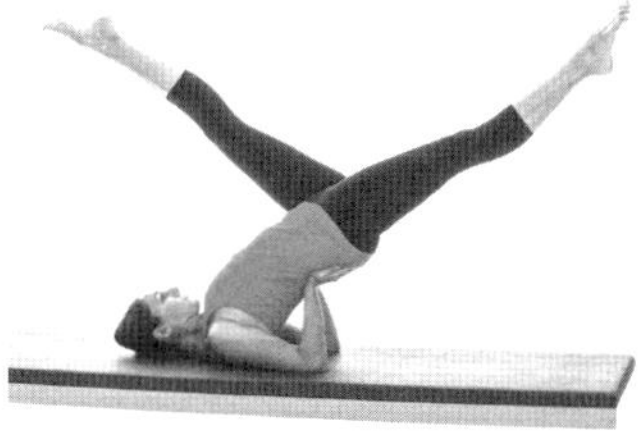
Scissors, page 91

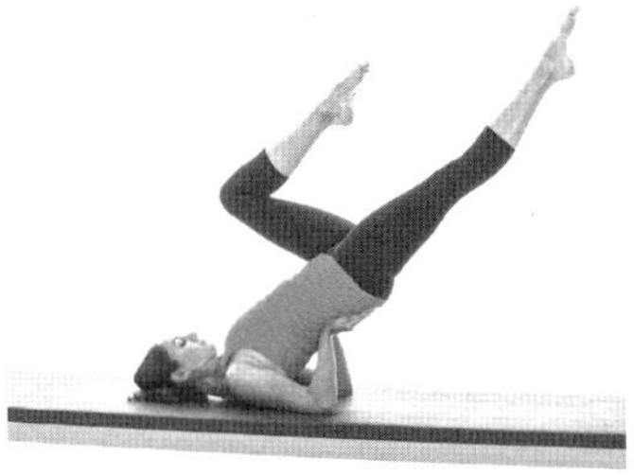
Bicycle, page 92

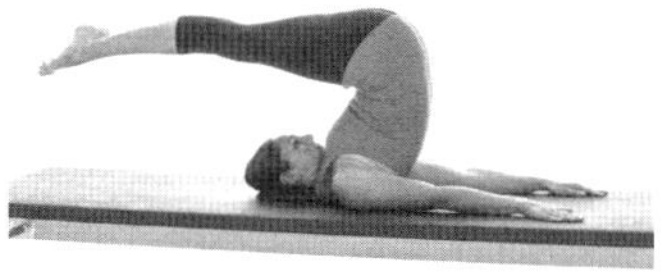
Jackknife, page 82

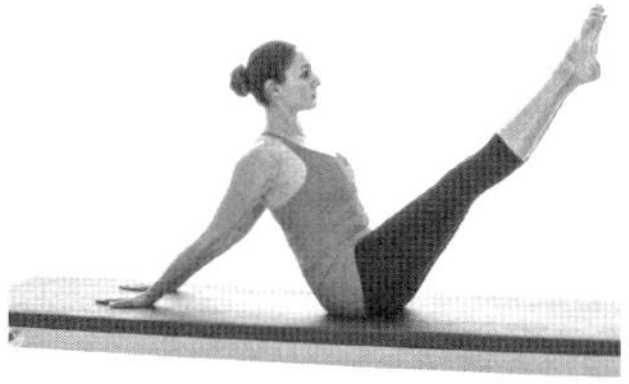
Hip Circle Prep, page 111

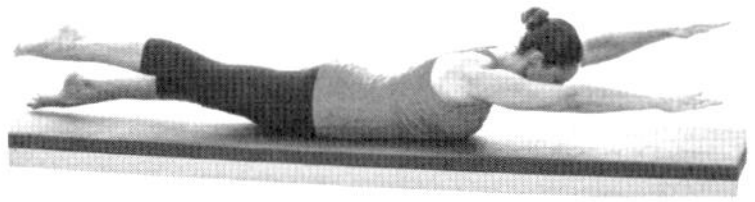
Swimming, page 118

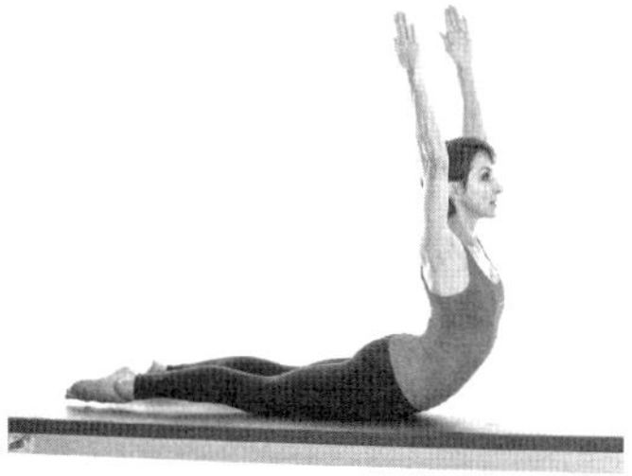
Swan Dive, page 120

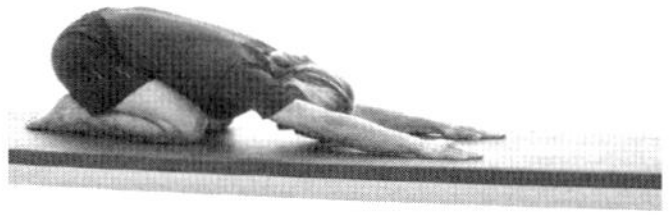
Rest Position, page 121

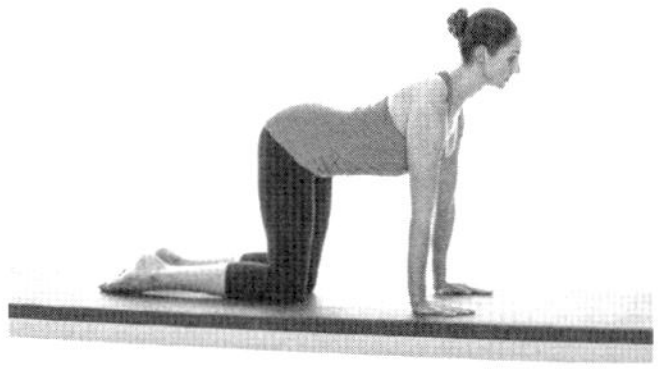
Cat Stretch, page 95

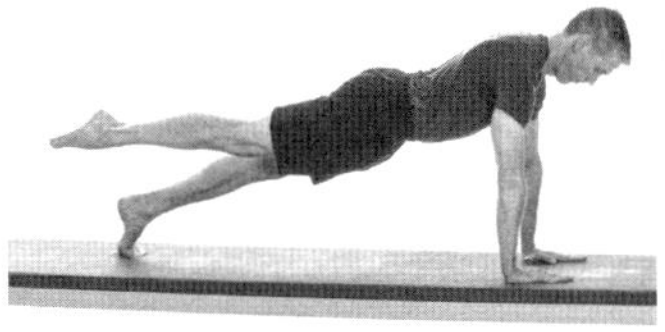
Leg Pull Front, page 97

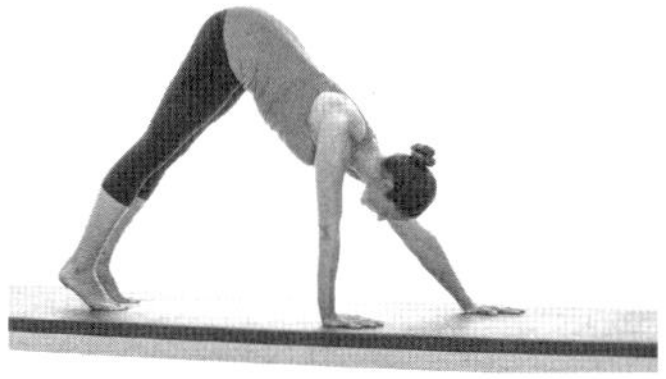
Push-Up, page 98

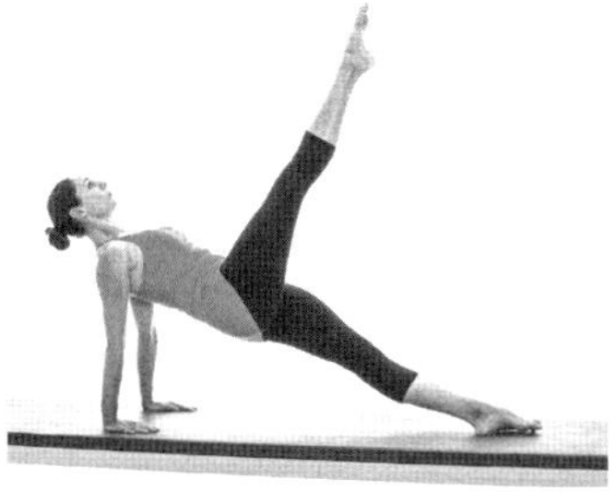
Leg Pull Back, page 94

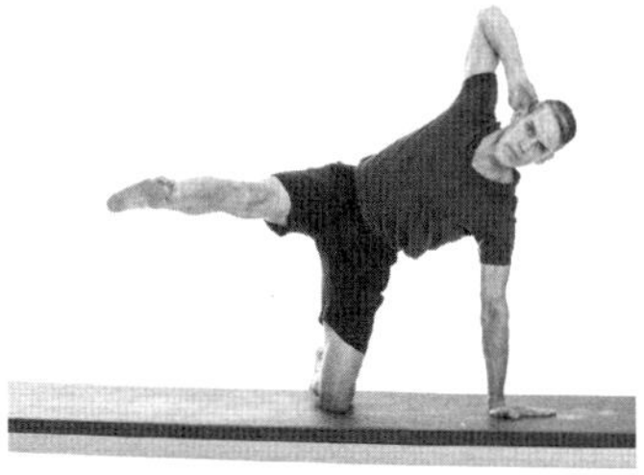
Side Kick—Kneeling, page 103

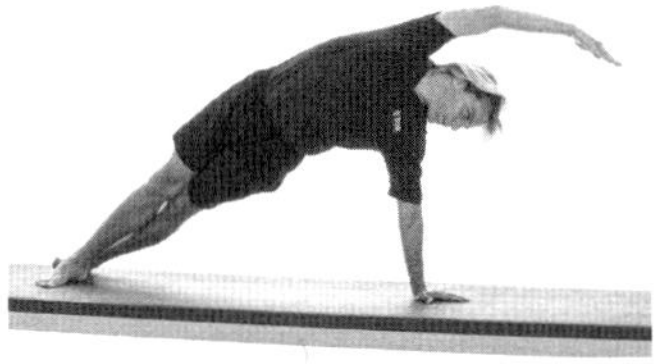
Side Bend, page 104

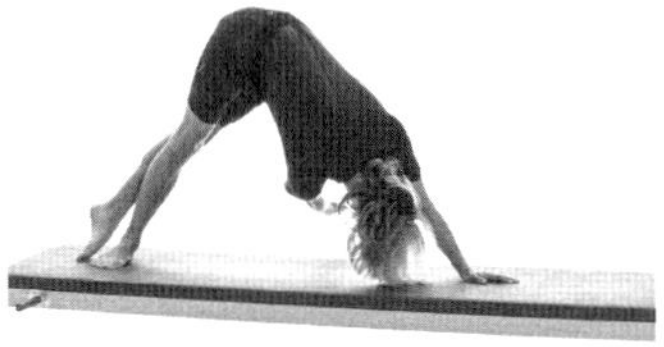
Twist, page 112

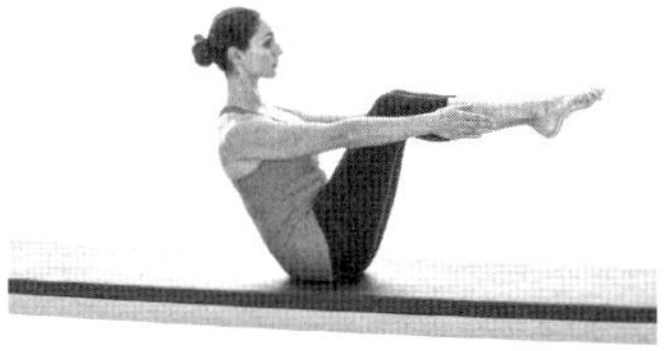
Teaser Prep, page 70

> *continued*

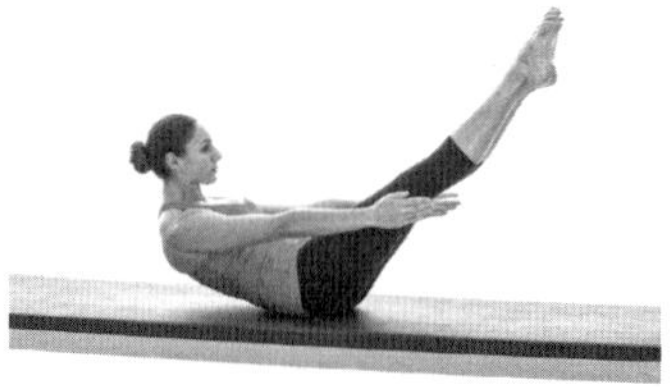

Teaser, page 71

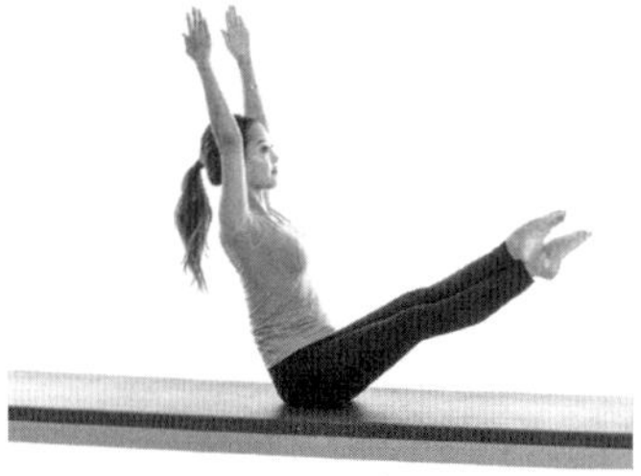

Boomerang, page 84

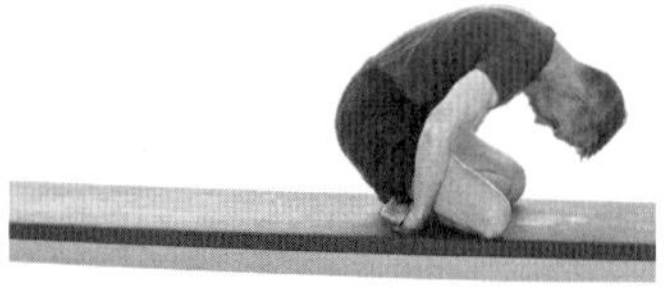

Crab, page 86

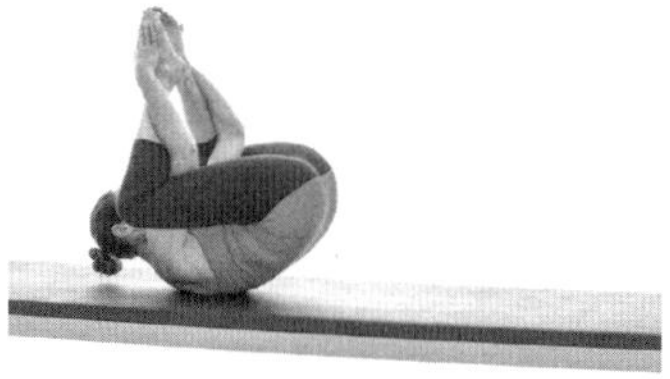

Seal Puppy, page 75

Apparatus Sequences

As stated previously, first and foremost in importance when using any of the Pilates apparatus is *safety*. I cannot stress this point enough. Second, the session should be comprehensive, just as the mat work is. Remember, the apparatus are tools we use to help us achieve our goals—they are not the system itself. I have always felt that I would rather work out using conventional gym equipment with an instructor who uses a Pilates approach than work on Pilates apparatus with a Pilates instructor who does not incorporate the principles of the work. The block system ensures that each session you do is a Pilates session and not merely a collection of exercises that happen to be done on Pilates apparatus.

I have offered three apparatus routines, one for each level (fundamental, intermediate, and advanced), which can be used as frameworks to build on. I have not offered any master-level programs in this book, because delving into this realm of the work takes years of practice and must involve professional instruction and guidance. One of the saddest outcomes of the Pilates boom is that the advanced- and master-level work is often used without adequate preparation, practice, or understanding, frequently resulting in subpar performance and outcomes, as opposed to a lifelong commitment.

I have provided alternative options for select exercises, illustrating how the repertoire within each block can be interchanged. As with the mat work routines, exercises may also be replaced with modifications, variations, or progressions as appropriate. As long as you adhere to the guidelines and principles in this book, you are guaranteed a positive outcome.

Fundamental Apparatus Routine

Exercises: 30; approximate time: 60 minutes

OPTIONAL

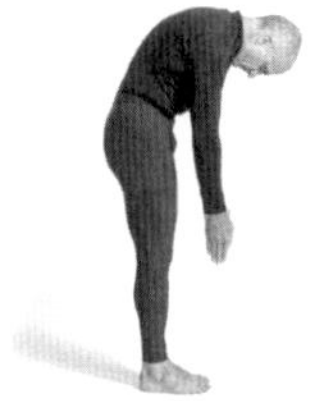

Mat: Roll-Down, page 26

WARM-UP

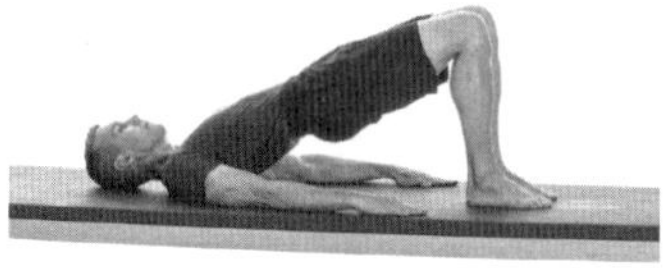

Mat: Pelvic Curl, page 49

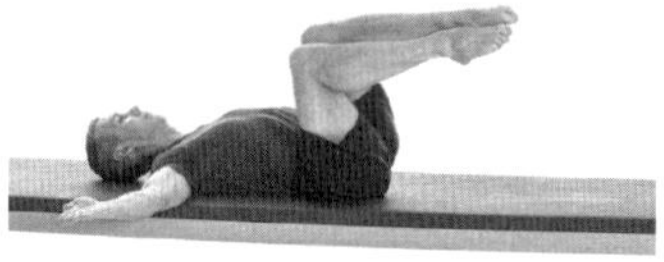

Mat: Spine Twist—Supine, page 50

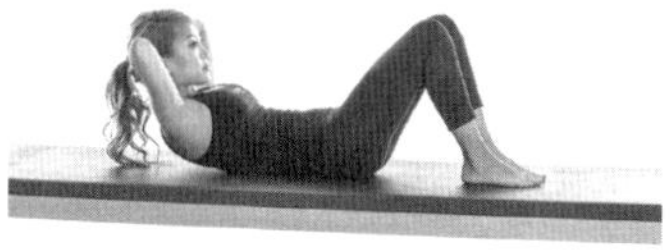

Mat: Chest Lift, page 51

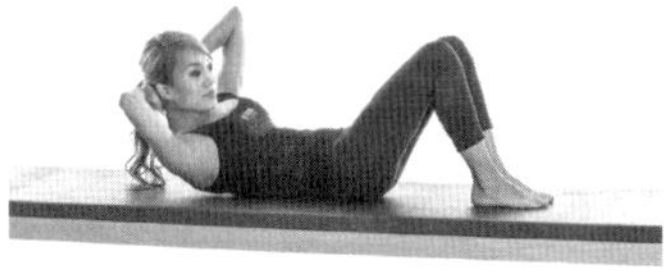

Mat: Chest Lift With Rotation, page 52

FOOT WORK

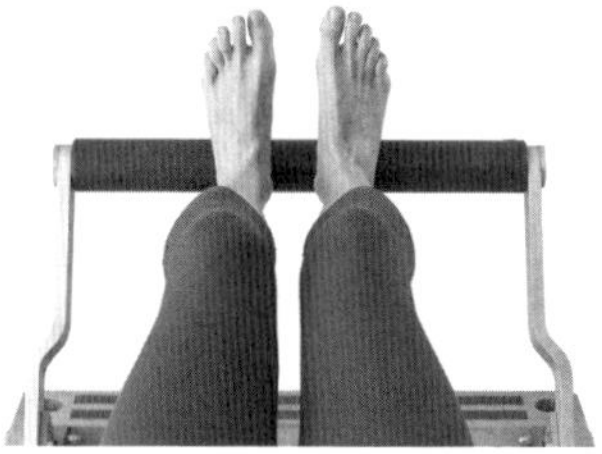

Reformer: Parallel Heels, page 127

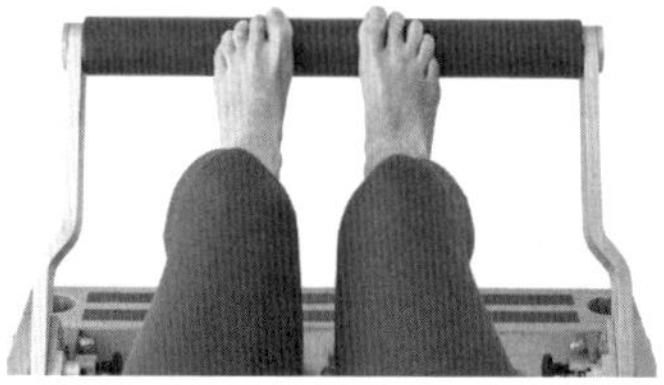

Reformer: Parallel Toes, page 128

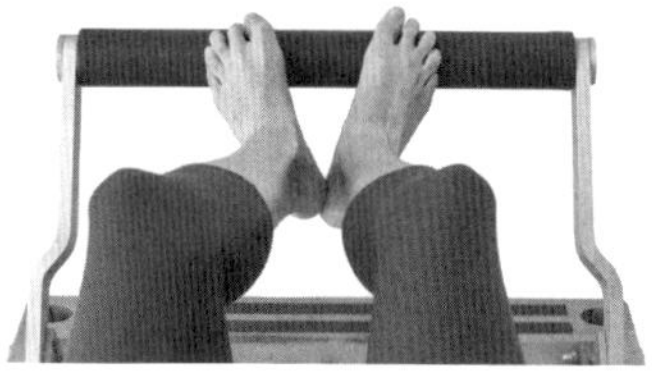

Reformer: V Position Toes, page 129

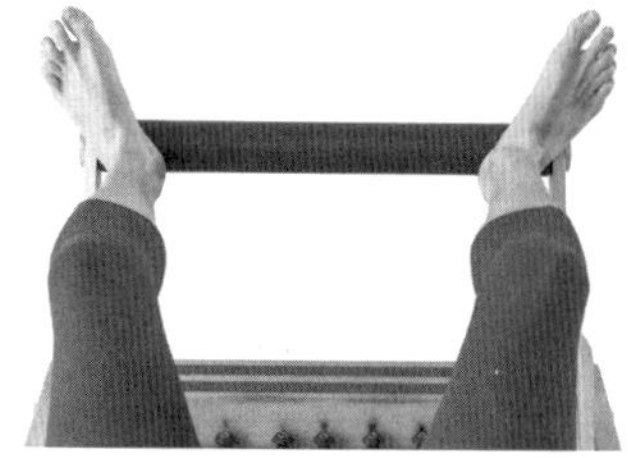

Reformer: Open V Position Heels, page 130

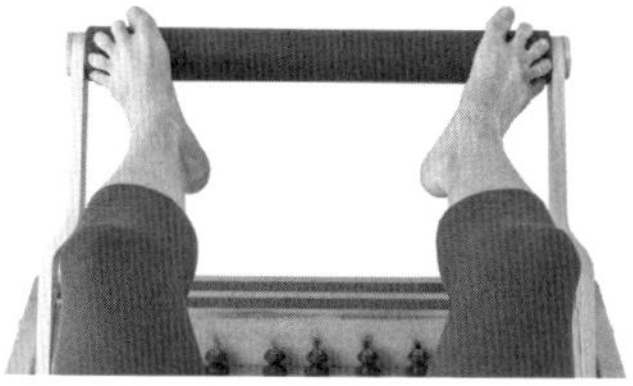

Reformer: Open V Position Toes, page 131

FOOT WORK

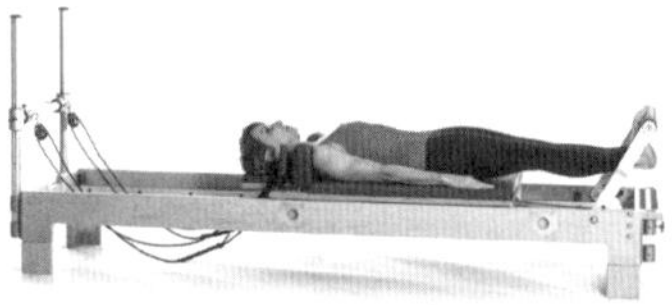

Reformer: Calf Raises, page 132

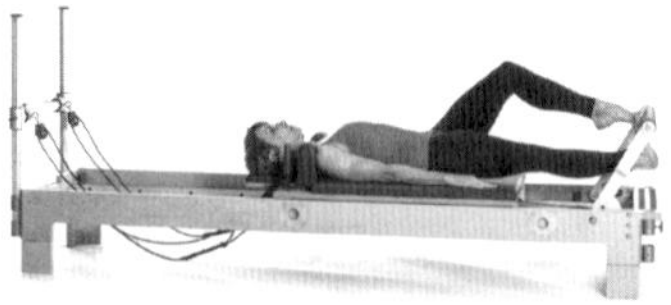

Reformer: Prances, page 133

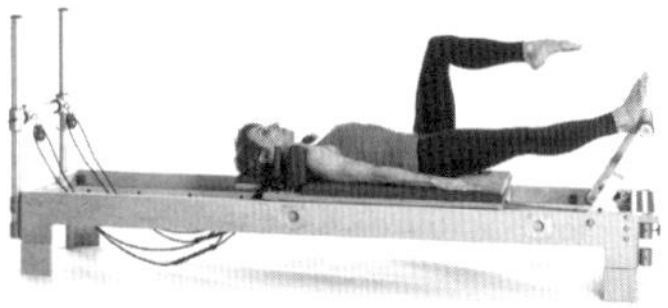

Reformer: Single-Leg Heel, page 135

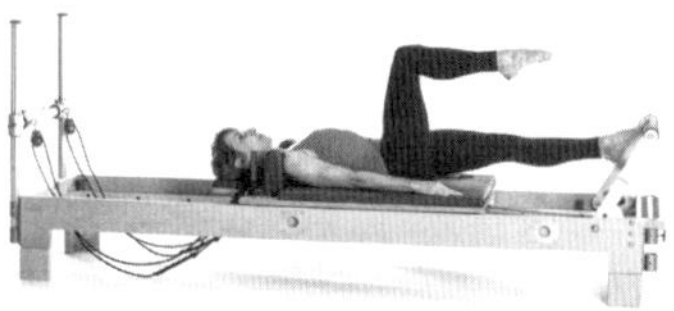

Reformer: Single-Leg Toes, page 136

ABDOMINAL WORK

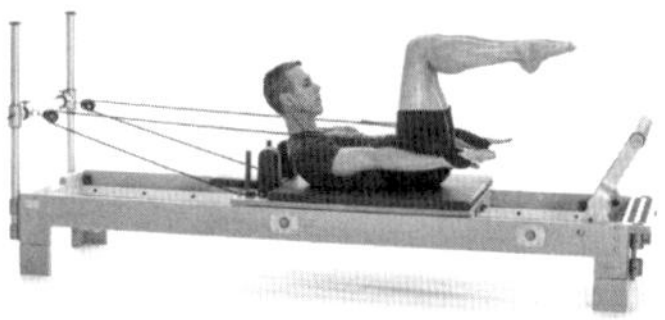

Reformer: Hundred Prep, page 138

HIP WORK

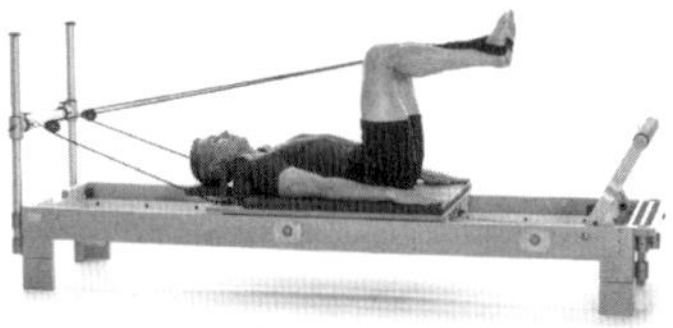

Reformer: Frog, page 153

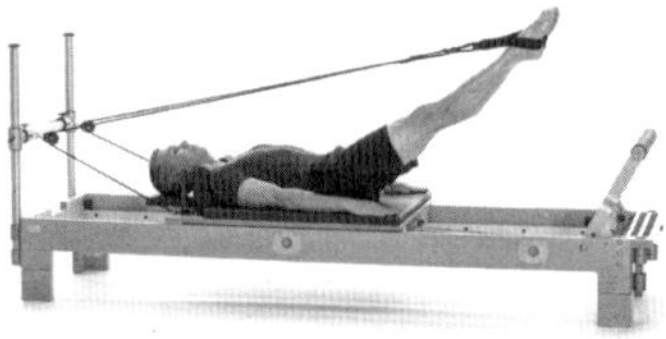

Reformer: Hip Circle Down, page 154

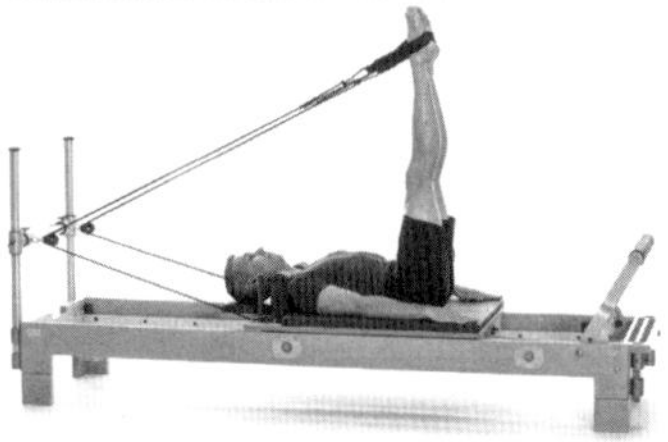

Reformer: Hip Circle Up, page 155

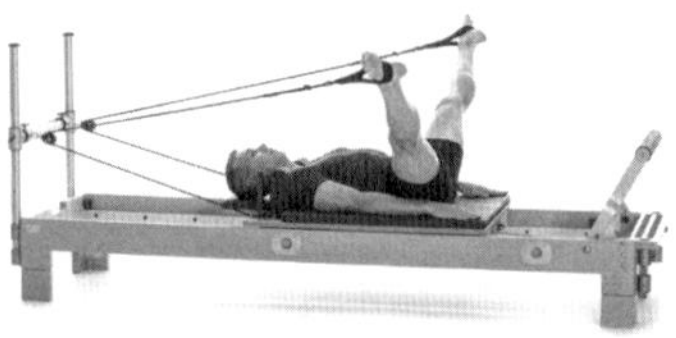

Reformer: Opening, page 156

SPINAL ARTICULATION

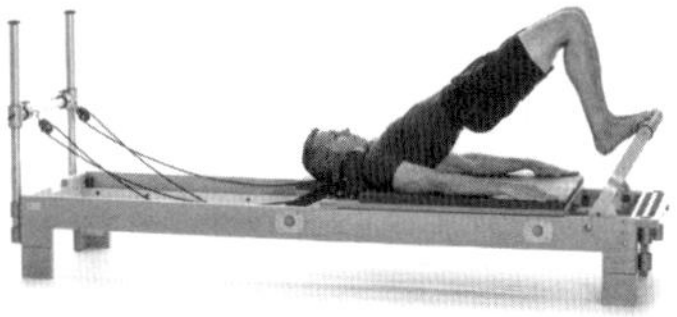

Reformer: Bottom Lift, page 160

STRETCHES

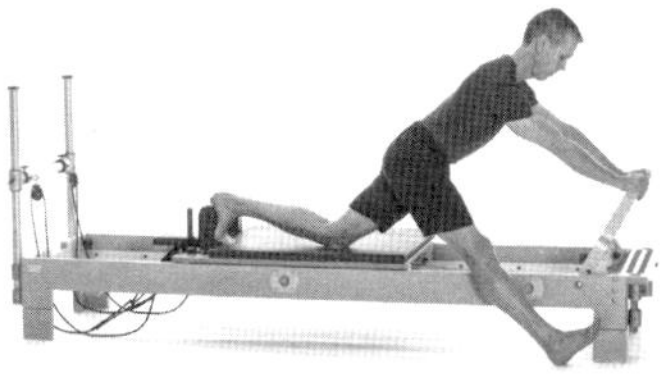

Reformer: Lunge—Standing, page 169

FULL BODY INTEGRATION I

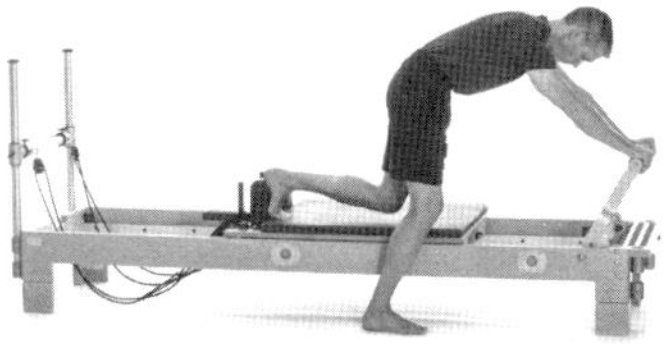

Reformer: Scooter, page 173

ARM WORK

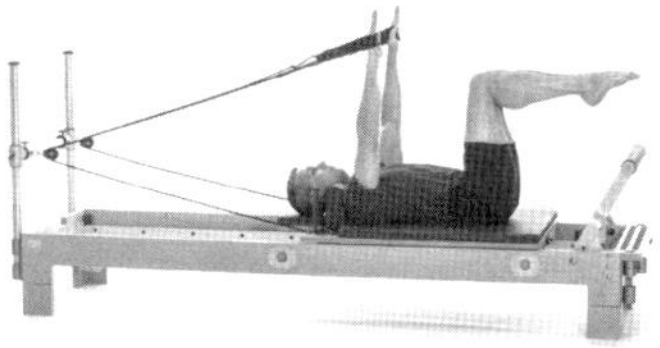

Reformer: Shoulder Extension—Supine, page 186
Alternate option: Ped-a-Pul: Extension, page 315

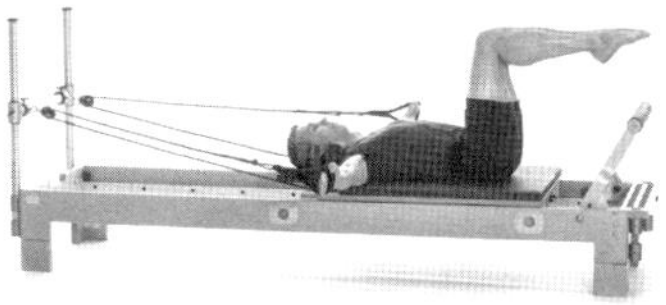

Reformer: Shoulder Adduction—Supine, page 187
Alternate option: Ped-a-Pul: Adduction, page 316

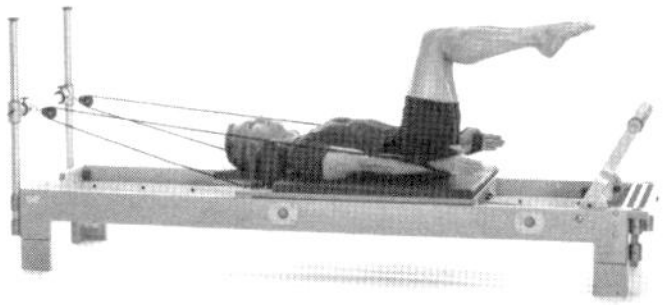

Reformer: Arm Circle Up—Supine, page 188
Alternate option: Ped-a-Pul: Circle, page 318

ARM WORK

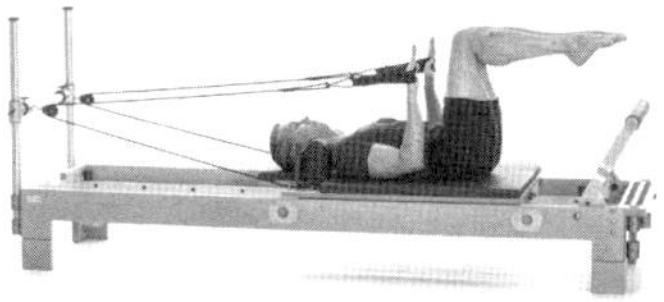

Reformer: Triceps—Supine, page 189
Alternate option: Ped-a-Pul: Triceps, page 317

LEG WORK

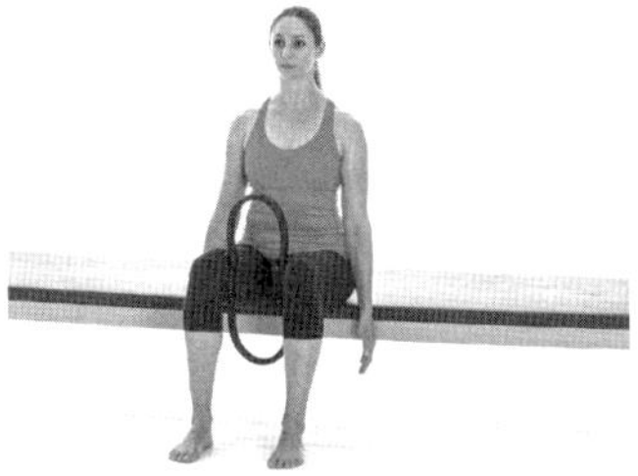

Magic Circle: Above Knees—Seated, page 335

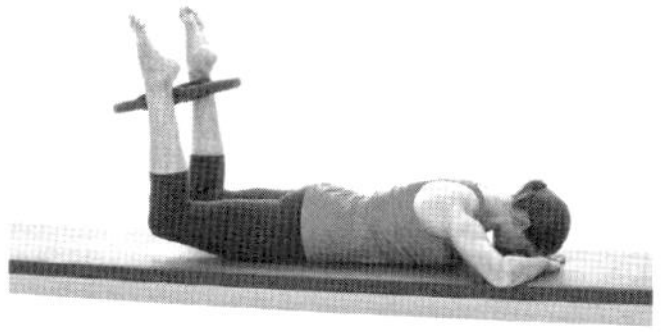

Magic Circle: Knees Bent—Prone, page 338

LATERAL FLEXION & ROTATION

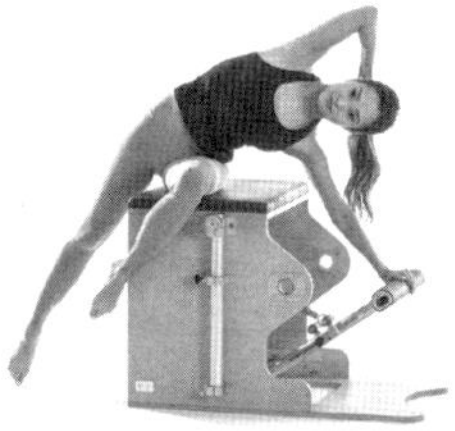

Wunda Chair: Side Over, page 288
Alternate option: Step Barrel: Side Over, page 310

BACK EXTENSION

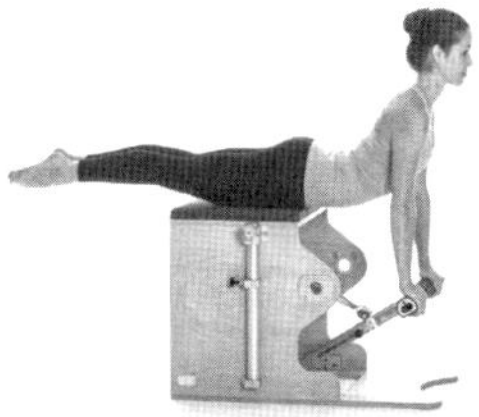

Wunda Chair: Swan, page 289
Alternate option: Step Barrel: Swan, page 311

OPTIONAL

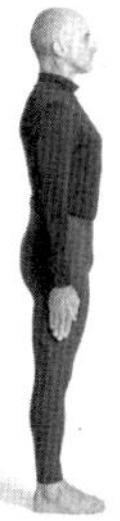

Mat: Roll-Down, page 26

Intermediate Apparatus Routine

Exercises: 32; approximate time: 60 minutes

OPTIONAL

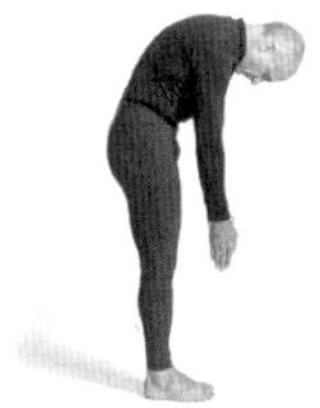

Mat: Roll-Down, page 26

WARM-UP

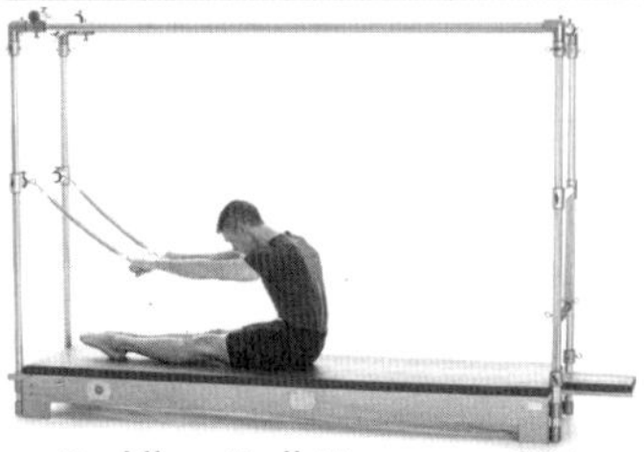

Cadillac: Roll-Up, page 236

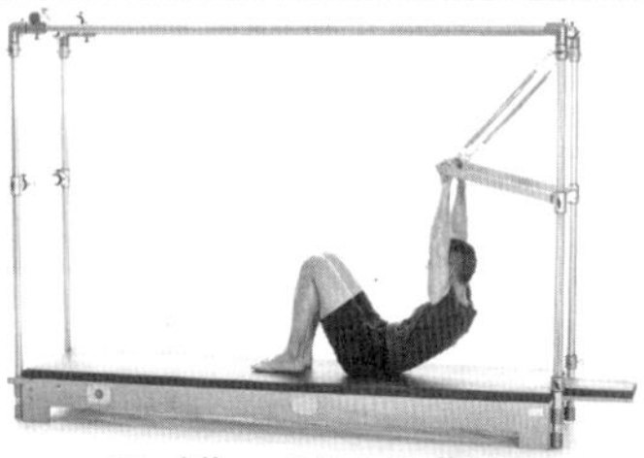

Cadillac: Mini Roll-Up, page 237

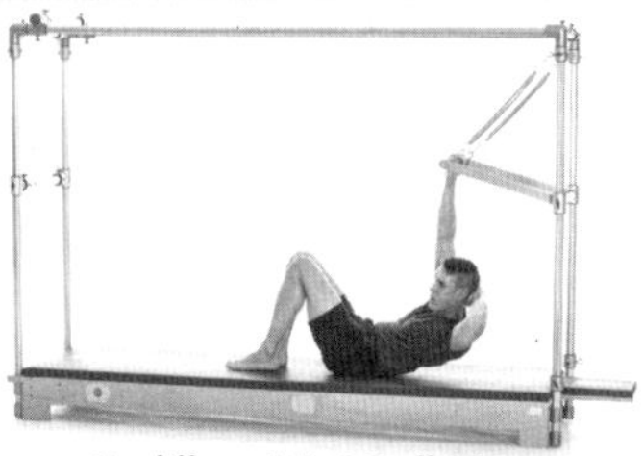

Cadillac: Mini Roll-Up—Oblique, page 238

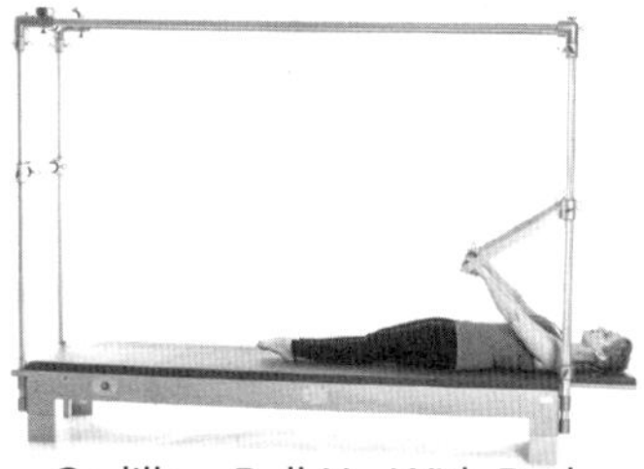

Cadillac: Roll-Up With Push Through Bar, page 240

FOOT WORK

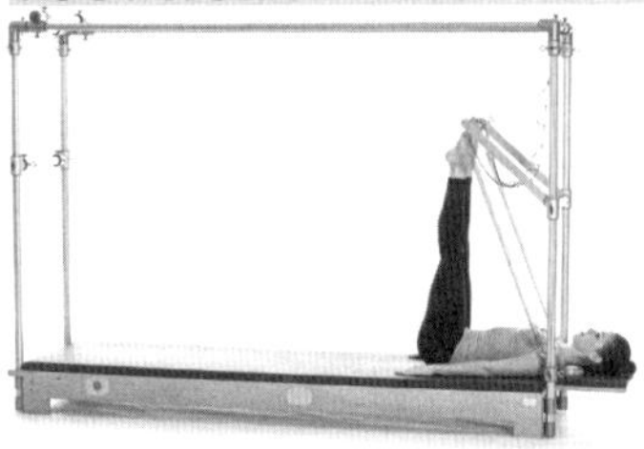

Cadillac: Parallel Heels and Toes, page 229

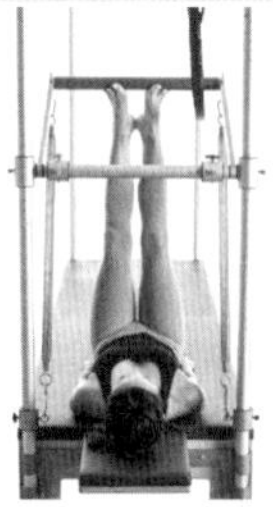

Cadillac: V Position Toes, page 230

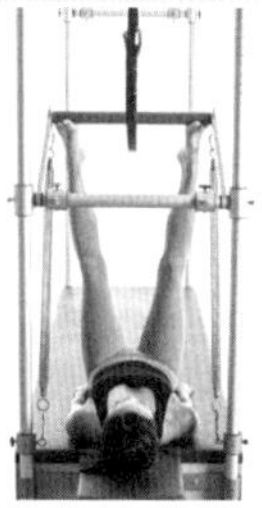

Cadillac: Open V Position Heels and Toes, page 231

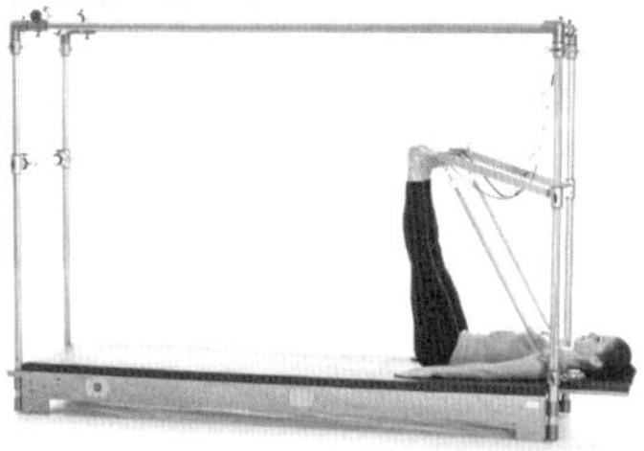

Cadillac: Calf Raises, page 232

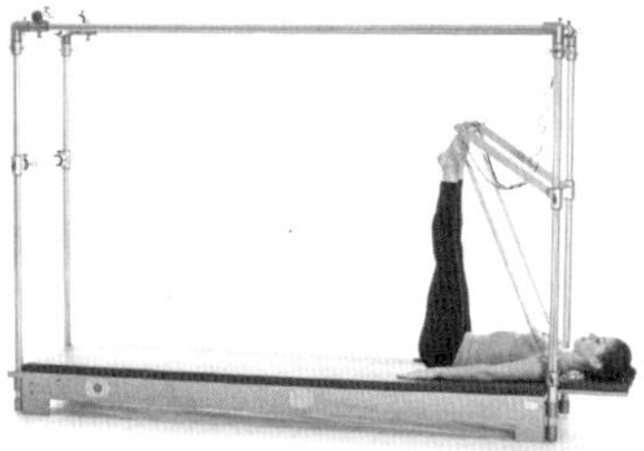

Cadillac: Prances, page 233

FOOT WORK

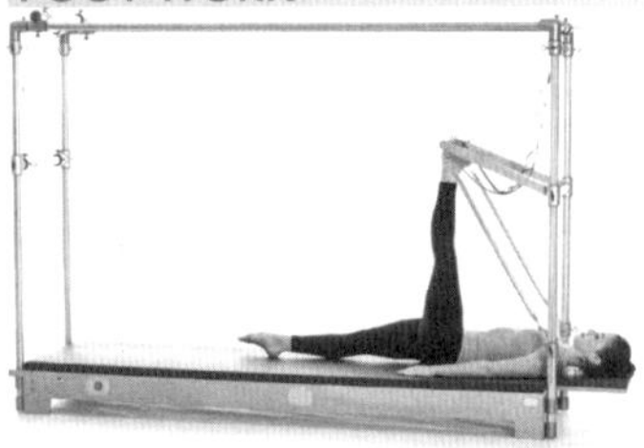

Cadillac: Single-Leg Heel, page 234

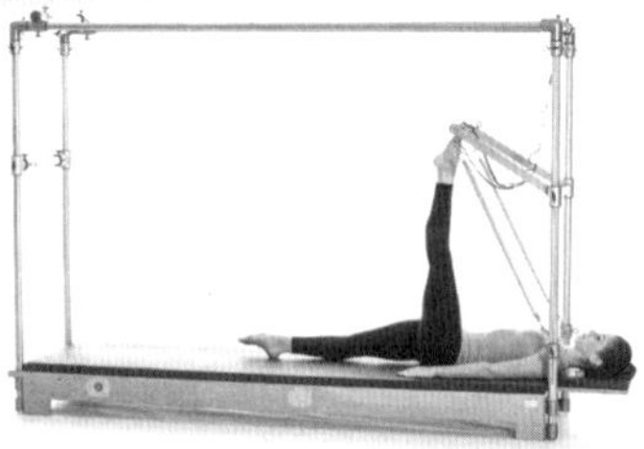

Cadillac: Single-Leg Toes, page 235

ABDOMINAL WORK

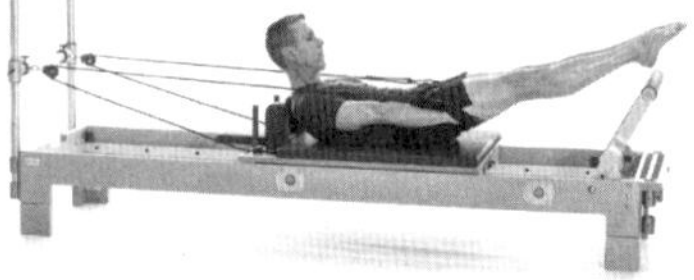

Reformer: Hundred, page 139

HIP WORK

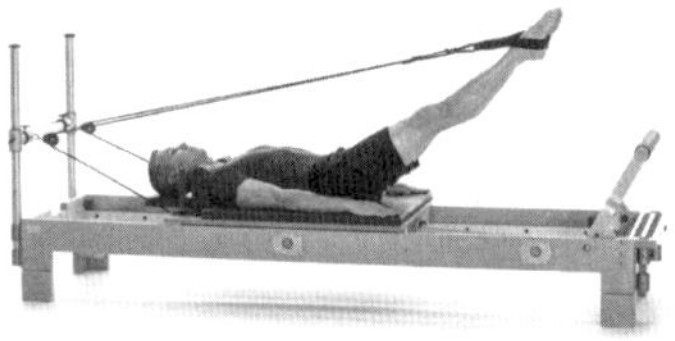

Reformer: Hip Circle Down, page 154

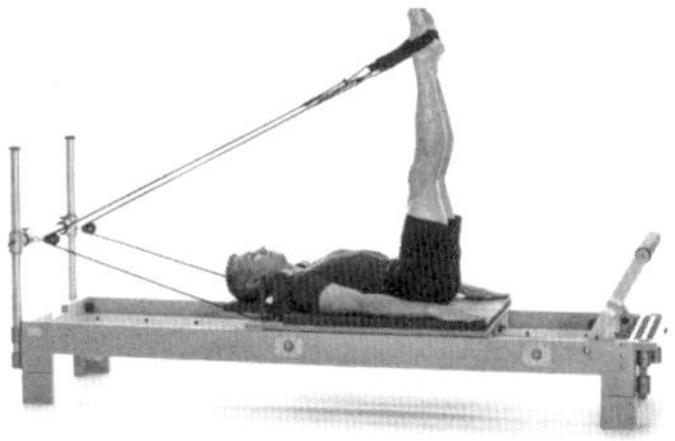

Reformer: Hip Circle Up, page 155

HIP WORK

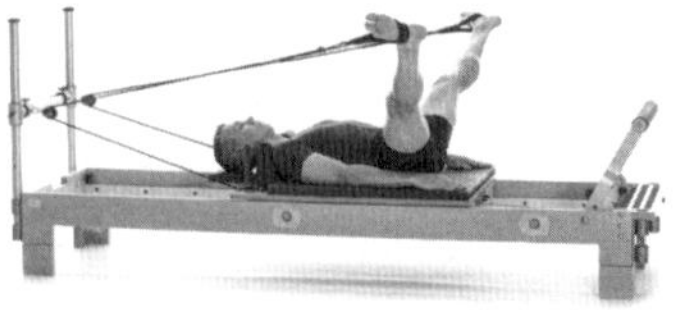

Reformer: Frog—Extended, page 157

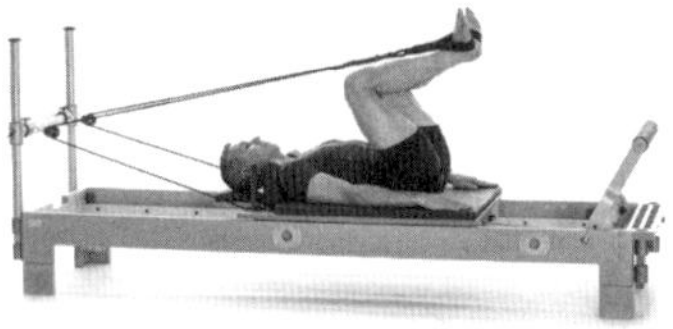

Reformer: Frog—Extended Reverse, page 158

SPINAL ARTICULATION

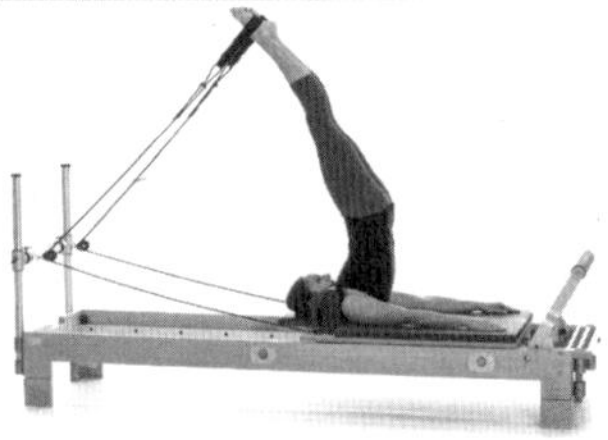

Reformer: Short Spine, page 164

STRETCHES

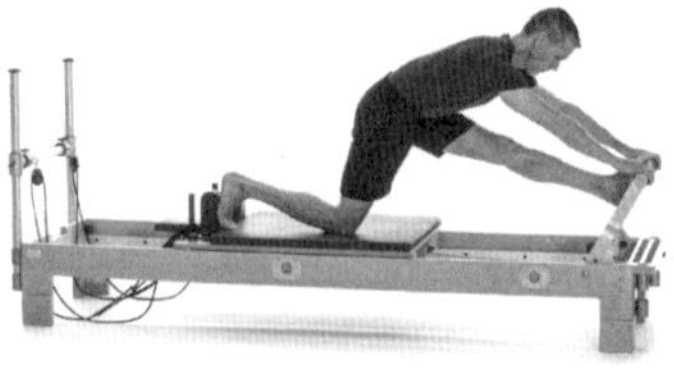

Reformer: Lunge—Kneeling, page 170

FULL BODY INTEGRATION I

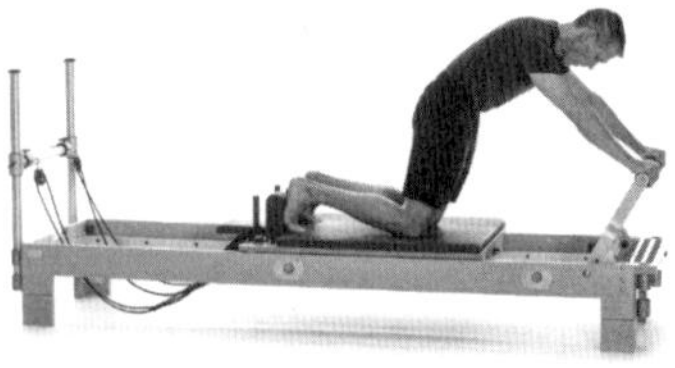

Reformer: Knee Stretch—Round Back, page 174

FULL BODY INTEGRATION I

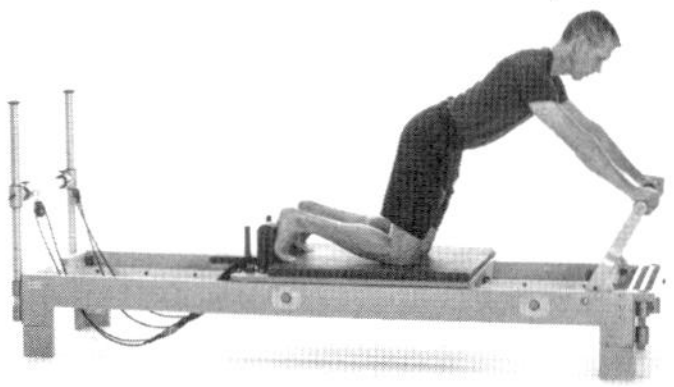

Reformer: Knee Stretch—Flat Back, page 175

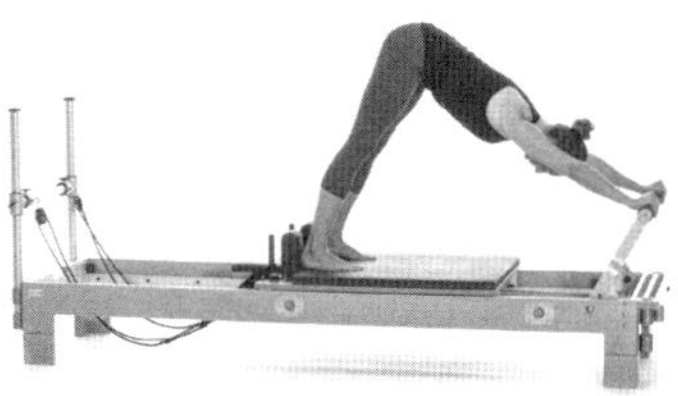

Reformer: Elephant, page 180

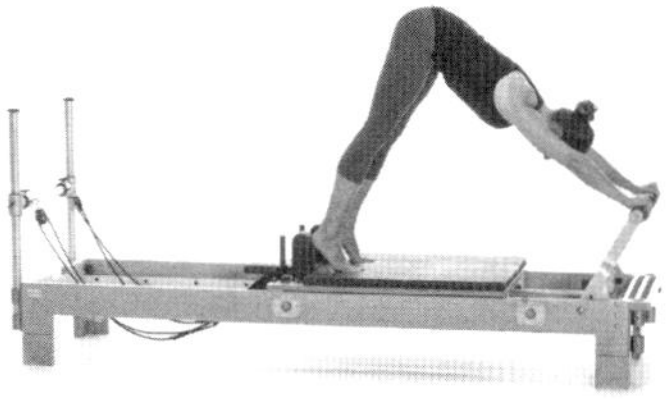

Reformer: Up Stretch, page 181

ARM WORK

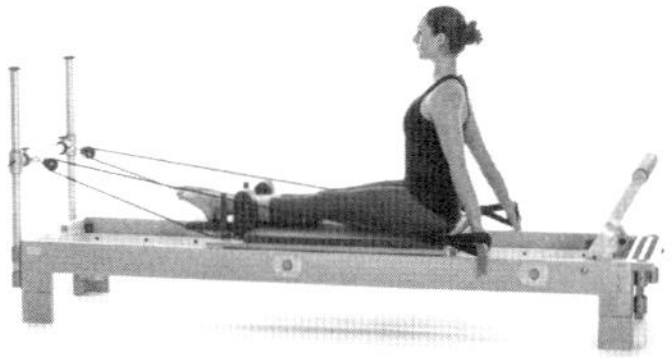

Reformer: Chest Expansion—Seated, page 190

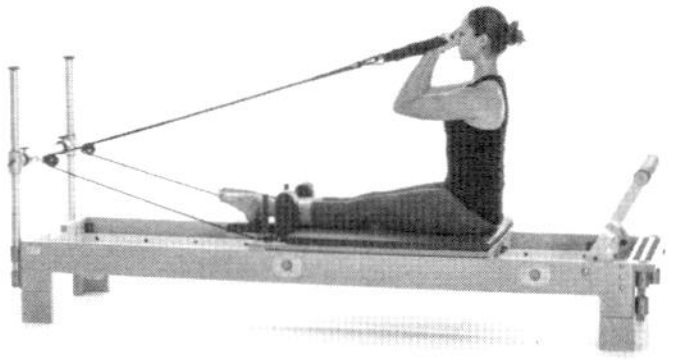

Reformer: Biceps—Seated, page 191

ARM WORK

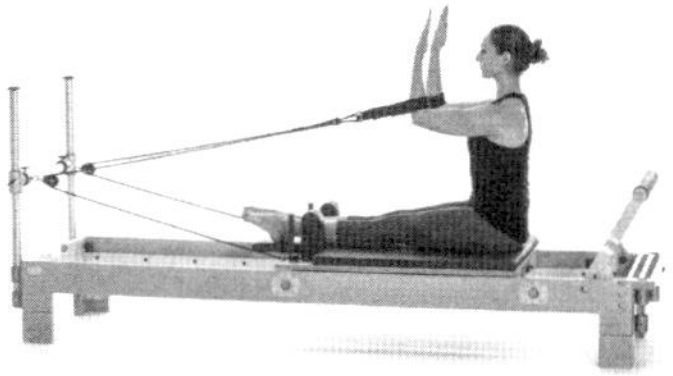

Reformer: Rhomboids—Seated, page 192

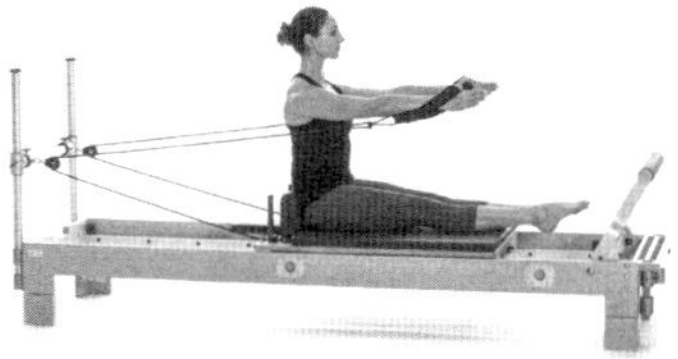

Reformer: Hug-a-Tree—Seated, page 193

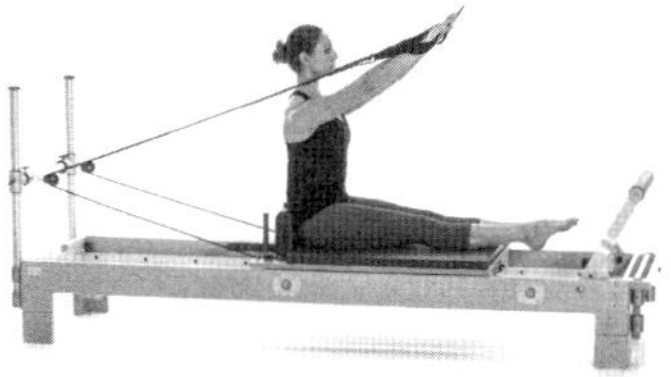

Reformer: Salute—Seated, page 194

LEG WORK

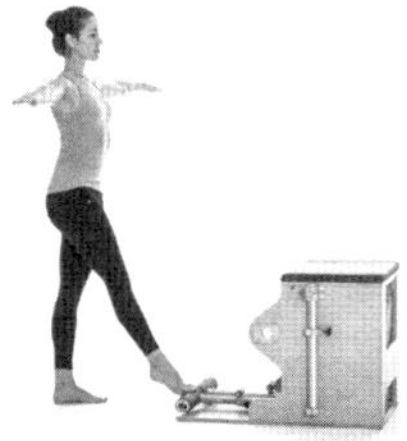

Wunda Chair: Leg Press—Standing, page 286

FULL BODY INTEGRATION II

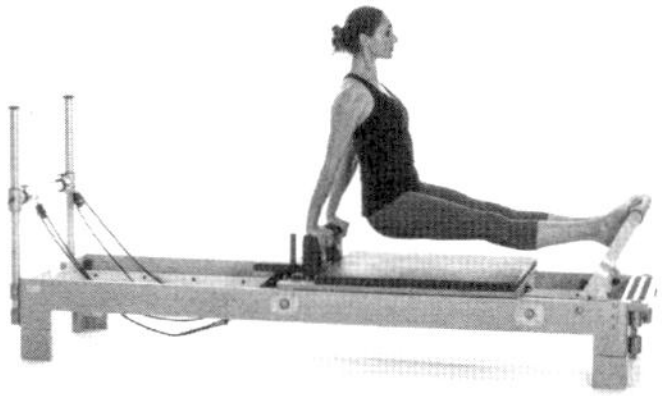

Reformer: Balance Control Back Prep, page 184

LATERAL FLEXION & ROTATION

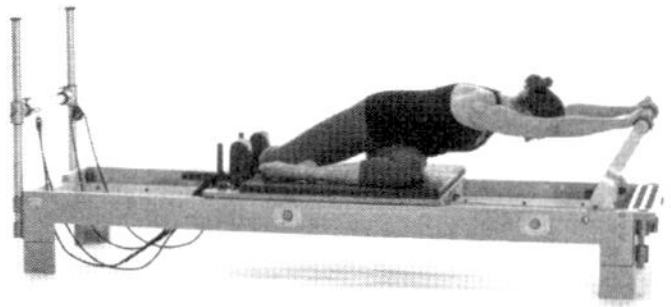

Reformer: Mermaid, page 218

BACK EXTENSION

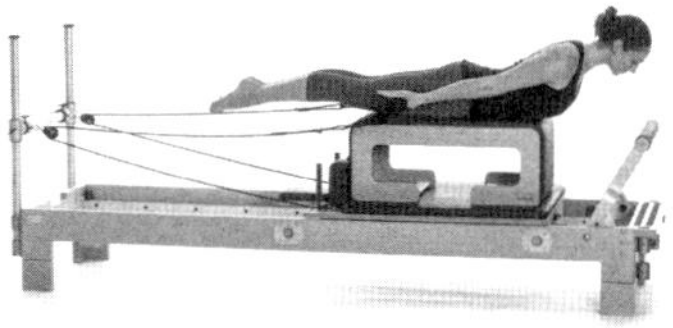

Reformer: Breaststroke, page 223

OPTIONAL

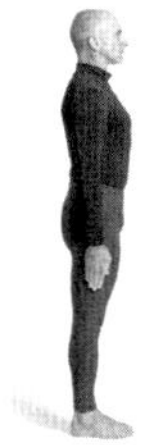

Mat: Roll-Down, page 26

Advanced Apparatus Routine

Exercises: 34; approximate time: 60 minutes

OPTIONAL

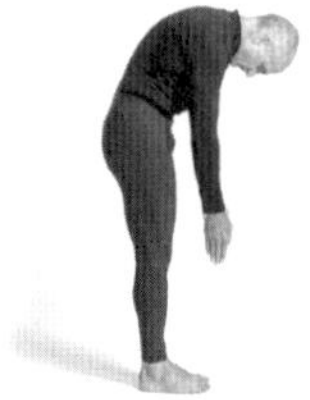

Mat: Roll-Down, page 26

WARM-UP

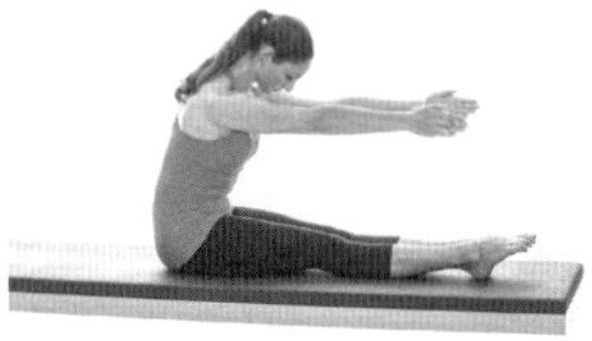

Mat: Roll-Up, page 58

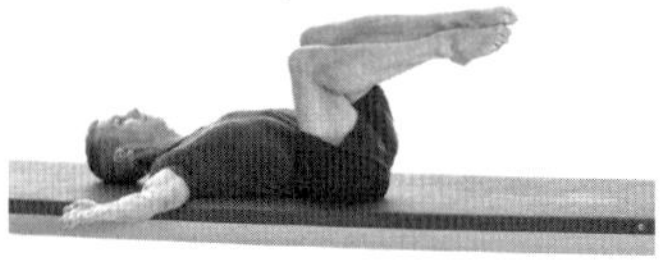

Mat: Spine Twist—Supine, page 50

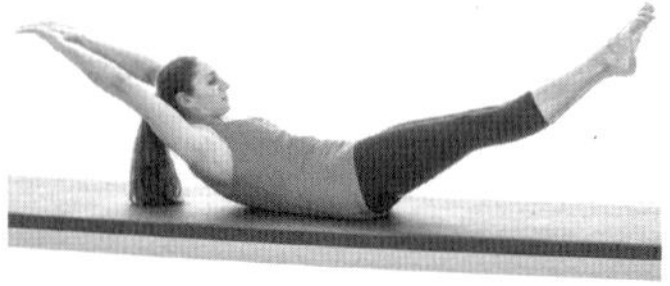

Mat: Double-Leg Stretch, page 66

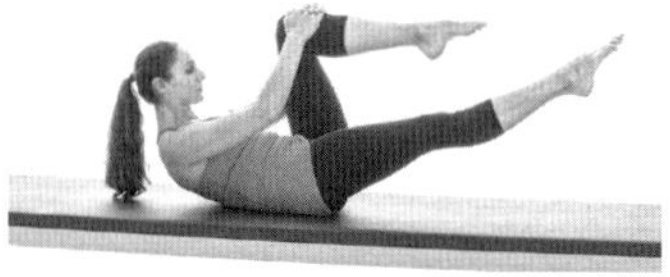

Mat: Single-Leg Stretch, page 62

WARM-UP

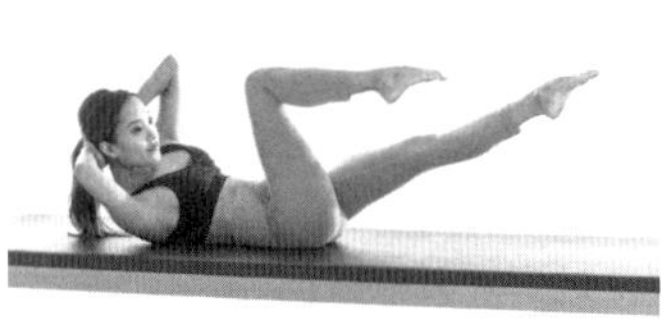

Mat: Criss-Cross, page 64

FOOT WORK

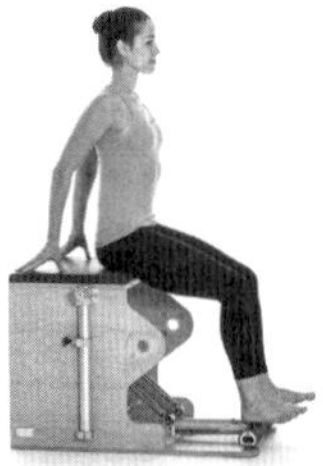

Wunda Chair: Parallel Heels and Toes, page 273

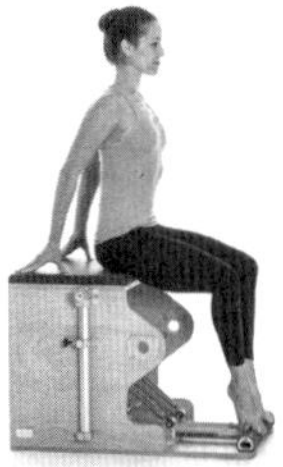

Wunda Chair: V Position Toes, page 274

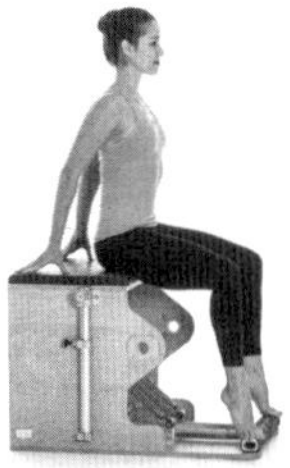

Wunda Chair: Open V Position Heels and Toes, page 275

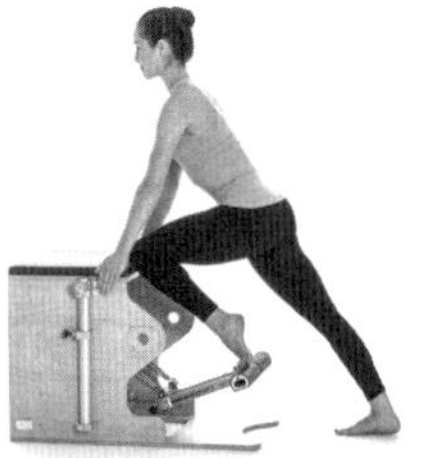

Wunda Chair: Calf Raises, page 276

FOOT WORK

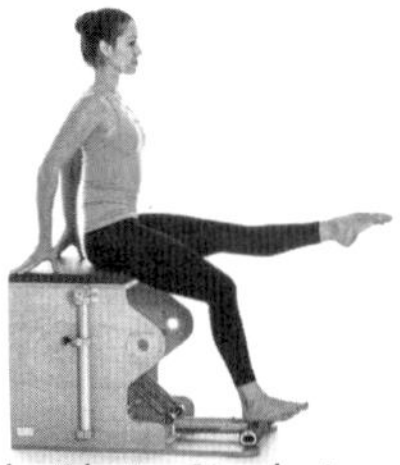

Wunda Chair: Single-Leg Heel and Toes, page 277

ABDOMINAL WORK

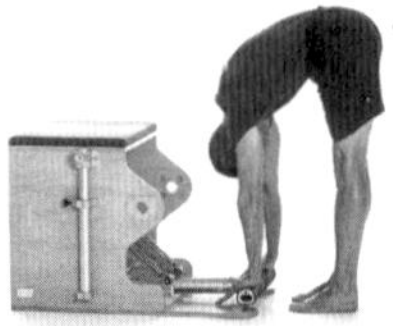

Wunda Chair: Pike—Standing, page 278
Alternate option: Wunda Chair: Pike—Forward, page 279

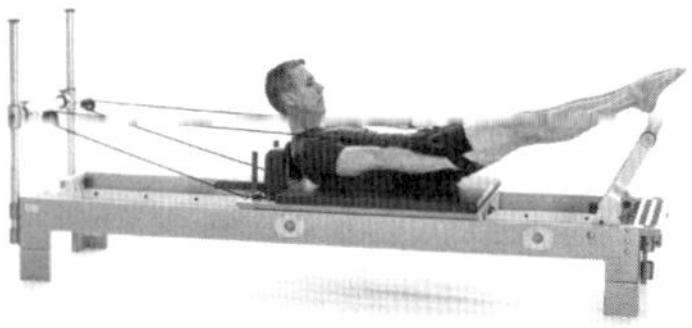

Reformer: Hundred, page 139
Alternate option: Reformer: Coordination, page 140

HIP WORK

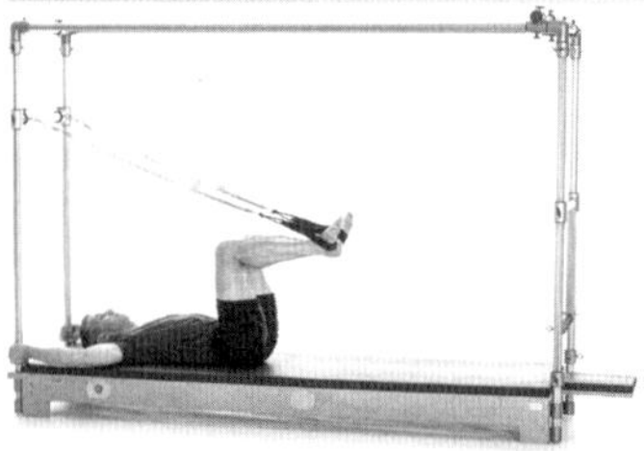

Cadillac: Frog, page 242

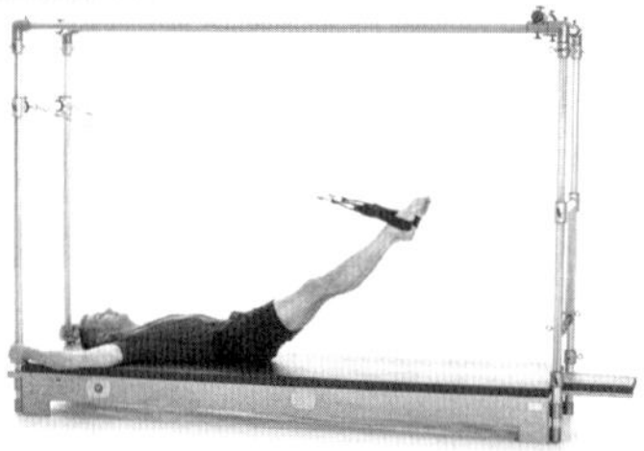

Cadillac: Hip Circle, page 243

HIP WORK

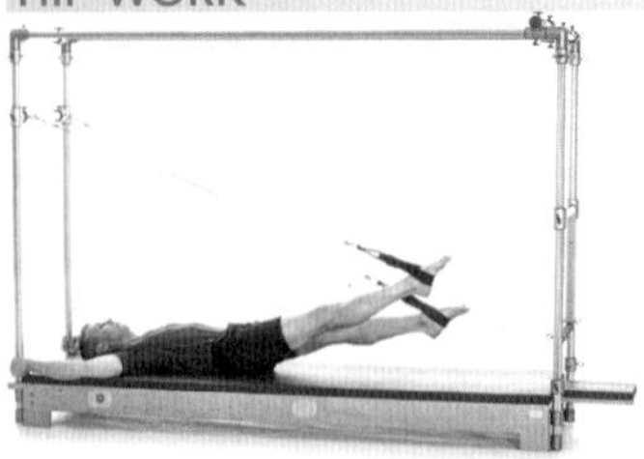

Cadillac: Walking, page 244

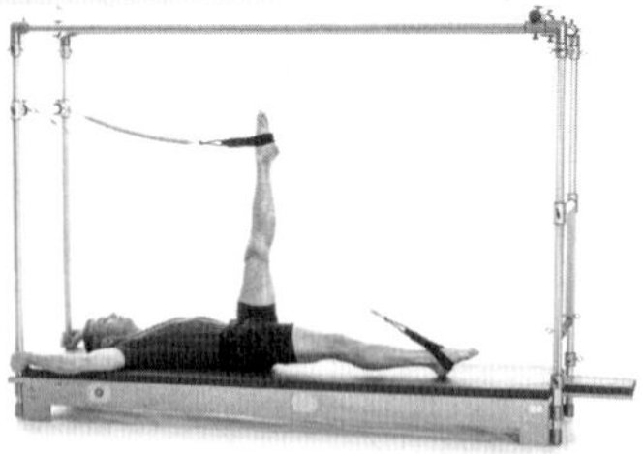

Cadillac: Bicycle, page 245

SPINAL ARTICULATION

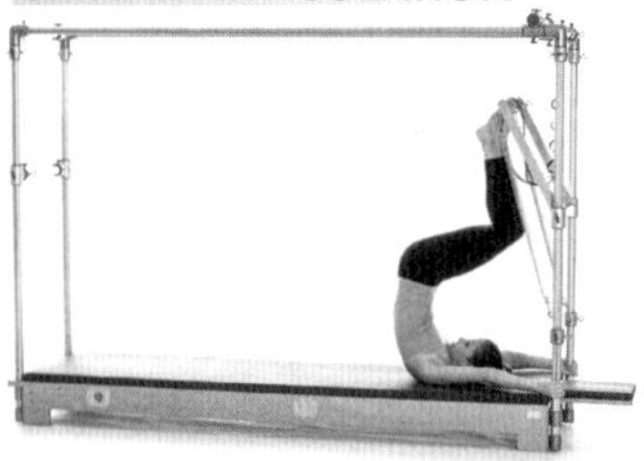

Cadillac: Tower, page 248

STRETCHES

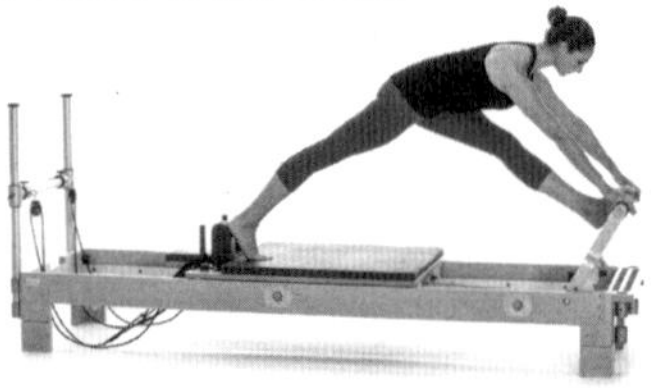

Reformer: Lunge—Forward, page 171

FULL BODY INTEGRATION I

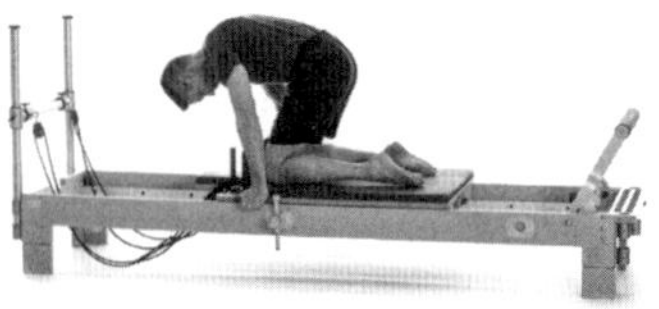

Reformer: Knee Stretch—Reverse, page 176

FULL BODY INTEGRATION I

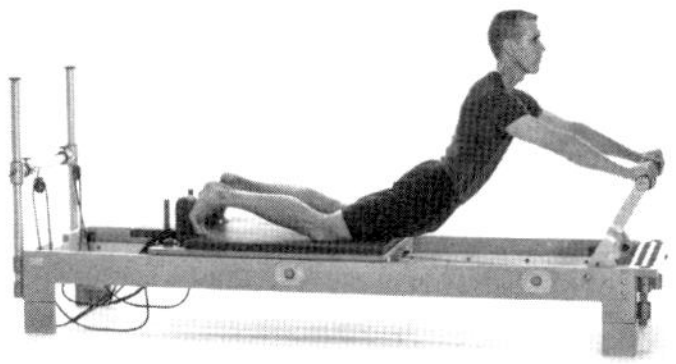

Reformer: Down Stretch, page 179

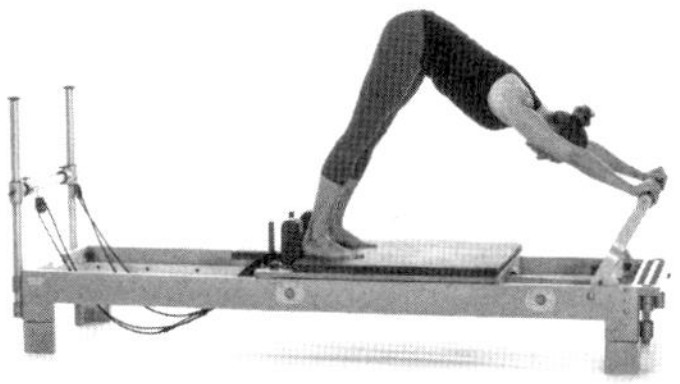

Reformer: Elephant, page 180

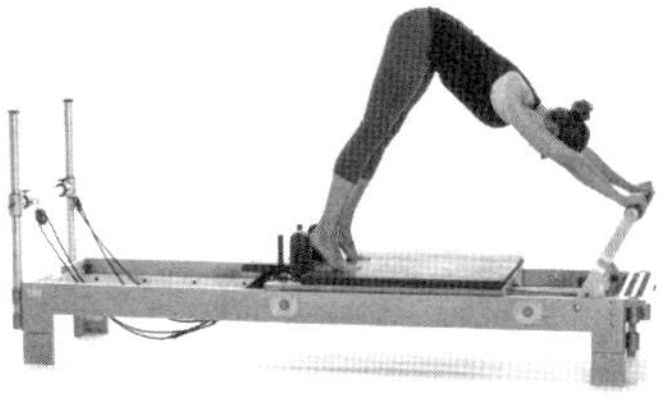

Reformer: Up Stretch, page 181

ARM WORK

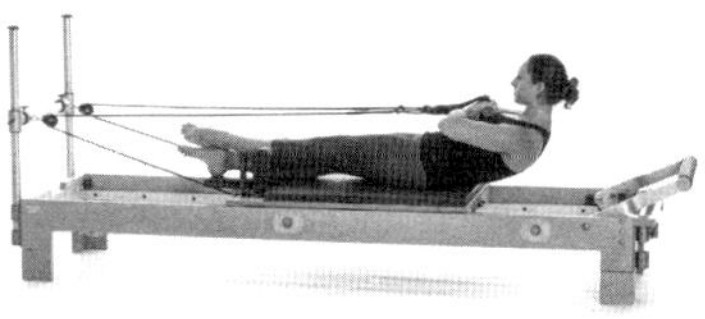

Reformer: Rowing Back 1, page 200

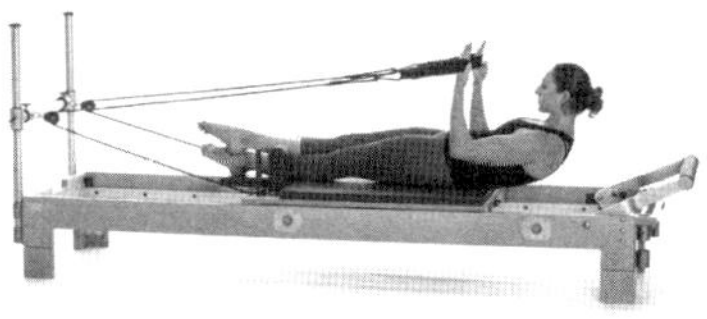

Reformer: Rowing Back 2, page 202

ARM WORK

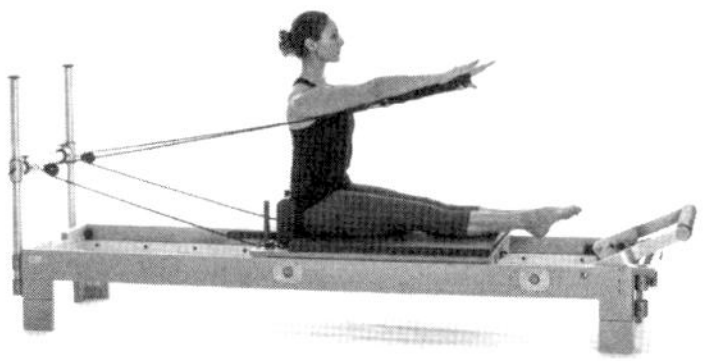

Reformer: Rowing Front 1, page 204

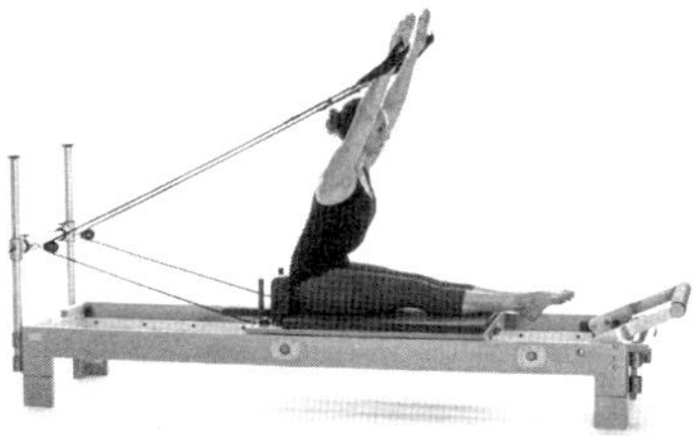

Reformer: Rowing Front 2, page 206

LEG WORK

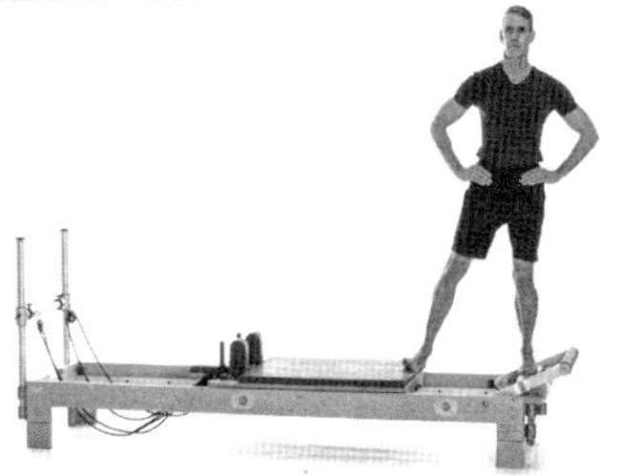

Reformer: Skating—Single Leg, page 210

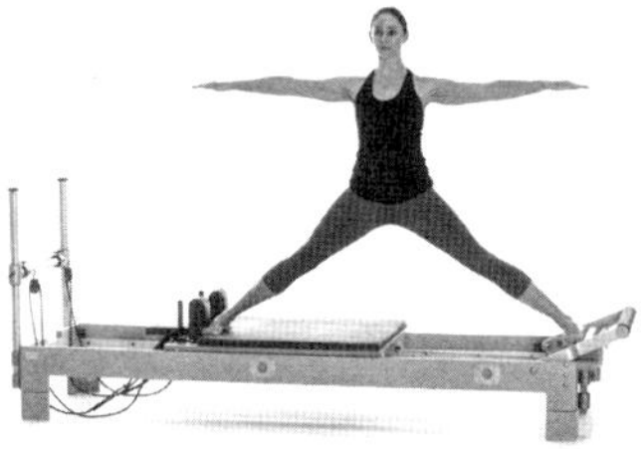

Reformer: Split—Side, page 209

FULL BODY INTEGRATION II

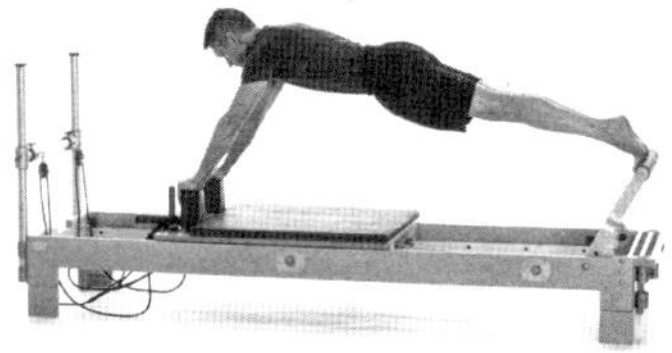

Reformer: Balance Control Front, page 183

FULL BODY INTEGRATION II

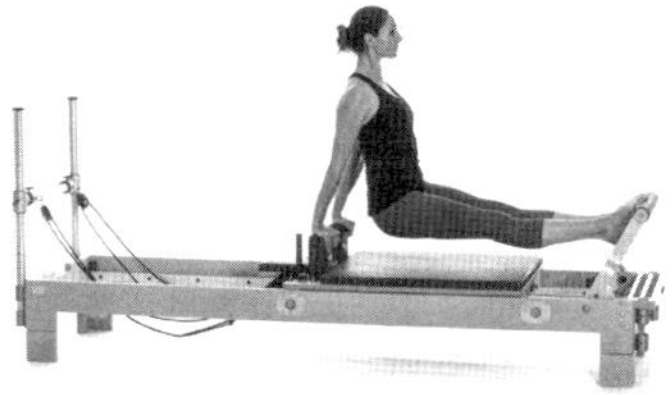

Reformer: Balance Control Back Prep, page 184

LATERAL FLEXION & ROTATION

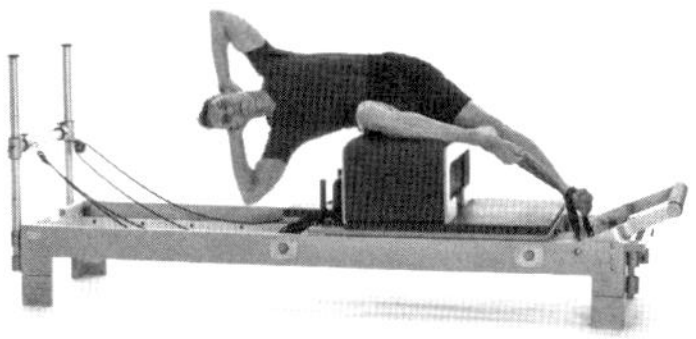

Reformer: Side Over, page 216
Alternate option: Ladder Barrel: Side Over, page 296

BACK EXTENSION

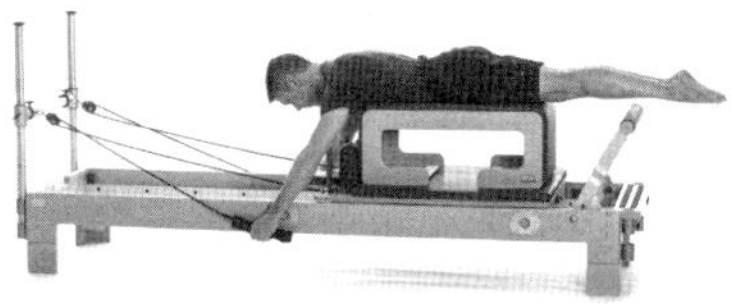

Reformer: Pulling Straps 1, page 224
Alternate option: Ladder Barrel: Swan, page 298

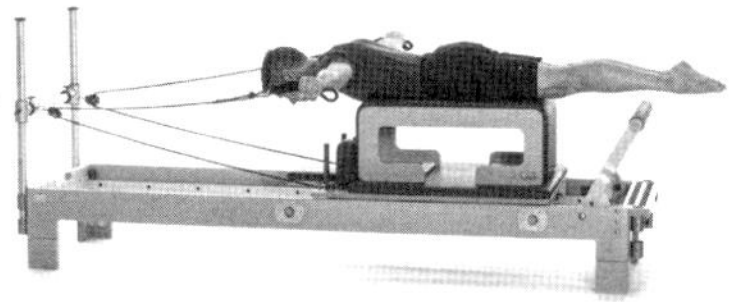

Reformer: Pulling Straps 2, page 225

OPTIONAL

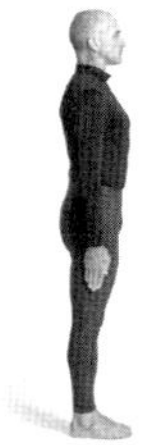

Mat: Roll-Down, page 26

As you embark on practice of Pilates, you can look forward to the positive changes that lie ahead. Joseph Pilates is quoted as having said, "in 10 sessions, you will feel the difference, in 20, you will see the difference, and in 30, you'll be on your way to having a whole new body." Certain changes—those relating to body awareness and alignment, muscle activation, the release of tension, rejuvenation, and inspiration—can occur immediately. However, for significant physiological changes to take place, the muscles must be challenged consistently for at least 6 weeks, meaning you should work out at least once every 72 hours. In *Return to Life Through Contrology,* Joseph Pilates wrote "if you faithfully perform [the] exercises regularly only four times a week for just three months . . . you will find your body development approaching the ideal, accompanied by renewed mental vigor and spiritual enhancement" (pp. 18-19). Without consistency and discipline, profound changes are unlikely to occur. Pilates is not a quick cure-all; it is a well-designed system of physical and mental conditioning that, when practiced with dedication and commitment, brings about positive changes and enhanced well-being.

As important as consistent practice is, Joseph Pilates intended for his system to be far more than the repetition of exercises. He considered it to be an approach to life that would imbue every daily activity with well-being. I have seen footage in which he went as far as to demonstrate how to shower correctly and wash every part of the body—that was Mr. Pilates, through and through! He was a man of strong opinions, who had unwavering belief in his system and a corresponding determination that it should be practiced universally.

Like the rest of us, Joseph Pilates had his shortcomings. Those who worked with him reported that he could be impatient, egotistical, and somewhat of a show-off. He may have been chauvinistic as well; he intended his method to be practiced mainly by men. It is ironic, therefore, that it is primarily women who have kept the flame alive all these years and that women still represent the majority of Pilates practitioners. Pilates, in its essence, is a wonderful balance of strength and grace, masculinity and femininity, yin and yang, complementary forces that make up the universe. It has much to offer both men and women.

Above all, Joseph Pilates was a "genius of the body," as renowned choreographer George Balanchine reportedly called him. He embraced the power of the mind–body connection early on, understanding that each human being is a complex entity. He viewed human movement as an intricate sequence of patterns. He was an unshakable idealist who believed that humankind deserved better than the status quo in terms of health and well-being. He spearheaded one of the greatest surges of popularity in a particular discipline in the history of the fitness industry. He promoted concepts that are only now being truly understood, embraced, and substantiated through research. Joseph Pilates' vast knowledge and creativity, which are even more apparent today than during his own lifetime, are a legacy that we can enjoy and use to enhance our lives.

In bidding farewell, I add my humble wish—that we generously share our knowledge and life experience so that we may all grow as individuals, as a global community, and as custodians of the planet itself. By sharing, practicing, and teaching, we keep the essence of Pilates alive. Enjoy this enlightening, lifelong journey—and most importantly, be safe!

Selected Resources

Books

Calais-Germain, Blandine. 1993. *Anatomy of Movement*. Seattle: Eastland Press.

Calais-Germain, Blandine, and Andrée Lamotte. 1996. *Anatomy of Movement Exercises*. Seattle: Eastland Press.

Cash, Mel. 1999. *Pocket Atlas of the Moving Body*. London: Ebury Press Random House.

Clippinger, Karen. 2015. *Dance Anatomy and Kinesiology*. 2nd ed. Champaign, IL: Human Kinetics.

Conraths-Lange, Nicola. 2004. *Survival Skills for Pilates Teachers*. Ann Arbor, MI: Logokinesis.

Corrigan, Brian, and G.D. Maitland. 1985. *Practical Orthopaedic Medicine*. Oxford, UK: Butterworth-Heinemann.

Csíkszentmihályi, Mihály. 1990. *Flow: The Psychology of Optimal Experience*. New York: Harper & Row.

Dowd, Irene. 1995. *Taking Root to Fly: Articles on Functional Anatomy*. 3rd ed. New York: Dowd.

Dufton, Jennifer. 2003. *The Pilates Difference*. London: Hamlyn.

Fitt, Sally S. 1988. *Dance Kinesiology*. New York: Schirmer.

Franklin, Eric. 2002. *Pelvic Power*. Hightstown, NJ: Princeton.

Friedman, Philip, and Gail Eisen. 1980. *The Pilates Method of Physical and Mental Conditioning*. Garden City, NY: Doubleday.

Gallagher, Sean P., and Romana Kryzanowska, eds. 2000. *The Joseph H. Pilates Archive Collection*. Philadelphia: Bainbridge.

Gladwell, Malcolm. 2000. *The Tipping Point*. New York: Little, Brown and Company.

Gladwell, Malcolm. 2008. *Outliers*. New York: Little, Brown and Company.

Hessel, Jillian. 2003. *Pilates Basics*. Emmaus, PA: Rodale.

Isacowitz, Rael. 2004. *Body Arts and Science International Movement Analysis Work Books: Mat, Reformer, Cadillac, Ladder Barrel and Wunda Chair, Auxiliary, Avalon*. Costa Mesa, CA: Author.

Isacowitz, Rael, and Karen Clippinger. 2019. *Pilates Anatomy*. 2nd ed. Champaign, IL: Human Kinetics.

Iyengar, B.K.S. 2001. *The Art of Yoga*. London: Allen & Unwin.

Juhan, Deane. 1998. *Job's Body: A Handbook for Body Work*. 3rd ed. Barrytown, NY: Station Hill Press.

Kaplanek, Beth, Brett Levine, and William Jaffe. 2011. *Pilates for Hip and Knee Syndromes and Arthroplasties*. Champaign, IL: Human Kinetics.

Kelly, Suzanne. 2005. *Pilates 4 Kidzz*. Bloomington, IN: Authorhouse.

Kendal, Florence P., Elizabeth K. McCreary, and Patricia G. Provance. 1993. *Muscles: Testing and Function*. 4th ed. Baltimore: Williams & Wilkins.

King, Bruce. 1991. *Rule of the Bones: Exercise Theory and Program for Correct Body Usage*. New York: Bruce King Foundation for American Dance.

Kounovsky, Nicholas. 1971. *The Joy of Feeling Fit*. Mattituck, NY: Amereon House.

Lett, Anthony. 2010. *Innovations in Pilates*. Eltham, VIC, Australia: Rebus Press.

Lingauer, Gabor. 2002. *Muscle Doctor*. Victoria, Canada: Trafford.

Myers, Thomas P. 2001. *Anatomy Trains*. London: Harcourt.

Netter, Frank H. 2011. *Atlas of Human Anatomy, Professional Edition*. 5th ed. Philadelphia, PA: Saunders/Elsevier.

Pilates, Joseph H. 1934. *Your Health: A Corrective System of Exercising That Revolutionizes the Entire Field of Physical Education*. Reprinted 1998. Incline Village, NV: Presentation Dynamics.

Pilates, Joseph H. 1945. *Return to Life Through Contrology*. Reprinted 2003. Miami: Pilates Method Alliance.

Robinson, Lynne. 2004. *The Body Control Pilates Pregnancy Book*. London: Pan Books.

Ruiz-Giménez Aguilar, Guady. 2021. *The Art of Aging Beautifully*. Self-published, Guady Ruiz-Giménez Aguilar.

San Miguel, Lolita. 2021. *An Enchanted Life: A Memoir*. Self-published, Lolita San Miguel.

Steel, John Howard. 2020. *Caged Lion*. Santa Barbara: Last Leaf Press.

Tardent, Helen. 2005. *Beautiful Pilates*. Camberwell, Australia: Penguin.

Thompson, Cem W., and R.T. Floyd. 2004. *Manual of Structural Kinesiology*. 15th ed. St. Louis: Times Mirror/Mosby.

Journals and Magazines

Health

IDEA Fitness Journal

Pilates Style

Yoga Journal

Videos and DVDs

Fletcher, Ron. *Ron Fletcher Workshop Tape*. The Ron Fletcher Company.

Gentry, Eve. 1991. *The Eve Gentry Technique*. Institute for the Pilates Method.

Isacowitz, Rael. 2003. *Rael Pilates System 7, 17, and 27*. Carlmarsh III Productions.

Liekens, Bob, Alycea Ungaro, and Peter Fiasca. 2003. *Classical Pilates Technique*. Classical Pilates Inc.

Pilates, Joseph H. *Demonstrating the principles of his method with Clara, students and friends, 1932-1945*. From Joseph and Clara Pilates personal collection. Attained by Evelyn de la Tour and bequeathed to Mary Bowen.

Trier, Carola. 1989. *Carola shares . . .* A Dadmehr Production.

Websites

BASI Interactive: www.basiinteractive.com

BASI Systems: www.basisystems.com

Body Arts and Science International: www.basipilates.com

Dynamic Chiropractic: www.chiroweb.com

Human Kinetics: www.humankinetics.com

Movement Anatomy: www.movementanatomy.com

Pilates Anytime: www.pilatesanytime.com

Pilates Method Alliance: www.pilatesmethodalliance.org

National Scoliosis Foundation: www.scoliosis.org

Scoliosis World: www.scoliosis-world.com

Somatics on the Web: www.somatics.com

Note: The italicized *f* following page numbers refers to figures.

About the Author

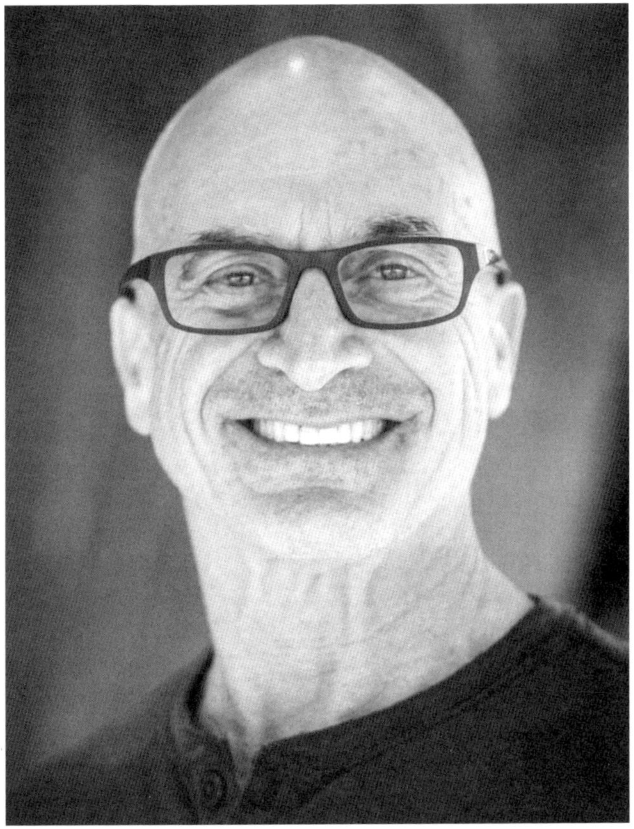

Rael Isacowitz received his bachelor of education degree from the Wingate Institute in Israel, where he was later invited to join the faculty, and his master of arts degree in dance from the University of Surrey in England. He worked extensively as a professional dancer and dance educator in Israel, England, Australia, and the United States. Rael was introduced to Pilates in the late 1970s and has since been practicing and teaching Pilates throughout the world.

In 1989, Rael founded BASI (Body Arts and Science International) Pilates, a comprehensive Pilates educational organization spanning the globe. Headquartered in Newport Beach, California, BASI Pilates is represented in more than 50 countries. Over 50,000 students have experienced the BASI teacher training programs, Learn From the Leaders conferences, and other advanced workshops and continuing education courses.

Rael spearheaded the development of BASI Interactive, a one-of-a-kind elearning platform, and he designed the original concepts for BASI Systems Pilates equipment. Rael has written two bestselling books that have been translated into multiple languages: *Pilates* (Human Kinetics) and *Pilates Anatomy* (Human Kinetics), the latter of which was coauthored by Karen Clippinger. He has published a series of comprehensive workbooks that serve as a road map for professionals. With over 1,000 pages of content, these workbooks (which are used in the BASI Legacy Program) cover everything from the basics to the most advanced repertoire. In the early 2000s, Rael was featured in a series of DVDs that remain universally popular today. He was a founding board member of Pilates Method Alliance. He has written for, and been featured in, professional publications such as *Pilates Style* magazine, for which he was the Q&A expert for over seven years.

Rael is honored to be part of the great legacy of Pilates teachers and mentors. He has studied from, and taught with, luminaries of the Pilates world, including several first-generation Pilates teachers. Among these Pilates elders was Kathy Grant, who Rael regards as his greatest teacher and mentor.

Rael's myriad contributions to Pilates as a teacher, author, and innovator are recognized and respected internationally. Passion, compassion, and excellence guide Rael in all he does. Creativity and commitment permeate his work and his daily practice. Rael brings to Pilates a unique athleticism—a synthesis of body, mind, and spirit.

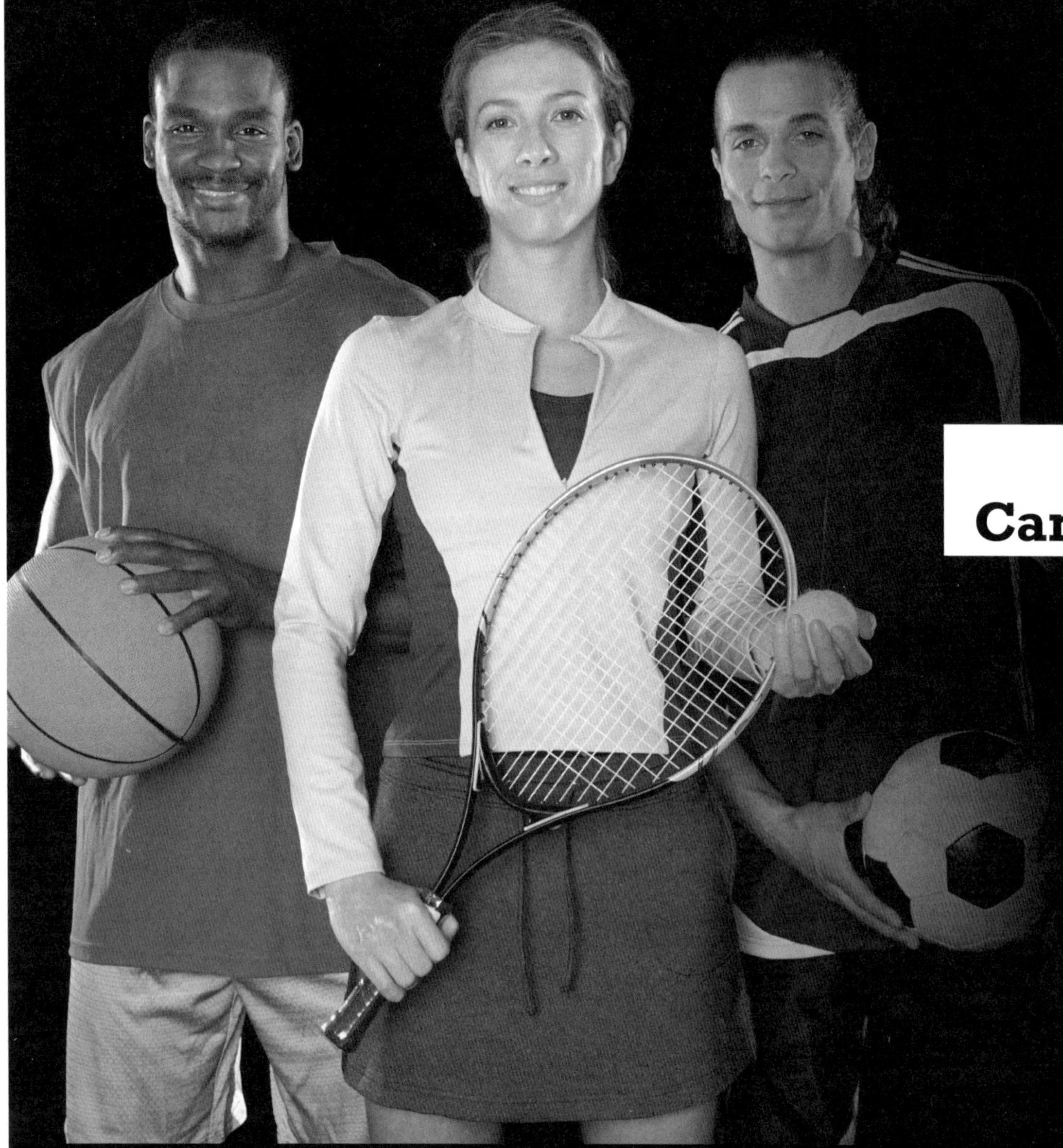